Accessing the E-book edition

Using the VitalSource® ebook

Access to the VitalBook™ ebook accompanying this book is via VitalSource® Bookshelf — an ebook reader which allows you to make and share notes and highlights on your ebooks and search across all of the ebooks that you hold on your VitalSource Bookshelf. You can access the ebook online or offline on your smartphone, tablet or PC/Mac and your notes and highlights will automatically stay in sync no matter where you make them.

1. **Create a VitalSource Bookshelf account at** *https://online.vitalsource.com/user/new* or log into your existing account if you already have one.

2. **Redeem the code provided in the panel below to get online access to the ebook.** Log in to Bookshelf and select **Redeem** at the top right of the screen. Enter the redemption code shown on the scratch-off panel below in the **Redeem Code** pop-up and press **Redeem**. Once the code has been redeemed your ebook will download and appear in your library.

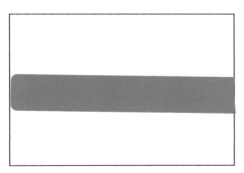

No returns if this code has been revealed.

DOWNLOAD AND READ OFFLINE

To use your ebook offline, download BookShelf to your PC, Mac, iOS device, Android device or Kindle Fire, and log in to your Bookshelf account to access your ebook:

On your PC/Mac
Go to *https://support.vitalsource.com/hc/en-us* and follow the instructions to download the free **VitalSource Bookshelf** app to your PC or Mac and log into your Bookshelf account.

On your iPhone/iPod Touch/iPad
Download the free **VitalSource Bookshelf** App available via the iTunes App Store and log into your Bookshelf account. You can find more information at *https://support.vitalsource.com/hc/en-us/categories/200134217-Bookshelf-for-iOS*

On your Android™ smartphone or tablet
Download the free **VitalSource Bookshelf** App available via Google Play and log into your Bookshelf account. You can find more information at *https://support.vitalsource.com/hc/en-us/categories/200139976-Bookshelf-for-Android-and-Kindle-Fire*

On your Kindle Fire
Download the free **VitalSource Bookshelf** App available from Amazon and log into your Bookshelf account. You can find more information at *https://support.vitalsource.com/hc/en-us/categories/200139976-Bookshelf-for-Android-and-Kindle-Fire*

N.B. The code in the scratch-off panel can only be used once. When you have created a Bookshelf account and redeemed the code you will be able to access the ebook online or offline on your smartphone, tablet or PC/Mac.

SUPPORT

If you have any questions about downloading Bookshelf, creating your account, or accessing and using your ebook edition, please visit *http://support.vitalsource.com/*

Obstetric Evidence Based Guidelines

SERIES IN MATERNAL-FETAL MEDICINE

Published in association with the
Journal of Maternal Fetal & Neonatal Medicine

Edited by
Gian Carlo Di Renzo and Dev Maulik

Howard Carp, *Recurrent Pregnancy Loss*, ISBN 9780415421300

Vincenzo Berghella, *Obstetric Evidence Based Guidelines*,
ISBN 9780415701884

Vincenzo Berghella, *Maternal-Fetal Evidence Based Guidelines*,
ISBN 9780415432818

Moshe Hod, Lois Jovanovic, Gian Carlo Di Renzo, Alberto de Leiva,
Oded Langer, *Textbook of Diabetes and Pregnancy, Second Edition*,
ISBN 9780415426206

Simcha Yagel, Norman H. Silverman, Ulrich Gembruch,
Fetal Cardiology, Second Edition, ISBN 9780415432658

Fabio Facchinetti, Gustaaf A. Dekker, Dante Baronciani,
George Saade, Stillbirth: *Understanding and Management*,
ISBN 9780415473903

Vincenzo Berghella, *Maternal-Fetal Evidence Based Guidelines,
Second Edition*, ISBN 9781841848228

Vincenzo Berghella, *Obstetric Evidence Based Guidelines, Second Edition*,
ISBN 9781841848242

Howard Carp, *Recurrent Pregnancy Loss: Causes, Controversies, and
Treatment, Second Edition*, ISBN 9781482216141

Moshe Hod, Lois G. Jovanovic, Gian Carlo Di Renzo, Alberto De Leiva,
Oded Langer, *Textbook of Diabetes and Pregnancy, Third Edition*,
ISBN 9781482213607

Vincenzo Berghella, *Maternal-Fetal Evidence Based Guidelines,
Third Edition*, ISBN 9781841848228

Vincenzo Berghella, *Obstetric Evidence Based Guidelines, Third Edition*,
ISBN 9781841848242

Obstetric Evidence Based Guidelines

Third Edition

Edited by

Vincenzo Berghella, MD, FACOG

Director, Division of Maternal-Fetal Medicine
Professor, Department of Obstetrics and Gynecology
Sidney Kimmel Medical College of Thomas Jefferson University
Philadelphia, Pennsylvania, USA

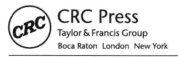

CRC Press is an imprint of the
Taylor & Francis Group, an **informa** business

CRC Press
Taylor & Francis Group
6000 Broken Sound Parkway NW, Suite 300
Boca Raton, FL 33487-2742

© 2017 by Taylor & Francis Group, LLC
CRC Press is an imprint of Taylor & Francis Group, an Informa business

No claim to original U.S. Government works

Printed on acid-free paper
Version Date: 20161111

International Standard Book Number-13: 978-1-4987-4746-2 (Pack - Book and Ebook)

This book contains information obtained from authentic and highly regarded sources. While all reasonable efforts have been made to publish reliable data and information, neither the author[s] nor the publisher can accept any legal responsibility or liability for any errors or omissions that may be made. The publishers wish to make clear that any views or opinions expressed in this book by individual editors, authors or contributors are personal to them and do not necessarily reflect the views/opinions of the publishers. The information or guidance contained in this book is intended for use by medical, scientific or health-care professionals and is provided strictly as a supplement to the medical or other professional's own judgement, their knowledge of the patient's medical history, relevant manufacturer's instructions and the appropriate best practice guidelines. Because of the rapid advances in medical science, any information or advice on dosages, procedures or diagnoses should be independently verified. The reader is strongly urged to consult the relevant national drug formulary and the drug companies' and device or material manufacturers' printed instructions, and their websites, before administering or utilizing any of the drugs, devices or materials mentioned in this book. This book does not indicate whether a particular treatment is appropriate or suitable for a particular individual. Ultimately it is the sole responsibility of the medical professional to make his or her own professional judgements, so as to advise and treat patients appropriately. The authors and publishers have also attempted to trace the copyright holders of all material reproduced in this publication and apologize to copyright holders if permission to publish in this form has not been obtained. If any copyright material has not been acknowledged please write and let us know so we may rectify in any future reprint.

Except as permitted under U.S. Copyright Law, no part of this book may be reprinted, reproduced, transmitted, or utilized in any form by any electronic, mechanical, or other means, now known or hereafter invented, including photocopying, microfilming, and recording, or in any information storage or retrieval system, without written permission from the publishers.

For permission to photocopy or use material electronically from this work, please access www.copyright.com (http://www.copyright.com/) or contact the Copyright Clearance Center, Inc. (CCC), 222 Rosewood Drive, Danvers, MA 01923, 978-750-8400. CCC is a not-for-profit organization that provides licenses and registration for a variety of users. For organizations that have been granted a photocopy license by the CCC, a separate system of payment has been arranged.

Trademark Notice: Product or corporate names may be trademarks or registered trademarks, and are used only for identification and explanation without intent to infringe.

Visit the Taylor & Francis Web site at
http://www.taylorandfrancis.com

and the CRC Press Web site at
http://www.crcpress.com

*To Paola, Andrea, Pietro, mamma, and papá,
for giving me the serenity, love, and strength at home now, then, and in the future
to fulfill my dreams and spend my talents as best as possible.
To all those who loved the 1st edition
To the health of mothers and babies
And, as I often toast: To the next generation!*

Contents

Introduction .... *ix*
How to "Read" This Book .... *xii*
List of Abbreviations .... *xiii*
List of Contributors .... *xv*

1. **Preconception care** 1
   Joanna Quist-Nelson

2. **Prenatal care** 15
   Gabriele Saccone and Kerri Sendek

3. **Physiologic changes** 35
   Jason Baxter and Colleen Horan

4. **Ultrasound** 49
   Lea M. Porche and Alfred Abuhamad

5. **Prenatal diagnosis and screening for aneuploidy** 59
   Dawnette Lewis

6. **Carrier screening for inherited genetic conditions** 75
   Lorraine Dugoff

7. **Before labor and first stage of labor** 85
   Serena Xodo

8. **Second stage of labor** 97
   Alexis Gimovsky

9. **Third stage of labor** 103
   Jennifer Salati and Jorge E. Tolosa

10. **Intrapartum fetal monitoring** 111
    Serena Xodo and Suneet P. Chauhan

11. **Analgesia and anesthesia** 125
    Kyle Jespersen and Michelle Mele

12. **Operative vaginal delivery** 137
    Adeeb Khalifeh

13. **Cesarean delivery** 143
    A. Dhanya Mackeen

14. **Trial of labor after caesarean delivery** 161
    Amen Ness and Amanda Yeaton-Massey

15. **Early pregnancy loss** 175
    Lisa K. Perriera, Beatrice A. Chen, and Aileen M. Gariepy

16. **Recurrent pregnancy loss** 183
    Reshama Navathe and Michela Villani

17. **Preterm birth prevention in asymptomatic women** 193
    Anju Suhag

18. Preterm labor 213
    B. Anthony Armson

19. Preterm premature rupture of membranes 227
    Anna Locatelli and Sara Consonni

20. Premature rupture of membranes at or near term 243
    Kimberly Ma and Sally Segel

21. Induction of labor 249
    Corina N. Schoen and Anthony C. Sciscione

22. Intra-amniotic infection... 265
    Elizabeth Liveright and Sara Campbell

23. Meconium 269
    Alessandro Ghidini

24. Malpresentation and malposition 273
    Alexis Gimovsky

25. Shoulder dystocia 281
    Sean C. Blackwell

26. Postpartum hemorrhage, retained placenta, and uterine inversion 289
    Jennifer Salati and Jorge E. Tolosa

27. Late-term and postterm pregnancies.............................. 295
    Rebecca Jackson

28. Placental disorders 299
    Moeun Son and William Grobman

29. Abruptio placentae 309
    John F. Visintine

30. Postpartum care.. 317
    Sarah K. Dotters-Katz and Alison M. Stuebe

31. The neonate.. 335
    Gary A. Emmett and Swati Murthy

32. The adnexal mass... 343
    Lauren Cooper Hand, George Patounakis, and Norman G. Rosenblum

33. Cervical cancer screening and management in pregnancy 349
    Talia M. Maas and Christine H. Kim

Index 355

Introduction

Welcome to the third edition of our evidence-based books on obstetrics and maternal-fetal medicine! I am indebted for your support! I can't believe how much praise we have gotten for these companion volumes. Your words of encouragement have kept me and all the collaborators past and present going now for well over a decade (we are indebted to contributors to previous editions of this text for their work). It has been extremely worthwhile, and fulfilling. You are making me happy! In return, I hope we are helping you and your patients toward ever better evidence-based care of pregnant women and their babies, and therefore better outcomes. Indeed, maternal and perinatal morbidities and mortalities throughout the world are improving.

To me, pregnancy has always been the most fascinating and exciting area of interest, as care involves not one, but at least two persons—the mother and the fetus—and leads to the miracle of a new life. I was a third-year medical student when, during a lecture, a resident said: "I went into obstetrics because this is the easiest medical field. Pregnancy is a physiologic process, and there isn't much to know. It is simple." I knew from my "classical" background that "obstetrics" means to "stand by, stay near," and that indeed pregnancy used to receive no medical support at all. After more than 25 years of practicing obstetrics, I now know that although physiologic and at times simple, obstetrics and maternal-fetal medicine can be the most complex of the medical fields: pregnancy is based on a different physiology than for nonpregnant women, can include any medical disease, require surgery, etc. It is not so simple. In fact, ignorance can kill, in this case with the health of the woman and her baby both at risk. Too often, I have gone to a lecture, journal club, rounds, or other didactic event to hear presented only one or a few articles regarding the subject, without the presenter reviewing the pertinent best review of the total literature and data. It is increasingly difficult to read and acquire knowledge of all that is published, even just in obstetrics, with about 3,000 scientific manuscripts published monthly on this subject. Some residents or even authorities would state at times that "there is no evidence" on a topic. We indeed used to be the field with the worst use of randomized trials [1]. As the best way to find something is to look for it, my coauthors and I searched for the best evidence. On careful investigation, indeed there are data on almost everything we do in obstetrics, especially on our interventions. Indeed, our field is now the pioneer for numbers of meta-analysis and extension of work for evidence-based reviews [2]. Obstetricians are now blessed with lots of data, and should make the best use of it.

The goals of this book are to summarize the best evidence available in the obstetrics and maternal-fetal medicine literature, and make the results of randomized controlled trials (RCTs) and meta-analyses of RCTs easily accessible to guide clinical care. The intent is to bridge the gap between knowledge (the evidence) and its easy application. To reach these goals, we reviewed all trials on effectiveness of interventions in obstetrics. Millions of pregnant women have participated in thousands of properly conducted RCTs. The efforts and sacrifice of mothers and their fetuses for science should be recognized at least by the physicians' awareness and understanding of these studies. Some of the trials have been summarized in over 600 Cochrane reviews, with hundreds of other meta-analyses also published in obstetrical topics (Table 1). All of the Cochrane reviews, as well as other meta-analyses and trials in obstetrics and maternal-fetal medicine, were reviewed and referenced. The material presented in single trials or meta-analyses is too detailed to be readily translated to advice for the busy clinician who needs to make dozens of clinical decisions a day. Even the Cochrane Library, the undisputed leader for evidence-based medicine efforts, has been criticized for its lack of flexibility and relevance in failing to be more easily understandable and clinically readily usable [3]. It is the gap between research and clinicians that needed to be filled, making sure that proven interventions are clearly highlighted, and are included in today's care. Just as all pilots fly planes under similar rules to maximize safety, all obstetricians should manage all aspects

Table 1 Obstetrical Evidence

- Over 600 current Cochrane reviews
- Hundreds of other current meta-analyses
- More than 1000 RCTs
- Millions of pregnant women randomized

of pregnancy with similar, evidenced-based rules. Indeed, only interventions that have been proven to provide benefit should be used routinely. On the other hand, *primum non nocere*: interventions that have clearly been shown to be not helpful or indeed harmful to mother and/or baby should be avoided. Another aim of the book is to make sure the pregnant woman and her unborn child are not marginalized by the medical community. In most circumstances, medical disorders of pregnant women can be treated as in nonpregnant adults. Moreover, there are several effective interventions for preventing or treating specific pregnancy disorders.

Evidence-based medicine is the concept of treating patients according to the best available evidence. While George Bernard Shaw said: "I have my own opinion, do not confuse me with the facts," this can be a deadly approach, especially in medicine, and compromise two or more lives at the same time in obstetrics and maternal-fetal medicine. What should be the basis for our interventions in medicine? Meta-analyses provide a comprehensive summary of the best research data available. As such, they provide the best guidance for "effective" clinical care [4]. It is unscientific and unethical to practice medicine, teach, or conduct research without first knowing all that has already been proven [4]. In the absence of trials or meta-analyses, lower level evidence is reviewed. This book aims at providing a current systematic review of all the best evidence, so that current practice and education, as well as future research can be based on the full story from the best-conducted research, not just the latest data or someone's opinion (Table 2).

These evidence-based guidelines cannot be used as a "cookbook," or a document dictating the best care. The knowledge from the best evidence presented in the guidelines needs to be integrated with other knowledge gained from clinical judgment, individual patient circumstances, and patient preferences, to lead to best medical practice. These are guidelines, not rules. Even the best scientific studies are not always perfectly related to any given individual, and clinical judgment must still be applied to allow the best "particularization" of the best knowledge for the individual, unique patient. Evidence-based medicine informs clinical judgment, but does not substitute it. It is important to understand though that greater clinical experience by the physician actually correlates with inferior quality of care if not integrated with knowledge of the best evidence [5]. The appropriate treatment is given in only 50% of visits to general physicians [5]. At times, limitations in resources may also limit the applicability of the guidelines, but should not limit the physician's knowledge. Guidelines and clinical pathways based on evidence not only point to the right management, but also can decrease medicolegal risk [6]. We aimed for brevity and clarity. Suggested management of the healthy or sick mother and child is stated as straightforwardly as possible, for everyone to easily understand and implement (Table 3). If you find the Cochrane reviews, scientific manuscripts, and other publications difficult to "translate" into care of your patients, this book is for you. We wanted to prevent information overload.

Table 2 Goals of This Book

- Improve the health of women and their children
- "Make it easy to do it right"
- Implement the best clinical care based on science (evidence), not opinion
- Education
- Develop lectures
- Decrease disease, use of detrimental interventions, and therefore costs
- Reduce medicolegal risks

Table 3 This Book Is For

- Obstetricians
- Midwives
- Family medicine and others (practicing obstetrics)
- Residents
- Nurses
- Medical students
- Maternal-fetal medicine attendings
- Maternal-fetal medicine fellows
- Other consultants on pregnancy
- Lay persons who want to know "the evidence"
- Politicians responsible for health care

On the other hand, "everything should be made as simple as possible, but not simpler" (A. Einstein). Key management points are highlighted at the beginning of each guideline, and in bold in the text. The chapters are divided in two volumes, one on obstetrics and one on maternal-fetal medicine; cross-references to chapters in *Maternal-Fetal Evidence Based Guidelines* have been noted in the text where applicable. Please contact us (vincenzo.berghella@jefferson.edu) for any comments, criticisms, corrections, missing evidence, etc.

I have the most fun discovering the best ways to alleviate discomfort and disease. The search for the best evidence for these guidelines has been a wonderful, stimulating journey. Keeping up with evidence-based medicine is exciting. The most rewarding part, as a teacher, is the dissemination of knowledge. I hope, truly, that this effort will be helpful to you, too.

REFERENCES

1. Cochrane AL. *1931–1971: A Critical Review, with Particular Reference to the Medical Profession.* In: *Medicines for the Year 2000.* London: Office of Health Economics, 1979:1–11. [Review]
2. Dickersin K, Manheimer E. The cochrane collaboration: Evaluation of health care and services using systematic reviews of the results of randomized controlled trials. *Clinic Obstet Gynecol.* 1998;41:315–331. [Review]
3. Summerskill W. Cochrane Collaboration and the evolution of evidence. *Lancet.* 2005;366:1760. [Review]
4. Chalmers I. Academia's failure to support systematic reviews. *Lancet.* 2005;365:469. [III]
5. Arky RA. The family business—To educate. *NEJM.* 2006;354:1922–1926. [Review]
6. Ransom SB, Studdert DM, Dombrowski MP, et al. Reduced medico-legal risk by compliance with obstetric clinical pathways: A case-control study. *Obstet Gynecol.* 2003;101:751–755. [II-2]

How to "Read" This Book

The knowledge from randomized controlled trials (RCTs) and meta-analyses of RCTs is summarized and easily available for clinical implementation. Key management points are highlighted at the beginning of each guideline, and in bold in the text. Relative risks and 95% confidence intervals from studies are quoted sparingly. Instead, the straight recommendation for care is made if one intervention is superior to the other, with the percent improvement often quoted to assess degree of benefit. If there is insufficient evidence to compare to interventions or managements, this is clearly stated.

References: Cochrane reviews with 0 RCT are not referenced, and, instead of referencing a meta-analysis with only one RCT, the actual RCT is usually referenced. RCTs that are already included in meta-analyses are not referenced, for brevity and because they can be easily accessed by reviewing the meta-analysis. If new RCTs are not included in meta-analysis, they are obviously referenced. Each reference was reviewed and evaluated for quality according to a modified method as outlined by the U.S. Preventive Services Task Force (http://www.ahrq.gov):

I	Evidence obtained from at least one properly designed randomized controlled trial.
II-1	Evidence obtained from well-designed controlled trials without randomization.
II-2	Evidence obtained from well-designed cohort or case-control analytic studies, preferably from more than one center or research group.
II-3	Evidence obtained from multiple time series with or without the intervention. Dramatic results in uncontrolled experiments could also be regarded as this type of evidence.
III (Review)	Opinions of respected authorities, based on clinical experience, descriptive studies, or reports of expert committees.

These levels are quoted after each reference. For RCTs and meta-analyses, the number of subjects studied is stated and, sometimes, more details are provided to aid the reader to understand the study better.

List of Abbreviations

Ab	antibody	DV	ductus venosus
AC	abdominal circumference	DVP	deepest vertical pocket
ACA	anticardiolipin antibody	DVT	deep vein thrombosis
ACOG	American College of Obstetricians and Gynecologists	ECV	external cephalic version
		EDC	estimated date of confinement
ACS	acute chest syndrome	EDD	estimated date of delivery (synonym of EDC)
ADR	autosomic dysreflexia		
AF	amniotic fluid	EKG	electrocardiogram
AFI	amniotic fluid index	FBS	fetal blood sampling
AFP	alpha-fetoprotein	FDA	Food and Drug Administration
AFV	amniotic fluid volume	FFN	fetal fibronectin
Ag	antigen	FGR	fetal growth restriction
AIDS	acquired immune deficiency syndrome	FHR	fetal heart rate
		FISH	fluorescent in situ hybridization
ALT	alanine aminotransferase	FLM	fetal lung maturity
ANA	antinuclear antibodies	FOB	father of baby
aPT	activated prothrombin time	FPR	false positive rate
APS	antiphospholipid syndrome	FTS	first-trimester screening
aPTT	activated partial thromboplastin time	FVL	factor V Leiden
AROM	artificial rupture of membranes	g	grams
ART	assisted reproductive technologies	GA	gestational age
ARV	antiretroviral therapy	GBS	group B streptococcus
ASA	aspirin	GDM	gestational diabetes
ASD	atrial septal defect	GI	gastrointestinal
AST	aspartate aminotransferase	HAART	highly active antiretroviral therapy
AT III	antithrombin III	HAV	hepatitis A virus
AZT	ziduvudine	HBV	hepatitis B virus
bid	"bis in die," i.e., twice per day	HBsAg	hepatitis B surface antigen
BPD	biparietal diameter	HCG	human chorionic gonadotroponin
BPD	bronchopulmonary dysplasia	Hct	hematocrit
BPP	biophysical profile	HCV	hepatitis C virus
BMI	body mass index	HG	hyperemesis gravidarum
BP	blood pressure	Hgb	hemoglobin
CAP	community-acquired pneumonia	HIE	hypoxic-ischemic encephalopathy
CBC	complete blood count	HIV	human immunodeficiency virus
CCB	calcium channel blocker	HR	heart rate
CDC	Centers for Disease Control	HSV	herpes simplex virus
CF	cystic fibrosis	HTN	hypertension
CHD	congenital heart defect	ICU	intensive care unit
CL	cervical length	IUGR	intrauterine growth restriction (synonym of FGR)
CMV	cytomegalovirus		
CNS	central nervous system	IV	intravenous
COX	cyclooxygenase	IVH	intraventricular hemorrhage
CRL	crown-rump length	L&D	labor and delivery floor
CSE	combined spinal epidural	LA	lupus anticoagulant
CSF	cerebrospinal fluid	Lab	laboratory
CT	computerized tomography	LFT	liver function tests
CVS	chorionic villus sampling	LMP	last menstrual period
DES	diethylstilbestrol	LBW	low birth weight (infants)
DIC	disseminated intravascular coagulation	LMW	low molecular weight
		LMWH	low-molecular-weight heparin
DM	diabetes mellitus	LR	likelihood ratio
DNA	deoxyribonucleic acid	MAS	meconium aspiration syndrome
DRVVT	dilute Russell's viper venom time	MCA	middle cerebral artery

MCV	mean corpuscular volume	PUBS	percutaneous umbilical blood sampling
MOM	multiple of the median	PVH	periventricular hemorrhage
MRI	magnetic resonance imaging	qd	once a day
MTHFR	methylenetetrahydrofolate reductase	qid	four times per day
MVP	maximum vertical pocket	qhs	before bedtime
NA	not available	QS	quadruple screen
NAIT	neonatal alloimmune thrombocytopenia	RBC	red blood cell
NEC	necrotizing enterocolitis	RCT	randomized controlled study
NIH	National Institutes of Health	RDS	respiratory distress syndrome
NIH	nonimmune hydrops	RNA	ribonucleic acid
NRFS	nonreassuring fetal status	ROM	rupture of membranes
NRFHR	nonreassuring fetal heart rate	RPR	rapid plasma reagin
NRFHT	nonreassuring fetal heart testing	RR	respiratory rate
NSAIDS	nonsteroidal anti-inflammatory drugs	Rx	treatment
NT	nuchal translucency	SAB	spontaneous abortion
NTD	neural tube defects	SC	subcutaneous
NST	nonstress test	SCI	spinal cord injury
n/v	nausea and/or vomiting	SDP	single deepest pocket
OR	operating room	SIDS	sudden infant death syndrome
ORA	oxytocin receptor agonist	SLE	systemic lupus erythematosus
PC	protein C	SPTB	spontaneous preterm birth
PCR	polymerase chain reaction	STD	sexually transmitted diseases (synonym of STI)
PE	pulmonary embolus	STI	sexually transmitted infections
PFT	pulmonary function tests	STS	second-trimester screening
PGM	prothrombin gene mutation	TB	tuberculosis
PID	pelvic inflammatory disease	TG	*Toxoplasma gondii*
PL	pregnancy loss	tid	three times per day
PNC	prenatal care	TOL	trial of labor
po	"per os," i.e., by mouth	TRAP	twin reversal arterial perfusion
PPH	postpartum hemorrhage	TRH	thyrotropin-releasing hormone
PRCD	planned repeat cesarean delivery	TSH	thyroid-stimulating hormone
PS	protein S	TSI	thyroid-stimulating immune globulins
PT	prothrombin time	TTTS	twin-twin transfusion syndrome
PTB	preterm birth	TVU	transvaginal ultrasound
PTT	partial thromboplastin time	UA	umbilical artery
PPROM	preterm premature rupture of membranes	UFH	unfractionated heparin
pRBC	packed red blood cells	U/S (or u/s)	ultrasound
PROM	preterm rupture of membranes	VBAC	vaginal birth after cesarean
PSV	peak systolic velocity	VDRL	venereal disease research laboratory
PTL	preterm labor	VSD	ventricular septal defect
PTU	propylthiouracil	VTE	venous thromboembolism
		WHO	World Health Organization

Contributors

Alfred Abuhamad Division of Maternal-Fetal Medicine, Eastern Virginia Medical School, Norfolk, Virginia

B. Anthony Armson Department of Obstetrics and Gynaecology, Dalhousie University, Halifax, Nova Scotia, Canada

Jason Baxter Department of Obstetrics and Gynecology, Maternal-Fetal Medicine, Sidney Kimmel Medical College of Thomas Jefferson University, Philadelphia, Pennsylvania

Sean C. Blackwell Division of Maternal-Fetal Medicine, University of Texas Health Science Center, Houston, Texas

Sara Campbell Department of Obstetrics and Gynecology, Sidney Kimmel Medical College of Thomas Jefferson University, Philadelphia, Pennsylvania

Suneet P. Chauhan Division of Maternal-Fetal Medicine, University of Texas Health Science Center, Houston, Texas

Beatrice A. Chen Department of Obstetrics, Gynecology, and Reproductive Sciences, University of Pittsburgh, Pittsburgh, Pennsylvania

Sara Consonni Department of Obstetrics and Gynecology, University of Milano-Bicocca School of Medicine, Milan, Italy

Sarah K. Dotters-Katz Department of Obstetrics and Gynecology, University of North Carolina School of Medicine, Chapel Hill, North Carolina

Lorraine Dugoff Department of Obstetrics and Gynecology, The Hospital of the University of Pennsylvania, Philadelphia, Pennsylvania

Gary A. Emmett Department of General Pediatrics, Thomas Jefferson University and AI DuPont Hospital for Children, Philadelphia, Pennsylvania

Aileen M. Gariepy Department of Obstetrics and Gynecology and Reproductive Sciences, Yale School of Medicine, New Haven, Connecticut

Alessandro Ghidini The Brock Perinatal Diagnostic Center, Inova Alexandria Hospital, Alexandria, Virginia, and Division of Maternal-Fetal Medicine, Georgetown University, Washington, D.C.

Alexis Gimovsky Division of Maternal-Fetal Medicine, Department of Obstetrics and Gynecology, The George Washington University School of Medicine and Health Sciences, Washington, DC

William Grobman Department of Obstetrics and Gynecology, Feinberg School of Medicine, Northwestern University, Chicago, Illinois

Lauren Cooper Hand Department of Obstetrics and Gynecology, Sidney Kimmel Medical College of Thomas Jefferson University, Philadelphia, Pennsylvania

Colleen Horan Department of Obstetrics and Gynecology, Central Vermont Medical Center, Berlin, Vermont

Rebecca Jackson Department of Obstetrics and Gynecology, Sidney Kimmel Medical College of Thomas Jefferson University, Philadelphia, Pennsylvania

Kyle Jespersen Department of Anesthesiology, Sidney Kimmel Medical College of Thomas Jefferson University, Philadelphia, Pennsylvania

Adeeb Khalifeh Department of Obstetrics and Gynecology, Sidney Kimmel Medical College of Thomas Jefferson University, Philadelphia, Pennsylvania

Christine H. Kim Division of Gynecologic Oncology, Department of Obstetrics and Gynecology, Sidney Kimmel Medical College of Thomas Jefferson University, Philadelphia, Pennsylvania

Dawnette Lewis Department of Obstetrics and Gynecology, Mount Sinai West, St Luke's Roosevelt Hospital, New York, New York

Elizabeth Liveright Department of Obstetrics and Gynecology, Sidney Kimmel Medical College of Thomas Jefferson University, Philadelphia, Pennsylvania

Anna Locatelli Department of Obstetrics and Gynecology, University of Milano-Bicocca School of Medicine, Milan, Italy

Kimberly Ma Division of Maternal-Fetal Medicine, Department of Obstetrics and Gynecology University of Washington Seattle, Washington

Talia M. Maas Department of Obstetrics and Gynecology, Sidney Kimmel Medical College of Thomas Jefferson University, Philadelphia, Pennsylvania

A. Dhanya Mackeen Division Maternal-Fetal Medicine, Geisinger Health System, Danville, Pennsylvania

Michelle Mele Department of Obstetrics and Gynecology, Sidney Kimmel Medical College of Thomas Jefferson University, Philadelphia, Pennsylvania

Swati Murthy Department of Neonatal Medicine, Sidney Kimmel Medical College of Thomas Jefferson University, Philadelphia, Pennsylvania

Reshama Navathe Department of Obstetrics and Gynecology, Sidney Kimmel Medical College of Thomas Jefferson University, Philadelphia, Pennsylvania

Amen Ness Department of Obstetrics and Gynecology, Stanford University Medical Center, Stanford, California

George Patounakis Department of Obstetrics and Gynecology, ART Institute of Washington, Bethesda, Maryland

Lisa K. Perriera Department of Obstetrics and Gynecology, Sidney Kimmel Medical College at Thomas Jefferson University, Philadelphia, Pennsylvania

Lea M. Porche Division of Maternal-Fetal Medicine, Eastern Virginia Medical School, Norfolk, Virginia

Joanna Quist-Nelson Department of Obstetrics and Gynecology, Sidney Kimmel Medical College of Thomas Jefferson University, Philadelphia, Pennsylvania

Norman G. Rosenblum Department of Obstetrics and Gynecology, Sidney Kimmel Medical College of Thomas Jefferson University, Philadelphia, Pennsylvania

Gabriele Saccone Department of Neuroscience, Reproductive Sciences, and Dentistry University of Naples Federico II, Naples, Italy

Jennifer Salati Department of Obstetrics and Gynecology, Maternal-Fetal Medicine, Oregon Health & Science University, Portland, Oregon

Corina N. Schoen Department of Obstetrics and Gynecology, Division of Maternal-Fetal Medicine, Baystate Medical Center, Springfield, Massachusetts

Anthony C. Sciscione Department of Maternal-Fetal Medicine, Delaware Center for Maternal & Fetal Medicine, Newark, Delaware

Sally Segel Department of Maternal-Fetal Medicine, The Vancouver Clinic, Portland, Oregon

Kerri Sendek Division of Maternal-Fetal Medicine, Department of Obstetrics and Gynecology, Sidney Kimmel Medical College of Thomas Jefferson University, Philadelphia, Pennsylvania

Moeun Son Department of Obstetrics and Gynecology, Feinberg School of Medicine, Northwestern University, Chicago, Illinois

Alison M. Stuebe Department of Obstetrics and Gynecology, University of North Carolina Hospitals, Chapel Hill, North Carolina

Anju Suhag Department of Obstetrics and Gynecology, University of Texas, Houston, Texas

Jorge E. Tolosa Department of Obstetrics and Gynecology, Division of Maternal-Fetal Medicine, Oregon Health and Science University, Portland, Oregon, and Departamento de Obstetricia y Ginecologia, Centro NACER, Salud Sexual y Reproductiva, Facultad de Medicina, Universidad de Antioquia, Medellin, Colombia

Michela Villani General Regional Hospital, Casa Sollievo della Sofferenza, San Giovanni Rotondo, Italy

John F. Visintine Division of Maternal-Fetal Medicine, Driscoll Children's Hospital, Corpus Christi, Texas

Serena Xodo Gynecology and Obstetrics Clinic, Santa Maria della Misericordia Hospital, Udine, Italy

Amanda Yeaton-Massey Department of Obstetrics and Gynecology, Stanford University Medical Center, Stanford, California

Preconception care

Johanna Quist-Nelson

KEY POINTS
- Preconception care is a **set of interventions that aim to identify and modify biomedical, behavioral, and social risks to a woman's health or pregnancy outcome through prevention and management.** The foundation of preconception care is prevention.
- Preconception care should occur any time if any health-care provider sees a reproductive-age woman (e.g., 15–44 years old).
- **Personal and family history, physical exam, laboratory screening, reproductive plan, nutrition, supplements, weight, exercise, vaccinations, and injury prevention** should be reviewed in all reproductive-age women.
- **Folic acid 400 µg/day,** as well as proper diet and exercise, should be encouraged.
- Regarding **vaccinations**, women should receive the **influenza** vaccine if planning pregnancy during flu season; the **rubella** and **varicella** vaccines if there is no evidence of immunity to these viruses; and **tetanus/diphtheria/pertussis** if lacking adult vaccination.
- **Specific interventions** to reduce morbidity and mortality for both the woman and her baby should be offered to those identified with chronic diseases or exposed to teratogens or illicit substances.

HISTORY
Preconception care has ancient origins. Plutarch (46–120 CE) wrote that the ancient Spartans "[...] ordered the maidens to exercise [...], to the end that the fruit they conceived might [...] take firmer root and find better growth" [1].

DEFINITION
Preconception care is a **set of interventions that aim to identify and modify biomedical, behavioral, and social risks to a woman's health or pregnancy outcome through prevention and management** [2,3]. This care has also been called prepregnancy, interpregnancy care, or periconceptional medicine [4].

AIM AND EFFECTIVENESS
The foundation of preconception care is prevention. Prevention of disease is the most effective form of medicine, and health care should shift from the delivery of procedure-based acute care to the provision of counseling-based preventive care [5,6]. For example, the two leading causes of death in the first year of life—birth defects and disorders caused by preterm birth (PTB)—can both be significantly reduced by preconception care. **Randomized controlled trials have corroborated that women are likely to incorporate change in modifiable health behaviors in response to preconception counseling** [7]. General practitioner-initiated preconception counseling not only decreases adverse pregnancy outcomes but also reduces anxiety in reproductive-age women [8].

TIMING AND TARGET POPULATION
The time that people should start caring for a pregnancy is not after, but before, conception. **Preconception care should occur any time any health-care provider sees a reproductive-age woman.** A reproductive-age woman is usually defined as between *15 and 44 years* of age, but occasionally even younger or older women contemplate, or at least are at risk of, pregnancy. The first prenatal visit is "months too late!" [9]. It often happens after first-trimester exposure to a potential teratogen has already occurred. There are about 1 billion reproductive-age women worldwide. In the United States, as an example, only about half of pregnancies are planned. As women get pregnant later in life, disease prevalence and medication exposures increase. Approximately 80% of reproductive-age U.S. women have dental disease, 66% are obese or overweight, 55% drink alcohol, 11% continue to smoke during pregnancy, 9% have diabetes, 6% asthma, 3% hypertension, and 3% cardiac disease [2]. The incidences of many of these conditions, even among pregnant women, are on the rise.

While some beneficial interventions could be started as soon as a pregnancy is diagnosed, this is unrealistic. Many of the preventive measures take time, often months, such as quitting smoking, losing weight, folic acid supplementation, and stabilization of medical conditions with effective and safe medications.

OPPORTUNITIES FOR PRECONCEPTION CARE
By age 25, about 50% of U.S. women have had at least one birth. The highest fertility rate occurs in 25- to 30-year-old women. By age 44, >85% have given birth at least once. About 84% of reproductive-age women, when asked, answer that they had a health-care visit within the prior year [6]. Therefore, **universal preconception care can be achieved if health-care providers make it a priority and plan for it at every opportunity** (Table 1.1). The approach should be **"every reproductive-age woman, every time" [6].** Every reproductive-age woman should be asked at every health-care encounter: **"Are you considering pregnancy?"** and **"Could you possibly become pregnant?"** Increased awareness of preconception care can be accomplished through improving health resources, public outreach, and advertising. Despite its great effectiveness, not all health-care plans cover preconception care. **A preconception visit (or often more than one) should be standard primary care,** as stated by the Center for Disease Control [2]. It should be as routine, if not more so, as prenatal care, as should the screening and interventions associated with it. A clear political will to drive the funding and insurance coverage for preconception care is required.

Therefore, providers of all specialties should be aware of the evidence-based recommendations (Tables 1.1–1.8).

Table 1.1 Visits That Are Opportunities for Preconception Care

- Adolescent (first gynecological exam)
- Any visit to a doctor during reproductive years (15–44 years old)
- College—graduate school health
- Family planning, contraception prescribing, and counseling
- Annual ob-gyn
- Postpartum
- Pregnancy test (especially if negative)
- Health maintenance
- Medical work
- Emergency visit
- Fertility
- (Pre)marriage

Table 1.2 Topics to Be Reviewed in Preconception Care

Screening for risk assessment
- Personal and family history, physical exam, and laboratory screening

Preventive health
- Reproductive plan
- Nutrition, supplements, weight, and exercise
- Vaccinations
- Injury prevention

Specific individual issues/"exposures"
- Chronic diseases
- Medications (teratogens)
- Substance abuse/environmental hazards and toxins

Sources: Modified from Johnson K et al., *MMWR Morb Mortal Wkly Rep*, 55(RR-6), 1–23, 2006; Henderson JT et al., *Women Health Issue*, 12, 138–149, 2002.

Organizations representing family and internal medicine, obstetrics and gynecology, nurse midwifery, nursing, public health, diabetes, neurology, cardiology, and many other associations have supported recommendations for preconception care. Unfortunately, practitioners seldom implement them [10], even though it is an opportunity to optimize the health of the woman independent of whether she is planning pregnancy [6]. Only one out of six obstetrician-gynecologists (ob-gyns) or family physicians provides preconception care to the majority of women for whom they provide prenatal care [11].

Preconception care may often need to be **multidisciplinary care**. Prior to pregnancy, a woman can have numerous different medical problems affecting different specialties, and her care should occur in close collaboration among the different fields involved. **Maternal physiology is different than nonpregnant adult physiology.** An entire field, **maternal-fetal medicine,** is dedicated to the care of pregnancies with maternal or fetal problems, and these specialists are particularly adept at directing best practices for preconception counseling. Preconception care occurs best if all practitioners, including primary and specialty care, either directly implement or appropriately refer for implementation of effective preconception screening and intervention. The worse scenario is the belief that a positive pregnancy test is a good reason to "stop all medicines" thereby stopping disease treatment. Prevent panic: get women ready for a healthy pregnancy before contraception is stopped.

CONTENT OF PRECONCEPTION CARE

Topics pertinent to optimizing preconception health and therefore future maternal and perinatal outcome should be discussed. Topics to be discussed in preconception care are listed in Table 1.2 [2,12]. Further research is needed to determine the best content of preconception care and the most effective way to implement it [13,14].

UNIVERSAL SCREENING AND RELATED INTERVENTIONS
History, Exam, and Laboratory Screen

Suggested preconception screening assessment is shown in Table 1.3 [12,15]. A **questionnaire should be completed ahead of time,** either on paper or online, to review this extensive list. A standardized form improves the completeness of preconception screening, which necessitates time and commitment [16]. This standardized preconception form should be integrated into the permanent record of all reproductive-age woman. In a randomized trial, women assigned to be screened with a preconception risk survey were found to have an average of nine risk factors, supporting the facts that even low-risk women may benefit from preconception screening [13].

History should be detailed, especially when pertinent positives are detected. **Prior inpatient and outpatient medical records should be reviewed**. Women should be empowered with easy access to their records (best if electronic), to facilitate multispecialty care coordination. Personal prenatal medical record access has been associated with increased maternal control, satisfaction during pregnancy, and increased availability of antenatal records during hospital attendance [17].

Prior **obstetrical and gynecological history,** including prior pregnancy complications, should be reviewed. Other reproductive issues should also be assessed: fertility, including the possibility of assisted reproductive technology needs, sexuality (in particular high-risk behaviors), contraception, partner selection, and sexual function. Several social issues need to be reviewed as well (Table 1.3).

All couples should have a basic screen for family history of **heritable genetic disorders,** with a pedigree to at least the second prior generation. Women belonging to an ethnic group at increased risk for a recessive condition (Table 1.4) should be offered appropriate screening. All couples should be made aware of the option for **cystic fibrosis** (CF) screening, especially those who have a family history of CF, are in a high-risk group, or are reproductive partners of individuals with CF [18]. Women with a specific indication for genetic testing should be referred for formal genetic counseling (see Chapters 5 and 6).

Physical exam details are shown in Table 1.3. Pelvic exam may include cytologic and sexually transmitted infection screening for women with certain risk factors. **Laboratory tests** are done routinely (Table 1.3) and depend on risk factors (Table 1.4) [12].

Reproductive Health Plan

Asking a reproductive-age woman, and therefore inducing her to think about, her reproductive health plan should be a **priority of any medical visit** [19]. Such a plan should address the desire (or not) for children; the optimal number, spacing, and timing of pregnancies; contraception to achieve this plan; opportunities to improve her health and therefore a successful reproductive life; and age-related changes in fertility [19]. Having a reproductive health plan reduces unintended pregnancies, age-related infertility, and fetal exposure to teratogens [2]. Very few women know that a **short interpregnancy interval (i.e., <6 months from the end of last pregnancy to** the next conception) is associated with increased incidence of both small-for-gestational-age and low-birth-weight neonates [20]. Folic acid depletion may be the etiology for these increased risks [21]. Education and **contraception advice** are necessary to aim for the wished reproductive plan, avoiding unplanned pregnancies, and optimizing the 18- to 24-month interpregnancy interval goal. In a nonrandomized study, preconception care decreased the number of unintended pregnancies [22].

Table 1.3 Preconception Screening Assessment for all Reproductive-Age Women (15–44 Years Old)

History
   Reason for visit
   Health status: obstetrical, gynecological, medical, surgical, and family history
   Use of prescription, over-the-counter, complementary, and alternative medicines
   Allergies (to medications or other)
   Tobacco, alcohol, other drug use
   Work-related exposures
   Dietary/nutrition assessment
   Physical activity
   Urinary and fecal incontinence

Physical examination
   Height, weight, body mass index (BMI)
   Blood pressure
   Head
   Neck: adenopathy and thyroid
   Breasts
   Heart, lungs
   Abdomen
   Pelvic examination
   Skin

Laboratory testing
   Rubella titer[a]
   Varicella titer[a]
   Human immunodeficiency virus (HIV) testing[b]
   Cervical cytology[c]
   Chlamydia testing (if aged 25 years or younger and sexually active)

Evaluation and counseling
   Sexuality and reproductive planning
      High-risk behaviors
      Discussion of a reproductive health plan
      Contraceptive options for prevention of unwanted pregnancy, including emergency contraception
      Genetic counseling
   Sexually transmitted diseases
      Partner selection
      Barrier protection
   Sexual function

Fitness and nutrition
   Dietary/Nutrition assessment
   Exercise program
   Folic acid supplementation (0.4 mg/day)
   Calcium intake

Psychosocial evaluation
   Abuse/neglect/violence (physical, sexual, and emotional)
   Sexual practices
   Lifestyle/stress
   Sleep disorders
   Home and work (including satisfaction, and environmental hazards)
   Interpersonal/family relationships; social support
   Depression (suicide)
   Criminality
   Education
   Language and culture
   Health insurance status; coverage; access; public programs

Table 1.3 Preconception Screening Assessment for all Reproductive-Age Women (15–44 Years Old) (Continued)

Cardiovascular risk factors
   Family history
   Hypertension
   Dyslipidemia
   Obesity
   Diabetes mellitus

Health/risk behaviors
   Hygiene (including dental)
   Injury prevention
      • Safety belts and helmets
      • Occupational hazards
      • Recreational hazards
      • Firearms
      • Hearing
      • Exercise and sports involvement
   Breast self-examination

Vaccinations
   See Table 1.5

Sources: Modified from Henderson JT et al., *Women Health Issue,* 12, 138–149, 2002; Jack BW et al., *Am J Obstet Gynecol,* 199(6B), S266–S279, 2008.
[a] Unless documented immunity.
[b] HIV screening should be offered as routine to all women of reproductive age, under an "opt-out" policy. Physicians should be aware of and follow their states'/countries' HIV screening requirements.
[c] Cervical cytology guidelines indicate that testing should begin at the age of 21, unless the patient is infected with HIV.

All women should be counseled that 2%–3% of babies are born with minor (usually) or major anomalies. Screening and diagnostic options to detect aneuploidy and birth defects should be reviewed so that women may consider their options in relation to their personal values.

Nutrition, Weight, and Exercise

Lifelong habits of healthy diet and regular exercise should be established preconceptionally [23]. Proper diet and exercise can prevent several complications of pregnancy, including gestational diabetes and hypertensive complications [24]. Some studies suggest a correlation between a diet high in fruits, vegetables, nuts, and legumes, less than two servings of meat weekly and at least two servings of fish weekly (the "Mediterranean Diet") with decreased rates of infertility and PTB [25–27].

In addition to following a healthy diet, issues of food safety are important to review. All meat, seafood, and shellfish should be **thoroughly cooked**. Eating at least 12 oz. of **fish** weekly is associated with several benefits, including a lower rate of PTB (see Chapter 17), but women must avoid >2 serving/week of shark, swordfish, king mackerel, some tuna, or tilefish, all of which may contain high concentrations of methyl mercury. Albacore (white) tuna has more mercury than canned, light tuna [28]. Other recommendations include **eating only pasteurized eggs and dairy products and washing raw fruits and vegetables** before eating. Women should try to obtain a minimum daily iodine intake of 150 mg/day. Education about proper hand, food, and cooking utensil hygiene is important, especially in developing countries.

Body mass index (BMI) should be calculated at least annually for reproductive-age women [29]. For women with a BMI that falls outside the normal range [28–34], preconception

Table 1.4 Preconception Laboratory Screening Depending on Risk Factors

Personal history:
  Age:
  - >35: fasting glucose

  Race:
  - African-American: fasting glucose; hemoglobin electrophoresis (for sickle cell disease)
  - Hispanic, Native American, Pacific Islander: fasting glucose
  - Mediterranean: mean corpuscular volume (MCV) screening (for thalassemia)
  - Ethnic testing: Ashkenazi—familial dysautonomia; Tay-Sachs; Canavan; Fanconi anemia type C; Niemann-Pick disease type A; Bloom's syndrome; Gaucher disease; glycogen storage 1a; maple syrup urine disease; mucolipidosis type IV

Prior obstetrical history:
  - Prior birth of a newborn weighting more than 9 lb or >4500 g (macrosomia): fasting glucose
  - History of gestational diabetes mellitus: fasting glucose
  - Prior unexplained fetal death: check autopsy and karyotype of fetal death; antiphospholipid antibody testing; fasting glucose
  - Prior infant with congenital anomaly (if not screened in that pregnancy): fasting glucose
  - Prior recurrent unexplained early pregnancy loss: antiphospholipid antibody testing; study of uterine anatomy; parental karyotype

Prior medical history:
  - Metabolic syndrome/obesity; family history of lipid or coronary disorders: cholesterol/lipid profile
  - Diabetes: lipid profile; hemoglobin A1c; cardiac and renal baseline function assessment; ophthalmologic exam
  - Hypertension: fasting glucose; baseline cardiac, renal, and liver functions
  - Multiple coronary heart disease risk factors (e.g., tobacco use, hypertension): lipid profile
  - High-density lipoprotein cholesterol level ≤35 mL/dL: fasting glucose
  - Triglyceride level ≥250 mg/dL: fasting glucose
  - History of impaired glucose tolerance or impaired fasting glucose: fasting glucose
  - Chronic use of steroids: fasting glucose
  - Polycystic ovary syndrome: fasting glucose
  - History of vascular disease: fasting glucose
  - Marfan syndrome: echocardiogram for assessment of aortic root; eye exam for lens
  - History of STD, drug abuse, etc.: HIV, Hep C
  - Recipients of blood from donors who later tested positive for HCV infection: Hep C
  - Recipients of blood or blood-component transfusion or organ transplant before July 1992: Hep C
  - Recipients of clotting factor concentrates before 1987: Hep C
  - Chronic (long-term) hemodialysis: Hep C
  - History of transfusion from 1978 to 1985: HIV
  - Invasive cervical cancer: HIV
  - HIV infection: STD screening; PPD
  - Medical risk factors known to increase risk of TB if infected: PPD
  - Not sure whether patient had varicella infection or vaccination in past: varicella titer

Social history:
  - HIV or TB contact, IV drug use, etc.: TB testing
  - History of injecting illegal drugs: Hep C; HIV; STD screening (chlamydia, gonorrhea, syphilis, etc.); PPD
  - Occupational percutaneous or mucosal exposure to HCV-positive blood: Hep C
  - More than one sexual partner since most recent HIV test or a sex partner with more than one sexual partner since most recent HIV test: HIV
  - Seeking treatment for STDs: HIV
  - History of prostitution: STD screening; HIV
  - Past or present sexual partner who is HIV positive or bisexual or injects drugs: HIV
  - Long-term residence or birth in an area with high prevalence of HIV infection: HIV
  - Adolescents who are or ever have been sexually active: HIV
  - Adolescents entering detention facilities: HIV; STD screening
  - Offer to women seeking preconception evaluation: HIV (all women should be screened)
  - History of multiple sexual partners or a sexual partner with multiple contacts: STD screening
  - Sexual contact with individuals with culture-proven STD: STD screening
  - History of repeated episodes of STDs: STD screening
  - Attendance at clinics for STDs: STD screening
  - All sexually active women aged 25 years or younger: chlamydia
  - All sexually active adolescents: gonorrhea
  - Close contact with individuals known or suspected to have TB: PPD
  - Born in country with high TB prevalence: PPD
  - Medically underserved: PPD
  - Low income: PPD
  - Alcoholism: PPD
  - Resident of long-term care facility (e.g., correctional institutions, mental institutions, and nursing homes and facilities): PPD
  - Health professional working in high-risk health-care facilities: PPD

Family history:
  - Family history of diabetes mellitus: fasting glucose
  - Family history of diabetes; history of gestational diabetes, overweight/obese, hypertension, high-risk ethnic group (African-American, Hispanic, Native American): fasting glucose every 3 years

Table 1.4 Preconception Laboratory Screening Depending on Risk Factors (*Continued*)

- Family history suggestive of familial hyperlipidemia: lipid profile
- Family history of premature (age < 50 years for men, age < 60 years for women) cardiovascular disease: lipid profile
- Colorectal cancer or adenomatous polyps in first-degree relative younger than 60 years or in two or more first-degree relatives of any ages; family history of familial adenomatous polyposis or hereditary nonpolyposis colon cancer: colonoscopy
- First-degree relative (i.e., mother, sister, or daughter) or multiple other relatives who have a history of premenopausal breast or breast or ovarian cancer: mammography
- Family history of Marfan syndrome: echocardiogram for assessment of aortic root; eye exam for lens
- Family history of breast cancer: mammography
- Family history of thyroid disease: TSH

Physical examination:
- Overweight (BMI ≥ 25): fasting glucose
- Hypertension: fasting glucose

Laboratory screening:
- Persistently abnormal alanine aminotransferase levels: Hep C
- Glycosuria: fasting glucose

Source: Modified from Henderson JT et al., *Women Health Issue*, 12, 138–149, 2002.
Abbreviations: STDs, sexually transmitted diseases; HIV, human immunodeficiency virus; Hep C, hepatitis C; HCV, hepatitis C virus; PPD, purified protein derivative; TB, tuberculosis; IV, intravenous; TSH, thyroid-stimulating hormone; BMI, body mass index.

counseling regarding the woman's increased risk of complications in pregnancy is extremely important. **Formal nutritional counseling should be offered and goals set to avoid pregnancy until optimal weight is achieved**. Women with low BMI should be screened for eating disorders. In overweight and obese women, **calorie and portion-size control** may be the most effective methods of sustained preconception weight loss. Unfortunately, there are no current evidence-based guidelines as to the most effective method of weight loss in the preconception period for obese and overweight patients [34]. Postpartum individual counseling on diet and physical activity increased the proportion of women returning to prepregnancy weight from 30% to 50% in one randomized trial [30].

An exercise routine that can be started preconceptionally and safely continued in pregnancy may include yoga; brisk walking (including hiking and backpacking); jogging; swimming; biking; cross-country skiing; and using fitness equipment such as an elliptical trainer, treadmill, or stationary bike. Women should be given standard advice for engaging in regular physical activity for 30–60 min/day for 5 or more days per week.

Supplements

The preconception intervention with the most evidence-based data to support its efficacy is **folic acid supplementation**. Folic acid supplementation is recommended, with a **minimum of 400 µg/day** for all women (93% decrease in neural tube defects [NTDs]), and **4 mg/day for women with prior children with NTDs** (69% decrease in recurrent NTDs) [32].

Supplementation should start at least 1 month before conception and continue until at least 28 days after conception (time of neural tube closure). Given the unpredictability of planned conception, all reproductive-age women should be on folic acid supplementation from menarche to menopause. Women taking antiseizure medications, other drugs that might interfere with folic acid metabolism, those with homozygous methylenetetrahydrofolate reductase (MTHFR) enzyme mutations, or those who are obese may need higher doses of folic acid supplementation. As increases in baseline serum folate level are directly proportional with a decrease in the incidence of NTD, some experts have advocated 5 mg of folic acid per day as optimal universal supplementation [33]. Folic acid supplementation has also been associated with a decrease in the risk of congenital anomalies other than NTDs (e.g., cardiac, facial clefts) [34,35].

The overall benefits or risks of fortifying basic foods such as grains with added folate have been associated with a 140–200 µg/day increase in supplementation and a 20%–50% decrease in incidence of NTD [33,36]. Education with provision of printed material [32,37], computerized counseling [38], and learner-centered nutrition education [39] all increase the awareness of the folate/NTDs association and the use of the folate supplements. These interventions may be effective in increasing the prophylactic use of additional preconception care activities.

There is insufficient evidence to justify the routine use of other supplements in reproductive-age women, especially in the developed world, unless a nutritional deficiency has been identified. It is important to obtain a **minimum daily iodine intake of 150 mg/day** and 10,000 IU daily of vitamin A (as beta-carotene) if deficiencies in these nutrients are identified. The use of certain supplements may be detrimental, especially if excessive amounts of lipid-soluble vitamins such as vitamin A (>10,000 IU/day) are taken, since they can be teratogenic. All supplements, including alternative and complementary medicines, should be reviewed (see also Chapter 2) [40,41].

Vaccines

Preconception vaccination for the prevention of fetal and maternal disease is an important preconception intervention (Table 1.5) (see also Chapter 38 in *Maternal-Fetal Evidence Based Guidelines*). **Maternal immunity to infections such as rubella and varicella** should be assessed for potential vaccination of nonimmune women, thus eliminating their risk for congenital syndromes associated with these viruses. Vaccination with live attenuated viruses should occur at least 4 weeks prior to conception due to theoretical risk of live virus affecting the fetus.

Annual influenza vaccination for women and their partners contemplating pregnancy will reduce the chance of maternal prenatal infection, a time during which higher morbidity has been documented. Influenza vaccination for new mothers and other close contacts of the newborn will reduce risk of infection for the child who is unable to receive vaccination until 6 months of age. Through this process of "cocooning," the newborn is protected from the high morbidity and mortality rates associated with influenza in the first year of life [42].

Table 1.5 Recommended Preconception Vaccinations

All reproductive-age women
- During flu season: Influenza
- No evidence of immunity to rubella: MMR
- No evidence of immunity to varicella: Varicella
- No adult Td vaccination in last 2 years: Tetanus/Diphtheria/Pertussis (Tdap)
- Hepatitis B nonimmune: Hepatitis B vaccine

Age
- All girls and women 9–26 years old: HPV
- All persons 18 years old and younger without immunity to hepatitis B infection: Hepatitis B

Occupational
- Health-care workers: Hepatitis B, Influenza, MMR, Varicella
- Public safety workers who have exposure to blood in the workplace: Hepatitis B
- Students in schools of medicine, dentistry, nursing, laboratory technology, and other allied health professions: Hepatitis B
- Staff of institutions for the developmentally disabled: Hepatitis B
- Individuals who work with HAV-infected nonhuman primates or with HAV in a research laboratory setting: Hepatitis A
- Military recruits: Meningococcus
- Microbiologists routinely exposed to *Neisseria meningitidis* isolates: Meningococcus

Social history/living situation
- Individuals with more than one sexual partner in the previous 6 months: Hepatitis B
- Household contacts and sexual partners of individuals with chronic hepatitis B infection: Hepatitis B
- Inmates of correctional facilities: Hepatitis B
- Clients of institutions for the developmentally disabled: Hepatitis B
- Illegal injected drug users: Hepatitis B
- Illegal drug users (injected and noninjected): Hepatitis A
- Exposure to environment where pneumococcal outbreaks have occurred: Pneumococcus
- Native Alaskan/Native American: Pneumococcus
- Alcohol abuse: Pneumococcus
- Tobacco smoking: Pneumococcus
- Residents of long-term care facilities: Influenza, Pneumococcus
- First-year college students living in dormitories: Meningococcus

Travel/immigration
- Individuals traveling to or working in countries that have high or intermediate endemicity of hepatitis A: Hepatitis A
- International travelers who will be in countries with high or intermediate prevalence of chronic hepatitis B infection for more than 6 months: Hepatitis B
- Travel to areas hyperendemic or epidemic for *Neisseria meningitides:* Meningococcus

Pulmonary conditions
- Chronic pulmonary disorders, including asthma: Pneumococcus

Cardiac conditions
- Chronic cardiovascular disorders (e.g., CHF, cardiomyopathies): Influenza, Pneumococcus

Renal conditions
- Chronic metabolic diseases, including renal dysfunction: Influenza, Pneumococcus
- Nephrotic syndrome: Pneumococcus
- End-stage renal disease including those on dialysis: Hepatitis B

Endocrine conditions
- Diabetes mellitus: Influenza, Pneumococcus

Hematologic/Immunologic conditions
- Prior transfusions: Hepatitis A, Hepatitis B
- Patients with clotting factor disorders (those who receive clotting factor concentrates): Hepatitis A
- Chronic illness, such as functional asplenia (e.g., sickle cell disease) or splenectomy: Pneumococcus
- Immunocompromised patients (e.g., HIV infection, hematologic or solid malignancies, chemotherapy, steroid therapy): Pneumococcus
- Adults with anatomic or functional asplenia: Pneumococcus, Meningococcus
- Terminal complement component deficiencies: Meningococcus

Infectious conditions
- Individuals with a recently acquired or recent evaluation for STI: Hepatitis B
- All clients in STD clinics: Hepatitis B
- HIV: Hepatitis B, Influenza, Pneumococcus, consider Meningococcus
- Individuals with Hepatitis C: Hepatitis A, Hepatitis B

GI/Hepatic conditions
- Chronic liver disease: Hepatitis A, Hepatitis B, Pneumococcus

Neurologic conditions
- Cerebrospinal fluid leaks: Pneumococcus

Source: Modified from Henderson JT et al., *Women Health Issue,* 12, 138–149, 2002 (see also Chapter 38 in *Maternal-Fetal Evidence Based Guidelines*).
Abbreviations: MMR, measles, mumps, and rubella; HPV, human papillomavirus; HAV, hepatitis A virus; CHF, congestive heart failure; HIV, human immunodeficiency virus; STI, sexually transmitted infection; STD, sexually transmitted disease; Td, tetanus diphteria.

Hepatitis B vaccination should be offered to all susceptible women of reproductive age in regions with intermediate and high rates of endemicity (where ≥2% of the population is hepatitis B surface antigen [HBsAg] positive). Perinatal transmission of hepatitis B results in 90% chance of chronic infection in the newborn, which places the child at risk for future cirrhosis and hepatocellular carcinoma. In regions of low prevalence, vaccination should be targeted to high-risk groups (Table 1.5).

Tetanus vaccination should remain up-to-date in reproductive-age women, particularly in regions of the world where maternal and neonatal tetanus is prevalent [43]. This has been shown to markedly reduce the incidence of tetanus related to parturition. Due to increasing prevalence and the high morbidity and mortality rates of neonatal pertussis, vaccination (in combination with tetanus and diphtheria) is recommended for all women and their partners of reproductive age who have not been immunized in their adult lives (since age 11 years) [44]. It is well documented that 75% of cases of neonatal pertussis have a family member as the index case [45]. Again, through the concept of cocooning, the incidence of neonatal pertussis can be reduced.

Other vaccination recommendations based on medical, occupational, or social risks are described in Table 1.5.

Injury Prevention

The second leading cause of death in reproductive-age women is accidents. Use of **seat belts** and **helmets** should be reviewed and strongly encouraged where appropriate. Inquiry should be made regarding occupational and recreational hazards. Possession and use of firearms should be evaluated. Possession and use of firearms should be evaluated, especially in individuals with a history of significant mental health diagnoses.

Universal Recommendations

Preconception recommendations for all women are listed in Table 1.6. Reproductive-age women should be aware of these evidence-based recommendations, both through their doctors and through public awareness campaigns. Several online resources are available [46–49]. Women and their partners should take more responsibility for their care and the future health of their offspring, and implement the health and lifestyle changes recommended.

SPECIFIC INDIVIDUAL ISSUES
History of PTB

There are currently no preconception recommendations for a woman with a history of PTB outside of the general recommendations for women trying to conceive. Randomized controlled trials examining preconception initiation of low-dose aspirin did not demonstrate an increased live birth rate or decrease in PTB [50,51]. Interval antibiotic treatment with azithromycin and metronidazole between pregnancies in women with a prior spontaneous PTB <34 weeks has not been associated with decreased risk of preterm delivery [52,53].

Advanced Maternal Age

In recent years, there has been a trend to delay childbearing. This trend is especially prevalent in developed countries, for example, in the United States where the birth rate in women age 40–44 has increased from 5.2 births per 1000 in 1990 to 10.4 births per 1000 women in 2013 [54]. It is well established that women of advanced maternal age (AMA) are at increased risks of poor obstetric outcomes, stillbirth, and fetal death [55–57]. Women of extreme AMA (>45 years old) have been found to increase the prevalence of preexisting chronic disease [58]. Although no Level I evidence exists for preconception testing in this population, it is reasonable to screen patients of extreme AMA for chronic hypertension, diabetes, hyperlipidemia, or heart disease with a cardiac echocardiogram.

Chronic Diseases

The incidences of several medical disorders such as obesity, diabetes mellitus, and hypertension are high and on the rise in reproductive-age women. There is literature for evidence-based recommendations on each disease or condition that can involve the reproductive-age woman and affect her reproductive health [3,4,15]. Full review of each is behind the scope of this chapter (see individual chapters in *Maternal-Fetal Evidence Based Guidelines*). Some common conditions are discussed for brief preconception management review (Table 1.7).

Diabetes
Diabetes (see Chapters 4 and 5 in *Maternal-Fetal Evidence Based Guidelines*) is associated with an increased risk of congenital anomalies, in particular cardiac defects and NTDs, if poorly controlled in the first weeks of pregnancy. The risk of congenital anomalies is related to long-term diabetic control, reflected in the level of glycosylated hemoglobin (**HgB A1c**): <7% = no increased risk (2%–3% baseline); 7%–9% = 15%; 9%–11% = 23%; >11% = 25% [32]. **It has been estimated that euglycemia (with normal HgB A1c) during the first trimester, which can only be achieved through attentive preconception counseling, could prevent >100,000 U.S. pregnancy losses or birth defects per year** [2]. Another cost analysis reported that universal preconception care could lead to averted lifetime costs for the affected cohort of children as high as $4.3 billion [59,60]. The benefits of preconception diabetes care have been previously demonstrated [61,62], even in teenagers [63]. Preconception care is also essential for counseling of the woman with conditions severe enough to make a successful pregnancy extremely

Table 1.6 Preconception Interventions for All Women

Intervention	Prevention of
Folic acid 400 µg/day[a]	NTDs, and also probably cardiac defects, facial clefts
Vaccinations	Maternal/perinatal infection[b] (Table 1.5)
Proper diet and exercise	Obesity, diabetes, hypertensive diseases, and their consequences
Injury prevention (e.g., seat belts, helmets)	Physical trauma
Screen for specific risk factors	See Table 1.7

[a]Consider higher dose, especially for women taking antiseizure medications, other drugs that might interfere with folic acid metabolism, those with homozygous MTHFR enzyme mutations, or those who are obese.
[b]By decreasing perinatal transmission, also decrease congenital defects caused by infection.
Abbreviations: NTDs, neural tube defects; STD, sexually transmitted disease; MTHFR, methylenetetrahydrofolate reductase.

Table 1.7 Preconception Care for Specific Maternal Medical Disorders

Disorder	Chapter in *MFM Evidence-Based Guidelines*	Brief preconception recommendations	Prevention of
Hypertensive disorders	1	- Discontinue ACE inhibitors and ARB; transition to another antihypertensive - Investigation into other etiologies - Baseline creatinine	Congenital anomalies, HTN complications, CD, IUGR, placental abruption, PTB, perinatal death
Cardiac disease	2	- Any necessary or possible cardiac interventions undergone prior to pregnancy - Patients with group III lesions or dilated cardiomyopathy are advised not to conceive	Worsening maternal cardiac condition, PTB, HTN
Obesity	3	- Counseling, diet and exercise to return to normal BMI - Evaluation of fasting lipids, fasting blood sugar - Screening for thyroid disease, OSA, HTN - If coexisting HTN or DM, obtain EKG and ECHO - Education about poor perinatal outcomes in obese patients - Motivational interviewing	Infertility, fetal NTDs, PTB, CD, HTN disorders, diabetes, VTE
Pregestational diabetes	4	- Optimize glycemic control with goal HgbA1c <7% - Screen for asymptomatic bacteriuria	Congenital anomalies, length of NICU admission, perinatal mortality and long-term health consequences in infant; miscarriage; maternal hospitalizations, maternal renal disease
Hypothyroidism	6	- Monitor TSH and FT4 to assure euthyroid state	Infertility, maternal HTN, miscarriage, preeclampsia, abruption, anemia, PTB, LBW, fetal death, possibly neurological problems in infant
Hyperthyroidism	7	- If radioiodine is required, should be completed 6–12 months before attempting conception - Emphasize minimum of 150 µg iodine daily (recommendation for all preconception women)	Spontaneous pregnancy loss, PTB, preeclampsia, fetal death, FGR, maternal congestive heart failure, and thyroid storm; neonatal Graves' disease
Prolactinoma	8	- Treat with dopamine agonist until decreasing size of adenoma to at least <1 cm, and normal prolactin	Risk of increasing size of maternal prolactinoma, possibly causing optic nerve impairment
History of hyperemesis gravidarum	9	- Start prenatal vitamins at 3 month prior to conception	Decreases risk of recurrence of hyperemesis
Inflammatory bowel disease	11	- Plan conception when disease is in remission >6 months - Discontinue MTX 3–6 months prior to conception - Screen for B12, vitamin D and iron deficiency	Birth defects
Liver transplantation	13	- Plan pregnancy when stable on immunosuppressive regimen >1 year - Assess baseline kidney/liver function, 24-hour urine - If patient is on mycophenolic acid products, assess fetal risks and consider switching to alternative immunosuppressant	PTB, HTN, preeclampsia, IUGR, GDM, graft rejection
Anemia	14	- Evaluation of etiology, assessment for iron, B12, and folate deficiency - In patients of African ancestry, hemoglobin electrophoresis - Genetic consult for patients with hereditable disorder	SGA, PTB, maternal CV compromise, need for transfusion
Sickle cell disease	15	- Start on 4 mg folic acid daily to optimize hemoglobin status - Vaccinate with pneumococcal and influenza - Discontinue teratogenic medications (ACE inhibitors, iron chelators)	Birth defects, crises
von Willebrand disease	16	- Consult hematology, genetics; administer Hepatitis B vaccine - Baseline labs (von Willebrand factor antigen, ristocetin cofactor activity, factor VIII, low-dose ristocetin-induced platelet aggregation, multimer assay)	Postpartum hemorrhage

Table 1.7 Preconception Care for Specific Maternal Medical Disorders (*Continued*)

Disorder	Chapter in *MFM Evidence-Based Guidelines*	Brief preconception recommendations	Prevention of
Renal disease/transplant	17	- Assess baseline creatinine, 24-hour proteinuria, intravenous pyelogram - Plan pregnancy when stable on immunosuppressive regimen, with drug therapies at maintenance levels if possible - Post transplant, await >1 year before conception	Preeclampsia
Seizures	19	- Recommend deferring conception until seizure-free on minimal medication, preferably monotherapy - Consult neurology to consider weaning medication if >2 years seizure-free - Start on folic acid 2–4 mg daily	Congenital anomalies
Spinal cord injury	20	- If cause is congenital, start on folic acid 4 mg daily and genetic counseling	Congenital anomalies
Mood disorders	21	- Counsel on the risks of discontinuing antidepressants in pregnancy - Stabilize mood on lowest effective dose prior to pregnancy - Avoid Paroxetine given risks of cardiac malformations	Cardiac malformations
Smoking	22	- Counsel regarding preventable pregnancy outcomes in patient who smoke - Encourage cessation with behavioral and educational interventions	PTB, LBW
Drug abuse	23	- Encourage patients to postpone conception until after completing detox	PTB, IUGR, neonatal withdrawal, etc. (Effect depends on drug of abuse)
Asthma	24	- Control of asthma with appropriate regimen through multidisciplinary care, set expectations to continue management throughout pregnancy	PTB, LBW, preeclampsia, perinatal mortality
Tuberculosis	24	- Screen high risk patients (hx of incarceration, TB exposure, international travel or immigration) with PPD or interferon gamma-release assay and treat accordingly	Active TB
Lupus	25	- Recommend conception when disease is in remission for >6 months - Screen for HTN, renal, heart, lung, or brain disease as well as antiphospholipid and SSA/SSB antibodies - Decrease meds to lowest possible effective dose - Replace mycophenolate mofetil and with other medications	HTN, preeclampsia, PTB, fetal death, IUGR, neonatal lupus
Venous thromboembolism and mechanical heart valves	28	- Screen all patients with history of VTE for thrombophilia - Perform any necessary valve replacements before pregnancy - If mechanical heart valve, consider continuing warfarin after full counseling of risks of warfarin embryopathy and under direction of cardiologist	Recurrence of venous thromboembolism
Hepatitis A	29	- Vaccinate patients who travel abroad, are at risk for contracting the disease, or who are infected with chronic hepatitis B or C prior to pregnancy; vaccine also safe in pregnancy	
Hepatitis B	30	- Administer HBV vaccine to any woman who is susceptible before pregnancy - If chronically infected, screen for Hepatitis A and vaccinate prior to pregnancy	Perinatal HBV transmission
Hepatitis C	31	- Screen high risk populations prior to pregnancy - Vaccinate against hepatitis A and B if non-immune - Consider treatment preconception	Cirrhosis, HCC, HCV infant transmission
HIV	32	- Initiate or modify antiretroviral therapy avoiding teratogenic agents (e.g., efavirenz) - CD4 count and indicated prophylaxis based on level - Screen for STIs - Advise how to optimize conception, yet minimizing risk of transmission	Perinatal HIV infection

(*Continued*)

Table 1.7 Preconception Care for Specific Maternal Medical Disorders (*Continued*)

Disorder	Chapter in *MFM Evidence-Based Guidelines*	Brief preconception recommendations	Prevention of
STI testing	33, 34, 35, 36	- Screen and treat for gonorrhea, chlamydia, syphilis and trichomonas in high risk patients (e.g., <25, prior STI, multiple sexual partners, inconsistent condom use, sex work, or drug use)	Ectopic pregnancy
PKU		- Low-phenylalanine diet	PKU-related mental retardation
Social issues (e.g., abuse)		- Counseling; Referral to appropriate agency	Physical and emotional trauma and their consequences
Alcohol		- Avoid all alcohol intake	Congenital anomalies, mental retardation
Supplements and over-the-counter medications		- Review and counsel: Avoid excess of recommended daily allowance (RDA) (see also Chapter 2)	Congenital anomalies

Abbreviations: ACE, angiotensin converting enzyme; ARB, angiotensin receptor blocker; HTN, hypertension; IUGR, intrauterine growth restriction; CD, cesarean delivery; PTB, preterm birth; LBW, low birth weight; NICU, neonatal intensive care unit; BMI, body mass index; DM, diabetes mellitus; EKG, electrocardiogram; ECHO, echocardiogram; OSA, obstructive sleep apnea; NTD, neural tube defects; VTE, venous thromboembolism; FGR, fetal growth restriction; TSH, thyroid-stimulating hormone; FT4, free thyroxine; CV, cardiovascular; MTX, methotrexate; TB, tuberculosis; PPD, purified protein derivative; SSA/SSB, Sjogren syndrome related antigen A and B; HIV, human immunodeficiency virus; STI, sexually transmitted infections; PKU, phenylketonuria.

unlikely. The diabetic woman with either ischemic heart disease, untreated proliferative retinopathy, creatinine clearance <50 mL/min, proteinuria >2 g/24 hours, creatinine >2 mg/dL, uncontrolled hypertension, or gastropathy should be told not to get pregnant before the above conditions can be improved, and counseled regarding adoption if the conditions cannot be improved [64]. The frequency of fetal/infant and maternal morbidity and mortality is reduced in diabetic women seeking consultation in preparation for pregnancy, but unfortunately only about one-third of these women receive such consultation [65]. The preconception consultation affords the opportunity to screen for vascular consequences of the diabetes, with **ophthalmologic, electrocardiogram (EKG), and renal evaluation via a 24-hour urine collection for total protein and creatinine clearance,** and determine ancillary pregnancy risks. Proliferative retinopathy should be treated with laser before pregnancy. *A thyroid-stimulating hormone (TSH)* level should be checked, as 40% of young women with type 1 diabetes have hypothyroidism. Of note, there is insufficient evidence to treat subclinical hypothyroidism [66].

Diabetes evaluation should emphasize the importance of tight glycemic control, with normalization of the HgB A1c to at least <7%. To achieve euglycemia, **diet, glucose monitoring, and exercise are always stressed. If euglycemia is not achieved with these means, oral hypoglycemic agents or insulins are utilized,** and their regimens should be optimized preconceptionally. Of the oral hypoglycemic agents, **glyburide and glucophage can be used,** and probably continued during pregnancy. The original safety data available for glyburide showed that it did not cross the placenta in appreciable amounts [67], but recent data have shown a 70% level in umbilical blood compared with maternal blood [68]. The other oral hypoglycemic agents should not be used for preconception glycemic control, as there is no sufficient evidence for their safety and efficacy in pregnancy. **A common insulin regimen currently used by diabetologists is long-acting (e.g., glargine) and short-acting (e.g., lispro).** This is a safe and effective regimen in pregnancy, too. Women compliant with insulin pumps should continue this regimen.

If a woman has a history of gestational diabetes, appropriate postpartum diabetes screening should be performed. Interconception counseling and lifestyle modifications may be beneficial for future pregnancies [69].

Hypertension

Hypertension (see Chapter 1 in *Maternal-Fetal Evidence Based Guidelines*) is associated with several maternal [worsening hypertension; superimposed preeclampsia; severe preeclampsia; eclampsia; hemolysis, elevated liver enzyme levels, and a low platelet count (HELLP) syndrome; cesarean delivery] and fetal (growth restriction; oligohydramnios; placental abruption; PTB; perinatal death) risks in pregnancy. **Serum creatinine, 24-hour urine for total protein and creatinine clearance, EKG, and ophthalmologic exam** are suggested, especially in women with long-standing or severe hypertension. It is important to identify cardiovascular risk factors and any reversible cause of hypertension, as well as assess for target organ damage or cardiovascular disease. If hypertension is newly diagnosed and has not been evaluated previously, a medical consult may be indicated to assess for any of these factors. Secondary hypertension, target organ damage (left ventricular dysfunction, retinopathy, dyslipidemia, microvascular disease, and prior stroke), maternal age >40, previous pregnancy loss, systolic blood pressure ≥180 mmHg, or diastolic blood pressure ≥110 mmHg are associated with higher risks in pregnancy. Abnormalities should be addressed and managed appropriately. If, for example, serum creatinine is >1.4 mg/dL, the woman should be aware of increased risks in pregnancy (pregnancy loss, reduced birth weight, PTB, and accelerated deterioration of maternal renal disease). Even mild renal disease (creatinine 1.1–1.4 mg/dL) with uncontrolled hypertension is associated with tenfold higher risk of fetal loss. Preconception prevention can be enormously effective. **Thirty minutes of exercise five times per week in all women with hypertension and weight reduction if overweight are recommended.** Restriction of sodium intake to the same <2.4 g sodium daily intake recommended for essential hypertension is beneficial in nonpregnant adults. If antihypertensive medical therapy is necessary, **angiotensin-converting enzyme (ACE) inhibitors and angiotensin II (AII) receptor antagonists should be discontinued** as they are associated with birth defects, fetal growth restriction, oligohydramnios, neonatal renal failure, and neonatal death in pregnancy. All other antihypertensive agents should be used at the lowest effective dose and are probably safe if started preconceptionally and continued in pregnancy.

Seizure Disorders

Conception should be deferred until seizures are well controlled on the minimum effective dose of medication (see Chapter 19 in *Maternal-Fetal Evidence Based Guidelines*). **Monotherapy** is preferable. Lamotrigine has been reported to be the first-line therapy for nonpregnant adults for partial seizures [70–72] and is associated with a low incidence of major malformations ([73], but not in all studies [74]. The best choice is the antiepileptic drug (AED) that best controls the seizures. The AEDs are usually U.S. Food and Drug Administration (FDA) category C (human risk unknown, but none proven yet) except for the following AEDs that are known potential teratogens: carbamazepine, primidone, phenytoin, and valproate (Table 1.8). These four AEDs should therefore be avoided if possible, by using a different therapy beginning in the preconception period. **Women who have been seizure-free for ≥2 years with a normal electroencephalogram (EEG) may be eligible to stop anticonvulsant therapy after consulting with a neurologist** [75].

Medications/Teratogens

Detailed discussion regarding prescribed and over-the-counter medications should occur at the preconception visit. The indication, safety, effectiveness, and necessity of each drug need to be reviewed. Often, women and their doctors stop efficacious and necessary medications as soon as the woman finds out she is pregnant, compromising the health of both the woman and her baby. **The vast majority of prescribed medications are safe in pregnancy, even in the first trimester. Only a few drugs, chemicals, infections, or radiation are proven teratogens** (Table 1.8) [76,77]. These should be avoided, except in rare circumstances (e.g., the woman with mechanical cardiac valves who accepts the teratogenic risk of warfarin). This medication counseling is often a crucial part of preconception care and can save and ameliorate significantly the health of a future offspring. Great resources exist on the Web for up-to-date teratologic information [78–80].

Substance Abuse/Environmental Hazards/Toxins

Tobacco smoking during pregnancy is associated with increased risks of several complications (see Chapter 22 in *Maternal-Fetal Evidence Based Guidelines*). The benefits of smoking cessation are tremendous: prevention of 10% of perinatal deaths, 35% of low-birth weight births, and 15% of preterm deliveries [81]. Smoking only one to five cigarettes per day is associated with a 55% higher incidence of low birth weight compared with nonsmokers. Reproductive-age women should be informed of other smoking-related diseases, such as ischemic heart disease, cancer, lung diseases, pneumonia, stroke, and congestive heart failure. Women at greatest risk for smoking are those <25 years old with less than a high school education. Smoking makes a major contribution to disparities in mortality [82]. Smoking cessation programs are associated with a 6% increase in smoking cessation, and decreases in incidences of low birth weight (by 19%) and PTB (by 16%) [83]. **Support and reward techniques** to help quit smoking are one of the best form of evidence-based medicine, supported by over 20 high-quality randomized trials. The "5 As" for screening and interventions to prevent smoking in pregnancy are **Ask, Advise, Assess, Assist, and Arrange** [67]. **Counseling with behavioral and educational interventions is associated with highest cessation rates. If necessary, most pharmacotherapies are effective preconception,** but contraindicated or with uncertain safety and efficacy during pregnancy. Nicotine replacement therapy (e.g., patch, gum, and bupropion) is safe and effective in reproductive-age women, but there is insufficient evidence for recommending them in pregnant smokers. Nicotine replacement therapy is associated with known adverse fetal effects, and nicotine is detected in breast milk. Possibly the best prevention of the adverse effects of smoking on pregnancy is achieved by avoiding sale of tobacco to young people, prohibition of smoking in public places, increase in tobacco taxation, workplace smoking cessation programs, and banning of tobacco sponsorship of sporting and cultural events.

Numerous recreational drug exposures have adverse pregnancy effects (see Chapter 23 in *Maternal-Fetal Evidence Based Guidelines*). This list is extensive and includes, but not limited to, common recreational drugs such as alcohol, cannabinoids, cocaine, heroin, and methamphetamines. Working to ensure that women with substance abuse issues engage in safe sex practices and family planning is a constant challenge, and these women are disproportionately overrepresented among women with unplanned pregnancies.

Table 1.8 Teratogens

Prescribed drugs
- Androgens and testosterone derivatives (e.g., danazol)
- Angiotensin-converting enzyme (ACE) inhibitors (e.g., enalapril, captopril) and angiotensin II receptor blockers
- Coumadin derivatives (e.g., warfarin)
- Carbamazepine
- Diethylstilbestrol
- Folic acid antagonists (methotrexate and aminopterin)
- HMG-CoA reductase inhibitors (statins)
- Lithium
- Phenytoin
- Primidone
- Streptomycin and kanamycin
- Tetracycline
- Thalidomide and leflunomide
- Trimethadione and paramethadione
- Valproic acid
- Vitamin A above RDA, and its derivatives (e.g., isotretinoin, etretinate, and retinoids)

Chemicals
- Lead
- Mercury

Drugs of abuse
- Alcohol
- Cocaine

Infections
- Cytomegalovirus
- Rubella
- Syphilis
- Toxoplasmosis
- Varicella

Radiation

Sources: Modified from Fretts RC et al., *N.Engl.J.Med.*, 333(15), 953–957, 1995; Reddy UM et al., *Am J Obstet Gynecol*, 195(3):764–770, 2006.
Abbreviations: HMG-CoA, 3-hydroxy-3-methyl-glutaryl-CoA reductase; RDA, recommended daily allowance.

REFERENCES

1. John D (Trans.). *Plutarch: Lycurgus 14.* New York, NY: Random House, 1932:59–60. [Historical reference]
2. Johnson K, Posner SF, Biermann J, et al. Recommendations to improve preconception health and health care—United States. A report of the CDC/ATSDR Preconception Care Work Group and the Select Panel on Preconception Care. *MMWR Morb Mortal Wkly Rep.* 2006;55(RR-6):1–23. Available at: http://www.cdc.gov/mmwr/PDF/rr/rr5506.pdf. Accessed on August 28, 2015. [Review]
3. Berghella V, Buchanan E, Pereira L, et al. Preconception care. *Obstet Gynecol Surv.* 2010;65(2):119–131. [Review]
4. Greer I, Steegers E. *Periconceptional Medicine.* London, UK, and New York, NY: Informa Healthcare, 2008. [Review]
5. The U.S. Preventative Services Task Forces' Guide to Clinical Preventive Services, 2006. Available at: http://www.ahrq.gov/clinic/uspstfix.htm. Accessed on January 18, 2009. [Guideline]
6. Atrash H, Jack BW, Johnson K, et al. Where is the "W"oman in MCH? *Am J Obstet Gynecol.* 2008;199(6B):S259–S265. [Review]
7. Whitworth M, Dowswell T. Routine pre-pregnancy health promotion for improving pregnancy outcomes. *Cochrane Database Syst Rev.* 2009;4:CD007536. [Meta-analysis; 4 RCTs, n = 2300]
8. de Jong-Potjer LC, Elsinga J, le Cessie S, et al. GP-initiated preconception counselling in a randomised controlled trial does not induce anxiety. *BMC Fam Pract.* 2006;7:66. [RCT]
9. Rabin R. That prenatal visit may be months too late. *The New York Times*, November 28, 2006. Available at: http://www.nytimes.com/2006/11/28/health/28natal.html. Accessed on March 13, 2009. [Magazine article]
10. Williams J, Abelman S, Fassett E, et al. Health care provider knowledge and practices regarding folic acid, United States 2002-03. *Matern Child Health J.* 2006;10(5 suppl):s67–s72. [II-3]
11. Henderson JT, Weisman CS, Grason H. Are two doctors better than one? Women's physician use and appropriate care. *Women Health Issue.* 2002;12:138–149. [III]
12. American College of Obstetricians and Gynecologists. Primary and preventive care: Periodic assessments. ACOG Committee Opinion No. 357. *Obstet Gynecol.* 2006;108:1615–1622. [Review]
13. Jack BW, Culpepper L, Babcock J, et al. Addressing preconception risks identified at the time of a negative pregnancy test: A randomized trial. *J Fam Pract.* 1998;47:33–38. [II-3]
14. Lumley J, Donohue L. Aiming to increase birth weight: A randomized trial of pre-pregnancy information, advice and counseling in inner-urban Melbourne. *BMC Public Health.* 2006;6:299–310. [RCT]
15. Jack BW, Atrash H, Coonrod DV, et al. The clinical content of preconception care: An overview and preparation of this supplement. *Am J Obstet Gynecol.* 2008;199(6B):S266–S279. [Review]
16. Bernstein PS, Sanghvi T, Merkatz IR. Improving preconception care. *J Repro Med.* 2000;45:546–552. [Review]
17. Brown HC, Smith HJ, Mori R, et al. Giving women their own case notes during pregnancy. *Cochrane Database Syst Rev.* 2015;(10): CD002856. [Meta-analysis]
18. American College of Obstetricians and Gynecologists and American College of Medical Genetics. *Preconception and Prenatal Carrier Screen for Cystic Fibrosis: Clinical and Laboratory Guidelines.* Washington, DC: ACOG/ACMG, 2001. [Guideline]
19. American College of Obstetricians and Gynecologists. The importance of preconception care in the continuum of women's health care. ACOG Committee Opinion No. 313. *Obstet Gynecol.* 2005;106:665–666. [Review]
20. Zhu B-P, Rolfs RT, Nangle BE, et al. Effect of interval between pregnancies on perinatal outcomes. *N Engl J Med.* 1999;340:589–594. [II-2]
21. Smits LJ, Essed GGM. Short interpregnancy intervals and unfavourable pregnancy outcome: role of folate depletion. *Lancet.* 2001;358:2074–2077. [Review]
22. Moos MK, Bangdiwala SI, Meibohm AR, et al. The impact of a preconceptional health promotion program on intendedness of pregnancy. *Am J Perinatol.* 1996;13:103–108. [II-3]
23. United States Department of Agriculture. MyPyramid.gov. Available at: http://www.mypyramid.gov/. Accessed on March 13, 2009. [Guideline]
24. Tieu J, Crowther CA, Middleton P. Dietary advice in pregnancy for preventing gestational diabetes mellitus. *Cochrane Database Syst Rev.* 2008;2:CD006674. [Meta-analysis]
25. Mikkelsen TB, Osterdal ML, Knudsen VK, et al. Association between a Mediterranean-type diet and risk of preterm birth among Danish women: A prospective cohort study. *Acta Obstet Gynecol Scand.* 2008;87(3):325–330. [II-1]
26. Vujkovic M, Steegers EA, Looman CW, et al. The maternal Mediterranean dietary pattern is associated with a reduced risk of spina bifida in the offspring. *BJOG.* 2009;116(3):408–415. [II-1]
27. Vujkovic M, de Vries JH, Lindemans J, et al. The preconception Mediterranean dietary pattern in couples undergoing in vitro fertilization/intracytoplasmic sperm injection treatment increases the chance of pregnancy. *Fertil Steril* 2010;94(6):2096-2101. [II-2].
28. Vujkovic M, de Vries JH, Lindemans J, et al. The preconception Mediterranean dietary pattern in couples undergoing in vitro fertilization/intracytoplasmic sperm injection treatment increases the chance of pregnancy. *Fertil Steril.* 2010;94(6):2096–2101 [Epub March 1, 2010]. [II-2]
29. U.S. Department of Health and Human Services and U.S. Environmental Protection Agency. What you need to know about mercury in fish and shellfish. 2004 EPA and FDA advice for women who might become pregnant, women who are pregnant, nursing mothers, young children. Washington, DC: U.S. Environmental Protection Agency, 2004. Available at: http://www.cfsan.fda.gov/~dms/admehg3.html. Accessed on February 23, 2009. [Review]
30. National Institute of Health Publication No. 98-4083. Clinical Guidelines on the Identification, Evaluation, and Treatment of Overweight and Obesity in Adults: The Evidence Report. NHLBI (National Heart, Lung, and Blood Institute), 1998. [Guideline]
31. Kinnunen TI, Pasanen M, Aittasalo M, et al. Reducing postpartum weight retention–A pilot trial in primary health care. *Nutr J.* 2007;6:21–30. [II-2]
32. De-Regil LM, Fernández-Gaxiola AC, Dowswell T, et al. Effects and safety of periconceptional folate supplementation for preventing birth defects. *Cochrane Database Syst Rev.* 2010;(10):CD007950 [Review]. [Meta-analysis]
33. Wald NJ. Folic acid and the prevention of neural-tube defects. *N Engl J Med.* 2004;350:101–103. [Review]
34. Opray N, Grivell RM, Deussen AR, et al. Directed preconception health programs and interventions for improving pregnancy outcomes for women who are overweight or obese. *Cochrane Database Syst Rev.* 2015;1:CD010932. [Meta-analysis]
35. Wilcox AJ, Lie RT, Solvoll K, et al. Folic acid supplements and risk of facial clefts: national population based case-control study. *BMJ.* 2007;334(7591):464. [II-3]
36. Honein MA, Paulozzi LJ, Mathews TJ, et al. Impact of folic acid fortification of the U.S. food supply on the occurrence of neural tube defects. *JAMA.* 2001;285:2981–2986. [II-1]
37. Watson MJ, Watson LF, Bell RJ, et al. A randomized community intervention trial to increase awareness and knowledge of the role of periconceptional folate in women of child-bearing age. *Health Expect.* 1999;2:255–265. [RCT]
38. Scwartz EB, Sobota M, Gonzales R, et al. Computerized counseling for folate and use: A randomized controlled trial. *Am J Prev Med.* 2008;35:606–607. [RCT]
39. Cena ER, Heneman K, Espinosa-Hall G, et al. Learner-centered nutrition education improves folate intake and food-related behaviors in non-pregnant, low-income women of childbearing age. *J Am Diet Assoc.* 2008;108:1627–1635. [RCT]
40. Mahomed K, Gulmezoglu AM. Maternal iodine supplements in areas of deficiency. *Cochrane Database Syst Rev.* 2009;1:CD000135. [Systematic review]

41. van den Broek N, Dou L, Othman M, et al. Vitamin A supplementation during pregnancy for maternal and newborn outcomes. *Cochrane Database Syst Rev.* 2010;(11):CD001996. [Meta-analysis]
42. Fiore AE, Shay DK, Broder K, et al. Prevention and control of influenza. *MMWR.* 2008;57(RR-7):1–60. [Guideline]
43. Tetanus vaccine: WHO position paper. *Wkly Epidemiol Rec.* 2006; 81:198–208. [Review]
44. Kretsinger K, Broder KR, Cortese MM, et al. Preventing tetanus, diphtheria, and pertussis among adults: Use of tetanus toxoid, reduced diphtheria toxoid and acellular pertussis vaccine. *MMWR Recomm Rep.* 2006;55(RR-17):1–37. [Guideline]
45. Bisgard KM, Pascual FB, Ehresmann KR, et al. Infant pertussis: Who was the source? *Ped Inf Dis J.* 2004;23(11):985–989. [Review]
46. Department of Health and Human Services Centers for Disease Control and Prevention (CDC). Available at: http://www.cdc.gov/ncbddd/preconception/default.htm. Accessed on March 13, 2009. [Guideline]
47. U.S. National Library of Medicine and the National Institutes of Health, Medline Plus. Available at: http://www.nlm.nih.gov/medlineplus/preconceptioncare.html. Accessed on March 13, 2009. [Guideline]
48. March of Dimes. Available at: http://www.marchofdimes.com. Accessed March 13, 2009. [Guideline]
49. The American College of Obstetricians and Gynecologists (ACOG). Available at: http://www.acog.org. Accessed on March 13, 2009. [Review]
50. Schisterman EF, Silver RM, Lesher LL et al. Preconception low-dose aspirin and pregnancy outcomes: Results from the EAGeR randomised trial. *Lancet.* 2014;384(9937):29–36. [RCT]
51. Silver RM, Ahrens K, Wong LF, et al. Low-dose aspirin and preterm birth: A randomized controlled trial. *Obstet Gynecol.* 2015;125(4):876–884. [RCT]
52. Tita AT, Cliver SP, Goepfert AR, et al. Clinical trial of interconceptional antibiotics to prevent preterm birth: Subgroup analyses and possible adverse antibiotic-microbial interaction. *Am J Obstet Gynecol.* 2007;197:367.e1–6. [RCT, n = 124]
53. Andrews WW, Goldenberg RL, Hauth JC, et al. Interconceptional antibiotics to prevent spontaneous preterm birth: A randomized clinical trial. *Am J Obstet Gynecol.* 2006;194:617–623. [RCT, n = 124]
54. *National Vital Statistics Reports*, Vol. 64, No. 1, January 15, 2015. [Database]
55. Fretts RC, Schmittdiel J, McLean FH, et al. Increased maternal age and the risk of fetal death. *N Engl J Med.* 1995 Oct 12;333(15):953–957.
56. Reddy UM, Ko CW, Willinger M. Maternal age and the risk of stillbirth throughout pregnancy in the United States. *Am J Obstet Gynecol.* 2006 Sep;195(3):764–770.
57. Salem Yaniv S, Levy A, Wiznitzer A, et al. A significant linear association exists between advanced maternal age and adverse perinatal outcome. *Arch Gynecol Obstet.* 2011 Apr;283(4):755–759. Epub 2010 Apr 8.
58. Yogev Y, Melamed N, Bardin R, et al. Pregnancy outcome at extremely advanced maternal age. *Am J Obstet Gynecol.* 2010 Dec;203(6):558.e1–7.
59. Peterson C, Grosse SD, Sharma AJ, et al. Preventable health and cost burden of adverse birth outcomes associated with pregestational diabetes in the United States. *Am J Obstet Gynecol.* 2015;212:74e1–9. [Economic Analysis]
60. Boggess KA, Berggren EK, Preconception care has the potential for high return on investment, *Am J Obstet Gynecol.* 2015;212:1–3. [Review]
61. Moos MK. *Preconception Health Promotion: A Focus for Women Wellness.* 2nd ed. White Plaines, NY: March of Dimes, 2003. [Review]
62. Pearson DWM, Kernahhan D, Lee R, et al. The relationship between pre-pregnancy care and early pregnancy loss, major congenital anamoly or perinatal death in type I diabetes mellitus. *Br J Obstet Gynecol.* 2007;114:104–107. [II-2]
63. Charron-Prochownik D, Ferons-Hannan M, Sereika S, et al. Randomized efficacy trial of early preconception counseling for diabetic teens. *Diabetes Care.* 2008; 31:1327–1330. [RCT]
64. American Diabetes Association. Preconception care of women with diabetes. *Diabetes Care.* 2004;27(suppl 1):S76–S78. [Review]
65. Korenbrot CC, Steinberg A, Bender C, et al. Preconception care: A systematic review. *Matern Child Health J* 2002;6(2):75–88. [Review]
66. Reid SM, Middleton P, Cossich MC, et al. Interventions for clinical and subclinical hypothyroidism prepregnancy and during pregnancy. *Cochrane Database Syst Rev.* 2013;CD007752. [Meta-analysis]
67. Langer O, Conway DL, Berkus MD, et al. A comparison of glyburide and insulin in women with gestational diabetes. *N Engl J Med.* 2000;343:1134–1138. [RCT]
68. Hebert MF, Ma X, Naraharisetti SB, et al. for the Obstetric-Fetal Pharmacology Research Unit Network. Are we optimizing gestational diabetes treatment with glyburide? The pharmacologic basis for better clinical practice. *Clin Pharmacol Ther.* 2009;85:607–614. [Review]
69. Tieu J, Bain E, Middleton P, et al. Interconception care for women with a history of gestational diabetes for improving maternal and infant outcomes. *Cochrane Database Syst Rev.* 2013;6:CD010211._ [Meta-analysis]
70. Marson AG, Al-Kharusi AM, Appleton R, et al. The SANAD study of effectiveness of carbamazepine, gabapentin, lamotrigine, oxcarbazepine, or topiramate for treatment of partial epilepsy: An unblended randomized controlled trial. *Lancet.* 2007;369:1000–1015. [RCT]
71. French JA. First-choice drug for newly diagnosed epilepsy. *Lancet.* 2007;369:970–971. [Review]
72. Meador KJ, Penovich P. What is the risk of orofacial clefts from lamotrigine exposure during pregnancy? *Neurology.* 2008; 71:706–707. [II-1]
73. Holmes LB, Baldwin EJ, Smith CR, et al. Increased frequency of isolated cleft palate in infants exposed to lamotrigine during pregnancy. *Neurology.* 2008;70:2152–2158. [II-2]
74. Report of the Quality Standards Subcommittee of the American Academy of Neurology. Practice parameter: management issues for women with epilepsy (summary statement). *Neurology* 1998;51(4):944–948. [Guideline]
75. American College of Obstetricians and Gynecologists. Teratology. ACOG Educational Bulletin No. 236. Washington, DC: ACOG, 1997. [Review]
76. Dunlop AL, Gardiner PM, Shellhaas CS, et al. The clinical content of preconception care: The use of medications and supplements among women of reproductive age. *Am J Obstet Gynecol.* 2008;12:s367–s372. [Review]
77. Thomson Reuters Healthcare. Available at: http://www.micromedex.com. Accessed March 13, 2009. [Review]
78. Reprotox. An Information System on Environmental Hazards to Human reproduction and Development. Available at: http://www.reprotox.org. Accessed March 13, 2009. [Review]
79. OTIS. Organization of Teratology Information Specialists. Available at: http://www.otispregnancy.org. Accessed March 13, 2009. [Review]
80. U.S. Department of Health and Human Services. The Health Benefits of Smoking Cessations: U.S. Department of Health and Human Services, Public Health Service, Centers for Disease Control, Center for Chronic Disease Prevention and Health Promotion, Office on Smoking and Health, 1990. [Review]
81. Wong MD, Shapiro MF, Boscardin WJ, et al. Contribution of major diseases to disparities in mortality. *N Engl J Med.* 2002; 347 (20):1585–1592. [Review]
82. Lumley J, Oliver SS, Chamberlain C, et al. Interventions for promoting smoking cessation during pregnancy. *Cochrane Database Syst Rev.* 2008;4:CD001055. [Meta-analysis]
83. Fiore MC, Bailey WC, Cohen SJ, et al. *Treating Tobacco Use and Dependence. Quick Reference Guide for Clinicians.* Rockville, MD: U.S. Department of Health and Human Services. Public Health Service, 2000. [Guideline]

Prenatal care

Gabriele Saccone and Kerri Sendek

KEY POINTS
- Prenatal care is of benefit to pregnant women, especially those with modifiable risk factors.
- **Most low-risk women can be offered midwife-led models of care**, and women should be encouraged to ask for this option. Continuity of care by midwives has been associated with improved patient satisfaction. Caution should be exercised in applying this advice to women with substantial medical or obstetric complications.
- **Group prenatal care should be promoted** as it has been associated reduction in preterm birth (PTB), greater satisfaction with care, and higher breastfeeding initiation. **In the developing world, participatory intervention with women's groups** is associated with **decreased maternal and neonatal mortality.**
- Women should be allowed to carry their record.
- Prenatal care usually consists of 7–12 visits per pregnancy, with a first prenatal visit soon after the pregnancy test is positive, and in time to establish location and number of embryo(s), usually at around 6–8 weeks, then at 11–14 weeks for aneuploidy screening, followed by visits about every 4 weeks approximately at 16, 20, 24, and 28 weeks; about every 2 weeks from 34 to 36 weeks, then weekly until delivery. **In settings with limited resources** where the number of visits is already low, **reduced visits programs of antenatal care (<5) are associated with an increase in perinatal mortality** compared with standard care.
- See Table 2.1 for screening and interventions at different times in pregnancy.
- **Early ultrasonography** should be used to determine the estimated date of confinement (EDC) if there is any uncertainty regarding last menstrual period (LMP).
- Content issues that should be included in prenatal care are lifestyle, nutrition, supplements, vaccinations, drugs, environment, prenatal education, and others.
- **Regular aerobic exercise for 35–90 minutes 3–4 times per week during pregnancy is beneficial to overall maternal fitness and sense of well-being,** as well as associated with prevention of excessive weight gain and higher chance of vaginal delivery.
- Most studies report that **sexual activity** is associated with **better pregnancy outcomes,** probably because women who are sexually active are healthier to begin with compared with women with less sexual activity.
- **Balanced nutrition and protein supplementation** is associated with modest increases in maternal weight gain and in mean birth weight, and **reduction in risk of small-for-gestational-age (SGA), stillbirth, and neonatal death.** High-protein and isocaloric protein supplementation should be avoided as they are associated with increased risk of SGA.
- Suggested weight gain in pregnancy is shown in Table 2.4. Women who are underweight are at increased risk for low birth weight (LBW) and PTB and have better outcomes with a higher total weight gain. Excessive weight gain in women with normal body mass index (BMI) can be prevented with dietary and lifestyle counseling.
- **Folic acid supplementation is recommended for neural tube defect (NTD) prevention,** with 400 μg/day for all women, and 4 mg/day for women with prior children with NTD. All reproductive-age women should be on folic acid (FA) supplementation.
- Immunity to **rubella, varicella, hepatitis B, influenza, tetanus, and pertussis should be assessed at the first prenatal visit.** Ideally needed vaccinations should be provided preconception. **Influenza vaccine** is recommended for pregnant women during flu season. **Tetanus, diphtheria, and acellular pertussis vaccine, also known as TDAP vaccine,** is recommended for all pregnant women after 28 weeks. Partners and family members should be encouraged to be vaccinated as well.
- **Prenatal education** directed at specific objectives has been demonstrated to be effective.
- **Implementation of community-based interventional care packages** is associated with a trend for **reduction in maternal mortality,** and with **significant reductions in maternal morbidity, neonatal mortality, stillbirths, and perinatal mortality.**
- **Perineal massage** with sweet almond oil for 5–10 minutes daily from 34 weeks until delivery is associated with a significantly higher chance of intact perineum in nulliparous women.
- **Antenatal classes with training to prepare for labor and delivery** are associated with **arriving to labor and delivery (L & D) ward more often in active labor,** and **less use of epidural analgesia**.
- Identifying mothers at risk for postpartum depression assists in prevention compared with intervening on the general population.
- **Breastfeeding is the best feeding method for most infants** and should be **strongly encouraged. Continued counseling and education** facilitate breastfeeding success.
- **Unsensitized RhD-negative women should be offered anti-D immunoglobulin prophylaxis.**
- **Sweeping or "stripping" of membranes** during cervical exam at ≥38 weeks **reduces the rate of postterm delivery**.
- **Magnesium lactate or citrate chewable tablets** 5 mmol in the morning and 10 mmol in the evening for 3 weeks for women with leg cramps are associated with **significant improvement in persistent leg cramps.**
- **Water gymnastics** for 1 hour weekly starting at <19 weeks **reduces back pain** in pregnancy and allows more women to continue to work, with no adverse effects. **Both**

Table 2.1 Suggested Prenatal Care Counseling, Screening, and Intervention

Initial visit ≤14 weeks	Visits at: 14–24 weeks	24–28 weeks	28–34 weeks	34–41 weeks
Assessments/procedures				
• Complete history and risk identification • Assessment of EDB by LMP and sizing; ultrasound if indicated • Baseline BP screening • Weight and BMI • Screening for domestic abuse • Vaccines according to risk status and season • Referral for specialist care according to history • Offer 11–13 6/7 weeks aneuploidy screening ultrasound	• Fetal heart tones • Fundal height • Fetal movement • BP • Weight • Screening ultrasound for anatomy	• Fetal heart tones • Fundal height • Fetal movement • BP • Weight • Rh immunoglobulin if indicated • Screening for domestic abuses	• Fetal heart tones • Fundal height • Fetal movement • BP • Weight	• Fetal heart tones • Fundal height/EFW • Fetal movement • Fetal presentation • BP • Weight • Sweeping of membranes starting at ≥38 weeks
Laboratory tests				
• Multiple-marker aneuploidy screen • CBC; blood type, Rh, antibody screen; Rubella IgG; RPR; HBsAg; HIV • Urine dipstick for protein and glucose • Urinalysis and urine culture • Gonorrhea/chlamydia[a] • Pap[a] • Additional testing as directed by history and PE[a]	• Multiple-marker aneuploidy screen • Urine dipstick for protein if indicated	• Gestational diabetes screen; repeat CBC and antibody screen • Antibody screen if indicated • Urine dipstick for protein	• Urine dipstick for protein	• Group B Strep • Urine dipstick for protein • HIV
Education/counseling				

• Cessation of harmful substances
• Exercise/activity
  • Nutrition
  • Weight gain
  • Supplements
  • Food safety
• Breastfeeding
	• Review and discuss results of testing	• Preterm labor s/sx	• Preterm labor s/sx
			• Preeclampsia s/sx
				• Labor symptoms/when to call
				• Preeclampsia s/sx
				• Post-dates management
				• Breastfeeding

Education/counseling not limited to specific weeks gestation				
• Danger signs • Dental care • Family planning • Labor preparation, options, s/sx to report • Travel • TOLAC				
Assessments/procedures				
• Complete history and risk identification • Assessment of EDB by LMP and sizing; ultrasound if indicated • Baseline BP screening • Weight and BMI • Screening for domestic abuse • Vaccines according to risk status and season • Referral for specialist care according to history • Offer 11–13 6/7 weeks aneuploidy screening ultrasound	• Fetal heart tones • Fundal height • Fetal movement • BP • Weight • Screening ultrasound for anatomy	• Fetal heart tones • Fundal height • Fetal movement • BP • Weight • Rh immunoglobulin if indicated • Screening for domestic abuses	• Fetal heart tones • Fundal height • Fetal movement • BP • Weight	• Fetal heart tones • Fundal height/EFW • Fetal movement • Fetal presentation • BP • Weight • Sweeping of membranes starting at 38 weeks

Sources: Adapted from a review of current prenatal care guidelines from four major groups: U.S. Veterans Health Administration, Department of Veteran Affairs, and Health Affairs, Department of Defense; Institute for Clinical Systems Improvement; the American Academy of Pediatrics and the American College of Obstetricians and Gynecologists; and the American Academy of Family Physicians; Hanson L et al., *J Midwifery Women's Health*, 54(6), 458–468, 2009.
[a]See text, only in certain circumstances.
Abbreviations: EDB, expected date of birth; LMP, last menstrual period; BP, blood pressure; BMI, body mass index; EFW, estimation of fetal weight; RPR, rapid plasma regain; HIV, human immunodeficiency virus; CBC, complete blood count; PE, physical exam; TOLAC, trial of labor after cesarean; s/sx, signs and symptoms.

physiotherapy and acupuncture starting <32 weeks for 10 sessions **might reduce back and pelvic pain**.
- **Exercise, increase in water intake, dietary counseling, and certain foods (e.g., prunes)** have shown relief in constipation. If these self-help measures are inadequate, the pregnant woman should then try **daily bran or wheat fiber supplements. Docusate sodium is an effective stimulant laxative.**

DEFINITION
Prenatal care is the care provided to pregnant women with the aim to prevent complications and decrease the incidence of perinatal and maternal morbidity and mortality [1]. This care consists of health promotion, risk assessment, and intervention linked to the risks and conditions uncovered. These activities require the cooperative and coordinated efforts of the woman, her family, her prenatal care providers, and other specialized providers. Prenatal care begins when conception is first considered and continues until labor begins. The objectives of prenatal care for the mother, infant, and family relate to outcomes through the first year following birth [1].

PURPOSE
Prenatal care developed, historically, to reduce the incidence of LBW and preterm infants [2]. It has evolved to encompass a broader purpose; to identify pregnancies with maternal or fetal conditions associated with morbidity/mortality, to provide interventions to prevent or treat such complications, and to provide education support and health promotion that can have lasting effects on the health of an entire family [3]. Care should be systematic, evidence based, and should result in informed shared decision making between the patient and the provider.

EFFECTIVENESS
Prenatal care is of benefit to pregnant women. Nonetheless, the value of prenatal care is controversial, as there is no definite evidence that prenatal care improves birth outcomes. **There are no randomized control trials (RCTs) of prenatal care versus no prenatal care.** Most studies are observational. Selection bias (women who self-select to prenatal care usually are more inclined to have better outcomes) leads to confounding bias (e.g., risk factors associated with LBW and neonatal death are also risk factors for inadequate prenatal care).

There are several RCTs on the number of prenatal care visits, which indirectly demonstrate the beneficial effects of prenatal care. **There is a higher incidence of perinatal mortality** (relative risk [RR] 1.14, 95% confidence interval [CI] 1.00–1.31) **in programs with significantly less (<5) numbers of prenatal visits, compared with the usual 8–12.** This is particularly significant for low- and middle-income countries [4]. Also, studies demonstrate **a reduction in poor outcomes in high-risk pregnancies with enhanced prenatal care** at no added cost [4] (see Section "Number and Timing of Visits"). In addition, **women are dissatisfied with a reduced schedule of prenatal visits** indicating a perceived benefit by women [4]. Specific interventions for specific risks may reduce morbidity and mortality. Prenatal care is probably of most benefit to medically high-risk women [2].

ORGANIZATIONAL ISSUES
Health-Care Provider
There is no evidence that physicians need to be involved in the prenatal care of every woman experiencing an uncomplicated pregnancy. The effect of midwife-led care compared with physician-led care or to other provider-led care has been evaluated mostly for the whole pregnancy, including together both antepartum care and care during labor and delivery (see also Chapter 7). Therefore it is difficult to assess the effect of midwife-led care just on antepartum care. From the evidence from both antepartum and L and D care, **most women can be offered midwife-led models of care and women should be encouraged to ask for this option. Caution should be exercised in applying this advice to women with substantial medical or obstetric complications.** In a meta-analysis, women, the vast majority low risk, who had midwife-led models of care, were **less likely to experience antenatal hospitalization, and less likely to experience fetal loss before 24 weeks' gestation** (RR 0.79, 95% CI 0.65–0.97), although there were no statistically significant differences in fetal loss/neonatal death of at least 24 weeks (RR 1.01, 95% CI 0.67–1.53) or in fetal/neonatal death overall (RR 0.83, 95% CI 0.70–1.00) [5] (see also Chapter 7). It is not clear whether these associations are due to **greater continuity of care or to midwifery care** [5].

Group Prenatal Care
In a meta-analysis, educational interventions were the focus of group prenatal care, and no consistent results were found. Sample sizes were very small to moderate. No data were reported concerning anxiety, breastfeeding success, or general social support. Knowledge acquisition, sense of control, factors related to infant-care competencies, and some labor and birth outcomes were measured. The largest of the included studies ($n = 1275$) examined an educational and social support intervention to increase vaginal birth after cesarean delivery. This high-quality study showed similar rates of vaginal birth after cesarean delivery in "verbal" and "document" groups (RR 1.08, 95% CI 0.97–1.21) [6]. One large RCT demonstrated significant **reduction in PTB, greater satisfaction with care, and higher breastfeeding initiation** at no added cost for group prenatal care over standard care in a group of medically low-risk (but socially at-risk) women in an urban clinic [7]. In this study, group care included, among other interventions, continuity of care from a single provider, patient keeping copies of their records, no waiting time at visits, about 20 hours of provider/patient time, with 8–10 women in each group session. **In the developing world, participatory intervention with women's groups** is associated with **decreased maternal and neonatal mortality** in several large cluster-randomized trials [8–10]. In one of these studies, participatory care involved a female facilitator convening nine women's group meetings every month. The facilitator supported groups through an action–learning cycle in which they identified local perinatal problems and formulated strategies to address them [8]. This strategy holds great promise in decreasing maternal and perinatal deaths among the most vulnerable in our world.

Group prenatal care may even be utilized in a higher risk population. In a non-RCT study, group prenatal care for women with gestational diabetes (GDM) is associated with decreased progression to A2 gestational diabetes and improved postpartum follow-up for appropriate diabetes screening without significantly affecting obstetrical or neonatal outcomes [11].

Group prenatal care should be promoted and further studied among more diverse populations.

Prenatal Record

A formal, structured record should be used for documenting care during the pregnancy. Structured records with reminder aids help ensure that providers incorporate evidence-based guidelines into clinical practice. There is no trial comparing different records. **Women should be allowed to carry their record.** A meta-analysis of three trials showed that carrying the record is **associated with increased maternal control and satisfaction during pregnancy, increased availability of antenatal records during hospital attendance, but also with more operative deliveries.** Importantly, all of the three trials included in the meta-analysis report that more women in the case notes group would prefer to hold their antenatal records in another pregnancy [12].

Number and Timing of Visits

There is insufficient evidence to recommend an ideal schedule of prenatal visits for all pregnant women. The most important visit to optimize pregnancy outcomes is the **preconception visit** (see Chapter 1). A visit early, soon after the pregnancy test is positive, and in time to establish location and number of embryo(s), usually around 6–8 weeks, is also desirable. At this early visit, each woman should be assessed for risk factors (see Tables 1.3 and 1.4 in Chapter 1). The frequency of subsequent visits can be determined based on risk factors.

In developed countries, **prenatal care usually consists of 7–12 visits per pregnancy, with a prenatal visit ideally at 10–14 weeks for aneuploidy screening** (see Chapters 5 and 6), **followed by visits about every 4 weeks approximately at 16, 20, 24, and 28 weeks; about every 2 weeks from 32 to 36 weeks, then weekly until delivery** (Table 2.1) [13]. Uncomplicated multiparous women may need fewer visits than uncomplicated nulliparous ones. Individual patient needs and risk factors should be assessed at the first prenatal visit and reassessed at each appointment thereafter.

A small reduction in the traditional number of prenatal visits in both developed and developing countries has *not* been associated with adverse biological maternal or perinatal outcomes, but **women may feel less satisfied with fewer visits** [4]. **But, in settings with limited resources where the number of visits is already low, reduced antenatal visits (<5) are associated with an increase in perinatal mortality compared with standard care, although admission to neonatal intensive care may be reduced** [4]. Women prefer the standard visits schedule. Where the standard number of visits is low, visits should not be reduced without close monitoring of fetal and neonatal outcome [4]. In addition, women in high-resource settings were more often dissatisfied with a reduced schedule of visits (defined as eight). The schedule of visits should be determined by the purpose of the appointment. A minimum of four prenatal care visits is recommended even for low-risk women [4].

STRUCTURE
Initial Visit

Ideally, this visit should occur prior to 12 weeks of gestation. Women should receive *written* information regarding their pregnancy care services, the proposed schedule of visits, screening tests that will be offered, and lifestyle issues, such as nutrition and exercise. Major parts of the visit include history, risk identification, physical examination, laboratory testing, education for health promotion, and a detailed plan of care for any risks identified (see Table 2.1) (see also Chapter 1, Tables 1.2–1.5).

History
A comprehensive history should be performed, preferably using standardized record forms (e.g., www.acog.org). Risk assessment should be performed with detailed review of systems. In particular, the woman who may require additional care or referral should be identified. **Early ultrasonography should be used to determine the EDC if there is any uncertainty regarding LMP** [14]. Accuracy of EDC is critical for timing of screening tests and appropriate interventions, managing complications, and consideration of delivery timing. It also provides early identification and chorionicity of multiple pregnancies (see Section "Ultrasonography" and Chapter 4). Content issues such as lifestyle, nutrition, supplements, drugs, environment, vaccinations, prenatal education, and others should be discussed (see Section "Content of Prenatal Care"). Prenatal diagnosis and screening for aneuploidy (Chapter 5) and genetic screening (Chapter 6) should be reviewed.

Physical Exam
The physical exam should be both general (Table 2.1) and directed by any risks identified in the history (see Chapter 1).

Weight and height should be determined at the initial prenatal visit in order to determine BMI (**BMI** = weight (kg)/height squared [m^2]). BMI should be based on weight at time of conception or the earliest known weight in pregnancy. Categories of BMI are in Table 2.2. Women with **obesity** are at increased risk for diabetes, shoulder dystocia, cesarean section, and other complications, and have better outcomes with a lower (or no) total weight gain. Women who are underweight (<50 kg or <120 lb.) also are at increased risk for LBW and PTB, and have better outcomes with a higher total weight gain (see Section "Nutrition").

Blood pressure is recommended at each prenatal visit. Initial blood pressure evaluation may help to identify women with chronic hypertension, while subsequent blood pressure readings aid in preeclampsia screening. A diastolic blood pressure of >80 at booking is associated with later risks of preeclampsia [15]. There are significant risks associated with both hypertension and preeclampsia in pregnancy. This simple, inexpensive, and widely accepted screening tool may help to identify abnormal trends in blood pressure over time. Blood pressure should be taken in the sitting position using an appropriately sized cuff and correct technique (see Chapter 1 in *Maternal-Fetal Evidence Based Guidelines*).

Pelvic Examination
Routine pelvic examination early in pregnancy is not as accurate for assessment of gestational age compared with ultrasound (see Chapter 4) and not a reliable predictive test of PTB

Table 2.2 Body Mass Index (BMI) Categories

Weight category	BMI
Underweight	<18.5
Normal weight	18.5–24.9
Overweight	25–29.9
Obesity (class I)	30–34.9
Obesity (class II)	35–39.9
Extreme obesity (class III)	>40

or cephalopelvic disproportion later in pregnancy (see also Chapters 7 and 17), and so it is not recommended for these assessments. Abdominal and pelvic examination to detect gynecologic pathology can be included in the initial examination, with no level 1 evidence for effectiveness of this screening test.

Laboratory Screening
Recommended initial universal laboratory screening is listed in Table 2.1. Other lab testing may be ordered if other risks/conditions are present.

ABO/Rh (D) type and antibody screen. Testing for blood group, Rh status, and atypical red cell antibodies at the initial visit is recommended. Unsensitized RhD-negative women should be offered anti-D immunoglobulin at 28 weeks (see Chapter 53 in *Maternal-Fetal Evidence Based Guidelines*). Anti-D immunoglobulin should also be offered for any invasive procedure (e.g., amniocentesis, chorionic villus sampling (CVS), percutaneous umbilical blood sampling [PUBS]), second- or third-trimester bleeding, partial molar pregnancies, spontaneous abortion, elective termination, and any condition that might be associated with fetal–maternal hemorrhage, such as abdominal trauma, external cephalic version, or placental abruption. It may also be offered for any first-trimester threatened abortion and ectopic pregnancy, although the evidence is not as strong, and it is probably not cost-effective or necessary unless the bleeding is significant. For the RhD-negative woman with a known RhD-negative father of the pregnancy, anti-D immunoglobulin can be deferred. Du-positive women do not need anti-D immunoglobulin (see Chapter 53 in *Maternal-Fetal Evidence Based Guidelines*).

Complete blood count. Recommended at the first prenatal visit to identify anemia (hemoglobin and hematocrit) and to screen for thalassemia (mean corpuscular volume [MCV]). Pregnant women identified with anemia (Hgb < 11.0 g/dL in first trimester) should be treated as per Chapter 14 in *Maternal-Fetal Evidence Based Guidelines*. Initial determination of platelet count (optimally also before pregnancy) may help identify chronic thrombocytopenias and aid in diagnosis of gestational thrombocytopenia or HEELP (hemolysis, elevated liver enzyme levels, and a low platelet count) syndrome later in pregnancy.

Rubella antibody. Screen all women at first encounter. Nonimmune pregnant women should be counseled to avoid exposure and seek immunization postpartum (see Chapter 38 in *Maternal-Fetal Evidence Based Guidelines*).

Syphilis screening. All pregnant women should be screened with a serologic test for syphilis at the first prenatal visit. Women who are at high risk, live in areas of high syphilis morbidity, or are previously untested should be screened at 28 weeks and again at delivery (see Chapter 35 in *Maternal-Fetal Evidence Based Guidelines*).

HBsAg. Screen at initial encounter, and rescreen high-risk populations in third trimester. Postnatal intervention is recommended in all HBsAg-positive women to reduce the risk of viral transmission to the neonate. Pregnancy and breastfeeding are not contraindications to immunization in women who are at risk for acquisition of the hepatitis B virus (see Chapter 30 in *Maternal-Fetal Evidence Based Guidelines*).

HIV serology. Screening is recommended for all pregnant women. The "opt-out" approach is recommended. It should be emphasized that testing not only provides the opportunity to maintain maternal health, but interventions can be offered to dramatically reduce the risk of viral transmission to the fetus (see Chapter 32 in *Maternal-Fetal Evidence Based Guidelines*).

Urine dipstick for protein. Screening for proteinuria should occur at the initial visit and routinely after 20 weeks in women at risk for preeclampsia. Urine dipsticks for protein do not reliably detect the variable elevations in albumin that may occur in preeclampsia and may not be indicated at each visit in low-risk women [16]. In women at high risk for preeclampsia, the 24-hour collection is a reasonable screen for proteinuria as a baseline at the first prenatal visit, and when other signs/symptoms of preeclampsia are present. The proteinuria/creatinine (P/C) ratio may be used as a screening test as a good predictor for remarkable proteinuria since it seems to be highly predictive for diagnosis to detect proteinuria over one gram but inadequate in detecting lower levels [17] (see Chapter 1 in *Maternal-Fetal Evidence Based Guidelines*).

Urine dipstick for glucose. Glycosuria ≥250 mg/dL (equivalent to 1+) on urine dipstick in the first or second trimester is associated with abnormal GDM screening later in pregnancy. Presence of significant glycosuria before 24–28 weeks is an indicator for earlier gestational glucose screening (see Chapters 4 and 5 in *Maternal-Fetal Evidence Based Guidelines*).

Urine culture for asymptomatic bacteriuria. Screening for bacteriuria is recommended at the first prenatal visit for all women. Pregnant women with asymptomatic bacteriuria are at increased risk for symptomatic infection and pyelonephritis. There is also as a positive relationship between untreated bacteriuria and LBW/PTB. Treatment of asymptomatic bacteriuria prevents these complications (see Chapter 17 in *Maternal-Fetal Evidence Based Guidelines*).

Cervical cancer screening. Cervical cancer screening should be obtained if not current according to guidelines. Pap smear screening should be initiated at age 21, regardless of onset of sexual activity. Routine screening intervals have also been extended to every 3 years for women in their 20s without human papillomavirus (HPV) co-testing and every 5 years in women over 30 with the addition of HPV co-testing. Colposcopy can be performed during pregnancy and a plan can be made for treatment postpartum (see Chapter 31).

Selective (Only Women with Risk Factors) Laboratory Screening
Hepatitis C serology. A test for hepatitis C antibodies should be performed in pregnant women at increased risk for exposure, such as those with a history of IV drug abuse, exposure to blood products or transfusion, organ transplants, kidney dialysis, etc. (see Chapter 31 in *Maternal-Fetal Evidence Based Guidelines*).

Chlamydia screening. All women of age <25 years (strongest risk factor), multiple sex partners, new partner within past 3 months, single marital status, inconsistent use of barrier contraception, previous or concurrent sexually transmitted infection (STI), vaginal discharge, mucopurulent cervicitis, friable cervix, or signs of cervicitis on physical examination should be screened. Some agencies advocate universal chlamydia screening. Rescreen in the third trimester if at increased risk for infection. Screening using polymerase chain reaction (PCR) technology is most accurate (see Chapter 34 in *Maternal-Fetal Evidence-Based Guidelines*).

Gonorrhea screening. All women of age <25 years, prior STI, multiple sexual partners, having a partner with a past history of any sexually transmitted disease (STD), sex work, drug use, and inconsistent condom use should be screened for gonorrhea. Some agencies advocate universal gonorrhea screening. Rescreen in the third trimester if at increased risk for infection. Screening using PCR technology is most accurate (see Chapter 33 in *Maternal-Fetal Evidence Based Guidelines*).

Bacterial vaginosis. There is **no benefit** to routine screening and treatment for asymptomatic bacterial vaginosis. Consideration can be given to screening and treating women with a prior PTB, but given the inconclusive evidence we do not recommended it as routine. However, those women who are symptomatic should be screened (see Chapter 17 in *Maternal-Fetal Evidence Based Guidelines*).

Genital herpes. Routine serologic or other screening for herpes simplex virus (HSV) in asymptomatic pregnant women is not recommended. In the absence of lesions during the third trimester, routine serial cultures are not indicated for women with a history of recurrent genital herpes (see Chapter 50 in *Maternal-Fetal Evidence Based Guidelines*).

Varicella. Screening is indicated if a woman has had neither past infection nor vaccination. Varicella vaccine (live attenuated) is not recommended during pregnancy, but seronegative women should be advised to take appropriate precautions (see Chapters 38 and 51 in *Maternal-Fetal Evidence Based Guidelines*).

Tuberculosis. Quantiferon gold or purified protein derivative (PPD) can be offered to high-risk women at any gestational age in pregnancy to screen for tuberculosis, and follow-up chest x-ray is recommended for recent converters. High-risk factors include human immunodeficiency virus (HIV) disease, homeless or impoverished women, prisoners, recent immigrants from areas where tuberculosis is prevalent, and others (see Chapter 24 in *Maternal-Fetal Evidence Based Guidelines*).

Cytomegalovirus (CMV). Routine testing is not recommended. Good hand washing and practicing universal precautions are recommended to prevent transmission [18] (see Chapter 47 in *Maternal-Fetal Evidence Based Guidelines*).

Parvovirus. Routine screening is not recommended, but can be considered for high-risk groups (see Chapter 48 in *Maternal-Fetal Evidence Based Guidelines*).

Toxoplasmosis. Universal screening is not recommended. Education regarding prevention of disease should be addressed (Table 2.3) (see Chapter 49 in *Maternal-Fetal Evidence Based Guidelines*).

Follow-Up Visits

Follow-up visits should provide for the following:

- Follow-up physical exam, laboratory screening, and testing as indicated
- Ongoing assessment of risk factors and plan for intervention as indicated
- Education and health promotion directed to individual plan of care
- Opportunity for discussion and questions

Follow-Up Physical Exam

- **Weight:** Usually done at each visit, as optimal weight gain (Table 2.4) is associated with better outcomes. Excessive fast weight gain can be a sign of preeclampsia.
- **Blood pressure:** Should be performed and recorded at each visit.
- **Fetal heart tones:** Should be performed and recorded at each visit after the first trimester.
- **Symphyseal-fundal height measurement:** Can be performed at each visit from the 24th through 41st weeks. Fundal height measurement may help to detect fetal growth restriction (FGR) and macrosomia, but there is poor intra- and interuser reliability. There is probably some value in evaluating trends and although it will not impact on the underlying condition, it may affect decision making on fetal surveillance. **There is insufficient evidence to show whether this measurement has any impact, beneficial or not, on pregnancy outcomes, with no effect in the only one trial** [19] (see also Chapter 45 in *Maternal-Fetal Evidence Based Guidelines*).
- **Cervical examination:** Routine digital examination of the cervix is not recommended as a screening measure for prevention of PTB (see Chapter 17 in *Maternal-Fetal Evidence Based Guidelines*).
  - **Sweeping or "stripping" of membranes during cervical exam at ≥ 38 weeks reduces the rate of late-term delivery** (see Chapter 21). Cervical examination may assist in the identification of abnormal presentation, and therefore the opportunity to offer appropriate intervention (i.e., version).
- **Fetal movement:** There is no evidence that formalized kick counts reduce the incidence of fetal death in the healthy singleton [20] (see Chapter 56 in *Maternal-Fetal Evidence Based Guidelines*). Nonetheless, women may be instructed to be aware of daily fetal movements from at or around 28 weeks.
- **Leopold's maneuvers:** Perform at each visit from 34 weeks to estimate fetal weight and determine presentation. Ultrasound can be used to confirm findings, and interventions may be offered [21,22].
- **Clinical pelvimetry:** Measurement of the bony birth canal is of limited, unproven value in predicting dystocia during delivery (see Chapters 7 and 8).
- **Routine evaluation for edema:** Edema has traditionally been a part of the evaluation for preeclampsia, but by itself, it is neither specific nor sensitive.

Table 2.3 Prevention of Food-Borne Illnesses

Food-borne illness to avoid	Preventive strategy
Listeriosis	Cook meat thoroughly including luncheon meats; avoid raw or smoked meats or fish, pates, unpasteurized cheese, and raw milk.
Toxoplasmosis	Cook meat and wash fruits and vegetables thoroughly; avoid cat litter; wear gloves when gardening outdoors.
Escherichia coli and *Salmonella*	Follow food-handling guidelines above.
Methylmercury	Avoid consumption of large, mercury-containing fish.

Table 2.4 Institute of Medicine Recommended Total Weight Gain in Pregnancy by Prepregnancy BMI (kg [lb.])

BMI	Singleton	Twin
<18.5	12.5–18 (27–40)	Insufficient information
18.5–24.9	11.5–16 (25–35)	17–25 (37–55)
25.0–29.9	7–11.5 (15–25)	14–23 (31–51)
≥30[a]	5–9 (11–20)	11–19 (24–41)

Source: Modified from Rasmussen KM and Yaktine AL, eds., *JAMA*, 302, 241–242, 2009.
[a] See Table 2.7 for our recommendations.

Follow-Up Laboratory Screening

- **10 6/7–13 6/7 weeks: Serum aneuploidy screening, with nuchal translucency screening by ultrasound** (see below), should be offered to every pregnant woman. Consider cell-free DNA aneuploidy testing (also called noninvasive prenatal testing, NIPT) in high-risk women (see Chapter 5) (Table 2.1).
- **14–21 weeks:** The second part of serum aneuploidy screening (best at 16–18 weeks) should be offered to all pregnant women interested in prenatal diagnosis of aneuploidy (see Chapter 5). Counseling regarding the variety of screening options and the limitations of testing should be made available to all pregnant women.
- **24–28 weeks:** Women with risk factors for GDM should be screened with either one-step or two-step tests, since intervention (diet, exercise, glucose monitoring, and, as necessary, medical therapy) prevents maternal and perinatal morbidities (see Chapter 5 in *Maternal-Fetal Evidence Based Guidelines*). Universal **glucose challenge screening for GDM** is the most sensitive approach, but the following women are at low risk and less likely to benefit from testing (must meet all of the following criteria): age <25 years; ethnic origin of low-risk (not Hispanic, African, Native American, South or East Asian, or Pacific Islander); BMI <25; no previous personal or family history of impaired glucose tolerance; and no previous history of adverse obstetric outcomes associated with GDM. Antibody screening and hemoglobin and hematocrit are also repeated. Repeat screening of rapid plasma reagin (RPR) (or venereal disease research laboratory [VDRL]) and HIV in the early third trimester and at delivery can be considered for high-risk populations (see Chapters 32 and 35 in *Maternal-Fetal Evidence Based Guidelines*).
- **35–37 weeks: Group B Streptococcus (GBS)** is a significant cause of morbidity and mortality in neonates. Approximately 10%–30% of pregnant women are asymptomatically colonized with GBS in the vagina or rectum. Vertical transmission of this organism from mother to fetus occurs most commonly after onset of labor or rupture of membranes. All women should be screened for GBS colonization by rectovaginal culture at 35–37 weeks of gestation. Colonized women should be treated with IV antibiotics (penicillin is first choice if not allergic) in labor or with rupture of membranes (see Chapter 37 in *Maternal-Fetal Evidence Based Guidelines*).

Ultrasonography

Ultrasound has not been proven harmful to mother or fetus (see Chapter 4).

- **First-trimester "fetal dating" ultrasonography (before 14 weeks):** First-trimester ultrasound is more accurate than LMP to determine gestational age. First-trimester ultrasound also allows earlier detection of multiple pregnancies, aneuploidy screening with nuchal translucency, and diagnosis of nonviable pregnancies.
- **Second-trimester "fetal anatomy" ultrasound:** Generally, women are offered an ultrasound at 18–22 weeks to screen for structural anomalies. Routine use of ultrasound reduces the incidence of postterm pregnancies and rates of induction of labor for postterm pregnancy, increases early detection of multiple pregnancies, increases earlier detection of major fetal anomalies when termination of pregnancy is possible, increases detection rates of fetal malformations, and decreases admission to special care nursery [23,24]. Given the benefits mentioned, all pregnant women should be offered a second-trimester ultrasound. No significant differences are detected for substantive clinical outcomes such as perinatal mortality, possibly because of insufficient data. Transvaginal ultrasound (TVU) cervical length (CL) screening of all singletons gestations, even those without a prior spontaneous PTB, can be offered (ACOG 2012, SMFM 2012), and is recommended by experts [25] (see also Chapter 17).
- **Third-trimester "fetal growth" ultrasound:** In low-risk or unselected populations, routine third-trimester ultrasound has not been associated with improvements in perinatal mortality [26]. Selective ultrasound in later pregnancy is of benefit in specific situations, such as calculation of interval growth for suspected FGR, assessment of amniotic fluid index for suspect oligohydramnios or hydramnios, and assessment of malpresentation (see Chapter 4). A large prospective cohort study showed that screening of nulliparous women with universal third-trimester fetal biometry roughly tripled the detection of SGA infants and that the combined analysis of fetal biometry and fetal growth velocity identified a subset of SGA fetuses that were at increased risk of neonatal morbidity [27].
- Routine umbilical artery or other Doppler ultrasound in low-risk or unselected patients has not been shown to be of benefit.

CONTENT OF PRENATAL CARE

The content of prenatal care is extensive and reviewed in detail not only in this chapter but also in most other chapters in this book, as well as its companion, *Maternal-Fetal Evidence Based Guidelines*. In Chapter 1, see Table 1.2 for topics to be reviewed, Table 1.3 for screening, Table 1.4 for laboratory tests, Table 1.5 for vaccinations, Table 1.6 for interventions for all women, and Table 1.7 for interventions for women with risk factors. Prenatal care usually incorporates, among other things, the following:

- **Prenatal education and reassurance** (regarding drugs, environment, lifestyle, nutrition, supplements, vaccinations, preventive measures, preparation for labor and delivery, depression, breastfeeding, etc.)
- Provision of evidence-based screening tests at appropriate intervals (Table 2.1)
- Risk assessment
- Problem-oriented visits as needed
- Condition-specific care for high-risk patients

Content issues that should be included in prenatal care such as drugs and environment, lifestyle, nutrition, supplements, vaccinations, prenatal education, and others are described below.

Drugs and Environment

Substance Abuse

Screening for use and counseling for cessation of tobacco, alcohol, and recreational or illicit drug use is recommended (see Chapters 22 and 23 in *Maternal-Fetal Evidence Based Guidelines*). Maternal smoking as well as exposure to secondhand smoke is dangerous to both the woman and her fetus. Provider support and educational material tailored to pregnancy are shown to increase smoking cessation by 70% and reduce LBW and PTB [28–30] as well as the number of women who continue to smoke in late pregnancy [30].

Alcohol use at any level in pregnancy cannot be supported although deleterious effects at low-moderate levels are difficult to quantify [31]. The evidence from the limited number of studies suggests that **psychological and educational interventions may result in increased abstinence from alcohol, and a reduction in alcohol consumption among pregnant women.** However, results were not consistent, and the paucity of studies, the number of total participants, the high risk of bias of some of the studies, and the complexity of interventions limit our ability to determine the type of intervention that would be most effective in increasing abstinence from, or reducing the consumption of, alcohol among pregnant women [32]. Counseling may be effective in reducing substance abuse in pregnancy, although women with addictions will need specialized interventions. **Screening and brief intervention (SBI)** for unhealthy alcohol use has demonstrated efficacy in some trials. There is some evidence regarding the acceptability and efficacy of computer-delivered SBI plus tailored mailings in women who screened positive for alcohol risk [33]. There is insufficient evidence to recommend the routine use of home visits for women with a drug or alcohol problem [34]. However, a cluster randomized controlled trial among urban South African mothers showed that a home-visiting intervention improved the emotional health of low-income mothers and that relative to standard care, intervention mothers were significantly less likely to report depressive symptoms and alcohol abuse [35].

Over-the-Counter, Alternative/Complementary, and Prescription Medications
Because of the possibility of adverse fetal effects, medication use, including alternative remedies, should be limited to circumstances where benefit outweighs risk. Beneficial medications should be continued in pregnancy when safe for both mother and fetus (see specific disease guidelines in *Maternal-Fetal Evidence Based Guidelines*).

Environmental/Occupational Risks and Exposures
In general, working is not associated with poor pregnancy outcome. Some workplace exposures, such as toxic chemicals, radiation (>5 rad), heavy repeated lifting, prolonged (>8 hours) standing, excessive (>80/week) work hours, and high fatigue score may be associated with pregnancy complications, but there is insufficient evidence on the effect of avoidance of these risks (see also Chapter 17). There is insufficient safety data for paint, solvents, hair dyes, fumes, anesthetic drugs, etc., with no absolute evidence of harm. Hot tubs, saunas should avoid temperatures >102°F to avoid risk of dehydration, especially in the first trimester.

Domestic Violence
Domestic violence against pregnant women is associated with an increased risk of PTB, LBW, second-and third-trimester bleeding, and fetal injury. Domestic violence may escalate during pregnancy. As such, providers need to be alert to signs and symptoms of abuse and provide opportunities for private disclosure. However, so far, there is insufficient evidence to assess the effectiveness of interventions for domestic violence on pregnancy outcome [36].

Lifestyle
Work
There is insufficient evidence to recommend exact work hours and when to take off from work before delivery (if at all). Work accommodations are often necessary and helpful to allow a pregnant woman to continue working and earning an income. Pregnant women should not be discriminated against by their employers just because they are pregnant. The website www.pregnantatwork.org provides online tools that health-care professionals can use to prepare notes drafted using language that increases the likelihood that a patient will receive the accommodations she needs to continue doing her job safely. Occupational lifting guidelines have been published [37].

Exercise
Regular exercise during low-risk pregnancies is beneficial as it increases overall maternal fitness and sense of well-being. Exercise is an effective tool in maternal weight gain control in pregnancy [38–40].

Aerobic exercise for 35–90 minutes 3–4 times per week can be safely performed by normal-weight women with singleton, uncomplicated gestations because this is not associated with an increased risk of PTB or with a reduction in mean gestational age at delivery [39], and was associated with a significantly higher incidence of vaginal delivery and a significantly lower incidence of cesarean delivery [39,40], with a significantly lower incidence of gestational diabetes mellitus and hypertensive disorders and therefore should be encouraged [39].

Structured physical exercise programs appear also to be safe for the neonate [41] and **reduce the risk of having a large newborn without a change in the risk of having a small newborn** [42]. Furthermore, there is some evidence that exercise may be *effective in treating depression* during pregnancy [43]. Diet or exercise, or both, during pregnancy can **reduce the risks of: excessive gestational weight gain (GWG), cesarean section, maternal hypertension, macrosomia, and neonatal respiratory morbidity,** particularly for high-risk women receiving combined diet and exercise interventions [39]. However, most of the studies included in the meta-analysis were carried out in developed countries and therefore it is not clear if these findings are widely applicable [44]. In another meta-analysis, exercise was associated with a lower (by 600 g) GWG [45]. Possible **maternal** benefits include **improved cardiovascular function, limited pregnancy weight gain, decreased musculoskeletal discomfort, reduced incidence of muscle cramps and lower limb edema, mood stability, and attenuation of GDM and gestational hypertension. Fetal benefits include decreased fat mass, improved stress tolerance, and advanced neurobehavioral maturation** [46]. **For most pregnant women, at least 30 minutes of moderate exercise is recommended on most days all of the week. There is no target heart rate that is right for every pregnancy woman. Walking, swimming, and other sports with low chance of loss of balance are recommended** (Table 2.5) [47]. Avoid contact sports and sports with high chance of loss of balance. Special considerations may be made for professional athletes at the patient and provider's discretion. Avoid hypoglycemia and dehydration. It is important to advise women to be careful while stretching, as the hormone relaxin can leave joints vulnerable to overstretching and injury [47]. It is important for clinicians to keep emphasizing that **exercise is medicine** [48].

Table 2.5 Examples of Safe and Unsafe Physical Activities During Pregnancy

The following activities are safe to initiate or continue:[a]
- Walking
- Swimming
- Stationary cycling
- Low-impact aerobics
- Yoga, modified[b]
- Pilates, modified
- Running or jogging[c]
- Racquet sports[c,d]
- Strength training[c]

The following activities should be avoided:
- Contact sports (e.g., ice hockey, boxing, soccer, and basketball)
- Activities with a high risk of falling (e.g., downhill snow skiing, water skiing, surfing, off-road cycling, gymnastics, and horseback riding)
- Scuba diving
- Sky diving
- "Hot yoga" or "hot pilates"

Source: Adapted from Committee Opinion No. 650, *Obstet Gynecols*, 126, 135–142, 2015. [Guideline]

[a] In women with uncomplicated pregnancies in consultation with an obstetric care provider.
[b] Yoga positions that result in decreased venous return and hypotension should be avoided as much as possible.
[c] In consultation with an obstetric care provider, running or jogging, racquet sports, and strength training may be safe for pregnant women who participated in these activities regularly before pregnancy.
[d] Racquet sports wherein a pregnant woman's changing balance may affect rapid movements and increase the risk of falling should be avoided as much as possible.

Yoga

Yoga in pregnancy is associated with lower pain and discomfort, as well as lower perceived stress and improved quality of life in physical domains in the three RCTs evaluating its effects [49].

Travel

Counseling should include the proper use of passenger restraint systems in automobiles with the lap belt below the abdomen, reduction of risk of venous thromboembolism during long-distance air travel by walking and exercise, and provision of care and prevention of illness during travel abroad.

Sex and Sexuality

Intercourse has not been associated with adverse outcomes in pregnancy. Some women have a progressive decrease in sexual desire during the pregnancy, most markedly in the third trimester. Couples are often concerned that intercourse may harm the pregnancy. This is associated with progressively decreasing frequency of sexual intercourse in pregnancy [50]. Most women desire more communication regarding sex in pregnancy by their care providers. Health-care provider counseling should be reassuring, in the absence of pregnancy complications. Semen is a source of prostaglandin, pyospermia is associated with preterm premature rupture of membranes (PPROM), and orgasms and nipple stimulation do increase contractions [51]. Therefore, sexual intercourse may be detrimental in women with cervical dilatation and/or shortening but this is not well studied. PTB and other complications of pregnancy do not seem increased in most studies of sex in pregnancy. **Most studies report that sexual activity is associated with better pregnancy outcomes,** probably because women who are sexually active are healthier to begin with compared with women with less sexual activity [52].

Nutrition

Energy (Calorie)/Protein Supplementation

A meta-analysis of 17 RCTs provided evidence that **antenatal nutritional education** with the goal of increasing energy and protein intake in pregnant women appears to be effective in **reducing the risk of PTB and of LBW** and effective in increasing the head circumference at birth and the birth weight **among undernourished women** [53]. **Balanced energy and protein supplementation seems to improve fetal growth, and may reduce the risk of stillbirth and infants born SGA.** However, **high-protein supplementation does not seem to be beneficial and may be harmful** to the fetus increasing the risk of SGA. Balanced-protein supplementation alone has no significant effects on perinatal outcomes [53].

Cholesterol-Lowering Diet

A cholesterol-lowering diet with omega-3 fatty acids and dietary counseling does not affect cord or neonatal lipids but is associated with a 90% reduction in PTB <37 weeks in one trial [54] (see also Chapter 17). More evidence is needed for a recommendation.

Low-Glycemic Index Diet

A low-glycemic index diet appears to be beneficial to both mother and child in reducing the incidence of abnormal glucose tolerance tests, large-for-gestational-age (LGA) infants, and ponderal indices. The numbers of studies and subjects are small, however, and therefore considered inconclusive [55]. Studies evaluating the effects of different types of dietary advice for women with gestational diabetes mellitus did not find any significant benefits for the diets investigated [56].

Antigen Avoidance Diet

Prescription of an antigen avoidance diet (e.g., avoiding chocolate or nuts) to a pregnant woman is unlikely to reduce her child's risk of atopic disease and such a diet may adversely affect maternal or fetal nutrition [57].

Probiotics

A probiotic capsule intervention among women with abnormal glucose tolerance had no impact on glycemic control [58].

Table 2.6 Food Safety in Pregnancy

Clean: Wash hands thoroughly with soap and water, before and after handling food, using the bathroom, changing diapers, or handling pets. Wash cutting boards, dishes, utensils, and countertops with soap and water. Rinse raw fruits and vegetables well, under running water.
Separate: Separate raw meats and seafood from fresh or prepared foods. Use a separate cutting board for raw meats and seafood. Place prepared food on a clean plate.
Cook: Cook foods thoroughly. Avoid allowing foods to sit at temperatures between 40°F and 140°F (4°C and 60°C). Discard foods left out at room temperature for more than 2 hours. Avoid foods made with raw eggs.
Chill: Maintain refrigerator temperature at 40°F (4°C) or below and the freezer at 0°F (−18°C).

Food Safety
Food safety and prevention of food-borne illness and infection are suggested in Tables 2.3 and 2.6.

BMI and Weight Gain
BMI is utilized in counseling a woman on optimal weight gain in pregnancy (Table 2.2) [59–71].

Suggested weight gain in pregnancy is shown in Table 2.4 [59]. **Women who are underweight are at increased risk for LBW and PTB and have better outcomes with a higher total weight gain** [67]. **Excessive weight gain in women with normal BMI can be prevented with dietary and lifestyle counseling** [62–69]. For example, a program of education on recommended GWG, application of personalized weight graph, formalized prescription of exercise, and regular monitoring of GWG at every antenatal visit is associated with a significant reduction in GWG [70]. Obesity is associated with cardiovascular disease, diabetes, hypertension, stroke, osteoarthritis, gallstones, endometrial, breast, and colon cancers, cardiomyopathy, fatty liver, obstructive sleep apnea, urinary tract infections, other complications, and most importantly, mortality. Prepregnancy obesity and excessive gestational weight gain are associated with increased risk of childhood obesity for the fetus. **Obese pregnant** women are specifically at increased risk for miscarriage, congenital malformations, GDM, hypertension, preeclampsia, stillbirth, cesarean birth, labor abnormalities, macrosomia, anesthesia complications, wound infection, and thromboembolism. These women **have better maternal outcomes with lower (or no) total weight gain** [60,61,67,68,71] (Table 2.7) (see also Chapter 3 in *Maternal-Fetal Evidence Based Guidelines*). Even if some studies have reported some small increased risk of SGA with weight loss in obese women, this is really NOT an increase. What happens is that obese women who gain weight have larger babies (incidence of SGA <5%), while those who lose weight have a normal incidence of SGA (i.e., ≤10%) [72]. Moreover, all other neonatal outcomes are the same or better with no weight gain or some moderate weight loss in obese pregnant women (Table 2.7) [61,72].

Caffeine
Moderate caffeine consumption (<200 mg/day) does not appear to be a major contributing factor in miscarriage or PTB.

Reducing the caffeine intake of regular coffee drinkers (3+ cups/day) during the second and third trimester by an average of 182 mg/day did not affect birth weight or length of gestation in one RCT [73]. A meta-analysis from two RCTs concluded that there is insufficient evidence to confirm or refute the effectiveness of caffeine avoidance on birth weight or other pregnancy outcomes; moreover, they found that reducing the caffeine intake of regular coffee drinkers (3+ cups/day) during the second and third trimester did not affect PTB or SGA rate [74].

Supplements
Multivitamin
There is **insufficient evidence** to suggest replacement of iron and folate supplementation with a multiple-micronutrient supplement. A reduction in the number of LBW and SGA babies and maternal anemia has been found with a multiple-micronutrient supplement compared with supplementation with two or less micronutrients or none or a placebo, but analyses revealed no added benefit of multiple-micronutrient supplements compared with iron and FA supplementation [75,76]. These results are limited by the small number of studies available. There is also insufficient evidence to identify which micronutrients are more effective, to assess adverse effects, and to say that excess multiple-micronutrient supplementation during pregnancy is harmful to the mother or the fetus [75,76]. Therefore, there is **insufficient evidence** to recommend routine multivitamin supplementation for all women, or even only for women who are underweight, have poor diets, smokers, substance abusers, vegetarians, multiple gestations, or others. **Excess (>1) prenatal vitamin intake per day should be avoided. No prenatal multivitamin supplement has been shown to be superior to another.** Use of multivitamin supplement not specific for pregnancy should be discouraged, as often excess doses can pose risks to the pregnancy. Each supplement, including each vitamin supplement, should be studied for safety and efficacy individually.

Folic Acid
Folic acid supplementation is recommended, with **minimum 400 µg/day for all women** (93% decrease in NTDs), and **5 mg/day for women with prior children with NTD** (69% decrease in NTD) [77,78]. Supplementation should **start at least 1 month before conception and continue until at least 28 days after conception** (time of neural tube closure). Given the unpredictability of conception and that 50% of pregnancies are unplanned, all reproductive-age women should be on FA supplementation. Because in several countries the baseline serum folate level is only 5 ng/mL, and increases in this level are directly proportional with a decrease in the incidence of NTD, some experts have advocated 5 mg of FA per day as optimal supplementation [79]. No increase in ectopic pregnancy, miscarriage, or stillbirth has been associated with folate supplementation, but it might increase (nonsignificant trend) the incidence of multiple gestations by 40% [77–82]. However, a multicenter prospective cohort study showed that children whose mothers used FA supplement dosages higher than 5 mg/mL had a lower mean psychomotor scale score than children whose mothers used a recommended FA supplements dosages (i.e., 400 µg/day) [82]. Folic acid supplementation has been associated (one non-RCT study) with decrease in severe language delay at 3 years of age [81]. **Fortifying basic foods such as grains** with added folate is associated with an increase in supplementation of only 140–200 µg/day, and with only a

Table 2.7 Weight Gain Suggestions for Overweight and Obese Women

Prepregnancy weight category	Our suggested total weight gain range (lb.)	IOM recommendations (lb.)
Overweight (BMI 25–29.9 kg/m^2)	6–20 (2.7–9.0 kg)	15–25 (6.8–11.4 kg)
Class I obesity (BMI 30–34.9 kg/m^2)	5–15 (2.3–6.8 kg)	11–20 (5–9.1 kg)
Class II obesity (BMI 35–39.9 kg/m^2)	−9–9 (−4.0–4.0 kg)	11–20 (5–9.1 kg)
Class III obesity (BMI >40 kg/m^2)	−15–0 (−6.8–0 kg)	11–20 (5–9.1 kg)

Source: Rasmussen KM and Yaktine AL, eds., *JAMA*, 302, 241–242, 2009.
Abbreviation: IOM, Institute of Medicine.

20%–50% decrease in incidence of NTD, with the potential for large-scale prevention [80]. Women taking antiseizure medications, other drugs that might interfere with FA metabolism, those with homozygous methylenetetrahydrofolate reductase (MTHFR) enzyme mutations, or those who are obese may need higher doses of folate supplementation. Women with first-trimester diabetes mellitus or exposure to valproic acid or high temperatures might not experience the decrease in NTD risk with folate supplementation due to these risks (see also Chapter 1).

Vitamin A
In pregnancy, some extra vitamin A is required for growth and tissue maintenance in the fetus, for providing fetal reserves, and for maternal metabolism. However, vitamin A in its synthetic form as well as in large doses as retinol (preformed vitamin A found in cod liver oil and chicken or beef liver) is teratogenic. It is recommended that pregnant women ingest vitamin A as β-carotene and limit the ingestion of retinol during pregnancy. In vitamin A-deficient populations (where night blindness is present), and in HIV-positive women, vitamin A supplementation reduces maternal night blindness and anemia. **Excess vitamin A intake can cause birth defects and miscarriages at doses >25,000 IU/day. Vitamin A supplements should be avoided, with maximum daily intake prior to and during pregnancy probably 5000 IU and certainly ≤10,000 IU, respectively. Vitamin A supplementation may be beneficial in women with vitamin A deficiency, especially in prevention of night blindness, in developing countries**. Optimal duration of supplement use cannot be evaluated. One large population-based trial in Nepal shows a possible beneficial effect on maternal mortality after weekly vitamin A supplements. Night blindness, associated with vitamin A deficiency, was assessed in a nested case–control study within this trial and found to be reduced but not eliminated [83]. There is insufficient evidence to support vitamin A supplementation as an intervention for anemia [83,84].

Vitamin B6 (Pyridoxine)
There is **insufficient evidence** to evaluate pyridoxine supplementation during pregnancy [85]. There are few trials, reporting few clinical outcomes and mostly with unclear trial methodology and inadequate follow-up. There is not enough evidence to detect clinical benefits of vitamin B6 supplementation in pregnancy and/or labor other than one trial suggesting protection against dental decay [86]. For the aim of decreasing dental decay or missing/filled teeth, pyridoxine supplementation 20 mg/day (lozenges or capsules) is associated with decreased incidence of these outcomes in pregnant women [86]. Pyridoxine has been used in the management of **nausea and vomiting** in pregnancy. It is now considered Category A in combination with doxylamine as "Diclegis" which is the only U.S. Food and Drug Administration (FDA) approved treatment for nausea and vomiting of pregnancy. Studies done for FDA approval of the drug showed no adverse outcomes and demonstrated safety and good tolerance by women when used in the recommended dose of up to 4 pills (10 mg/10 mg) per day (see Chapter 9 in *Maternal-Fetal Evidence Based Guidelines*).

Vitamin C
The **data are insufficient** to assess if vitamin C supplementation either alone or in combination with other supplements is beneficial during pregnancy for either low-or high-risk women. There may be an associated increased risk of PTB with vitamin C supplementation (RR 1.38, 95% CI 1.04–1.82, 3 trials, 583 women) [87]. No other difference in outcome is noted between vitamin C supplementation and no treatment or placebo. There are very limited trials available to assess whether vitamin C supplementation may be useful for all pregnant women. Usually the women involved in the trials were either at high risk of preeclampsia or PTB or the women had established severe early-onset preeclampsia (see also Chapter 1 in *Maternal-Fetal Evidence Based Guidelines*). No difference is seen between women supplemented with vitamin C alone and those supplemented with vitamin C in combination with other supplements compared with placebo for the risk of stillbirth, neonatal death, LBW, or intrauterine growth restriction (IUGR) [87].

Vitamin D
There is **insufficient evidence** to evaluate the effects of vitamin D supplementation during pregnancy [88–92]. Vitamin D 1000 IU/day in the third trimester is associated with no consistent effect on incidence of LBW [88]. **Neonatal hypocalcemia is less common** with vitamin D supplementation compared with placebo [88]. Vitamin D supplementation during pregnancy is associated with increase circulating 25(OH)D levels, birth weight and birth length but with no effects on maternal-fetal outcomes [89]. There are limited data to assess any benefit of vitamin D supplements for complete vegetarians and women with extremely limited exposure to sunlight. Vitamin D supplementation of vitamin D deficient pregnant women prevents neonatal vitamin D deficiency [90]. Vitamin D plus calcium have no effect on duration of pregnancy, type of delivery, and infant anthropometric indicators [91]. However, low maternal vitamin D levels in pregnancy ≤50 nmol/L may be associated with an increased risk of preeclampsia, gestational diabetes, PTB, and SGA [92].

Vitamin E
There is **insufficient evidence** to assess if vitamin E supplementation either alone or in combination with other supplements is beneficial during pregnancy [93]. All evidence tested women at high risk of preeclampsia or with established preeclampsia and assessed vitamin E in combination with other supplements (usually vitamin C) (see Chapter 1 in *Maternal-Fetal Evidence Based Guidelines*). There is no convincing evidence that vitamin E supplementation alone or in combination with other supplements results in other important benefits or harms [93].

Magnesium
Numerous studies demonstrate an association between magnesium supplementation and decreased incidences of LBW, SGA, antenatal hospitalization, and antenatal hemorrhage. The majority of RCTs are of poor quality, except one judged to be of high quality which did not support these associations. There is **insufficient high-quality evidence** to show that dietary magnesium supplementation during pregnancy is beneficial [94]. Including high- and low-quality trials, oral magnesium treatment from before the 25th week of gestation is associated with a lower frequency of PTB, a lower frequency of LBW, and fewer SGA infants compared with placebo [87]. In addition, magnesium-treated women have less hospitalization during pregnancy and fewer cases of antepartum hemorrhage than placebo-treated women. Incidences

of preeclampsia and all other outcomes are similar. In the analysis of one high-quality trial, no differences between magnesium and placebo groups are seen. Poor-quality trials are likely to have resulted in a bias favoring magnesium supplementation.

Calcium
Calcium supplementation is associated with a **reduction of the incidence of preeclampsia in pregnancy in all women, particularly for women at high risk of hypertension and in women with low dietary calcium intake** (e.g., <600 mg/day) [95]. The minimum dose in the Cochrane review was 1 g/day. Further research is needed to determine whether dietary sources of calcium confer the same benefit and at what amount. There is insufficient evidence to determine optimum dosage and the effect on other important maternal and fetal outcomes. There is no overall reduction in PTB, although there is **reduction in PTB among women at high risk of developing hypertension**. Benefits are considered to outweigh an anomalous increase in the risk of HELLP syndrome, which was small in absolute numbers. There is no evidence of any effect of calcium supplementation on stillbirth or death before discharge from hospital. In women at high risk of hypertension, calcium supplementation is associated with fewer babies with birth weight <2500 g. In one study, childhood systolic blood pressure >95th percentile was reduced [95] (see also Chapter 1 in *Maternal-Fetal Evidence Based Guidelines*).

Iron
There is no evidence to advice against a policy of routine iron and folate supplementation in pregnancy. Iron supplementation is associated with **prevention of low hemoglobin at birth or at 6 weeks postpartum** [96]. Iron supplementation, however, has no detectable effect on any substantive measures of either maternal or fetal outcome. One trial, with the largest number of participants of selective versus routine supplementation, shows an increased likelihood of cesarean section and postpartum blood transfusion, but a lower perinatal mortality rate (up to 7 days after birth). There are few data derived from communities where iron deficiency is common and anemia is a serious health problem. There is limited evidence for daily versus intermittent supplementation. High-dose supplementation (80 mg daily) has no clinical advantage over low-dose supplementation (20 mg daily) and is associated with more gastrointestinal (GI) side effects. One RCT suggests adverse effects of hemoconcentration from iron supplementation in nonanemic women. For iron supplementation for women with anemia, see chapter 14 in *Maternal-Fetal Evidence Based Guidelines*.

Zinc
There is insufficient evidence to evaluate fully the effect of zinc supplementation during pregnancy [97]. Zinc supplementation is associated with **significant reduction in PTB** (RR 0.86, 95% CI 0.76–0.98; 13 RCTs; 6854 women). These studies were primarily from a low social-economic population and **may reflect overall poor nutrition**. Reductions in induction of labor and cesarean delivery are from small studies, with no other differences detected between groups of women who had zinc supplementation and those who had either placebo or no zinc during pregnancy. There is insufficient evidence to assess the best dose, gestational age and duration, and population for zinc supplementation in pregnancy [97].

Iodine
Iodine is essential for normal fetal thyroid and brain development. Iodine supplementation **in populations with low iodine intake and high levels of endemic cretinism** results in an important reduction in the incidence of the condition with no apparent adverse effects. Iodine supplementation is associated with **a reduction in deaths during infancy and early childhood, with decreased endemic cretinism at the age of 4 years and better psychomotor development scores between 4 and 25 months of age** [98]. There is little data, however, on the safety of routine iodine supplementation in populations with normal or low normal iodine levels. Some data suggest an increased risk of fetal and maternal hypothyroidism from iodine supplementation. The upper levels of safety have not been established [98,99].

Omega-3
Pregnancy is a time of increased risk for omega-3 deficiency as omega-3 is used for the developing fetus. Thirty-four RCTs have been performed to assess whether omega-3 supplementation during pregnancy affects maternal-fetal outcomes. Pooled results from the 34 studies [100] show lack of evidence to support the routine use of omega-3 supplementation during pregnancy, as omega-3 supplementation did not affect PTB, preeclampsia, IUGR, gestational diabetes, SGA, post-partum depression, children development or other maternal or fetal outcomes. Meta-analyses also found that omega-3 supplementation during pregnancy did not prevent PTB in low-risk women [101], or in women with prior PTB [102], and did not prevent recurrent IUGR [103].

Oral Health Care

Oral health care is an important component of general health and therefore should be maintained during pregnancy and through a woman's lifespan. However, although some studies have shown a possible association between periodontal infection and pregnancy outcome such as PTB and preeclampsia, the evidence shows **no improvement in obstetric or perinatal outcomes after dental treatment** during pregnancy. A meta-analysis from 13 RCTs showed that providing periodontal treatment to pregnant women was not associated with reduction in PTB, or perinatal mortality, except for a significant reduction in PTB and LBW in populations with high occurrence (>20%) of PTB and LBW [104].

Vaccinations

Immunity to **rubella, varicella, hepatitis B, influenza, tetanus, and pertussis should be assessed at the first prenatal visit. Ideally, needed vaccinations would be provided preconception.** There is no vaccine that is more dangerous to a pregnant woman or her fetus than the disease it is designed to prevent. Recombinant, inactivated, and subunit vaccines, as well as toxoids, and immunoglobulins pose no threat to a developing fetus. Inactivated influenza vaccine should be given (by injection, as killed virus) to all pregnant women during the influenza season. The live attenuated form of the vaccine (intranasal spray) should not be given during pregnancy. Hepatitis B vaccine can be safely given in pregnancy. TDAP or "whooping cough" vaccine is recommended for all pregnant women after 28 weeks (see Table 1.5 in Chapter 1, and Chapter 38 in *Maternal-Fetal Evidence Based Guidelines*).

Abdominal Decompression

Abdominal decompression consists of a rigid dome placed about the abdomen and covered with an airtight suit, with the space around the abdomen decompressed to −50 to −100 mmHg for 15–30 seconds out of each minute for 30 minutes once to thrice daily, or with uterine contractions during labor. This is thought to "pump" blood through the intervillous space. There is no evidence to support the use of abdominal decompression in normal pregnancies. There is no difference between the abdominal decompression groups and the control groups for LBW, admission for preeclampsia, low Apgar score, perinatal mortality, and childhood development [105].

Prevention of Complications

Please see specific diseases in each chapter of this book, and its companion, *Maternal-Fetal Evidence Based Guidelines*. Here are reported only some general, nonspecific interventions.

Antibiotic prophylaxis of pregnant women with no specific risk factor or infection is associated with similar incidence of PPROM, PTB, and postpartum endometritis [106,107] (see also Chapter 17).

Programs offering **additional social support** (caring family members, friends, and health professionals) for at-risk (e.g., for PTB and LBW) pregnant women are not associated with improvements in any perinatal outcomes, but there is a **reduction in the likelihood of antenatal hospital admission** (RR 0.79, 95% CI 0.68–0.92) and **cesarean birth** (RR 0.87, 95% CI 0.78–0.97) [108].

For issues such as mild hypertension or preeclampsia, small studies suggest that there are no major differences in clinical outcomes for mothers or babies between antenatal day units and hospital admission, but women may prefer day care [109] (see also Chapter 1 in *Maternal-Fetal Evidence Based Guidelines*).

Prenatal Education

There is insufficient evidence to assess the effectiveness of formal prenatal education programs. **Prenatal education directed at specific objectives (e.g., promoting breastfeeding and avoiding planned induction of labor) has been demonstrated to be effective** [110–113]. Individualized prenatal education directed toward avoidance of a cesarean delivery does not increase the rate of vaginal birth after cesarean section. As a part of prenatal care, women should be provided with information and instruction regarding their health, including risk avoidance, breastfeeding, what to expect during labor and birth (see Section "Preparation for Labor and Delivery"), how to obtain care when labor begins, and the value of a support person during the labor process (see Chapters 7 and 8).

Community Interventions

There is encouraging evidence of the value of integrating maternal and newborn care in community settings through a range of interventions that can be packaged effectively for delivery through a range of community health workers and health promotion groups. Such evidence-based available interventions as immunization to mothers, clean and skilled care at delivery, newborn resuscitation, exclusive breastfeeding, clean umbilical cord care, and management of infections in newborns require facility-based and outreach services. **Implementation of community-based interventional care packages is associated with a trend for reduction in maternal mortality** (RR 0.77, 95% CI 0.59–1.02) **and with significant reductions in maternal morbidity** (RR 0.75, 95% CI 0.61–0.92), **neonatal mortality** (RR 0.76; 95% CI 0.68–0.84), **stillbirths** (RR 0.84, 95% CI 0.74–0.97), **and perinatal mortality** (RR 0.80; 95% CI 0.71–0.91). It also increases the referrals to health facility for pregnancy-related complication by 40% and improves the rates of early breastfeeding by 94% [113].

Preparation for Labor and Delivery

Perineal massage with sweet almond oil for 5–10 minutes daily from 34 weeks until delivery is associated with a significantly higher chance of intact perineum compared with no massage in nulliparous, but probably not multiparous women [114–116]. The type of the oil used during the second stage of labor for prevention of perineal tears has no effect on the integrity of the perineum; accordingly it seems that there is no perfect oil [117]. For perineal massage in labor, see Chapter 8.

Women should be provided with written information and instruction regarding what to expect during labor and delivery, how to obtain care when labor begins, and the value of a support person during the labor process (see Chapters 7 and 8).

Labor and delivery classes should be encouraged. Compared with no such training, 9 hours of **antenatal classes with training to prepare for labor and delivery are associated with arriving to L and D ward more often in active labor** (RR 1.45, 95% CI 1.26–1.65) **and using less epidural analgesia** (RR 0.84, 95% CI 0.73–0.97) [118].

Compared with standard antenatal education, antenatal education focusing on natural childbirth preparation with training in breathing and relaxation techniques is not associated with any effects on maternal or perinatal outcomes, including similar incidences of epidural analgesia, childbirth, or parental stress, in nulliparous women and their partners [119].

Compared with conventional therapy, intensive counseling therapy for fear of childbirth does not affect the incidence of cesarean but is associated with reduced pregnancy-and birth-related anxiety and concerns, and shorter labors in one RCT [120].

In a small RCT, **a specific antenatal education program is associated with a reduction in the mean number of visits to the labor suite before the onset of labor** [4]. It is unclear whether this results in fewer women being sent home because they are not in labor [120] (see also Chapter 7). One trial study, comparing the use of an educational technique based on patient participation with routine instructions to prepare patients to recognize the onset of active labor, showed that, without any increase in time, nurses can prepare patients to make judgments about the need for hospitalization [121].

Depression in Pregnancy and the Postpartum Period

Between 14% and 23% of pregnant women will experience a depressive mood disorder while pregnant [122–129]. Maternal anxiety, life stress, history of depression, lack of social support, unintended pregnancy, public insurance, domestic violence, lower income, lower education, smoking, single status, and poor relationship quality were associated with a greater likelihood of antepartum depressive symptoms in bivariate analyses. Life stress, lack of social support, and domestic violence continued to demonstrate a significant association in multivariate analyses [123,124]. Identification of risk factors and screening for depression will facilitate referral for treatment (see Chapter 21 in *Maternal-Fetal Evidence Based Guidelines*).

Between 5% and 7% of women will experience postpartum depression. Risk factors include antenatal depressive symptoms, a history of major depressive disorder, or previous postpartum major depression [123]. If left untreated, postpartum major depression can lead to poor mother–infant bonding, delays in infant growth and development, and an increased risk of anxiety or depressive symptoms in the infant later in life. **Identifying mothers at-risk assists the prevention of postpartum depression compared with intervening on the general population.** The provision of **Intensive postpartum support provided by public health nurses or midwives** is associated with 32% less postpartum depression. Interventions with **only a postnatal component** appeared to be more beneficial than interventions that also incorporated an antenatal component. **Individual-based interventions** may be more effective than those that are group based. Women who received multiple-contact intervention are just as likely to experience postpartum depression as those who received a single-contact intervention [125]. **There is insufficient evidence to assess the effectiveness of antidepressants given immediately postpartum in preventing postnatal depression in all women or just in high-risk women** [126]. Norethisterone enanthate, a synthetic progestogen, 200 mg intramuscularly (IM) administered once within 48 hours of delivery to unselected women is associated with a significantly higher risk of developing postpartum depression at 6 weeks [127]. A pilot randomized controlled trial showed that **prenatal yoga** may be of benefit in **prevention of postpartum depression** in low-risk women [128]. Moreover, prenatal yoga was also found to be a feasible and acceptable intervention and was associated with reductions in symptoms in women with symptoms of anxiety and depression [129] (see Chapter 21 in *Maternal-Fetal Evidence Based Guidelines*).

Breastfeeding
Breastfeeding is the best feeding method for most infants and should be strongly encouraged (see Chapter 30). **Counseling and education during pregnancy have been shown to facilitate breastfeeding success** [130]. Breastfeeding education and/or support increased exclusive breastfeeding rates and decreased no breastfeeding rates at birth and at 1–5 months. Combined individual and group counseling appeared to be superior to either individual counseling alone or group counseling alone. Attitudes of the health-care provider are highly associated with breastfeeding success. Antigen avoidance diet during lactation by high-risk women may reduce the child's risk of developing atopic eczema, and may reduce atopic eczema in children already with atopic eczema during the first 12–18 months, although more trials are needed.

INTERVENTIONS FOR COMMON PREGNANCY COMPLAINTS
Itching
The differential diagnosis of itching in late pregnancy (>32 weeks) is presented in Chapter 10 in *Maternal-Fetal Evidence Based Guidelines*. If the itching is not due to liver disease, and if there is no rash, aspirin (600 mg qid) has been reported to decrease itching [124], but because of potential detrimental fetal effects (closure of ductus arteriosus and oligohydramnios) should not be used. If there are both itching and a rash, chlorpheniramine 4 mg tid decreased itching in a small trial [131]. However, aspirin 600 mg four times a day appears to be more effective than chlorpheniramine 5 mg three times a day for relief of itching when no rash is present in a small crossover trial [132].

Stretch Marks
Some stretch marks (striae gravidarum) develop in about 50% of women by the end of pregnancy. **There is no-high quality evidence to support the use of any topical preparation in the prevention of stretch marks during pregnancy** [133,134]. There is also no proven treatment for stretch marks once they have developed [134]. **Olive oil is not effective in preventing the occurrence of striae gravidarum or affecting its severity** [134]. There is no available product that has been definitively shown to prevent the formation of SG. Massage with either **Trofolastin cream** or **Verum ointment** is associated in small RCTs with a decrease in the development of SG [134]. A small randomized trial showed that a specific anti-stretch mark cream (emollient and moisturizer containing hydroxyprolisilane C, rosehip oil, *Centella asiatica*, triterpenes, and vitamin E) had a small effect in reducing severity (but not the incidence) of striae during pregnancy [135] (see Chapter 43 in *Maternal-Fetal Evidence Based Guidelines*).

Leg Cramps
Leg cramps are reported to occur in a reported 34% of pregnant women in the midtrimester [136,137]. **Magnesium lactate or citrate chewable tablets 5 mmol in the morning and 10 mmol in the evening for 3 weeks are associated with one-third of women not having persistent leg cramps** compared with 94% of placebo controls having persistent cramps. Multivitamin with mineral supplement might decrease leg cramps, but it is unclear which one of the 12 ingredients (or combination) is beneficial. Sodium chloride is associated with a slight reduction although consideration must be given to potential effect on blood pressure. **Calcium supplements do not decrease leg cramps compared with placebo.** However, it is unclear whether any of the interventions studied (i.e., oral magnesium, oral calcium, oral vitamin B or oral vitamin C) provide an effective treatment for leg cramps due to poor study design and trials being too small to address the question satisfactorily.

Calf stretching prior to bedtime does not decrease nocturnal leg cramps in nonpregnant patients [137].

Back and Pelvic Pain
Back pain is common in pregnancy, given weight gain and its uneven distribution as well as the softening effects of pregnancy hormones on the musculature.

There is evidence that *exercise* (any exercise on land or in water) may reduce pregnancy-related low-back pain, improve functional disability and reduce sick leave. **Water gymnastics for 1 hour weekly starting at <19 weeks reduces back pain in pregnancy and allows more women to continue to work, with no adverse effects** [138].

Pregnancy-specific exercises, physiotherapy, and acupuncture starting <32 weeks for 10 sessions appear to reduce back and pelvic pain; individual acupuncture sessions are more beneficial than group physiotherapy sessions. Education, other exercises, massage, heat therapy, support belts, analgesic therapy, etc. have not been studied in a trial in pregnancy for back pain relief.

Constipation

Constipation is common in pregnancy, probably because of decreased bowel peristalsis (possibly related to increased progesterone). It is reported by nearly 70% of women in the midtrimester. In nonpregnant adults, **exercise, increase in water intake, dietary counseling, and certain foods (e.g., prunes)** have been shown to relieve constipation. If these self-help measures are inadequate, the pregnant woman should then try daily bran or wheat fiber supplements. There is insufficient evidence to comprehensively assess the effectiveness and safety of interventions (pharmacological and nonpharmacological) for treating constipation in pregnancy, due to limited data (few studies with small sample size and no meta-analyses). Compared with bulk-forming laxatives, stimulant laxatives (e.g., Senna 14 mg, or dioctyl sodium succinate 120 mg and dihydroxyanthroquinone 100 mg—Normax) appear to be more effective in improvement of constipation (moderate quality evidence), but are accompanied by an increase in diarrhea and abdominal discomfort. **Docusate sodium** is a similar **stimulant laxative**, and it is widely available. Additionally, **dietary fiber supplements** (e.g., 10 mg/day of either corn-based biscuits—"Fibermed"—or 23 g wheat bran) increase the frequency of defecation and are associated with softer stools [139]. These findings in pregnant women are consistent with nonpregnant evidence.

Varicosities and Leg Edema

A small RCT ($n = 69$) shows that rutoside capsules improve leg edema symptoms; however, there are insufficient data to confirm rutoside safety in pregnancy. Another small RCT ($n = 43$) demonstrates a reduction in leg edema with **reflexology**. Compression stockings are not effective compared with simple resting, but studies do not compare compression stockings to no compression stockings. Leg elevation, compression hosiery, and swimming have not been studied for leg edema/varicosities relief in pregnancy [140].

Hemorrhoids

Hemorrhoids are common during pregnancy with 13% of women complaining of them in the midtrimester. **Oral hydroxyethylrutosides decrease symptoms compared with placebo group in women with hemorrhoids and reduce the signs identified by the health-care provider** [141]. Rutosides are associated with mild side effects such as GI discomfort, and their safety data in pregnancy are still insufficient. Constipation is a predisposing factor for hemorrhoids and should be treated. Sitz baths, ice, or ointments have been insufficiently studied for treatment of hemorrhoids in pregnancy. A small RCT showed that Hai's Perianal Support toilet seat device reduced the symptoms of hemorrhoids in pregnancy and improved the well-being of pregnant women [142].

Heartburn

Heartburn is common during pregnancy with 53% of women complaining of it in the midtrimester. There is no large-scale RCT to assess heartburn relief in pregnancy [143].

A consensus document has recommended that **lifestyle and dietary modifications** should remain the first-line treatment for heartburn in pregnancy. The measures include reducing and avoiding intake of reflux-inducing foods (e.g., greasy and spicy foods, tomatoes, highly acidic citrus products, and carbonated drinks) and substances such as caffeine. Nonsteroidal anti-inflammatory drugs (NSAIDs) should also be avoided. Other lifestyle changes to reduce the risk of reflux, such as avoiding lying down within 3 hours after eating, are advised. However, if heartburn is severe enough to warrant this action, medication should begin after consultation with a health-care professional. **Antacids, H_2 blockers, and proton pump inhibitors** all have acceptable safety profiles for the pregnant woman [143–145].

REFERENCES

1. Rosen MG, Merkatz IR, Hill JG. Caring for our future: A report by the expert panel on the content of prenatal care. *Obstet Gynecol*. 1991;77(5):782–787. [Review] [III]
2. Alexander GR, Kotelchuck M. Assessing the role and effectiveness of prenatal care: History, challenges, and directions for future research. *Public Health Rep*. 2001;116(4):306–316. [II-3]
3. Novick G. Centering pregnancy and the current state of prenatal care. *J Midwifery Women's Health*. 2004; 49(5):405–411. [III]
4. Dowswell T, Carroli G, Duley L, et al. Alternative versus standard packages of antenatal care for low-risk pregnancy. *Cochrane Database Syst Rev*. 2015;16:CD:000934. [Meta-analysis; 7 RCTs, $n = >60,000$]
5. Ickovics JR, Kershaw TS, Westdahl C, et al. Group prenatal care and perinatal outcomes: A randomized controlled trial. *Obstet Gynecol*. 2007;110(2 pt 1):330–339. [RCT, $n = 1047$]. [I]
6. Hatem M, Sandall J, Devane D, et al. Midwife-led versus other models of care for childbearing women. *Cochrane Database Syst Rev*. 2008;1: CD004667. [Meta-analysis; 11 RCTs, $n = 12,276$]
7. Gagnon AJ, Sandall J. Individual or group antenatal education for childbirth or parenthood, or both. *Cochrane Database Syst Rev*. 2007;18:CD002869. [Meta-analysis; 9 RCTs, $n = 2,284$]
8. Manandhar DS, Osrin D, Shrestha BP, et al. Effect of participatory intervention with women's groups on birth outcomes in Nepal: Cluster-randomized controlled trial. *Lancet*. 2004;364:970–979. [RCT, $n = 6212$] [I]
9. Mushi D, Mpembeni R, Jahn A. Effectiveness of community based safe motherhood promoters in improving the utilization of obstetric care. The case of Mtwara Rural District in Tanzania. *BMC Pregnancy Childbirth*. 2010;10:14. [II-1] [II-A]
10. Bhutta ZA, Lassi ZS. Empowering communities for maternal and newborn health. *Lancet*. 2010;375(9721):1142–1144. [Review] [III]
11. Mazzoni SE, Hill PK, Webster KW et al. Group prenatal care for women with gestational diabetes. *J Matern Fetal Neonatal Med*. 2015 Nov 23:1–5. [II-2]
12. Brown HC, Smith HJ. Giving women their own case notes to carry during pregnancy. *Cochrane Database Syst Rev*. 2004;2:CD002856. [Meta-analysis; 3 RCTs, $n = 675$]
13. Hanson L, VandeVusse L, Roberts J, et al. A critical appraisal of guidelines for antenatal care: Components of care and priorities in prenatal education. *J Midwifery Women's Health*. 2009;54(6):458–468. [Review]
14. The American College of Obstetricians and Gynecologists. Committee opinion no 611: Method for estimating due date. *Obstet Gynecol*. 2014;124:863–866
15. Duckitt K, Harrington D. Risk factors for pre-eclampsia at antenatal booking: Systematic review of controlled studies. *BMJ*. 2005;330(7491):565. [II-2]
16. Alto WA. No need for glycosuria/proteinuria screen in pregnant women. *J Fam Pract*. 2005;54(11):978–983. [II-2]
17. Sanchez-Ramos L, Gillen G, Zamora J, et al. The protein-to-creatinine ratio for the prediction of significant proteinuria in patients at risk for preeclampsia: A meta-analysis. *Ann Clin Lab Sci*. 2013 Spring;43(2):211–220. [Meta-analysis]
18. Yinon Y, Farine D, Yudin MH, et al. Cytomegalovirus infection in pregnancy. *J Obstet Gynaecol Can*. 2010;32(4):348–354. [Review]
19. Lindhard A, Nielsen PV, Mouritsen LA, et al. The implications of introducing the symphyseal-fundal height measurement.

A prospective randomized controlled trial. *BJOG*. 1990;97: 675–680. [RCT, *n* = 1,639] [I]
20. Kamysheva BA, Wertheim EH, Skouteris H, et al. Frequency, severity, and effect on life of physical symptoms experienced during pregnancy. *J Midwifery Women's Health*. 2009;54: 43–49. [II-2]
21. Nahum GG. Predicting fetal weight. Are Leopold's maneuvers still worth teaching to medical students and house staff? *J Reprod Med*. 2002;47(4):271–278. [II-3]
22. McFarlin BL, Engstrom JL, Sampson MB, et al. Concurrent validity of Leopold's maneuvers in determining fetal presentation and position. *J Nurse Midwifery*. 1985;30(5):280–284. [II-3]
23. Whitworth M, Bricker L, Neilson JP, et al. Ultrasound for fetal assessment in early pregnancy. *Cochrane Database Syst Rev.* 2010;(4):CD007058. [Meta-analysis; 11 RCTs, *n* = 37,505]
24. Neilson JP. Ultrasound for fetal assessment in early pregnancy. *Cochrane Database Syst Rev.* 2010;(4):CD000182. [Meta-analysis; 9 RCTs]
25. Khalifeh A, Berghella V. Ten reasons why universal cervical length screening should be recommended. *AJOG*. 2016 (in press). [III]
26. Bricker L, Neilson JP, Dowswell T. Routine ultrasound in late pregnancy (after 24 weeks' gestation). *Cochrane Database Syst Rev.* 2015;6:CD001451. [Meta-analysis; 13 RCTs, *n* = 34,980]
27. Savio U, White IR, Dacey A, et al. Screening for fetal growth restriction with universal third trimester ultrasonography in nulliparous women in the Pregnancy Outcome Prediction (POP) study: A prospective cohort study. *Lancet*. 2015 Sep 8. [II-2]
28. Mullen PD. Maternal smoking during pregnancy and evidence-based intervention to promote cessation. *Prim Care*. 1999;26 (3):577–589. [Review]
29. Naughton F, Prevost AT, Sutton S. Self-help smoking cessation interventions in pregnancy: A systematic review and meta-analysis. *Addiction*. 2008;103(4):566–579. [Meta-analysis; 11 RCTs, *n* = 6,208]
30. Lumley J, Chamberlain C, Dowswell T, et al. Interventions for promoting smoking cessation during pregnancy. *Cochrane Database Syst Rev.* 2009;(3):CD001055. [Meta-analysis; 72 RCTs, *n* = >20,000]
31. Henderson J, Gray R, Brocklehurst P. Systematic review of effects of low-moderate prenatal alcohol exposure on pregnancy outcome. *BJOG*. 2007;114(3):243–252. [II-1]
32. Stade BC, Bailey C, Dzendoletas D, et al. Psychological and/or educational interventions for reducing alcohol consumption in pregnant women and women planning pregnancy. *Cochrane Database Syst Rev.* 2009;(2):CD004228. [Meta-analysis; 4 RCTs, *n* = 715]
33. Ondersma SJ, Beatty JR, Svikis DS et al. Computer-delivered screening and brief intervention for alcohol use in pregnancy: A pilot randomized trial. *Alcohol Clin Exp Res*. 2015;39:1219–1226. [RCT, *n* = 48]
34. Doggett C, Burrett SL, Osborn DA. Home visits during pregnancy and after birth for women with an alcohol or drug problem. *Cochrane Database Syst Rev.* 2005;(4):CD004456. [Meta-analysis; 6 RCTs, *n* = 709]
35. Rotheram-Borus MJ, Tomlinson M, Roux IL, Stein JA. Alcohol use, partner violence and depression: A cluster randomized controlled trial among urban South African mothers over 3 years. *Am J Prev Med*. 2015 Jul 28. [RCT, *n* = 1,238]
36. Jahanfar S, Howard LM, Medley N. Interventions for preventing or reducing domestic violence against pregnant women. *Cochrane Database Syst Rev.* 2014;11:CD009414. [Meta-analysis; 10 RCTs, *n* = 3,417]
37. MacDonald LA, Waters TR, Napolitano PG et al. Clinical guidelines for occupational lifting in pregnancy: Evidence summary and provisional recommendations. *Am J Obstet Gynecol* 2013;209:80–88. [Review]
38. Lamina S, Agbanusi E. Effect of aerobic exercise training on maternal weight gain in pregnancy: A meta-analysis of randomized controlled trials. *Ethiop J Health Sci*. 2013;23:59–64. [Meta-analysis; 11 RCTs, *n* = 1,177]
39. Di Mascio D, Magro-Malosso ER, Saccone G, Marhefka GD, Berghella V. Exercise during pregnancy in normal-weight women and risk of preterm birth: A systematic review and meta-analysis of randomized controlled trials. *Am J Obstet Gynecol*. 2016 Jun 16;pii: S0002-9378(16)30344-1 [Epub ahead of print]. [Meta-analysis; 9 RCTs, n= 2,059]
40. Poyatos-Leon R, Garcia-Hermoso A, Poyatos-Leon R, et al. Effects of exercise during pregnancy on mode of delivery: A meta-analysis. *Acta Obstet Gynecol Scand*. 2015;94:1039–1047. [Meta-analysis; 13 RCTs, *n* = 2,873]
41. Sanabria-Martinez G, Garcia-Hermoso A, Poyatos-Leon R et al. Effects of exercise-based interventions on neonatal outcomes: A meta-analysis. *Am J Health Promot*. 2015 May 14, 06;3:CD000180. [Meta-analysis; 13 RCTs, *n* = 2,873]
42. Wiebe HW, Boule NG, Chari R, Davenport MH. The effect of supervised prenatal exercise on fetal growth: A meta-analysis. *Obstet Gynecol*. 2015;125:1185–1194. [Meta-analysis; 13 RCTs, *n* = 2,873]
43. Daley AJ, Foster L, Long G, et al. The effectiveness of exercise for the prevention and treatment of antenatal depression: Systematic review with meta-analysis. *BJOG*. 2015;122:57–62. [Meta-analysis 6 RCTs, *n* = 406]
44. Muktabhant B, Lawrie TA, Lumbiganon P, et al. Diet or exercise, or both, for preventing excessive weight gain in pregnancy. *Cochrane Database Syst Rev.* 2015;6:CD007145. [Meta-analysis, 49 RCTs, *n* = 11,444]
45. Streuling I, Beyerlein A, Rosenfeld E, et al. Physical activity and gestational weight gain: A meta-analysis of intervention trials. *BJOG*. 2010;118(3):278–284. [Meta-analysis; 12 RCTs]
46. Melzer K, Schutz Y, Boulvain M, et al. Physical activity and pregnancy: Cardiovascular adaptations, recommendations and pregnancy outcomes. *Sports Med*. 2010;40(6):493–507. [Review]
47. ACOG. Committee Opinion No.650: Physical activity and exercise during pregnancy and the postpartum period. *Obstet Gynecol*. 2015;126:135–142. [Guideline]
48. Eijsvolgels TM, Thompson PD. Exercise is medicine: At any dose? *JAMA*. 2015;10:314:1915–1916. [Review]
49. Babbar S, Parks-Savage AC, Chauhan SP. Yoga during pregnancy: A review. *Am J Perinatol*. 2012;29:459–464. [Meta-analysis; 3 RCTs, *n* = 298]
50. Serati M, Salvatore S, Siesto G, et al. Female sexual function during pregnancy and after childbirth. *J Sex Med*. 2010;7(8):2782–2790. [Review]
51. Kavanagh J, Kelly AJ, Thomas J. Sexual intercourse for cervical ripening and induction of labour. *Cochrane Database Syst Rev.* 2001;(2):CD003093. [Meta-analysis; 1 RCT, *n* = 28]
52. Berghella V, Klebanoff M, McPherson C, et al. Sexual intercourse association with asymptomatic bacterial vaginosis and trichomonas vaginalis treatment in relationship to preterm birth. *Am J Obstet Gynecol*. 2002;187:1277–1282. [II-2]
53. Ota E, Hori H, Mori R, et al. Antenatal dietary education and supplementation to increase energy and protein intake. *Cochrane Database Syst Rev.* 2015;6:CD0000032. [Meta-analysis; 17 RCTs, *n* = 9,030]
54. Khoury J, Henriksen T, Christophersen B, et al. Effect of a cholesterol-lowering diet on maternal, cord, and neonatal lipids, and pregnancy outcome: A randomized clinical trial. *Am J Obstet Gynecol*. 2005;193:1292–1301. [RCT, *n* = 290] [I]
55. Meta-analysis, RCTBain E, Crane M, et al. Diet and exercise interventions for preventing gestational diabetes mellitus. *Cochrane Database Syst Rev.* 2015;4:CD010443. [Meta-analysis; 13 RCTs, *n* = 4,983]
56. Han S, Crowther CA, Middleton P, et al. Different types of dietary advice for women with gestational diabetes mellitus. *Cochrane Database Syst Rev.* 2013;CD009275. [Meta-analysis; 9 RCTs, *n* = 429]

57. Kramer MS, Kakuma R. Maternal dietary antigen avoidance during pregnancy or lactation, or both, for preventing or treating atopic disease in the child. *Cochrane Database Syst Rev.* 2012;9:CD000133. [Meta-analysis; 5 RCTs, n = 952]
58. Lindsay KL, Brennan L, Kennelly MA, et al. Impact of probiotics in women with gestational diabetes mellitus on metabolic health: A randomized controlled trial. *Am J Obstet Gynecol.* 2015;212:496e1–496e11. [RCT, n = 149)
59. Rasmussen KM, Yaktine AL, eds. Committee to reexamine IOM pregnancy weight guidelines. Weight gain during pregnancy: Reexamining the guidelines. Institute of Medicine; National Research Council. *JAMA.* 2009;302:241–242. [Guideline]
60. Kiel DW, Dodson EA, Artal R, et al. Gestational weight gain and pregnancy outcomes in obese women. How much is enough? *Obstet Gynecol.* 2007;110:752–758. [II-2]
61. Davies GA, Maxwell C, McLeod L, et al. Obesity in pregnancy. *J Obstet Gynaecol Can.* 2010;32(2):165–173. [Review]
62. Asbee SM, Jenkins TR, Butler JR, et al. Preventing excessive weight gain during pregnancy through dietary and lifestyle counseling–A randomized controlled trial. *Obstet Gynecol.* 2009;113:305–312. [RCT, n = 100] [I]
63. Polley BA, Wing RR, Sims CJ. Randomized controlled trial to prevent excessive weight gain in pregnant women. *Intern J Obesity.* 2002;26:1494–1502. [RCT, n = 120] [I]
64. Siega-Riz AM, Viswanathan M, Moos M-K, et al. A systematic review of outcomes of maternal weight gain according to the Institute of Medicine recommendations: Birthweight, fetal growth, and postpartum weight retention. *Am J Obstet Gynecol.* 2009;201:339.e1–339.e14. [Systematic review of 35 studies from 1990 to 2007]
65. Committee to Reexamine IOM Pregnancy Weight Guidelines, Food and Nutrition Board, and Board on Children, Youth, and Families. *Weight Gain During Pregnancy: Reexamining the Guidelines.* Washington, DC: Institute of Medicine, 2009. [Consensus report]
66. Oken E, Kleinman KP, Belfort MB, et al. Association of gestational weight gain with short-and longer-term maternal and child health outcomes. *Am J Epidemiol.* 2009;170:173–180. [II-2: project viva, Massachusetts 1999–2002 U.S. observational study, n = 2012]
67. Cedergren MI. Optimal gestational weight gain for body mass index categories. *Obstet Gynecol.* 2007;110(4):759–764. [II-2: Swedish Medical Birth Register, population-based cohort study, n = 298,648]
68. Nohr EA, Vaeth M, Baker JL, et al. Pregnancy outcomes related to gestational weight gain in women defined by their body mass index, parity, height, and smoking status. *Am J Clin Nutr.* 2009;90:1288–1294. [II-2: Danish population-based observational study, n = 59,147]
69. Dietz PM, Callaghan WM, Smith R, et al. Low pregnancy weight gain and small for gestational age: A comparison of the association using 3 different measures of small for gestational age. *Am J Obstet Gynecol.* 2009;201:53.e.1–53.e.7. [II-2: retrospective cohort study, Pregnancy Risk Assessment Monitoring System (PRAMS), n = 104,980]
70. Ronnberg AK, Ostlund I, Fadl H, et al. Intervention during pregnancy to reduce excessive gestational weight gain—A randomised controlled trial. *BJOG.* 2015;122:537–544. [RCT, n = 445]
71. Bianco AT, Smilen SW, Davis Y, et al. Pregnancy outcome and weight gain recommendations for the morbidly obese woman. *Obstet Gynecol.* 1998;91:97–102. [II-2, U.S. retrospective cohort study, n = 11,926]
72. Catalano PM, Mele L, Landon MB, et al. Eunice Kennedy Shriver National Institute of Child Health and Human development Materna-Fetal Medicine Units Network. Inadequate weight gain in overweight and obese pregnant women: What is the effect on fetal growth? *Am J Obstet Gynecol.* 2014;211:137.e1–7. [II-2]
73. Bech BH, Obel C, Henriksen TB, et al. Effect of reducing caffeine intake on birth weight and length of gestation: Randomised controlled trial. *BMJ.* 2007;334:409. [RCT, n = 1198] [I]
74. Jahanfar S, Jaafar SH. Effects of restricted caffeine intake by mother on fetal, neonatal and pregnancy outcomes. *Cochrane Database Syst Rev.* 2015;6:CD006965. [Meta-analysis; 2 RCTs, n = 1,197]
75. Shah PS, Ohlsson A. Effects of prenatal multimicronutrient supplementation on pregnancy outcomes: A meta-analysis. *CMAJ.* 2009;180(12):1188–1189. [Meta-analysis]
76. Haider BA, Bhutta ZA. Multiple-micronutrient supplementation for women during pregnancy. *Cochrane Database Syst Rev.* 2006;(4):CD004905. [Meta-analysis; 9 RCTs, n = 15,378]
77. Lumley L, Watson L, Watson M, et al. Periconceptional supplementation with folate and/or multivitamins for preventing neural tube defects. *Cochrane Database Syst Rev.* 2005;(3). [Meta-analysis; 4 RCTs, 6425 women]
78. De-Regil LM, Fernández-Gaxiola AC, Dowswell T, et al. Effects and safety of periconceptional folate supplementation for preventing birth defects. *Cochrane Database Syst Rev.* 2010;(10):CD007950. [Meta-analysis; 5 RCTs, n = 6105]
79. Wald NJ. Folic acid and the prevention of neural-tube defects. *N Engl J Med.* 2004;350:101–103. [Editorial] [III]
80. Honein MA, Paulozzi LJ, Mathews TJ, et al. Impact of folic acid fortification of the US food supply on the occurrence of neural tube defects. *JAMA.* 2001;285:2981–2986. [Observational] [II-2]
81. Valera-Gran D, Garcia de la Hera M, Navarrete-Munoz EM, et al. Folic acid supplements during pregnancy and child psychomotor development after the first year of life. *JAMA Pediatr.* 2014;168:e142611. [II-1]
82. Roth C, Magnus P, Schjolberg S, et al. Folic acid supplements in pregnancy and severe language delay in children. *JAMA.* 2011;306:1566–1573. [II-1]
83. van den Broek N, Dou L, Othman M, et al. Vitamin A supplementation during pregnancy for maternal and newborn outcomes. *Cochrane Database Syst Rev.* 2010;(11):CD008666. [Meta-analysis]
84. Barger MK. Maternal nutrition and perinatal outcomes. *J Midwifery Women's Health.* 2010;55(6):502–511. [II-3]
85. Thaver D, Saeed MA, Bhutta ZA. Pyridoxine (vitamin B6) supplementation in pregnancy. *Cochrane Database Syst Rev.* 2006;(2):CD000179. [Meta-analysis; 5 RCTS, n = 1646]
86. Hillman RW, Cabaud PG, Schenone RA. The effects of pyridoxine supplements on the dental caries experience of pregnant women. *Am J Clin Nutr.* 1962;10:512–515. [1 RCT, n = 371]
87. Rumbold A, Ota E, Nagata C, et al. Vitamin C supplementation in pregnancy. *Cochrane Database Syst Rev.* 2015;9:CD004072.
88. Mahomed K, Gulmezoglu AM. Vitamin D supplementation in pregnancy. *Cochrane Database Syst Rev.* 2011;2:CD000228. [Meta-analysis; 2 RCTs, n = 232]
89. Perez-Lopez FR, Pasupuleti V, Mezones-Holguin E et al. Effect of vitamin D supplementation during pregnancy on maternal and neonatal outcomes: A systematic review and meta-analysis of randomized controlled trials. *Fertil Steril* 2015;103:1278–1288. [Meta-analysis; 13 RCTs, n = 2,299]
90. Rodda CP, Benson JE, Vincent AK, Whitehead CL, Polykov A, Vollenhoven B. Maternal vitamin D supplementation during pregnancy prevents vitamin D deficiency in the newborn: An open-label randomized controlled trial. *Clin Endocrinol (Oxf).* 2015;83:363–368. [RCT, n = 78] [I]
91. Mohammad-Alizadeh-Charandabi S, Mirghafourvand M, Mansouri A, et al. The effect of vitamin D and calcium plus vitamin D during pregnancy on pregnancy and birth outcomes: A randomized controlled trial. *J Caring Sci.* 2015;4:35–44. [RCT, n = 126] [I]
92. Wei SQ, Qi HP, Luo ZC, et al. Maternal vitamin D status and adverse pregnancy outcomes: A systematic review and meta-analysis. *J Matern Fetal Neonatal Med.* 2013;26:889–899. [Meta-analysis of 24 cohort studies]
93. Rumbold A, Ota E, Hori H, et al. Vitamin E supplementation in pregnancy. *Cochrane Database Syst Rev.* 2015;9:CD004069. [Meta-analysis; 21 RCTs, n = 22,129]

94. Makrides M, Crosby DD, Brain E, et al. Magnesium supplementation in pregnancy. *Cochrane Database Syst Rev.* 2014;4:CD000937. [Meta-analysis, 10 RCTs, $n = 9,090$]
95. Hofmeyr JG, Lawrie TA, Atallah AN, et al. Calcium supplementation during pregnancy for preventing hypertensive disorders and related problems. *Cochrane Database Syst Rev.* 2010;(8):CD001059. [Meta-analysis; 13 RCTs, $n = 15,730$]
96. Pena-Rosas JP, Viteri FE. Effects and safety of preventive oral iron or iron+folic acid supplementation for women during pregnancy. *Cochrane Database Syst Rev.* 2015;7:CD004736. [Meta-analysis, 49 RCTs, $n = 23,200$]
97. Mahomed K, Bhutta ZA, Middleton P. Zinc supplementation for improving pregnancy and infant outcome. *Cochrane Database Syst Rev.* 2007;(2):CD000230. [Meta-analysis; 17 RCTs, $n = >9000$]
98. Rebagliato M, Murcia M, Espada M, et al. Iodine intake and maternal thyroid function during pregnancy. *Epidemiology.* 2010;21(1):62–69. [II-2]
99. Pearce EN. What do we know about iodine supplementation in pregnancy? *J Clin Endocrinol Metab.* 2009;94(9):3188–3190. [Review]
100. Saccone G, Saccone I, Berghella V. Omega-3 long chain polyunsaturated fatty acids and fish oil supplementation during pregnancy: Which evidence? *J Matern Fetal Neonatal Med.* 2015. [Meta-analysis; 34 RCTs, $n = 16,684$]
101. Saccone G, Berghella V. Omega-3 long chain polyunsaturated fatty acids to prevent preterm birth: A systematic review and meta-analysis. *Obstet Gynecol.* 2015;3:663–672. [Meta-analysis; 9 RCTs, $n = 3,854$]
102. Saccone G, Berghella V. Omega-3 supplementation to prevent recurrent preterm birth: A systematic review and meta-analysis. *Am J Obstet Gynecol.* 2015 Mar 7. doi: 10.1016/j.ajog.2015.03.013. [Meta-analysis; 2 RCTs, $n = 1,080$]
103. Saccone G, Berghella V, Maruotti GM, et al. Omega-3 supplementation during pregnancy to prevent recurrent intrauterine growth restriction: A systematic review and meta-analysis of randomized controlled trials. *Ultrasound Obstet Gynecol.* 2015 May 29. doi: 10.1002/uog.14910. [Meta-analysis; 3 RCTs, $n = 575$]
104. Schwendicke F, Karimbux N, Allareddy V, et al. Periodontal treatment for preventing adverse pregnancy outcomes: A meta- and trial sequential analysis. *PLOS One.* 2015;10:e0129060. [Meta-analysis; 13 RCTs, $n = 6,283$]
105. Hofmeyr JG, Kulier R. Abdominal decompression in normal pregnancy. *Cochrane Database Syst Rev.* 2012; 6:CD001062. [Meta-analysis; 3 RCTs, $n = 951$]
106. Thinkhamrop J, Hofmeyr GJ, Adetoro O, et al. Prophylactic antibiotic administration in pregnancy to prevent infectious morbidity and mortality. *Cochrane Database Syst Rev.* 2002;(4):CD002250. [Meta-analysis; 6 RCTs, $n = 2189$, both low- and high-risk women]
107. McGregor JA, French JI, Richter R, et al. Cervicovaginal microflora and pregnancy outcome: Results of a double-blind, placebo-controlled trial of erythromycin treatment. *Am J Obstet Gynecol.* 1990;163:1580–1591. [RCT, $n = 229$]
108. Hodnett ED, Fredericks S, Weston J. Support during pregnancy for women at increased risk of low birthweight babies. *Cochrane Database Syst Rev.* 2010;(6):CD000198. [Meta-analysis; 17 RCTs, $n = 12,264$]
109. Dowswell T, Middleton P, Weeks A. Antenatal day care units versus hospital admission for women with complicated pregnancy. *Cochrane Database Syst Rev.* 2009;(4):CD001803. [Metaanalysis; 3 RCTs, $n = 504$]
110. Dyson L, McCormick F, Renfrew MJ. Interventions for promoting the initiation of breastfeeding. *Cochrane Database Syst Rev.* 2005;(2):CD001688. [Meta-analysis; 7 RCTs, $n = 1,388$]
111. Palda VA, Guise JM, Wathen CN. Interventions to promote breast-feeding: Applying the evidence in clinical. *CMAJ.* 2004;170(6):976–978. [II-2]
112. Gagnon AJ. Individual or group antenatal education for childbirth/parenthood. *Cochrane Database Syst Rev.* 2005;(3). [Meta-analysis; 6 RCTs, 1443 women]
113. Lassi ZS, Haider BA, Bhutta ZA. Community-based intervention packages for reducing maternal and neonatal morbidity and mortality and improving neonatal outcomes. *Cochrane Database Syst Rev.* 2010;(11):CD007754. [Meta-analysis; 18 cluster-randomized studies]
114. Labrecque M, Marcoux S, Pinault JJ, et al. Prevention of perineal trauma by perineal massage during pregnancy: A pilot study. *Birth.* 1994;21:20–25. [RCT, $n = 46$] [I]
115. Labrecque M, Eason E, Marcoux S, et al. Randomized controlled trial of prevention of perineal trauma by perineal massage during pregnancy. *AJOG.* 1999;180:593–600. [RCT, $n = 1,527$] [I]
116. Shipman MK, Boniface DR, Tefft ME, et al. Antenatal perineal massage and subsequent perineal outcomes: A randomized controlled trial. *BJOG.* 1997;104:787–791. [RCT, $n = 861$] [I]
117. Harlev A, Parient G, Kessous R et al. Can we find the perfect oil to protect the perineum? A randomized-controlled double-blind trial. *J Matern Fetal Neonatal Med.* 2013;26:1328–1331. [RCT, $n = 164$] [I]
118. Maimburg RD, Vaeth M, Durr J, et al. Randomized trial of structured antenatal training sessions to improve the birth process. *BJOG.* 2010;117:921–928. [RCT, $n = 1193$] [I]
119. Bergstrom M, Kieler H, Waldenstrom U. Effects of natural childbirth preparation versus standard antenatal education on epidural rates, experience of childbirth and parental stress in mothers and fathers: A randomized controlled trial. *BJOG.* 2009;116:1167–1176. [RCT, $n = 1087$] [I]
120. Saisto T, Salmela-Aro K, Nurmi J-E, et al. A randomized controlled trial of intervention in fear of childbirth. *Obstet Gynecol.* 2001;98:820–826. [RCT, $n = 176$] [I]
121. Bonovich L. Recognizing the onset of labour. *J Obstet Gynecol Neonatal Nurs.* 1990;19(2):141–145. [RCT, $n = 245$; 208 analyzed] [I]
122. Yonkers KA, Wisner KL, Stewart DE, et al. The management of depression during pregnancy: A report from the American Psychiatric Association and the American College of Obstetricians and Gynecologists. *Obstet Gynecol.* 2009;114(3):703–713. [Review]
123. Lancaster CA, Gold KJ, Flynn HA, et al. Risk factors for depressive symptoms during pregnancy: A systematic review. *Am J Obstet Gynecol.* 2010;202(1):5–14. [Systematic review]
124. Hirst KP, Moutier CY. Postpartum major depression. *Am Fam Physician.* 2010;82(8):926–933. [Review]
125. Dennis CL, Creedy D. Psychosocial and psychological interventions for preventing postpartum depression. *Cochrane Database Syst Rev.* 2013;2:CD001134. [Meta-analysis; 28 RCTs, $n = 17,000$]
126. Howard LM, Hoffbrand S, Henshaw C, et al. Antidepressant prevention of postnatal depression. *Cochrane Database Syst Rev.* 2005;(2):CD004363. [Meta-analysis; 2 RCTs, $n = 73$]
127. Lawrie TA, Hofmeyr GJ, de Jager M, et al. A double-blind randomised placebo controlled trial of postnatal norethisterone enanthate: The effect on postnatal depression and serum hormones. *Br J Obstet Gynaecol.* 1998;105:1082–1090. [RCT, $n = 180$] [I]
128. Uebelacker LA, Battle CL, Sutton KA, et al. A pilot randomized controlled trial comparing prenatal yoga to perinatal health education for antenatal depression. *Arch Womens Ment Health.* 2015 Sep 18. [RCT, $n = 46$] [I]
129. Davis K, Goodman SH, Leiferman J, et al. A randomized controlled trial of yoga for pregnant women with symptoms of depression and anxiety. *Complement Ther Clin Pract.* 2015;21:166–172. [RCT, $n = 46$] [I]
130. Haroon S, Das JK, Salam RA, et al. Breastfeeding promotion interventions and breastfeeding practices: A systematic review. *BMC Public Health.* 2013;13:S20.
131. Read MD. A new hypothesis of itching in pregnancy. *Practitioner.* 1977;218:845–847. [RCT, $n = 36$] [I]

132. Young G, Jewell D. Antihistamines versus aspirin for itching in late pregnancy. *Cochrane Database Syst Rev.* 2010;11:CD0000027. [Meta-analysis, 1 RCT, $n = 38$]
133. Brennan M, Young G, Devane D. Topical preparations for preventing stretch marks in pregnancy. *Database Syst Rev.* 2012;11:CD000066. [Meta-analysis, 6 RCTs, $n = 800$]
134. Soltanipour F, Delaram M, Taavoni S, et al. The effect of olive oil and the Saj cream in prevention of striae gravidarum: A randomized controlled clinical trial. *Complement Ther Med.* 2014;22:220–225. [I]
135. Garcia Hernandez JA, Madera Gonzalez D, Padilla Castillo M, et al. Use of a specific anti-stretch mark cream for preventing or reducing the severity of striae gravidarum. Randomized double-blind controlled trial. *Int J Cosmet Sci.* 2013;35:233–237. [I]
136. Zhou K, West HM, Zhang J, et al. Intervention for leg cramps in pregnancy. *Cochrane Database Syst Rev.* 2015;8:CD010655. [Meta-analysis, 6RCTs, $n = 390$]
137. Coppin RJ, Wicke DM, Little PS. Managing nocturnal leg cramps-calf-stretching exercises and cessation of quinine treatment: A factorial randomized controlled trial. *Br J Gen Pract.* 2005;55:186–199. [RCT, $n = 191$ women] [I]
138. Liddle SD, Pennick V. Interventions for preventing and treating low-back and pelvic pain during pregnancy. *Cochrane Database Syst Rev.* 2015;9:CD001139. [Meta-analysis, 34 RCTs, $n = 5,121$]
139. Rungsiprakarn P, Laopaiboon M, Sangkomkamhand US, et al. Interventions for treating constipation in pregnancy. *Cochrane Database Syst Rev.* 2015;9:CD011448. [Meta-analysis; 2 RCTs, $n = 180$]
140. Bamigboye AA, Smyth RMD. Interventions for varicose veins and leg oedema in pregnancy. *Cochrane Database Syst Rev.* 2007;(1):CD001066. [Meta-analysis; 3 RCTs, $n = 159$]
141. Quijano CE, Abalos E. Conservative management of symptomatic and/or complicated haemorrhoids in pregnancy and the puerperium. *Cochrane Database Syst Rev.* 2005;(3):CD004077. [Meta-analysis, 2 RCTs, $n = 150$]
142. Lim SS, Yu CW, Aw LD. Comparing topical hydrocortisone cream with Hai's perianal support in managing symptomatic hemorrhoids in pregnancy: A preliminary trial. *J Obstet Gynaecol Res.* 2015;42:238–247. [RCT, $n = 23$] [I]
143. Phupong V, Hanprasertopong T. Interventions for heartburn in pregnancy. *Cochrane Database Syst Rev.* 2015;9:CD011379. [Meta-analysis, 4 RCTs, $n = 358$]
144. Gill SK, O'Brien L, Einarson TR, et al. The safety of proton pump inhibitors (PPIs) in pregnancy: A meta-analysis. *Am J Gastroenterol.* 2009;104:1541–1545. [Meta-analysis]
145. Gill SK, O'Brien L, Koren G. The safety of histamine 2 (H2) blockers in pregnancy: A meta-analysis. *Dig Dis Sci.* 2009;54(9):1835–1838. [II-1]

Physiologic changes

Jason Baxter and Colleen Horan

KEY POINTS
- The normal physiologic changes of pregnancy are several and listed in part in Table 3.1.
- Normal laboratory values for pregnant women are presented in Table 3.2.
- Failure to understand these physiologic changes of pregnancy may result in both undue alarm and costly evaluation of normal symptoms of pregnancy or in the neglect of pathologic conditions due to which the presentation is dismissed as another "discomfort of pregnancy."
- The physician should carefully address the pregnant patient **keeping in mind the question "how is this presentation affected by the physiology of pregnancy?"**

BACKGROUND
Over the course of human pregnancy, the significance of physiologic changes that occur is such that it often becomes no longer appropriate for the physician to evaluate her according to standards that have been set through the observation and study of men and nonpregnant women. Some of these physiologic changes are advantageous to the growth and survival of the fetus. Others enhance the ability of the maternal system to compensate for demands of pregnancy, prepare for stress of delivery, and recover from delivery.

Understanding physiologic changes in pregnancy is important in evaluating common symptoms associated with pregnancy, interpreting laboratory values in the parturient, and understanding pathologic conditions to which pregnant women are susceptible. **Failure to understand the normal physiologic changes of pregnancy may result in both undue alarm and costly evaluation of normal symptoms of pregnancy or in the neglect of pathologic conditions due to which the presentation is dismissed as another discomfort of pregnancy.** The patient will most likely be better served by the physician who carefully addresses her symptoms while **keeping in mind the questions "how is this presentation affected by the physiology of pregnancy?"** and "what pathologic conditions may be represented by this scenario?" than by the physician who uncritically memorizes laboratory values and makes a diagnosis without considering the interplay between pregnancy and underlying pathophysiology.

Two summary tables are provided. Table 3.1 summarizes the commonly accepted pregnancy-related changes in various physiologic parameters and their importance in the evaluation and management during pregnancy [1]. Table 3.2 provides a summary of laboratory values in each trimester of pregnancy versus in the nonpregnant state based on a recent systematic review [2]. The reader will note that some values show significant overlap between pregnant and nonpregnant states. Some show little change between pregnant and nonpregnant states. Others show trends that clearly increase or decrease with pregnancy. In most cases, it is not possible to consider the effect of pregnancy on laboratory values in a simplistic or formulaic way. Rather, it is the understanding of the underlying physiology that these laboratory values reflect that is the most important in their evaluation during pregnancy.

CARDIOVASCULAR/HEMODYNAMIC
An understanding of pregnancy-related hemodynamic changes is crucial in the management of both benign and life-threatening complications of pregnancy ranging from near-syncopal episodes experienced by many pregnant women to hypotension from obstetric hemorrhage and gestational hypertension, both of which are leading causes of maternal intensive care unit admissions and mortality [3]. Even the ultimate clinical emergency of cardiac arrest is complicated by hemodynamic changes which are unique to pregnancy.

Hemodynamic changes in pregnancy that have been well established include an **increase in cardiac output and a decrease in both systemic and pulmonary vascular resistance. There is an overall increase in the heart rate and a decrease in the blood pressure. Blood volume, plasma volume, and erythrocyte volume increase, with a greater relative increase in the plasma volume resulting in a dilution lowering of hematocrit and other blood indices.** There is also a redistribution of cardiac output with an increase in flow to the uterus, kidneys, skin, and breasts [1]. The increase in stroke volume and cardiac output creates a more audible physiologic flow murmur and splitting of the S2 sound during pregnancy, which may be striking upon physical examination.

One longitudinal study followed maternal hemodynamics as measured by thoracic electrical bioimpedance monitoring in 50 healthy pregnant women [4]. The results showed an increase in the mean heart rate from 87 ± 2 beats per minute (bpm) at 10–18 weeks to 92 ± 1 bpm at 34–42 weeks. Mean arterial pressure (MAP) decreased significantly after 14 weeks and increased after 29 weeks. Systemic vascular resistance (SVR) increased during the last trimester. This study also found a significantly higher mean cardiac output in nulliparous women compared with multiparous women. Mean cardiac output and stroke volume, which show an overall increase during pregnancy, were found to decrease in the third trimester in this study [4]. However, the change in cardiac output during the third trimester showed significant individual variation and has not been consistent in other longitudinal studies, demonstrating the need for further research for a more conclusive understanding of how this parameter changes across gestation [5].

Another longitudinal study performed serial echocardiography studies on 35 healthy pregnant women from the early second trimester to 6–12 weeks postpartum [6]. This study showed a significant increase in the cardiac output that peaked in the early third trimester and was maintained until term.

Table 3.1 Summary of Physiologic Adaptations during Pregnancy

Parameter	Expected change	Comments
Cardiovascular system		
Heart size	Increases 12%	Increased diastolic filling and muscle hypertrophy
Murmurs	Physiologic systolic	Ejection murmurs attributable to increased stroke volume usually occur in early or midsystole and are best heard along the left sternal edge
EKG	Positional heart shifts result in changes that resemble ischemia	Heart is pushed upward and forward, deviating electrical axis to the left by 15°–20°, causing flattened or inverted T in lead III
Cardiac output	Increases 30%–50% From 4.5 to about 6.0 L/min (by 1.5 L/min) Influenced by maternal position	Greatest increase occurs immediately after delivery with redistribution of blood flow from uterus. Cardiac output then decreases
Rhythm	Increases atrial and ventricular extrasystole	SVT not infrequent
Heart rate	Increases	Onset of change is first trimester
Stroke volume	Increases	Significant change in second half of pregnancy
Mean arterial pressure	Decreased soon after beginning of pregnancy and midpregnancy (100–110/60–70 mean levels); then returns to prepregnant values by third trimester and term	Supine hypotension—decreased venous return due to compression from gravid uterus; increased blood flow through alternative pathways such as paravertebral azygous veins
Pulse pressure	Increases	
Venous pressure	Increases in femoral system; unchanged in arms	
Systemic vascular resistance	Decreases	
Pulmonary BP	Unchanged	
Blood flow to uterus	Increases by 500 mL/min Increases from 1% to 3% of CO to 17%–20%	No autoregulation
Blood flow to kidneys	Increases by 400 mL/min	
Blood flow to skin	Increases by 300–400 mL/min	
Blood flow to breasts	Increases by 200 mL/min	
Respiratory system		
Anatomy	Increases subcostal angle from 68° to 103° → 3 cm increase in transthoracic diameter	Increased upper respiratory capillary engorgement can cause increased congestion, epistaxis, and intubation trauma
Tidal volume	Increases by 300 mL or 40%	
Expiratory reserve volume	Decreases by 200 mL	Cephalad displacement of diaphragm
Inspiratory capacity	Increases by 300 mL	
Functional residual volume	Decreases by 500 mL	
Minute volume	Increases by 40% or 3 L/min beginning in first trimester	Increased rate of induction of, and emergence from, inhaled anesthetics
Maximum breathing capacity	Unchanged	
Forced expiratory volume	Unchanged	
Peak expiratory flow rate	Unchanged	
Pulmonary diffusing capacity	Decreases by 4 mL/min/mmHg	
Oxygen requirement	Increases by 30–40 mL/min	
Carbon dioxide output	Increases; expressed as respiratory quotient	
Carbon dioxide pressure	Decreases from 35–40 mmHg to 28–30 mmHg	
Oxygen pressure	Increases	
pH	Mild increase (7.40–7.44 is normal)	Compensated respiratory alkalosis
PCO_2	Decrease (30–31 mmHg is normal)	
PO_2	Mild increase (100–104 mmHg is normal)	
Renal system and homeostasis		
GFR	Increases from 97 mL/min to 128 mL/min by 10 weeks	Increased renal clearance of certain drugs and vitamins
Glucose excretion	Increased	Random glycosuria
Protein excretion	Increased (up to 300 mg/24 hours is normal)	
Renin, angiotensins I and II	Increased	Diminished vascular response causes less pressor effect from angiotensin
Anatomic changes	Dilation of renal calyces and ureters to pelvic brim; "physiologic" hydronephrosis, right > left	Increased risk of pyelonephritis; screen for asymptomatic bacteriuria
Potassium	Increased retention	
Sodium	Increased retention	
Urine output	No significant change	

(Continued)

Table 3.1 Summary of Physiologic Adaptations during Pregnancy (*Continued*)

Parameter	Expected change	Comments
Vitamin excretion	Increased loss of folate, B12, and ascorbic acid	
Osmolality	Decreases 10 mOsm/kg first trimester, then stable	
Sodium	Decreases 3 mEq/L first trimester, then stable	
Potassium	Decreases 0.5 mEq/L	
Calcium	Decreased total and ionized	Increased intestinal absorption of calcium and increased bone turnover
Magnesium	Decreases 10%–20% in first half of pregnancy	
Chloride	Unchanged	
Bicarbonate	Decreases markedly (18–22 mEq/L is normal)	Compensates for decrease in PCO_2
Total protein	Decreases from 72 to 62 g/L	
Albumin	Decreases from 47 to 36 g/L	
Urea, creatinine, and uric acid	Decrease in first trimester; stabilize in second trimester; increase toward term	
Vitamin B6	Decreases	
Blood glucose	Fasting levels *decrease* in first trimester, then unchanged	Postprandial levels remain elevated longer, prolonging return to fasting state. Increased glucose levels allow passive diffusion across placenta to fetus
Folate	Decreases 50% toward term	
Vitamin B12	Decreases 50% or more	B12 levels in folate-deficient women will increase with folate supplementation alone
Endocrine system		
Pituitary gland	Increases to 50% greater than adult male	Attributable to increase of prolactin-secreting cells in anterior lobe
Prolactin	Increases from 300 to 5000 mIU/L	Estrogen stimulates hyperplasia and hypertrophy of pituitary lactotrophs
Follicle-stimulating hormone and luteinizing hormone	Decrease to nearly undetectable	
Melanocyte-stimulating hormone	Increased	Likely responsible for linea nigra, chloasma, and increased areolae pigmentation
Thyroid-stimulating hormone	Normal range is unchanged	May be suppressed during late first to early second trimester due to hCG-mediated increase in TH production—subtle effect may be exacerbated by conditions that increase hCG levels, such as hyperemesis, molar pregnancies, and multiples
Thyroid-binding globulin	Increases—doubles by end of first trimester; triples by term	Due to estrogen effect on liver
Thyroxine (T_4) and triiodothyronine (T_3)	Increased total circulating amount; unchanged free fraction	Fetal thyroid hormone production commences at 18 weeks
Reverse T_3	Unchanged in maternal circulation; increased in cord blood	
Cortisol	Increased to 3 × nonpregnant values	Episodic pattern of release is maintained
Aldosterone	Increased twofold by term	
Deoxycorticosterone	Increased by 20–100 times	
Testosterone	Increased total amount; decreased free fraction	
Androstenedione	Increases	Tenfold increase rate of transformation to estradiol and estrone
DHEA	Unchanged or small decrease	Precursor for steroid hormone synthesis by placenta
Pancreas	Hypertrophy of islets due to hyperplasia of B cells	
Insulin	Increases fasting levels toward term; hyperplasia of pancreatic B cells	Proportionally less increase of glucagons compared with insulin; so insulin:glucagon ratio is increased
Glucagon	Increases fasting levels	
Glucose	Slight decrease	Especially fasting levels
Parathyroid hormone	Increased during end of pregnancy	Maintains calcium levels in face of increased renal absorption and transfer to fetus
Progesterone	Markedly increases	Production originates in corpus luteum over first 7–8 weeks; then placenta takes over
Estradiol	Markedly increases	
17-Hydroxyprogesterone	Increases	
Estriol	Increases	
Human placental lactogen (hPL)	Increases 5000-fold from 0.002 μU/mL to 10 mU/mL	
hCG	Increases to maximum values by 8–10 weeks	Peak 93 U/mL; term 14 U/mL
Relaxin	Peaks at 10 weeks	

(*Continued*)

Table 3.1 Summary of Physiologic Adaptations during Pregnancy (*Continued*)

Parameter	Expected change	Comments
Gastrointestinal system		
Appetite	Increases	
Gastric reflux	Increases	Cardiac sphincter laxity and anatomic displacement; treated during labor and delivery/anesthetic procedures with nonparticulate oral antacids
Gastric secretion	Decreased acidity; increased volume	"Full stomach" effect increases risk of aspiration
Gastric motility	Decreases	
Intestinal absorption	Increased	
Intestinal transit time	Delayed	
Large intestine	Greater absorption; slower transit time	
Gallbladder	Larger due to passive dilation	
Hematologic system		
Plasma volume	40%–60% *increase* from 12 to 36 weeks; 70%–100% increase in multiple gestations	Offsets blood loss at delivery
Total erythrocyte volume	Increases 15%–30%	Greater increase with iron supplementation
Hematocrit	Decreases 3%–5% by 36 weeks	Physiologic anemia due to greater proportionate increase plasma volume compared with erythrocyte volume; less change with iron supplementation
Hemoglobin	Decreases	
Mean corpuscular volume	Unchanged	Best indicator of iron status. Slight increase with iron supplementation
Erythrocyte sedimentation rate	Significantly increased	Provides little diagnostic value; combined with increase in white blood cell (WBC) can cause false suspicion for infection
WBC count	Increases 8% by term and may increase further postpartum	Predominantly due to increase in neutrophils
Serum iron	Decreases 35% by term	
Serum transferrin	Increases by 100% or more by second trimester	TIBC markedly increased
TIBC	Increases by 25%–100%	
Serum ferritin	Decreases markedly (even with iron supplementation)	Nadir 30% or less of normal values. Best test to assess iron-deficiency anemia in pregnancy
Erythropoietin	Increases fourfold	
α-Fetoprotein	Increases	Larger increase in neural tube defects, abdominal wall defects, and fetal death
Glutamic-oxaloacetic transaminase and glutamic-pyruvic transaminase	Unchanged	
Alkaline phosphatase	Increases	Heat stable fraction formed by placenta
Lipids	Increase	Triglycerides, cholesterol, phospholipids, and free fatty acids each increase progressively
Fibrinogen	Increases 2 g/L by term	Overall increased tendency toward thrombosis
Factors VII, VIII, IX, and X	Increase	
Factors XI and XIII	Decrease by about 30%	
Antithrombin III	Decreases	
Fibrin, FDP	Increase progressively	
Protein C	Unchanged	
Protein S	Decreases	Protein S–binding protein levels fluctuate in pregnancy, making screening more reliable in nonpregnant women

Source: Modified from Lind T, *Maternal Physiology: CREOG Basic Science Monograph in Obstetrics and Gynecology*, CREOG, Washington, DC, 1985.
Abbreviations: BP, blood pressure; CO, cardiac output; TH, thyroid hormone; DHEA, dehydroepiandrosterone; FDP, fibrin degradation products; TIBC, total iron binding capacity.

The detected 46%–51% increase in the cardiac output was attributed to a 15% increase in heart rate and a 24% increase in stroke volume [6]. **The changes in heart rate occur early in pregnancy, whereas those of stroke volume occur later, with the net effect of a progressively increasing cardiac output as gestation progresses.** Again, significant variation in cardiac output changes in the late third trimester was attributed to patient factors, precluding confident conclusions regarding the behavior of cardiac output at the very end of pregnancy. Maternal cardiac output was found to correlate with maternal body surface area and with fetal birth weight. Left ventricular mass and left ventricular mass index increased to maximal levels at term but remained well below the cutoff for a diagnosis of left ventricular hypertrophy. This increase corresponded to an increase in the mean blood pressure at term as well as to an increase in the left atrial size and a decrease in the left ventricular diastolic filling value. These changes may explain some of the variations in cardiac output in the third trimester and may be relevant to the

Table 3.2 Normal Reference Ranges in Pregnant Women

	Nonpregnant adult	First trimester	Second trimester	Third trimester
Hematology				
Erythropoietin (U/L)	4–27	12–25	8–67	14–222
Ferritin (ng/mL)	10–150	6–130	2–230	0–116
Folate, red blood cell (ng/mL)	150–450	137–589	94–828	109–663
Folate, serum (ng/mL)	5.4–18	2.6–15	0.8–24	1.4–20.7
Hemoglobin (g/dL)	12–15.8	11.6–13.9	9.7–14.8	9.5–15
Hematocrit (%)	35.4–44.4	31–41	30–39	28–40
Iron, total binding capacity (µg/dL)	251–406	278–403		359–609
Iron, serum (µg/dL)	41–141	72–143	44–178	30–193
Mean corpuscular hemoglobin (pg/cell)	27–32	30–32	30–33	29–32
Mean corpuscular volume (µm³)	79–93	81–96	82–97	81–99
Platelet (×10⁹/L)	165–415	174–391	155–409	146–429
Mean platelet volume (µm³)	6.4–11	7.7–10.3	7.8–10.2	8.2–7.4
Red blood cell count (×10⁶/mm³)	4–5.2	3.42–4.55	2.81–4.49	2.71–4.43
Red cell distribution width (%)	<14.5	12.5–14.1	13.4–13.6	12.7–15.3
White blood cell count (×10³/mm³)	3.5–9.1	5.7–13.6	5.6–14.8	5.9–16.9
Neutrophils (×10³/mm³)	1.4–4.6	3.6–10.1	3.8–12.3	3.9–13.1
Lymphocytes (×10³/mm³)	0.7–4.6	1.1–3.6	0.9–3.9	1–3.6
Monocytes (×10³/mm³)	0.1–0.7	0.1–1.1	0.1–1.1	0.1–1.4
Eosinophils (×10³/mm³)	0–0.6	0–0.6	0–0.6	0–0.6
Basophils (×10³/mm³)	0–0.2	0–0.1	0–0.1	0–0.1
Transferrin (mg/dL)	200–400	254–344	220–441	288–530
Transferrin, saturation without iron (%)	22–46		10–44	5–37
Transferrin, saturation with iron (%)	22–46		18–92	9–98
Coagulation				
Antithrombin III, functional (%)	70–130	89–114	88–112	82–116
D-dimer (µg/mL)	0.22–0.74	0.05–0.95	0.32–1.29	0.13–1.7
Factor V (%)	50–150	75–95	72–96	60–88
Factor VII (%)	50–150	100–146	95–153	149–211
Factor VIII (%)	50–150	90–210	97–312	143–353
Factor IX (%)	50–150	103–172	154–217	164–235
Factor XI (%)	50–150	80–127	82–144	65–123
Factor XII (%)	50–150	78–124	90–151	129–194
Fibrinogen (mg/dL)	233–496	244–510	291–538	373–619
Homocysteine (µmol/L)	4.4–10.8	3.34–11	2–26.9	3.2–21.4
International normalized ratio	0.9–1.04	0.89–1.05	0.85–0.97	0.80–0.94
Partial thromboplastin time, activated (seconds)	26.3–39.4	24.3–38.9	24.2–38.1	24.7–35
Prothrombin time (seconds)	12.7–15.4	9.7–13.5	9.5–13.4	9.6–12.9
Protein C, functional (%)	70–130	78–121	83–133	67–135
Protein S, total (%)	70–140	39–105	27–101	33–101
Protein S, free (%)	70–140	34–133	19–113	20–65
Protein S, functional activity (%)	65–140	57–95	42–68	16–42
Tissue plasminogen activator (ng/mL)	1.6–13	1.8–6	2.4–6.6	3.3–9.2
Tissue plasminogen activator inhibitor-1 (ng/mL)	4–43	16–33	36–55	67–92
von Willebrand factor (%)	75–125			121–260
Blood chemical constituents				
Alanine transaminase (U/L)	7–41	3–30	2–33	2–25
Albumin (g/dL)	4.1–5.3	3.1–5.1	2.6–4.5	2.3–4.2
Alkaline phosphatase (U/L)	33–96	17–88	25–126	38–229
α1-Antitrypsin (mg/dL)	100–200	225–323	273–391	327–487
Amylase (U/L)	20–96	24–83	16–73	15–81
Anion gap (mmol/L)	7–16	13–17	12–16	12–16
Aspartate transaminase (U/L)	12–38	3–23	3–33	4–32
Bicarbonate (mmol/L)	22–30	20–24	20–24	20–24
Bilirubin, total (mg/dL)	0.3–1.3	0.1–0.4	0.1–0.8	0.1–1.1
Bilirubin, unconjugated (mg/dL)	0.2–0.9	0.1–0.5	0.1–0.4	0.1–0.5
Bilirubin, conjugated (mg/dL)	0.1–0.4	0–0.1	0–0.1	0–0.1
Bile acids, (µmol/L)	0.3–4.8	0–4.9	0–9.1	0–11.3
Calcium, ionized (mg/dL)	4.5–5.3	4.5–5.1	4.4–5	4.4–5.3
Calcium, total (mg/dL)	8.7–10.2	8.8–10.6	8.2–9	8.2–9.7
Ceruloplasmin (mg/dL)	25–63	30–49	40–53	43–78
Chloride (mEq/L)	102–109	101–105	97–109	97–109
Creatinine (mg/dL)	0.5–0.9	0.4–0.7	0.4–0.8	0.4–0.9
γ-Glutamyl transpeptidase (U/L)	9–58	2–23	4–22	3–26
Lactate dehydrogenase (U/L)	115–221	78–433	80–447	82–524
Lipase (U/L)	3–43	21–76	26–100	41–112

(Continued)

Table 3.2 Normal Reference Ranges in Pregnant Women (*Continued*)

	Nonpregnant adult	First trimester	Second trimester	Third trimester
Magnesium (mg/dL)	1.5–2.3	1.6–2.2	1.5–2.2	1.1–2.2
Osmolality (mOsm/kg H_2O)	275–295	275–280	276–289	278–280
Phosphate (mg/dL)	2.5–4.3	3.1–4.6	2.5–4.6	2.8–4.6
Potassium (mEq/L)	3.5–5	3.6–5	3.3–5	3.3–5.1
Prealbumin (mg/dL)	17–34	15–27	20–27	14–23
Protein, total (g/dL)	6.7–8.6	6.2–7.6	5.7–6.9	5.6–6.7
Sodium (mEq/L)	136–146	133–148	129–148	130–148
Urea nitrogen (mg/dL)	7–20	7–12	3–13	3–11
Uric acid (mg/dL)	2.5–5.6	2–4.2	2.4–4.9	3.1–6.3
Metabolic and endocrine tests				
Aldosterone (ng/dL)	2–9	6–104	9–104	15–101
Angiotensin-converting enzyme (U/L)	9–67	1–38	1–36	1–39
Cortisol (µg/dL)	0–25	7–19	10–42	12–50
Hemoglobin A1c (%)	4–6	4–6	4–6	4–7
Parathyroid hormone (pg/mL)	8–51	10–15	18–25	9–26
Parathyroid hormone-related protein (pmol/L)	<1.3	0.7–0.9	1.8–2.2	2.5–2.8
Renin, plasma activity (ng/mL/hour)	0.3–9		7.5–54	5.9–58.8
TSH (µIU/mL)	0.34–4.25	0.6–3.4	0.37–3.6	0.38–4.04
Thyroxine-binding globulin (mg/dL)	1.3–3	1.8–3.2	2.8–4	2.6–4.2
Thyroxine, free (ng/dL)	0.8–1.7	0.8–1.2	0.6–1	0.5–0.8
Thyroxine, total (µg/dL)	5.4–11.7	6.5–10.1	7.5–10.3	6.3–9.7
Triiodothyronine, free (pg/mL)	2.4–4.2	4.1–4.4	4–4.2	
Triiodothyronine, total (ng/dL)	77–135	97–149	117–169	123–162
Vitamins and minerals				
Copper (µg/dL)	70–140	112–199	165–221	130–240
Selenium (µg/L)	63–160	116–146	75–145	71–133
Vitamin A (retinol) (µg/dL)	20–100	32–47	35–44	29–42
Vitamin B12 (pg/mL)	279–966	118–438	130–656	99–526
Vitamin C (ascorbic acid) (mg/dL)	0.4–1			0.9–1.3
Vitamin D, 1,25-dihydroxy (pg/mL)	25–45	20–65	72–160	60–119
Vitamin D, 24,25-dihydroxy (ng/mL)	0.5–5	1.2–1.8	1.1–1.5	0.7–0.9
Vitamin D, 25-hydroxy (ng/mL)	14–80	18–27	10–22	10–18
Vitamin E (α-tocopherol) (mg/mL)	5–18	7–13	10–16	13–23
Zinc (µg/dL)	75–120	57–88	51–80	50–77
Autoimmune and inflammatory mediators				
C3 complement (mg/dL)	83–177	62–98	73–103	77–111
C4 complement (mg/dL)	16–47	18–36	18–34	22–32
C-reactive protein (mg/L)	0.2–3		0.4–20.3	0.4–8.1
Erythrocyte sedimentation rate (mm/hour)	0–20	4–57	7–47	13–70
Immunoglobulin A (mg/dL)	70–350	95–243	99–237	112–250
Immunoglobulin G (mg/dL)	700–1700	981–1267	813–1131	678–990
Immunoglobulin M (mg/dL)	50–300	78–232	74–218	85–269
Sex hormones				
Dehydroepiandrosterone sulfate (µmol/L)	1.3–6.8	2–16.5	0.9–7.8	0.8–6.5
Estradiol (pg/mL)	<20–443	188–2497	1278–7192	6137–3460
Progesterone (ng/mL)	<1–20	8–48		99–342
Prolactin (ng/mL)	0–20	36–213	110–330	137–372
Sex hormone-binding globulin (nmol/L)	18–114	39–131	214–717	216–724
Testosterone (ng/dL)	6–86	26–211	34–243	63–309
17-Hydroxyprogesterone (nmol/L)	0.6–10.6	5.2–28.5	5.2–28.5	15.5–84
Lipids				
Cholesterol, total (mg/dL)	<200	141–210	176–299	219–349
High-density lipoprotein cholesterol (mg/dL)	40–60	40–78	52–87	48–87
Low-density lipoprotein cholesterol (mg/dL)	<100	60–153	77–184	101–224
Very-low-density lipoprotein cholesterol (mg/dL)	6–40	10–18	13–23	21–36
Triglycerides (mg/dL)	<150	40–159	75–382	131–453
Apolipoprotein A-I (mg/dL)	119–240	111–150	142–253	145–262
Apolipoprotein B (mg/dL)	52–163	58–81	66–188	85–238
Cardiac				
Atrial natriuretic peptide (pg/mL)			28.1–70.1	
B-type natriuretic peptide (pg/mL)	<167		13.5–29.5	
Creatine kinase (U/L)	39–238	27–83	25–75	13–101
Creatine kinase-MB (U/L)	<6			1.8–2.4
Troponin I (ng/mL)	0–0.8			0–0.064 (intrapartum)

(*Continued*)

Table 3.2 Normal Reference Ranges in Pregnant Women (*Continued*)

	Nonpregnant adult	First trimester	Second trimester	Third trimester
Blood gas				
pH	7.38–7.42 (arterial)	7.36–7.52 (venous)	7.4–7.52 (venous)	7.41–7.53 (venous) 7.39–7.45 (arterial)
PO_2 (mmHg)	90–100	93–100	90–98	92–107
PCO_2 (mmHg)	38–42			25–33
Bicarbonate (HCO_3^-) (mEq/L)	22–26			16–22
Renal function tests				
Effective RPF (mL/min)	492–696	696–985	612–1170	595–945
GFR (mL/min)	106–132	131–166	135–170	117–182
Filtration fraction (%)	16.9–24.7	14.7–21.6	14.3–21.9	17.1–25.1
Osmolarity, urine (mOsm/kg)	500–800	326–975	278–1066	238–1034
24-hour albumin excretion (mg/24 hours)	<30	5–15	4–18	3–22
24-hour calcium excretion (mmol/24 hours)	<7.5	1.6–5.2	0.3–6.9	0.8–4.2
24-hour creatinine clearance (mL/min)	91–130	69–140	55–136	50–166
24-hour creatinine excretion (mmol/24 hours)	8.8–14	10.6–11.6	10.3–11.5	10.2–11.4
24-hour potassium excretion (mmol/24 hours)	25–100	17–33	10–38	11–35
24-hour protein excretion (mg/24 hours)	<150	19–141	47–186	46–185
24-hour sodium excretion (mmol/24 hours)	100–260	53–215	34–213	37–149

Source: Adapted from Abbassi-Ghanavati M et al., *Obstet Gynecol*, 114(6), 1326–1331, 2009.

vulnerability of pregnant women to pulmonary edema during hypertensive crisis [6].

Perhaps the most common hemodynamic complaint that must be evaluated during pregnancy is that of **syncope or near-syncope,** which provides a useful example of how an understanding of pregnancy physiology is useful in clinical evaluation. Syncope is defined as a transient loss of consciousness and posture, caused by decreased cerebral perfusion that may result from hypotension, changes in heart rate, or changes in blood volume or redistribution. The decreased SVR of pregnancy makes pregnant women particularly susceptible to this condition, with 28% of gravidas experiencing at least one episode of presyncope, 10% experiencing recurrent presyncopal episodes, and 5% experiencing outright syncope [7]. The overwhelming majority of syncopal episodes are benign neurocardiogenic syncope but there are also several potentially dangerous conditions in the differential diagnosis of syncope. An understanding of the vasovagal reflex at the root of most syncopal episodes helps the clinician to manage benign syncopal episodes while being alert for signs and symptoms that may point to a more serious underlying condition. The most common trigger of syncope is venous pooling that results in a drop in venous return and a subsequent drop in cardiac output. This results in stimulation of arterial baroreceptors which trigger catecholamine stimulation of atria and ventricles. The resultant vigorous cardiac contraction in volume-depleted chambers stimulates cardiac mechanoreceptors or C-fibers which, in susceptible individuals, can result in paradoxical stimulation of the dorsal vagal nucleus. This stimulation is paradoxical because, in the face of low SVR and cardiac output, there is a further decrease in sympathetic tone and an increase in vagal tone causing vasodilation and bradycardia and the clinical presentation of presyncope or syncope [7]. The reflex may be initiated by emotional stimuli in some individuals or may be initiated by compression of the inferior vena cava by the gravid uterus causing a decrease in venous return and intracardiac pressure. Less common conditions that may present with symptoms of syncope include cerebrovascular accidents, seizures, cardiac arrhythmias or valvular disease, cardiomyopathy, pericardial tamponade, myocardial infarction, congenital heart defects, thromboembolic phenomenon, anemia, hypoglycemia, or electrolyte disorders [7]. Further evaluation for such conditions should be prompted when an apparent syncopal episode is accompanied by focal neurologic findings, prolonged loss of consciousness or postictal confusion, carotid or subclavian bruits, a pathologic cardiac murmur, or electrocardiogram (EKG) or laboratory abnormalities [7].

The above events that are precipitated by a decrease in venous return can also explain the occurrence of **supine hypotension** in pregnancy. The commonly recommended "leftward tilt" position is intended to displace the uterus off of the inferior vena cava, which runs to the right of midline. This position should be used to avoid supine hypotension when recumbent as well as when performing surgery on the parturient in the second half of pregnancy. A more extreme application of this physiology comes in the performance of perimortem cesarean section during maternal cardiac arrest. The procedure is purported to allow fetal survival and also the evacuation of the uterus, which may allow an increase in venous return and cardiac output that may increase the chance of maternal survival [8]. In order to optimize maternal and fetal survival, it is recommended that the procedure should be performed within 4 minutes of cardiac arrest due to the inadequacy of chest compressions in producing adequate cardiac output during pregnancy and the susceptibility of both mother and fetus to anoxic brain injury [8] (see also Chapters 1 and 2 in *Maternal-Fetal Evidence Based Guidelines*).

RESPIRATORY

During pregnancy the respiratory system undergoes alterations that are reflected in pulmonary function tests and in acid–base balance. These are important in the evaluation of dyspnea in pregnancy, the management of pregnancy with coexisting pulmonary diseases such as asthma, and the recognition of acute pulmonary complications of pregnancy.

Pregnancy is associated with a significant increase in ventilatory drive both at rest and during exercise [9]. **Minute ventilation increases** mostly due to an **increase in tidal volume** with little or no increase in respiratory rate [3,9,10]. Alveolar ventilation increases, along with an **increase in arterial partial pressure of oxygen (PaO_2) and alveolar partial** pressure of oxygen (PAO_2), and a decrease in arterial partial pressure of carbon dioxide ($PaCO_2$), with a compensatory decrease in serum bicarbonate with an overall mild increase in pH, reflecting a state of compensated respiratory alkalosis [9]. These changes occur early in pregnancy and are almost fully established by 7–8 weeks' gestation [9]. This may be due to stimulation of the ventilatory drive by progesterone and/or estrogen. Ventilatory equivalents for CO_2 and O_2 are increased both at rest and during exercise throughout pregnancy. The underlying mechanism for the increased ventilatory drive during pregnancy is not fully understood, but theories have included an increased sensitivity to chemoreflexive drives to breathe (due to hypercapnia or hypoxia) versus a hormone-mediated increase in the neural drive to breathe [9].

Uterine enlargement and abdominal distension result in a 4- to 5-cm cephalad displacement of the diaphragm and a 5- to 7-cm increase in thoracic circumference. This results in a **decrease in expiratory reserve volume, residual volume, and functional residual capacity.** There is a compensatory increase in inspiratory capacity, while total lung capacity and vital capacity do not change [9]. Chest wall compliance is increased but inspiratory muscle strength is preserved with an overall increase in the oxygen cost of breathing [9]. However, it is important to recognize that there is **no significant change in the parameters of forced vital capacity, peak expiratory flow rate (PEFR), or forced expiratory volume in 1 second (FEV_1) during pregnancy.**

Physiologic **dyspnea** of pregnancy, experienced by 60%–70% of healthy pregnant women, must be clinically distinguished from more serious respiratory conditions. Physiologic dyspnea tends to be an isolated symptom that begins in early pregnancy, plateaus, or improves as pregnancy progresses, and does not interfere with daily activities [11]. The mechanism for physiologic dyspnea has not been conclusively defined, but pregnant women with dyspnea have been demonstrated to have an increase in minute ventilation and tidal volume and a decrease in end-tidal CO_2 pressure compared with pregnant women who do not report dyspnea [11]. The perception of physiologic dyspnea during pregnancy has been associated with increased sensitivity to hypoxia and hypercapnia, suggesting an increased chemosensitivity causing an increased central inspiratory drive in pregnant women who experience dyspnea. However, the chemical stimuli of hypoxia and hypercapnia are both reduced in pregnancy, causing others to suggest a neural mechanism [9]. Despite the common symptom of physiologic dyspnea, **pregnancy has not been found to be associated with a decrease in aerobic work capacity or with an increased perception of breathlessness during exercise** [9].

While measurement of FEV_1 requires a spirometer, measurement of PEFR correlates well with FEV_1 and can be measured with a relatively inexpensive spirometer (peak flow meter), which patients can be taught to use at home. Again, these parameters do not change due to pregnancy, so any detected worsening should be treated appropriately and not attributed to pregnancy or to physiologic dyspnea. In the evaluation of severe acute asthma exacerbations with the potential for impending respiratory arrest, knowledge of physiologic changes of pregnancy is particularly important in the interpretation of blood gases (Table 3.1). The normal parturient lives in a state of compensated respiratory alkalosis with a lower partial pressure of carbon dioxide (PCO_2) compared with that of nonpregnant patients. Thus, significant CO_2 retention may be present despite values that are high normal for nonpregnant patients.

While physiologic dyspnea and asthma exacerbation are two of the most common causes of dyspnea in pregnancy, the obstetrician must also be alert to other pulmonary complications to which the parturient is susceptible such as pulmonary embolism and pulmonary edema. Pulmonary edema may occur as a result of preeclampsia, peripartum cardiomyopathy, or the use of certain tocolytics. It is important that the prevalence of pulmonary symptoms in pregnancy should not be met with complacency by the obstetrician, for it may signify a life-threatening condition for the pregnant woman.

ENDOCRINE

Pregnancy-related endocrine alterations include the production of hormones that are specific to pregnancy, an increase in other reproductive hormones, and alterations in the level and function of nonreproductive hormones, especially of thyroid hormones. There is a significant contribution of steroid hormone secretion by the fetal-placental unit. This section provides a brief description of the changes in reproductive hormones during gestation followed by a more in-depth review of the behavior and clinical application of thyroid hormones during pregnancy.

Pregnancy-specific hormones include human chorionic gonadotropin (hCG) and relaxin. **Relaxin** is detectable in maternal serum by the time of missed menses and peaks at 10 weeks' gestation then declines over the course of the second and third trimesters [12]. Relaxin is secreted by the corpora lutea of pregnancy and thought to have an important role in early pregnancy maintenance that has not yet been clearly elucidated [13]. **hCG** also peaks at approximately 10 weeks' gestation. The reproductive hormones **estradiol, progesterone, testosterone, prolactin, and 17-hydroxyprogesterone,** all increase significantly during gestation. Initially the corpus luteum and maternal ovarian tissue make the greatest contribution to steroid hormone concentrations, but as of 9 weeks' gestation aromatization of dehydroepiandrosterone sulfate by the placenta becomes the predominant source of maternal steroids [14]. The elevated estradiol levels stimulate increased hepatic production of sex hormone–binding globulin and thyroxin-binding globulin. Estrogen also induces hypertrophy and hyperplasia of pituitary lactotrophs with a resultant increase in prolactin levels corresponding to the increase in estradiol levels throughout gestation [14]. Meanwhile, there is a reflexive decrease in follicle-stimulating hormone and luteinizing hormone to almost undetectable levels, as would be expected.

One longitudinal study assayed reproductive hormone levels in the blood of 60 healthy women drawn during the first, second, and third trimesters of uncomplicated pregnancies [14]. Mean progesterone levels increased steadily from 49 nmol/L at 5 weeks' gestation to 584 nmol/L at term. Mean 17-hydroxyprogesterone levels are more stable during the first and second trimesters at 12.2 nmol/L but then increase threefold to 36 nmol/L by term. Mean testosterone increased from 3.3 nmol/L at 5 weeks to 5.7 nmol/L at 40 weeks. Mean serum estradiol levels increased during the first trimester from 1.64 nmol/L at 5 weeks to 11.13 nmol/L at 16 weeks and then increased fivefold to 53.44 nmol/L at 40 weeks. Mean sex hormone-binding globulin levels increase rapidly during the first half of gestation from 71 nmol/L at 5 weeks to 392 nmol/L at 25 weeks, and then remain relatively constant until 40 weeks. Mean levels of dehydroepiandrosterone sulfate decreased from 5.8 mmol/L at 5 weeks to 2.7 mmol/L at midgestation, which remained constant until term. Mean prolactin concentration rose from 294 milli-international units (mIU) to 1106 mIU at 16 weeks. Prolactin levels then continued to increase to a mean of 4092 mIU at 35 weeks and to 4293 mIU at 40 weeks. Mean androstenedione levels increase gradually from 8.1 nmol/L at 5 weeks to 10.6 nmol/L at 40 weeks [14].

Other hormonal alterations include an increase in aldosterone, cortisol, parathyroid hormone, parathyroid-related hormone, and renin [2]. Deoxycorticosterone increases. Androstenedione increases with an increase in the transformation to estrone and estradiol [1]. Fasting levels of both insulin and glucagon increase [1]. There is an increase in melanocyte-stimulating hormone to which can be attributed the pregnancy-related increases in pigmentation seen in the areola, the linea nigra, and in chloasma [1].

The function of the **thyroid gland** is crucial to a healthy gestation (see also Chapters 6 and 7 in *Maternal-Fetal Evidence Based Guidelines*). The interplay between maternal and fetal thyroid function can cause confusion for the obstetrician. Early fetal development is dependent on maternal thyroid function, and both hypothyroidism and hyperthyroidism can have important maternal and fetal effects and risks of thyroid dysfunction extend well into the postpartum period. The effects of subclinical thyroid disease are more controversial. Symptoms of hyperthyroidism and hypothyroidism can mimic symptoms of normal pregnancy. For example, symptoms such as fatigue, muscle cramps, palpitations, thyromegaly, and constipation can be common in normal pregnancy, but progressive symptoms of insomnia, intellectual slowness, or weight loss should be evaluated [15].

Thyroid-binding globulin increases due to stimulation of synthesis by estrogen as well as decreased hepatic clearance. **Total thyroxine (TT_4) and total triiodothyronine (TT_3) both increase while resin triiodothyronine uptake (RT_3U) decreases.** Structural similarities between hCG and thyroid-stimulating hormone (TSH) may result in an hCG-mediated increase in free thyroxine (FT_4) and the free thyroxine index as well as a decrease in TSH in the first trimester. However, these changes, sometimes referred to as gestational transient thyrotoxicosis, are typically self-limited and do not tend to result in values that are outside the normal range for nonpregnant individuals [16] (see also Chapters 6 and 7 in *Maternal-Fetal Evidence Based Guidelines*).

Iodine requirements during pregnancy increase by greater than 50% due to increased maternal thyroxine production to maintain maternal and fetal euthyroidism and increased renal iodine clearance [17]. Plasma iodine levels decrease. This is associated with an increase in the size of the maternal thyroid gland. Longitudinal studies of thyroid ultrasonography in pregnancy show a mean increase in the thyroid size of 18%, which is noticeable in most women but not associated with abnormalities in thyroid function tests [16]. Iodine supplementation results in a less substantial increase in the thyroid gland size [17]. While ultrasound or laboratory evaluation is not necessary in the pregnant patient with a mild diffuse increase in the thyroid size, a significant goiter or thyroid nodule must be evaluated as in any patient. A woman who is marginally iodine deficient may be able to compensate with increased thyrotropin stimulation of the thyroid to achieve euthyroidism, but become hypothyroid when faced with the increasing iodine requirements of pregnancy [17].

Thyroid homeostasis is important for healthy fetal development. The fetal thyroid begins to concentrate iodide at 10–12 weeks. Thyroid hormone necessary for fetal brain development before this time is provided by the maternal system [15,18]. Thyroid hormone synthesis in the fetus is controlled by the fetal pituitary gland by 20 weeks. **Small amounts of T_4 and T_3 pass the placenta but TSH does not cross the placenta. Thyroid-releasing hormone (TRH) and iodide do cross the placenta** [16]. Maternal hypothyroidism has been associated with abnormal intelligence quotient testing and pediatric neurodevelopment in offspring, particularly when untreated [18]. While severe maternal iodine deficiency can lead to cretinism in the offspring, it is less clear whether mild-to-moderate iodine deficiency leads to more subtle cognitive or neurologic dysfunction. Iodine supplementation in iodine-deficient populations has been found to substantially reduce the relative risk of cretinism and to improve psychomotor and cognitive test scores in the offspring [17].

Hyperemesis gravidarum is associated with elevated levels of hCG, an increase in FT4, and a decrease in TSH (biochemical hyperthyroidism). However, this is largely transitory and rarely associated with clinical hyperthyroidism. Thus, routine measuring of thyroid function in hyperemesis is not indicated in the absence of other signs of hyperthyroidism such as weight loss or persistent tachycardia [16]. Furthermore, treatment of transient hyperthyroidism associated with elevated hCG and hyperemesis should not be undertaken in the absence of evidence of intrinsic thyroid disease [19] (see also Chapter 9 in *Maternal-Fetal Evidence Based Guidelines*). A large prospective observational study of 25,765 pregnant women who underwent thyroid screening in pregnancy showed no difference in pregnancy complications or in perinatal morbidity and mortality in women with subclinical hyperthyroidism [20].

HEMATOLOGIC

Pregnancy is characterized by both quantitative and qualitative changes in the hematologic system. These changes can be adaptive to normal pregnancy but can also put the pregnant women at increased risk for certain pathologic conditions. Anemia and thrombocytopenia are commonly diagnosed during pregnancy, as will be discussed below. Measurements of the acute phase response such as erythrocyte sedimentation rate, C-reactive protein, and white blood cell count have been found to increase during pregnancy. This presents a challenge in the evaluation of pregnant women suspected to have various infectious or inflammatory conditions, but careful clinical assessment allows the practitioner to distinguish between physiologic and pathologic abnormalities in these tests. Pregnancy also has important effects on the coagulation system, with the creation of an overall **hypercoagulable state.** This section also reviews the theories and limitations of the evidence surrounding the diagnosis of thrombophilia during pregnancy.

Anemia is usually defined as a hemoglobin less than 11 g/dL and hematocrit less than 33% in the first trimester, hemoglobin less than 10.5 g/dL and hematocrit less than 32% in the second trimester, and hemoglobin less than 11 g/dL and hematocrit less than 33% in the third trimester [21] (see also Chapter 14 in *Maternal-Fetal Evidence Based Guidelines*). Anemia may be caused by decreased production of red blood cells, by increased destruction of red blood cells, or by blood loss. Anemia in pregnancy is complicated by increased iron requirements and an expanded blood volume. Blood volume increases by about 50% while red blood cell mass increases by about 25%, resulting in an anemia of dilution, as measured by hemoglobin and hematocrit, that is physiologic in pregnancy. **Iron requirements increase** in order to support the increase in red blood cell mass, support the requirements of the fetus and placenta, and prepare for blood loss during delivery. **Iron-deficiency anemia** is characterized by microcytosis and hypochromatosis. Iron studies reveal a decrease in total iron and ferritin and an increase in total iron-binding capacity (TIBC). **Ferritin levels** have the highest sensitivity and specificity for iron deficiency, with levels less than 10–15 µg/dL being diagnostic of iron deficiency [21]. Iron supplementation as well as screening for iron deficiency during pregnancy is recommended by the Centers for Disease Control and Prevention (CDC). The typical diet contains 15 mg of elemental iron per day, while the recommended dietary daily allowance during pregnancy is 27 mg/day [21]. Iron-deficiency anemia in pregnancy has been associated with an increased risk of low birth weight, prematurity, perinatal mortality, postpartum depression, and poor mental and psychomotor testing in offspring. Severe anemia (less than 6 g/dL) has been associated with abnormal fetal oxygenation, abnormal fetal heart rate patterns, reduced amniotic fluid volumes, cerebral vasodilation, and fetal death. Transfusion may be indicated for fetal indications in the case of anemia of this severity [21]. Iron supplementation has been found to decrease the incidence of anemia at delivery, although its effect on healthy, non-iron-deficient women is not clear. Factors that increase the risk for iron deficiency in pregnancy include young maternal age, heavy menses, short interpregnancy interval, low socioeconomic status, and non-Hispanic black race [21]. Dietary factors can have a significant effect on iron levels, not only due to levels of consumption of iron-rich foods but also due to consumption of foods that significantly enhance or inhibit iron absorption.

Megaloblastic macrocytic anemia may be caused by deficiency of folic acid and vitamin B12 and by pernicious anemia. Nonmegaloblastic macrocytic anemia may be caused by alcoholism, hypothyroidism, liver disease, aplastic anemia, or increased reticulocyte count. The most common cause of onset of macrocytic anemia during pregnancy in the United States is folic acid deficiency [21]. During pregnancy, daily folic acid requirements increase from 50 to 400 µg [21]. Women who have had gastric surgery and those with Crohn's disease may be at risk of vitamin B12 deficiency in pregnancy [21].

The performance of complete blood counts as a part of routine prenatal screening results in a frequent diagnosis of **thrombocytopenia** in asymptomatic pregnant women. The mean platelet count in pregnant women is lower than in nonpregnant women, with about 8% of pregnant women meeting criteria for the diagnosis of thrombocytopenia [22]. Manifestations of thrombocytopenia include epistaxis, petechiae, and ecchymosis, although frequently there are no clinically significant effects. Clinically significant spontaneous bleeding is rare as long as platelet counts are greater than 10,000/µL and even excessive bleeding associated with trauma or surgery is unlikely with platelet counts greater than 50,000/µL [22]. **The most common cause of thrombocytopenia in pregnancy is gestational thrombocytopenia**, which is an apparently benign condition whose underlying physiology is not well understood. However, thrombocytopenia in pregnancy may also be caused by more severe underlying conditions such as preeclampsia, human immunodeficiency virus infection, immune thrombocytopenic purpura (ITP), systemic lupus erythematosus, antiphospholipid antibody syndrome, hypersplenism, disseminated intravascular coagulation, thrombotic thrombocytopenic purpura, hemolytic uremic syndrome, congenital thrombocytopenia, or medication effect [22]. Most of these conditions can be ruled out by history, physical exam, and exclusion of underlying diagnoses.

The most difficult differential usually comes down to gestational thrombocytopenia versus **ITP**. These conditions cannot be reliably differentiated with antiplatelet antibody testing or any other diagnostic test. Differentiation can be obtained by documenting platelet counts less than 70,000/µL, which suggests ITP, or by documenting a return to normal platelet counts after delivery, suggestive of gestational thrombocytopenia [22]. To be classified as gestational thrombocytopenia, there are several conditions that must be satisfied. Gestational thrombocytopenia is mild, with platelet counts greater than 70,000/µL. There is no history of significant bleeding and no history of thrombocytopenia prior to pregnancy. Platelet counts generally return to normal within 2–12 weeks following delivery, and there is an extremely low risk of fetal or neonatal thrombocytopenia. Many women with ITP have a history of abnormal bleeding prior to pregnancy, although this is not universal. Findings suggestive of ITP include persistent platelet counts less than 100,000/µL, normal or increased megakaryocytes in the bone marrow, absence of splenomegaly, and exclusion of other systemic disorders known to be associated with thrombocytopenia [22].

Women with gestational thrombocytopenia are not at risk for maternal or fetal hemorrhage or bleeding complications [22]. Immunologic thrombocytopenia such as ITP and neonatal alloimmune thrombocytopenia (NAIT) have the potential for fetal complications. Both are characterized by increased platelet destruction. Twelve to fifteen percent of neonates born to mothers with ITP may develop platelet counts less than 50,000/µL. This may result in findings such as purpura, ecchymosis, or melena. Less commonly, fetal intracranial hemorrhage may develop, unrelated to mode of delivery. The incidence of serious bleeding complications in neonates of women with ITP is estimated at 3% and the rate of intracranial hemorrhage at 1% [22].

Onset of thrombocytopenia during the third trimester should prompt consideration of gestational hypertensive disorders, which are associated with about 20% of maternal thrombocytopenia, and decreasing platelet count is considered a sign of worsening of disorders of this spectrum (see also Chapter 1 in *Maternal-Fetal Evidence Based Guidelines*). When combined with hemolytic anemia and elevated liver tests, thrombocytopenia is indicative of the diagnosis of hemolysis, elevated liver enzymes, and low platelet count (HELLP) syndrome. These disorders are associated with an increase in platelet destruction but the underlying physiology is not known. Platelet function may be reduced even if platelet counts are normal, and thrombocytopenia may occur prior to other manifestations of gestational hypertension. Hemorrhage is uncommon in the absence of disseminated intravascular coagulation. Neonatal thrombocytopenia following gestational hypertension is increased in premature infants but not in term infants [22].

Pregnancy is associated with significant alterations in the **coagulation system. There is a decrease in protein S levels as well as in coagulation factors XI and XIII. There is an increase in coagulation factors I, VII, VIII, IX, and X. D-dimer and fibrinogen levels** also increase. The overall result is the creation of a **hypercoagulable state** that is exacerbated by venous stasis and compression of the inferior vena cava and pelvic veins by the enlarging uterus [3,23]. This places the pregnant women at increased risk for such phenomena as deep venous thrombosis and pulmonary embolism, which are further elevated when pregnancy is associated with other high-risk states such as obesity, prolonged immobility (bed rest), or surgery (see also Chapter 28 in *Maternal-Fetal Evidence Based Guidelines*). Consideration of these risks is important in the evaluation of the pregnant patient with unilateral lower extremity edema or acute dyspnea. They also warrant caution and the responsibility to practice evidence-based medicine rather than erroneously recommending "bed rest" for treatment of conditions ranging from threatened abortion to preterm contractions to gestational hypertension.

GASTROINTESTINAL

Changes in gastrointestinal physiology lead to some of the most commonly described discomforts of pregnancy ranging from nausea and vomiting in early pregnancy to more persistent symptoms of gastroesophageal reflux and constipation. However, gastrointestinal symptoms may reflect coexisting diseases or may even herald life-threatening complications of pregnancy such as severe preeclampsia and HELLP syndrome or acute fatty liver of pregnancy (AFLP). Once again, it becomes crucial for the obstetric care provider to be skilled in recognizing signs and symptoms that result from normal pregnancy physiology and distinguishing those of more serious conditions.

There are several recognizable effects of pregnancy on gastrointestinal function. Gastric secretion acidity declines but volume increases and relaxation of the cardiac sphincter leads to greater esophageal reflux [1]. Combined with a **decrease in gastric and intestinal motility**, this leads to the "full stomach" effect that puts pregnant women at increased risk of aspiration. This, combined with increased airway edema, increases the risks of general endotracheal anesthesia during pregnancy. Thus, for anesthesia purposes, all pregnant women are considered to have a full stomach. Precautions to reduce aspiration risk include the use of nonparticulate oral antacids prior to induction of anesthesia, the use of rapid sequence induction methods, and the use of a cuffed endotracheal tube [1].

During pregnancy there is a decrease in colonic motility and an increase in water absorption, leading to **constipation** as a common complaint among pregnant women. A prospective study of constipation in pregnancy found that one in two women reports constipation at some point in pregnancy, with rates of 24%, 26%, 16%, and 24% in first, second, third trimesters, and postpartum, respectively. Constipation is more likely in women with a prior history of constipation and in women taking iron supplements. The study did not include nonpregnant controls, but historic controls indicate a constipation rate of 7% in a similar age group [24].

The most common gastrointestinal symptom of pregnancy is **nausea and vomiting** (see also Chapter 9 in *Maternal-Fetal Evidence Based Guidelines*). As many as 80% of women report nausea during pregnancy and it is also the most common reason for hospitalization in the first trimester [19,25]. Nausea is generally considered a normal symptom of early pregnancy, and morning sickness has been associated with improved pregnancy outcomes such as reduced risk of miscarriage, preterm birth, low birth weight, and perinatal death. This is theorized to be due to a placental etiology for nausea and vomiting, which is increased by early development of a healthy and robust placenta [19]. However, the exact etiology of this symptomatology is not known. It has been hypothesized that nausea and restricted intake in the mother create an environment that is favorable for early placental development [26] or that it confers an evolutionary advantage by causing the mother to avoid the ingestion of foods that may be dangerous to the developing fetus [19]. Numerous psychological theories have also been proposed to explain the phenomenon of nausea and vomiting in pregnancy. Nausea in pregnancy is commonly attributed to hCG levels, but conclusive evidence of the underlying physiology is lacking. Experience of nausea is also correlated with elevated estradiol levels and inversely correlated with prolactin levels [25]. Estrogens in oral contraceptive pills have shown a dose-related effect of nausea and vomiting. Smoking decreases both hCG and estrogen, and a reduced rate of nausea and vomiting of pregnancy has been demonstrated in smokers [19]. Increased placental mass, as found in multiple gestations and gestational trophoblastic disease, has been found to increase the risk of nausea and vomiting and of hyperemesis gravidarum.

It is important for nausea and vomiting of pregnancy to be distinguished from that resulting from other pathologic conditions. Complacency in the evaluation of pregnant patients with nausea and vomiting may result in undertreatment of distressing symptoms, development of hyperemesis gravidarum, or failure to diagnose a coexisting underlying disease. Nausea and vomiting of pregnancy typically start before 9 weeks' gestation and are not accompanied by fever, abdominal pain, or headache [19]. Deviation from this presentation should prompt evaluation for other etiologies. The differential diagnosis includes gastrointestinal disorders such as gastroenteritis, gastroparesis, achalasia, biliary tract disease, hepatitis, intestinal obstruction, peptic ulcer disease, pancreatitis, and appendicitis. Genitourinary conditions that may cause nausea and vomiting include pyelonephritis, uremia, ovarian torsion, kidney stones, and degenerating myoma. Nausea and vomiting may also be due to metabolic disorders such as diabetic ketoacidosis, porphyria, Addison's disease, and hyperthyroidism or neurologic disorders such as pseudotumor cerebri, vestibular lesions, migraines, or central nervous system tumors. Finally, drug-related toxicity, psychologic factors, or pregnancy-related complications such as preeclampsia and AFLP may present with nausea and vomiting [19].

Patients who are taking a multivitamin at the time of conception have reduced rates of nausea and vomiting [21]. There is good evidence to support the use of vitamin B6 alone or combined with doxylamine for the treatment of nausea and vomiting in pregnancy. Ginger supplements have also been shown to reduce severity of nausea and vomiting [19,27]. Numerous antiemetics have also shown acceptable safety and efficacy against nausea and vomiting. Hospitalization, intravenous fluids, and enteral nutrition may be used in rare cases of continued weight loss in spite of these therapies (see also Chapter 9 in *Maternal-Fetal Evidence Based Guidelines*).

RENAL SYSTEM AND HOMEOSTASIS

Pregnancy-related changes in the urinary tract include dilation of calyces, pelvis, and ureters. Ureteral dilatation may be noted as early as the first trimester and is present in 90% of gravidas by term. Obstructive and humoral mechanisms have been proposed for this dilatation, with obstruction by the gravid uterus and ovarian venous plexus likely causing the dilatation above the pelvic brim [28]. Dextrorotation of the gravid uterus, likely due to the sigmoid colon on the left and posterior to the uterus, causes the mechanical obstruction at the pelvic brim on the right more than the left. One important adverse consequence of this ureterocalyceal dilatation is the increased incidence of pyelonephritis among gravidas with asymptomatic bacteriuria.

There are significant increases in renal blood flow and in glomerular filtration rate (GFR) in pregnancy [1]. Indeed, GFR increases up to 50% higher than in the nonpregnant state. As a result, serum urea and creatinine levels decline in pregnancy [29]. This can have significant effects on renal clearance of vitamins and pharmaceutical agents. There is a lowering of the threshold for glucose excretion, which may result in significant random glucosuria even in the absence of gestational diabetes. This glycosuria may also contribute to the increased susceptibility of pregnant women to urinary tract infections.

There is also a marked increase in ureteral pressure in the third trimester while standing or sitting that is decreased when in the lateral recumbent position [28]. This has implications for collection of 24-hour urine samples, as retention of urine in the dilated collecting system may result in an incomplete sample. This may be alleviated by instructing the patient to lie in the lateral recumbent position for about 45 minutes before the discard void prior to starting the collection and again before the final void of the sample [28]. Proteinuria is considered abnormal if excessive of 300 mg/24 hours in pregnant patients [28].

Relaxin and nitric oxide (NO) have been implicated as key factors in mediating the renal vasodilation and glomerular hyperfiltration that is characteristic of normal human pregnancy. In vivo, relaxin administration to male and nonpregnant female rats produced physiologic changes that mimicked normal pregnancy, with decrements in SVR along with significant increases in effective renal plasma flow (RPF) and, hence, GFR [29].

Pregnancy is associated with altered tubular function and therefore altered reabsorption of protein, glucose, amino acids, and uric acid. In contrast to tubular function, our knowledge of the factors that govern gestational changes in serum electrolytes is somewhat more definitive. Total body sodium increases on an average by 3–4 mEq/d, ultimately producing a net balance of 900–1000 mEq, and total body potassium also increases by up to 320 mEq by the end of gestation [29]. Despite the net increase in body stores of sodium and potassium Table 3.1, serum levels of both electrolytes decrease during pregnancy Table 3.2. Therefore, pregnancy is characterized by increments in total body electrolyte stores, albeit with decrements in serum levels. Clinicians must recognize that increments in serum electrolytes that still fall within the range of normal may constitute meaningful aberrations in electrolyte balance. Furthermore, conditions prone to either electrolyte retention or loss may be exacerbated during pregnancy [29].

PHARMACOKINETICS

It may be helpful to conclude with a final clinical topic that illustrates many of the previously described physiologic changes: that of pharmacokinetics. **The four major events involved in pharmacokinetics (absorption, distribution, metabolism, and excretion) are potentially altered by physiologic change of pregnancy in a number of organ systems.** Absorption is affected by changes in gastric pH, gastric emptying, and small intestine motility. Increased cardiac output and heightened blood flow to the stomach and small intestine can increase absorption [30]. Changes in plasma volume, body fat, and total body water affect drug distribution; the proportion of unbound fraction of certain drugs may increase due to a decrease in protein concentration. Metabolism is affected by upregulation or downregulation of various enzymes. For example, liver cytochrome p-450 activities increase while CYP1A2 activity decreases while extrahepatic cholinesterase activity decreases [30]. Drug excretion is affected by the increased renal blood flow and elevated GFR of pregnancy as well as by increased respiratory elimination [30]. This has important implications for both the maintenance of therapeutic drug levels and the avoidance of toxicity. **Clinical evidence to guide pharmacologic therapy in pregnancy is limited,** in part due to the frequent elimination of women of reproductive age from pharmacokinetic trials. A review of the **National Library of Medicine database shows that there are a very limited quantity of pharmacokinetic data for pregnancy,** and thus evidence-based recommendations for dosing and scheduling of drugs during pregnancy are sparse [30].

REFERENCES

1. Lind T. *Maternal Physiology: CREOG Basic Science Monograph in Obstetrics and Gynecology.* Washington, DC: CREOG, 1985. [Review]
2. Abbassi-Ghanavati M, Greer L, Cunningham F. Pregnancy and laboratory studies: A reference table for clinicians. *Obstet Gynecol.* 2009;114(6):1326–1331. [Review]
3. American College of Obstetricians and Gynecologists. ACOG Practice Bulletin No. 100: critical care in pregnancy. *Obstet Gynecol.* 2009;113:443–450. [III]
4. Van Oppen A, Van Der Tweel I, Alsbach GPJ, et al. A longitudinal study of maternal hemodynamics during normal pregnancy. *Obstet Gynecol.* 1996;88:40–46. [II-3]
5. Van Oppen A, Stigter R, Bruinse H. Cardiac output in normal pregnancy: A critical review. *Obstet Gynecol.* 1996;87:310–318. [Review]
6. Desai D, Moodley J, Naidoo D. Echocardiographic assessment of cardiovascular hemodynamics in normal pregnancy. *Obstet Gynecol.* 2004;104:20–29. [II-2]
7. Yarlagadda S, Poma P, Green L, et al. Syncope during pregnancy. *Obstet Gynecol.* 2010;115(2 pt 1):377–380. [Review]
8. Katz V, Dotters D, Droegemueller W. Perimortem cesarean delivery. *Obstet Gynecol.* 1986;68:571–576. [Review]
9. Jensen D, Webb K, O'Donnell D. Chemical and mechanical adaptations of the human respiratory system at rest and during exercise in human pregnancy. *Appl Physiol Nutr Metab.* 2007;32:1239–1250. [Review]
10. Dombrowski M. Asthma and pregnancy. *Obstet Gynecol.* 2006;108:667–681. [Review]
11. Garcia-Rio F, Pino J, Gómez L, et al. Regulation of breathing and perception of dyspnea in healthy pregnant women. *Chest.* 1996;110(2):446–453. [II-2]
12. Bell R, Eddie L, Lester A, et al. Relaxin in human pregnancy serum measured with homologous radioimmunoassay. *Obstet Gynecol.* 1987;69:585–589. [II-2]
13. Quagliarello J, Steinetz B, Weiss G. Relaxin secretion in early pregnancy. *Obstet Gynecol.* 1979; 53:62–63. [II-3]
14. O'Leary P, Boyne P, Flett P, et al. Longitudinal assessment of changes in reproductive hormones during normal pregnancy. *Clin Chem.* 1991; 37(5):667–672. [II-3]
15. Casey B, Leveno K. Thyroid disease in pregnancy. *Obstet Gynecol.* 2006;108(5):1283–1292. [III]

16. American College of Obstetricians and Gynecologists. ACOG Practice Bulletin No. 37: Thyroid disease in pregnancy. *Obstet Gynecol*. 2002;100:387–396. [III]
17. Zimmermann M. Iodine deficiency in pregnancy and the effects of maternal iodine supplementation in the offspring: A review. *Am J Clin Nutr*. 2009;89(suppl):668S–672S. [Review]
18. Gyamfi C, Wapner R, D'Alton M. Thyroid dysfunction in pregnancy: The basic science and clinical evidence surrounding the controversy in management. *Obstet Gynecol*. 2009;113:702–707. [Review]
19. American College of Obstetricians and Gynecologists. ACOG Practice Bulletin No. 52: Nausea and vomiting of pregnancy. *Obstet Gynecol*. 2004;103:803–815. [III]
20. Casey BM, Dashe JS, Wells CE, et al. Subclinical hyperthyroidism and pregnancy outcomes. *Obstet Gynecol*. 2006;107:337–341. [II-2]
21. American College of Obstetricians and Gynecologists. ACOG Practice Bulletin No. 95: Anemia in pregnancy. *Obstet Gynecol*. 2008;112:201–207. [III]
22. American College of Obstetricians and Gynecologists. ACOG Practice Bulletin No. 6: Thrombocytopenia in pregnancy. *Obstet Gynecol*. 1999; reaffirmed 2009. [III]
23. American College of Obstetricians and Gynecologists. Practice Bulletin No. 113: Inherited thrombophilias in pregnancy. *Obstet Gynecol*. 2010;116:212–222. [III]
24. Bradley C, Kennedy C, Turcea AM, et al. Constipation in pregnancy: Prevalence, symptoms, and risk factors. *Obstet Gynecol*. 2007;110:1351–1357. [II-3]
25. Lagiou P, Tamimi R, Mucci LA, et al. Nausea and vomiting in pregnancy in relation to prolactin, estrogens, and progesterone: A prospective study. *Obstet Gynecol*. 2003;101:639–644. [II-3]
26. Huxley R. Nausea and vomiting in early pregnancy: Its role in placental development. *Obstet Gynecol*. 2000; 95:779–782. [III]
27. Vutyavanich T, Kraisarin T, Ruangsri R. Ginger for nausea and vomiting of pregnancy: Randomized, double-masked, placebo controlled trial. *Obstet Gynecol*. 2001;97:577–582. [I]
28. Lindheimer M, Kanter D. Interpreting abnormal proteinuria in pregnancy: The need for a more pathophysiological approach. *Obstet Gynecol*. 2010;115:365–375. [III]
29. Odutayo A, Hladunewich M. Obstetric nephrology: Renal hemodynamic and metabolic physiology in normal pregnancy. *Clin J AM Soc Nephrol*. 2012;7(12):2073–2080. [Review]
30. Little B. Pharmacokinetics during pregnancy: Evidence-based maternal dose formulation. *Obstet Gynecol*. 1999;93:858–868. [II-2]

Ultrasound

Lea M. Porche and Alfred Abuhamad

KEY POINTS

- There is **no evidence that ultrasound examination during pregnancy is harmful.** Prenatal exposure to ultrasound is not associated with adverse influence on school performance, physical or neurological function.
- Ultrasound should be performed by **trained and experienced professionals,** with continuing education and ongoing quality-monitoring programs.
- **Routine use of ultrasound** in pregnancy increases early detection of **multiple pregnancies, and major fetal anomalies.**
- **Ultrasound examination is the best method to estimate accurate gestational dating in pregnancy.**
- **Ultrasound** dating in the first trimester is most accurate for gestational age assessment. **Ultrasound examination at first prenatal visit (usually *first trimester*) versus at 18–20 weeks provides more precise estimate of gestational age, and may be associated with less maternal worry.** First trimester ultrasound **allows earlier detection of multiple pregnancies, screening for Down's syndrome with nuchal translucency, and diagnosis of nonviable pregnancies.**
- **All pregnant women should be offered a *second trimester* ultrasound for optimal anatomy evaluation.** If only one ultrasound will be done in pregnancy, it should be done in the second trimester at about 18–22 weeks.
- In low-risk or unselected populations, *routine third trimester* (>24 weeks) pregnancy ultrasound has not been associated with improvements in perinatal mortality. Routine use of ultrasound in the third trimester is associated with higher detection of small-for-gestational-age babies.
- In **low-risk or unselected populations, routine Doppler ultrasound examination** in the third trimester does **not result in reduced perinatal mortality.**
- In high-risk pregnancies with **fetal growth restriction, umbilical artery Doppler assessment** is associated with a **reduction in perinatal deaths and obstetric interventions.**
- Measurement of **cervical length** (CL) by transvaginal ultrasound (TVU) has been shown to be an effective predictor of preterm birth (PTB). When a short CL is detected before 24 weeks, interventions such as vaginal progesterone in singletons without prior PTB (using TVU CL ≤ 20 mm), and cerclage in singletons with prior PTB (using TVU CL ≤ 25 mm), have been associated with decrease in PTB and perinatal morbidity and mortality.

SAFETY OF ULTRASONOGRAPHY

The main concern about the safety of ultrasound is about tissue temperature elevation from energy transfer and its possible effect of cavitations, or the formation of microbubbles in the tissues exposed to ultrasound waves. The effect of ultrasound on tissues has been studied with animal experimentation and has suggested an adverse effect. In humans, however, the information comes from epidemiological data and population studies. **No epidemiologic studies have shown harmful effects in humans.**

There is no consistent evidence that ultrasound examination during pregnancy is harmful. Studies have shown that prenatal exposure to ultrasound is not associated with adverse effects on children's physical or cognitive development [1]. Even multiple ultrasound exams during pregnancy were not shown to adversely affect speech, language, behavior or neurologic function on postnatal follow up at 8 years of age [2]. In a randomized trial comparing those receiving a second trimester ultrasound to those who remained unexposed, there was no significant difference in school performance up to age 15–16 [3]. Overall, ultrasound in pregnancy is not associated with adverse maternal or perinatal outcome, however, there may be a weak association between exposure to ultrasound and nonright handedness in boys [4].

Despite the lack of evidence suggesting harmful effect, ultrasound is a form of energy and may produce secondary effects in the tissues it traverses. Obstetrical ultrasound in pregnancy should be considered a medical procedure for the evaluation of the fetus and maternal pelvic organs. Current expert consensus recommends that **ultrasound be only performed with valid medical indications, with the shortest duration possible and at the lowest settings. Adhering to the as low as reasonably achievable (ALARA) principle helps to avoid unnecessary exposure to ultrasonic waves.** Sonographers and sonologists should familiarize themselves with the mechanical and thermal indices during ultrasound examinations. **Exposing the fetus to ultrasonography with no anticipation of medical benefit is thus not justified [5,6].**

QUALITY

Levels of expertise vary between different health care centers. Since ultrasound efficiency is operator dependent, **continuing education and ongoing quality-monitoring programs are important** strategies in each center offering ultrasound diagnosis. The ongoing risks of "false-negative" tests and/or misinterpretation of the images obtained (either false-positives, or wrong diagnoses) can be minimized if those examinations are carried out and interpreted by **trained and experienced professionals.** Sensitivity of ultrasound screening for pregnancy varies widely. **Appropriate ultrasound laboratory accreditation, certification of staff, documentation of findings, and continuous careful quality control are important components** of ultrasound competency [5,6].

INFORMED CONSENT AND PATIENTS' EXPECTATIONS

Even though a formal written informed consent is not always needed **before the examination, every pregnant woman should be informed on expectations about the obstetric** ultrasound, as well as its benefits and risks. The patients should know that ultrasound evaluation is a screening test with wide variations in detection rates for fetal anomalies, and that all ultrasound diagnoses, especially false-positive and false-negative ones, can put both mother and fetus at risk.

Whether the sex of the fetus should be revealed to the patient with a singleton gestation should be addressed. It may be harmful for the physician–patient relationship to withhold this information, especially if the patient previously requested it. Although a moral conflict may exist in some cultures around the world where this information is used by the patient for voluntary abortions based on sex selection and sex preferences [7], **in general disclosing fetal gender during ultrasound can benefit not only the doctor–patient relation but also parent–child relationship** [8].

During high-feedback ultrasound scans, women can see the screen and they receive detailed explanations of the images. In low-feedback ultrasound scans, only the operator can see the screen and the women are told the results at the end of the scan. Compared with low-feedback ultrasound, women who had high-feedback fetal ultrasound are significantly more likely to stop smoking and avoid alcohol during pregnancy, with a trend favoring the women's increased use of positive adjectives to describe their feelings after the ultrasound [9].

ROUTINE VERSUS SELECTIVE USE OF ULTRASOUND

Routine (i.e., performed on every pregnant woman) ultrasound examination is associated with the following, compared with **selective** ultrasound examination (i.e., performed only on women with specific indications) [1]:

1. **Increases the early detection of multiple pregnancies.**
2. **Increases detection of major fetal anomalies.**
3. **Reduces the incidence of late-term and post-term pregnancies and rates of induction of labor for late-term pregnancy** by allowing a more precise estimation of gestational age.
4. **No significant differences are detected for clinical outcomes such as perinatal mortality.** The effect of ultrasound on perinatal mortality is dependent on the detection rate of fetal malformations and on the uptake of pregnancy termination for anomalies in the population at study.

If one routine ultrasound examination is done, it is usually performed at 18–22 weeks (<24 weeks). Earlier examination provides more accurate assessment of gestational age; later examination (e.g., 20–22 weeks) allows more complete inspection of fetal anatomy. **In the obese population, transabdominal ultrasound screening may have better completion rates if delayed by 2 weeks** (20–22 weeks gestation) [10] and TVU at 12–16 weeks may offer better fetal anatomy screening (see later in this chapter).

GESTATIONAL AGE DATING IN PREGNANCY

Precise estimation of gestational age is extremely important for optimal obstetric care, including evaluation of fetal growth, interpretation of maternal screening markers, choosing the appropriate gestational age to perform interventions, and management of preterm and late-term pregnancies.

For gestational age estimation, cardinal numbers should be preferred to ordinal numbers to avoid confusion. So week 1 is 1–7 days after LMP, week 2 is 8–14 days, etc. In clinical practice, gestational weeks are used to estimate dating, and not months. If a lay person asks "How many months am I?," then 6 weeks of gestation can be equated approximately to 1 month, etc., and 38 weeks = 9 months. **Definitions of gestational age, while not uniformly accepted, are shown in Table 4.1** [10].

Ultrasound examination is the best method to determine gestational age and estimated due date (EDD) [10]. The first day of the last menstrual period (LMP) should be asked of all pregnant women to determine when the dating ultrasound should be performed. Compared with LMP, ultrasound-based gestational age is more precise due to errors in patient recall, and variations in cycle length and timing of ovulation [10,11]. The error, even with certain LMP, is due often to late ovulation (>14 days after LMP). Some have stated that there is no reason to use LMP for dating when adequate ultrasound data is available by 24 weeks [10,11].

Ultrasound-based gestational age estimates are lower than LMP-based gestational age estimates, and generate a higher rate of PTB and lower rate of post-term birth. The Naegele rule (add 7 days to first day of LMP, add 1 year, take back 3 months), manual assessment of uterine size, quickening, etc., should not be used unless ultrasound dating is unavailable.

In general, **the earlier the ultrasound, the more accurate the dating**. Multiple parameters and equations have been evaluated to estimate gestational age. **The crown-rump length is associated with the most accurate estimation up to and including 13 6/7 weeks of gestation with an accuracy of ± 2–7 days.** For pregnancies in the second trimester, beyond 14 weeks gestation, the head circumference (HC) or biparietal diameter (BPD) appear to be the best single-measurement predictor of gestational dating. BPD is most accurate for dating early, between 12 and 14 weeks. Combining three or more parameters improved dating slightly over single biometric parameter [12]. A combination of BPD, HC, abdominal circumference (AC), and femur length (FL) is commonly used for dating by ultrasound in the second and third trimesters [13]. Repeated examinations improve the prediction only marginally, and the EDD should always be set by the earliest ultrasound due to a smaller prediction error. While prediction of gestational age by ultrasound can be very accurate, prediction of date of delivery remains less accurate, with an error of usually ≥7–8 days, given other biologic factors.

Other parameters that may play a role in estimating gestational age include trans-cerebellar diameter (TCD) and long bone measurements. The TCD is an accurate predictor of gestational age, and can be used between 14 and 28 weeks reliably with the use of nomograms. There is some reliability in gestational age prediction even up to 35 weeks, and TCD is spared effects from intrauterine growth restriction, so can be used to assess pregnancies at risk for this complication [14]. The presence of epiphyses in the lower extremities usually signifies a gestational age (GA) of >32 weeks [15].

Table 4.1 Definition of Gestational Age Periods in Pregnancy

Period	Gestational age (weeks)
First trimester	0–13 6/7
Second trimester	14 0/7–27 6/7
Third trimester	28 0/7 to delivery
Preterm	20 0/7–36 6/7
Late preterm	34 0/7–36 6/7
Term	37 0/7–41 6/7
Early term	37 0/7–38 6/7
Full-term	39 0/7–40 6/7
Late-term	41 0/7–41 6/7
Post-term	≥42 0/7

Table 4.2 Gestational Age Dating by Ultrasound

Gestational age by ultrasound (weeks)	Best ultrasound parameter(s)	EDD changed if discrepancy from LMP-dates more than (days)
<9	CRL	5
9 0/7–13 6/7	CRL	7
14 0/7–15 6/7	BPD, HC, AC, FL	7
16 0/7–21 6/7	BPD, HC, AC, FL	10
22 0/7–27 6/7	BPD, HC, AC, FL	14
≥28 0/7	BPD, HC, AC, FL	21

Source: Adapted from American College of Obstetricians and Gynecologists. Method for estimating due date. ACOG Committee Opinion No. 611. American College of Obstetricians and Gynecologists, Washington, DC, 2014.
Note: IVF pregnancies can be dated by the date of embryo transfer minus 14 days to obtain LMP, and then EDC by Naegele's rule. There is no need to ever change dating in these pregnancies.

The American College of Obstetricians and Gynecologists (ACOG) have published specific guidelines to guide amendment of dating when ultrasound and LMP are discrepant. Ultrasound dating is adopted when discrepancy is noted. Knowledge about LMP, regularity of cycles, OCP use and unusual bleeding are clinically helpful, but imprecise regarding dating. **Ultrasound dating is best**, and often corrects dating by even a "certain" LMP [16]. Table 4.2 shows dating criteria based on ultrasound results.

ULTRASOUND EXAMINATIONS BY TRIMESTER
First Trimester

Ultrasonographic evaluation in the first trimester (0–13 6/7 weeks) is the most accurate method to determine exact gestational age, as discussed above. **Ultrasound examination at the first prenatal visit versus at 18–20 weeks provides more precise estimate of gestational age, and may be associated with less maternal worry. First trimester ultrasound also allows earlier detection of multiple pregnancies, nonviable pregnancies, certain fetal anomalies, and screening for Down's syndrome and other aneuploidy with nuchal translucency (NT)** [1,6,17]. No other important maternal or perinatal outcome differences are detected, with insufficient data to accurately assess some rare outcomes such as perinatal mortality. Current guidelines do not recommend the routine use of ultrasound in the first trimester in the absence of indications [10], but several experts advocate its routine use for the benefits listed above.

Transvaginal scanning is preferred for dating early in the first trimester. It is also useful in cases of a pregnancy resulting from ovulation induction or other assisted reproductive technologies, first trimester bleeding, or increased risk of aneuploidy, and should be used if transabdominal examination is inconclusive for diagnosis. First trimester screening for congenital defects by TVU is an option for pregnant women who meet certain criteria, such a very high risk for congenital anomalies (e.g., very elevated hemoglobin A1c) and who may elect termination based on abnormal results. It should be done by experienced sonographers and findings confirmed at 18–22 weeks [10]. In a randomized control trials (RCT), 38% of major malformations and 69% of lethal malformations were detected by a 12- to 14-week ultrasound [18]. In a meta-analysis, 51% of malformations were found to have been detected by 11- to 14-week ultrasound [19].

The NT is a physiologic fluid-filled space at the back of the fetal neck measured for aneuploidy screening between weeks 10 6/7 and 13 6/7 of gestation. Increase in NT has been associated with chromosomal and anatomic abnormalities in the fetus. First trimester screening for aneuploidy between 10 6/7 and 13 6/7 weeks (or crown–rump length or CRL 45–84 mm) combines NT measurement with maternal serum markers to provide individualized risk assessment. Early risk determination permits choosing the most appropriate definitive diagnostic procedures like chorionic villus sampling, allowing women to prepare for a child with health problems and also providing the option of earlier pregnancy termination [6] (see Chapter 5).

Indications by ACOG and American Institute of Ultrasound in Medicine (AIUM) for first trimester ultrasound are shown in Table 4.3 and essential elements of first trimester ultrasound in Table 4.4 [5,6].

Ultrasound Diagnosis of Anembryonic Pregnancy or Embryonic Demise

Diagnostic criteria for the diagnosis of nonviable pregnancy in the first trimester is a subject that has undergone recent revision. Balancing risk of harming a viable intrauterine pregnancy must be balanced with intervention for a nonviable one. Some criteria are routinely used (Table 4.5), usually based on **TVU**: absence of cardiac activity with an embryo of certain length, absence of embryo with gestational sac of a certain size, and absence of embryo by a certain time in pregnancy [20].

A gestational sac is normally noted within the uterus by 5 weeks of gestation. Shortly thereafter at approximately 5 ½ weeks in a normal pregnancy, the yolk sac appears, followed by the fetal pole at 6 weeks. When measuring the gestational sac, dimensions are recorded in three orthogonal planes; the average of the measurements is the mean sac diameter. **A mean gestational sac diameter of ≥25 mm without an embryo** is diagnostic of pregnancy failure (e.g., anembryonic pregnancy, or blighted ovum) with positive predictive value approaching 100% [21]. An intrauterine gestational sac should be visible by TVU with a serum beta-human chorionic gonadotropin (B-HCG) of >1500 mIU/mL. If this is not the case, ectopic pregnancy should be suspected.

Fetal cardiac activity is usually seen once the fetal pole is visible around 6 weeks of gestation. A CRL cutoff of 5 mm without cardiac activity was previously used to diagnose nonviable pregnancy, but literature review showed that there have been pregnancies that met this criterion that went on to be viable [21,22]. Interobserver variability in measurements can also lead to inaccurate diagnosis of failed pregnancy. Adopting a **CRL cutoff of 7 mm with no visible cardiac activity** brings the specificity of this finding for diagnosing failed pregnancy (e.g., embryonic demise, or missed abortion) close to 100% [20].

Since the presence of intrauterine structures in a viable pregnancy appear in a predictable sequence at standard time intervals [23], aberrations in this sequence can indicate abnormal pregnancy. Abnormal pregnancy should thus be suspected in the **absence of an embryo with a heartbeat ≥14 days**

Table 4.3 Indications for First Trimester Ultrasound

- To confirm the presence of an intrauterine pregnancy
- To evaluate suspected ectopic pregnancy
- To define the cause of vaginal bleeding
- To evaluate pelvic pain
- To estimate gestational age
- To diagnose or evaluate multiple gestations
- To confirm cardiac activity and identify nonviable pregnancies
- As an adjunct to chorionic villus sampling, embryo transfer, and localization and removal of an intrauterine device
- To evaluate maternal pelvic masses and/or uterine anomalies
- To evaluate suspected hydatiform mole
- To screen for certain anomalies such as anencephaly in patients at high risk
- To measure NT when part of a screening program for fetal aneuploidy

Sources: American Institute of Ultrasound in Medicine, *J Ultrasound Med*, 32(6), 1083–1101, 2013; American College of Obstetricians and Gynecologists. Ultrasonography in pregnancy. ACOG Practice Bulletin No. 101. American College of Obstetricians and Gynecologists, Washington, DC, 2009.

Table 4.4 Essential Elements of First Trimester Ultrasound

- Gestational sac (location, mean diameter).
- Yolk sac (diameter).
- CRL of embryo[a].
- Development of fetal anatomy in early pregnancy.
- Fetal viability (cardiac activity should be seen in embryo >7 mm).
- Fetal number (amnionicity and chorionicity has to be reported for multiples).
- Ultrasound features of early pregnancy failure, e.g., ectopic pregnancy, hydatidiform mole.
- Uterus, adnexa, cervix, and cul de sac.
- If possible, the appearance of the nuchal region should be assessed, and specific measurement of Nuchal translucency (NT) measured as part of desired screening.
- Any other abnormalities (e.g., leiomyomata).

Sources: American Institute of Ultrasound in Medicine, *J Ultrasound Med*, 32(6), 1083–1101, 2013; American College of Obstetricians and Gynecologists. Ultrasonography in pregnancy. ACOG Practice Bulletin No. 101. American College of Obstetricians and Gynecologists, Washington, DC, 2009; Doubilet PM et al., *N Engl Med*, 369(15),1443–1451, 2013
[a]CRL is a more accurate indicator of gestational age than gestational sac size.

Table 4.5 Criteria for Diagnosis of Embryonic or Anembryonic Demise

Diagnosis	Criteria
Anembryonic pregnancy	Mean gestational sac diameter ≥ 25 mm without an embryo
Embryonic demise	CRL ≥7 mm with no visible cardiac activity
Anembryonic pregnancy	No embryo with cardiac activity: ≥14 days after gestational sac without yolk sac Or ≥11 days after gestational sac with yolk sac

after seeing a gestational sac without a yolk sac, or ≥11 days after presence of a gestational sac with a yolk sac [20]. The presence of normal embryonic cardiac activity in the uterine cavity in the first trimester has a >90% prediction for a live birth in both symptomatic and asymptomatic pregnancies.

Precautions and Pitfalls

Physiologic midgut herniation is normal at 7–11 weeks; it resolves ≥12 weeks; do not confuse with omphalocele. The rhomboencephalon can appear as a cystic mass up until 8–10 weeks, and should not be confused with a central nervous system (CNS) anomaly; ventriculomegaly cannot be assessed well in the first trimester. The amnion and chorion are expected to be fused by 14 weeks.

Second Trimester (aka "Anatomy," "Morphology," or "Standard" Ultrasound)

If just a single exam is to be done during pregnancy, the best timing for such ultrasound screening of the fetal anatomy and dating is the early to mid-second trimester (18–22 weeks) [1], to obtain an accurate estimation of gestational age and a satisfactory inspection of the fetal anatomy. This is therefore usually called the anatomy, morphology, or standard ultrasound examination (nomenclature such as Levels I, II, etc. ultrasound is controversial and less descriptive). All **pregnant women should be offered a second trimester ultrasound,** whether or not they have had a first trimester ultrasound. **The estimated sensitivity to detect fetal anomalies varies widely,** with higher rates of detection for major anomalies than for minor anomalies, and some organs (e.g., neural tube defect) versus others (e.g., heart) [19]. The detection of major fetal anomalies is often reported at about 50%–70% even in the best centers [18]. The detection of fetal cardiac malformations is particularly poor, with often not more than 20%–30% of major heart malformations detected [24]. A **"detailed" ultrasound** can be performed with the aim to detect anomalies or markers associated with fetal aneuploidy [25].

While the best time for detection of most malformations is around 20–24 weeks it is important for women to obtain this information as early as possible. In some circumstances more than one second trimester ultrasound is necessary, especially if the first second trimester ultrasound is performed at 18–19 weeks. Experts have suggested essential elements for second trimester ultrasound (Table 4.6) [5,6].

There can be other types of follow-up ultrasounds. **Limited ultrasound examination** is performed when a specific question requires investigation. Examples include assessment of amniotic fluid volume, fetal viability, biophysical profile, to guide amniocentesis, to localize the placenta in antepartum bleeding, or to evaluate fetal position. A limited ultrasound is only appropriate if a prior complete standard ultrasound examination has been done. A **detailed ultrasound examination** should be considered for a patient who, by history, clinical evaluation, or prior scanning evaluation, is at an increased risk for a fetal anatomic or physiological abnormality. This ultrasound examination must be done by personnel with expertise in obstetric ultrasonography, and maternal and fetal diseases [25].

Other specialized examinations include but are not limited to fetal Doppler studies, biophysical profile, CL, three-dimensional (3D) imaging, and fetal echocardiography (see the section Fetal Echocardiography).

Third Trimester

The potential benefit of a third trimester ultrasound examination greatly depends on the quality of prior ultrasounds and maternal indications. If the first and only ultrasound is in the third trimester, it probably has similar benefits to the routine second trimester ultrasound, with the exception of accurate dating and early anomaly detection of the latter. Ultrasound evaluations in the third trimester generally involve assessments of fetal growth,

Table 4.6 Essential Elements for Second Trimester Ultrasound[a]

- Fetal cardiac activity (abnormal heart rate or rhythm should be documented).
- Fetal number (multiple pregnancies require additional information: chorionicity, amnionicity, comparison of fetal sizes, estimation of amniotic fluid volume at each side of the membranes, and fetal gender).
- Presentation.
- A qualitative or semi quantitative assessment of amniotic fluid (e.g., amniotic fluid index, single deepest pocket, 2-diameter pocket) (see Chapter 57 in *Maternal Fetal Evidence Based Guidelines*).
- The placental location, appearance and relationship to the internal cervical os should be recorded.[b]
- The umbilical cord should be imaged to confirm number of vessels. Placental cord insertion site should be documented when technically feasible.
- TVU may be offered for detection of short CL (see Chapter 17).
- Gestational age assessment.[c]
- Fetal weight estimation can be calculated by obtaining measurements, such as BPD, HC, AC, and FL.[d]
- Evaluation of the maternal uterus and adnexal structures should be performed.
- Fetal anatomy survey: Fetal anatomy is best assessed by ultrasound ≥18 weeks. Essential elements of a standard examination:
  - Head and neck: Cerebellum, choroids plexus, cisterna magna, lateral cerebral ventricles, midline falx, cavum septi pellucidi, upper lip.
  - Chest: The basic cardiac inspection includes a four-chamber view of fetal heart with visualization of the right and left ventricular outflow tracts.
  - Abdomen: stomach (presence, size, situs), kidneys, bladder, umbilical cord (insertion site into fetal abdomen and vessel number).
  - Spine: Cervical, thoracic, lumbar, and sacral spine.
  - Extremities: Legs and arms (presence or absence).
  - Gender: For evaluation of multiple gestations and when medically indicated.

Sources: American Institute of Ultrasound in Medicine, *J Ultrasound Med*, 32(6), 1083–1101, 2013; American College of Obstetricians and Gynecologists. Ultrasonography in pregnancy. ACOG Practice Bulletin No. 101. American College of Obstetricians and Gynecologists, Washington, DC, 2009.

[a]If not performed in second trimester, a third trimester ultrasound is indicated.
[b]The apparent position early in pregnancy may not correlate well with its location at the time of delivery. Therefore, if low-lying placenta or placenta previa are suspected early in gestation, a TVU is indicated, with verification in the third trimester by a TVU if previa or placental edge within 20 mm of internal os is found.
[c]First trimester CRL measurement is the most accurate means for sonographic dating.
[d]None of the several equations for estimating fetal weight based on such fetal biometric measurements is superior to others; ideally, the equations should be derived by actual fetal weights of the local or institutional population. Results can be compared with fetal weight percentiles from published nomograms. Consecutive ultrasound examinations for growth evaluation should typically be performed no less than 3 weeks apart.

amniotic fluid volume, evaluation of the placenta, and evaluation of fetal wellbeing (possibly biophysical profile or Doppler studies). Examples of possible indications for third trimester ultrasound based on maternal and fetal risk factors are shown in Table 4.7.

In low risk women, ultrasound examinations at 30–32 weeks and at 36–37 weeks **significantly decrease the likelihood of newborns with growth restriction**, though they do increase the rate of antenatal intervention. This randomized controlled trial included 1998 women, and investigators calculate over 30,000 women are required for a trial to show a significant decrease in neonatal mortality [26]. In a meta-analysis, there was no difference in antenatal, obstetric and neonatal intervention in women screened with >24 weeks (late) ultrasound versus those not screened. There was a slightly higher caesarean section rate in women screened with late ultrasound, but this difference did not reach statistical significance. Routine late pregnancy ultrasound was not associated with improvements in overall perinatal mortality [27]. In a recent RCT, performing a growth ultrasound at 36 versus 32 weeks is **more sensitive** (61% vs. 32%) **in detecting severe FGR, but not associated with significant differences in perinatal outcomes** [28]. Routine screening for fetal growth restriction in the third trimester has been investigated also in a large prospective cohort study and may increase detection of fetuses that will go on to be small for gestational age infants, to 57% in routine screening from 20% in selected screening [29]. **Currently there is insufficient data to recommend routine screening for growth restriction in the third trimester without indication, but many experts advocate its routine use based on the data just described.** There is insufficient data about the potential psychological effects of routine ultrasound in late pregnancy, and limited data about its effects on both short- and long-term neonatal and childhood outcome.

Placental grading as an adjunct to third trimester ultrasound examination was associated with a significant reduction in the stillbirth rate in one trial [30]. In one study 15,122 patients were evaluated for Grannum grade III placental calcifications prior to 28 weeks of gestation. Grade III placental appearance prior to term was independently associated with increased risk of stillbirth after controlling for tobacco use [31]. **More research is needed in placental grading before recommendation can be made for its routine use for prediction of poor perinatal outcome.**

DOPPLER
Umbilical Artery

In low-risk or unselected populations, routine Doppler ultrasound examination, usually of the umbilical artery and fetal vessels at around 28–34 weeks, does not result in increased antenatal, obstetric and neonatal interventions, and no overall differences are detected for substantive short term clinical outcomes such as perinatal mortality [32]. On the other hand, **the use of umbilical artery Doppler ultrasound in pregnancies with fetal growth restriction is associated with a reduction in perinatal deaths and obstetric interventions** [33]. Guidelines published by the Society for Maternal Fetal Medicine confirm a decrease in induction of labor, cesarean delivery and perinatal death with use of umbilical artery Doppler assessment in high-risk pregnancies with fetal growth restriction. Surveillance with umbilical artery Doppler studies should be started once growth restriction is

Table 4.7 Suggested Ultrasound Surveillance for Specific Conditions

Condition	Start of ultrasounds (weeks)	Frequency of ultrasounds (every x week)
Chronic HTN on medications	24	4
Gestational HTN	At diagnosis	4
Preeclampsia	At diagnosis	4
GDMA1	30–32	once
GDMA2	At diagnosis	4
Pregestational DM on medications	24	4
Fetal growth restriction	At diagnosis	3
Maternal age at delivery ≥35 years	30–32	once
Concordant, non-IUGR di/di twins	24	4
Mono/di twins	24	4
Mono/mono twins	24	3
Prior unexplained IUFD	28	4
SLE or renal disease	24	4
Organ transplant	28	4
Hypothyroidism or Hyperthyroidism	30–32	once
Maternal Cardiac disease	28	4
Oligohydramnios (MVP < 2 cm)	At diagnosis	3–4
Polyhydramnios (MVP > 8 cm)	At diagnosis	3–4
Sickle cell disease	24	4
Fetal arrhythmia	At diagnosis	4

Abbreviations: HTN, hypertension; GDMA, gestational diabetes mellitus; DM, diabetes mellitus; di/di, dichorionic diamniotic; mono/di, monochorionic diamniotic; mono/mono, monochorionic monoamniotic; IUFD, intrauterine fetal demise; SLE, systemic lupus erythematosus; MVP, maximum vertical pocket. For an expanded version of this chapter, including suggestions for antepartum fetal testing (e.g., NST, BPS, etc.) and timing of delivery, see Chapter 56.

suspected in the viable fetus [34]. Guidelines for the technical aspects of Doppler use in pregnancy are available [35] (see Chapter 45 in *Maternal-Fetal Evidence Based Guidelines*).

Middle Cerebral Artery

Fetal middle cerebral artery (MCA) peak systolic velocity (PSV) Doppler has been used to evaluate fetal anemia in cases of maternal red cell alloimmunization, parvovirus infection, or twin-twin transfusion syndrome in monochorionic twins. Fetal MCA Dopplers are considered a screening test that requires a confirmatory test for diagnosis (fetal blood sampling) at the initiation of therapy (transfusion). **MCA-PSV is regarded as the best noninvasive screening test for fetal anemia** [36,37] (see Chapter 53 in *Maternal-Fetal Evidence Based Guidelines*).

Ductus Venosus

The ductus venosus (DV) is a vascular shunt that connects the umbilical vein to the inferior vena cava in the fetus. This waveform is reflective of downstream pressure in the right atrium. In high resistance states (increased uteroplacental resistance), the DV shows absent or reversed flow in late diastole. A small retrospective study showed that reversed flow in the DV in addition to increased MCA is associated with perinatal mortality in fetuses less than 32 weeks gestation [38]. A meta-analysis including data from 2267 patients confirmed these data, showing moderate predictive value for fetal outcomes in high-risk pregnancies with placental insufficiency [39]. A randomized trial did not show significant perinatal benefit from adding DV screening to fetal heart rate monitoring alone for antepartum monitoring of the growth restricted fetus [40]. Therefore, there insufficient data to currently recommend the use of DV Doppler in the routine evaluation and management of the fetus with intrauterine growth restriction (IUGR) [34] (see Chapter 45 in *Maternal-Fetal Evidence Based Guidelines*).

Uterine Artery

The Doppler waveform of the uterine artery has been shown to reflect high impedance placental circulation by the presence of a waveform notch and low diastolic flow in association with hypertension and preeclampsia. Studies have shown an association between abnormal uterine artery Doppler and early onset preeclampsia, but predictive value is low. Current evidence has not shown a benefit to performing routine mid-pregnancy utero-placental Doppler ultrasound for prevention of preeclampsia, intrauterine growth restriction or adverse pregnancy outcome [41,42] (see Chapter 45 in *Maternal-Fetal Evidence Based Guidelines*). Furthermore, there is currently paucity of data to recommend the use of uterine artery Doppler in the clinical management of hypertensive pregnancies [42].

BIOPHYSICAL PROFILE

A fetal biophysical profile score (BPS) is a specialized obstetric ultrasound consisting of monitoring of fetal movements, tone and breathing, and assessment of amniotic fluid volume, with or without fetal heart rate monitoring. BPS has been used to identify fetuses that may be at high risk of poor pregnancy outcome. While information gained from a biophysical profile (BPP) regarding fetal status can help guide clinical management, available evidence from randomized trials does not support the use of BPS as an isolated test of fetal well-being in high-risk pregnancies. Additional evidence from larger trials is needed [43] (see Chapter 56 in *Maternal-Fetal Evidence Based Guidelines*).

CERVICAL LENGTH

TVU for the measurement of CL has been shown to be predictive of spontaneous PTB in all populations studied so far, including singletons and multiple gestations, either asymptomatic or with symptoms of preterm labor (PTL). TVU CL can be effective in evaluating the need for such interventions as cervical cerclage or progesterone supplementation, as well as more effective management of women with symptoms of PTL [44–47].

TVU CL screening is considered **universal** when offered routinely to singleton gestations without a prior spontaneous PTB at the time of the anatomy ultrasound, i.e., 18–24 weeks. Both ACOG and Society for Maternal-Fetal Medicine (SMFM) have published guidelines indicating that universal

TVU CL screening **is deemed reasonable,** but not mandatory [48,49]. About 1% of singletons without a prior spontaneous PTB develop a TVU CL ≤ 20 mm before 24 weeks [50], and should be started on vaginal progesterone daily until 36 weeks [51,52]. Over two-thirds of academic maternal-fetal medicine units in the United States perform universal CL screening [53].

Women with history of spontaneous PTB prior to 37 weeks gestation should be offered intramuscular progesterone supplementation [54]. In addition, current recommendations are for screening of these high risk women (history of spontaneous PTB) with serial TVU CL ultrasounds every 2 weeks from 16 to 24 weeks gestation. In those (about 40%) with TVU CL ≤ 25 mm, a cerclage can be offered [55].

TVU CL screening of singletons presenting between 24 and 34 weeks with symptoms of PTL has been associated with both lower evaluation and triage time, and significantly less incidence of PTB [56] (see Chapter 17).

THREE-DIMENSIONAL ULTRASOUND

3D ultrasound examination is not considered a required modality for all pregnant women at this time [4], but it can add accuracy in the assessment of the fetus identified to have anomalies by 2D ultrasound (especially facial anomalies, neural tube defects, and skeletal malformations). 3D ultrasound allows the acquisition of volume measurements, which can depict topographic anatomy not able to be seen on 2D imaging. New technology allows for 3D reconstruction of vascular structures, further characterizing vessel relationship [57], vascular malformations and vascular invasion. It has not been shown to have a clear clinical advantage over traditional ultrasound in routine settings [6].

Routine 3D ultrasound (versus the traditional 2D ultrasound) among low-risk women has not shown a significant impact on maternal-fetal bonding [58]. Additionally, 3D/4D ultrasound in women at risk for having a fetus with congenital anomalies does not reduce maternal anxiety compared with conventional 2D ultrasound alone [59].

FETAL ECHOCARDIOGRAPHY

The incidence of moderate to severe congenital heart disease (CHD) has been reported at 6–13 per 1000 live births [60,61], with most affected infants born to pregnancies without identifiable risk factors [62]. Fetal cardiac evaluation is an important part of the prenatal ultrasound examination. Basic cardiac screening to be completed during the mid-trimester ultrasound during every pregnancy includes the four-chamber view and evaluation of the right and left outflow tracts [5,10]. An in depth evaluation of fetal cardiac structures should be performed if the screening exam is abnormal or incomplete, or when there are maternal or fetal indications (Table 4.8) [63,64]. Fetal echocardiography is usually performed between 18 and 22 weeks. Main areas of evaluation include visceral situs, atrial and ventricular anatomy, valvular structure and function, and the orientation and morphology of the great vessels. Gray scale and color Doppler imaging are required while spectral Doppler and M-mode should be used as needed to evaluate suspected anomalies [65]. These structures are usually best seen in the second trimester, but experienced technicians and sonologists may be able to detect cardiac anomalies in the first trimester. One prospective observational study showed a sensitivity and specificity of 88% and 100%, respectively, for detection of cardiac anomalies when using the four-chamber view, three-vessel view, and three-vessel trachea view to screen an unselected patient population in the first trimester [66].

Table 4.8 Indications for Fetal Echocardiography

Maternal indications
- Autoimmune antibodies, anti-Ro/anti-La
- Familial inherited disorders (e.g., 22q11.2 deletion syndrome)
- In vitro fertilization
- Metabolic disease (e.g., diabetes mellitus and phenylketonuria)
- Teratogen exposure (e.g., retinoids, lithium)

Fetal indications
- Abnormal cardiac screening exam
- First degree relative of a fetus with CHD
- Abnormal heart rate or rhythm
- Fetal chromosome anomaly
- Extracardiac anomaly
- Hydrops
- Increased nuchal translucency
- Monochorionic twins

Source: Adapted from American Institute of Ultrasound in Medicine, *J Ultrasound Med*, 2(6):1067–1082, 2013.

REFERENCES

1. Whitworth M, Bricker L, Neilson JP, Dowswell T. Ultrasound for fetal assessment in early pregnancy. *Cochrane Library.* 2015. [Meta-analysis; 11 RCTs, n = >37,505]
2. Newnham JP, Doherty DA, Kendall GE, et al. Effects of repeated prenatal ultrasound examinations on childhood outcome up to 8 years of age: Follow-up of a randomized trial. *Lancet.* 2004;364:2038–2044. [Follow-up at 8 yrs of RCT of 5 vs. 1 ultrasounds in pregnancy]
3. Stalberg K, Axelsson O, Haglund B, et al. Prenatal ultrasound exposure and children's school performance at age 15–16: Follow-up of a randomized controlled trial. *Ultrasound Obstet Gynecol.* 2009;34:297–2303. [RCT, n = 4458]
4. Torloni M, Vedmedovska N, Merialdi M, et al. Safety of ultrasonography in pregnancy: WHO systematic review of the literature and meta-analysis. *Ultrasound Obstet Gynecol.* 2009;33:599–608. [Meta analysis, of which RCT = 16]
5. American Institute of Ultrasound in Medicine. AIUM practice guideline for the performance of obstetric ultrasound examination. *J Ultrasound Med.* 2013 Jun; 32(6):1083–1101. [Review]
6. American College of Obstetricians and Gynecologists. Ultrasonography in pregnancy. ACOG Practice Bulletin No. 101. Washington, DC: American College of Obstetricians and Gynecologists; 2009. [Review]
7. Gonzaga MA. An exploratory study of the views of Ugandan women and health practitioners on the use of sonography to establish fetal sex. *Pan Afr Med J.* 2011;9:6. [II-2]
8. Raphael T. Disclosing the sex of the fetus: A view from the UK. *Ultrasound Obstet Gynecol.* 2002;20:421–424. [Review]
9. Nabhan AF, Aflaifel N. High feedback versus low feedback of prenatal ultrasound for reducing maternal anxiety and improving maternal health behaviour in pregnancy. *Cochrane Rev.* 2015. [Meta-analysis, 4 RCTs, n = 365]
10. Reddy UM, Abuhamad AZ, Levine D, Saade GR. Imaging. *J Ultrasound Med.* 2014;33:745–757. [Review]
11. Gardosi J. Dating of pregnancy: Time to forget the last menstrual period. *Ultrasound Obstet Gynecol.* 1997;9(6):367–368. [Review]
12. Chervenak FA, Skupski DW, Romero R, et al. How accurate is fetal biometry in the assessment of fetal age? *Am J Obstet Gynecol.* 1998 Apr;178(4):678–687. [II-2]

13. Taipale P, Hilesmaa V. Predicting delivery date by ultrasound and last menstrual period in early gestation. *Obstet Gynecol.* 2001;97:189–194. [II-3]
14. Chavez MR, Ananth CV, Smulian JC, et al. Transcerebellar measurement with particular emphasis on the third trimester: A reliable predictor of gestational age. *AJOG.* 2004;191: 979–984. [II-2]
15. Delle Donne H, Faiúndes A, Tristão EG, et al. Sonographic identification and measurement of the epiphyseal ossification centers as markers of fetal gestational age. *J Clin Ultrasound.* 2005 Oct;33(8):394–400. [II-2]
16. American College of Obstetricians and Gynecologists. Method for estimating due date. ACOG Committee Opinion No. 611. Washington, DC: American College of Obstetricians and Gynecologists; 2014. [III]
17. Abuhamad A (ed.). Ultrasound in Obstetrics and Gynecology: A Practical Approach. *GLOWM.* 2014. Online. [III]
18. Saltvedt S, Almström H, Kublickas M, et al. Detection of malformations in chromosomally normal fetuses by routine ultrasound at 12 or 18 weeks of gestation—A randomised controlled trial in 39 572 pregnancies. *BJOG.* 2006;113:664–674. [RCT, $n = 39,572$]
19. Rossi AC, Prefumo F. Accuracy of ultrasonography at 11–14 weeks of gestation for detection of fetal structural anomalies. *AJOG.* 2013;122:1160–1167. [meta-analysis, 19 articles]
20. Doubilet PM, Benson CB, Bourne T, et al. Diagnostic criteria for nonviable pregnancy early in the first trimester. *N Engl J Med.* 2013 Oct 10;369(15):1443–1451. [Review]
21. Abdallah Y, Daemen A, Krik E, et al. Limitations of current definitions of miscarriage using mean gestational sac diameter and crown-rump length measurements: A multicenter observational study. *Ultrasound Obstet Gynecol.* 2011;38:497–502. [II-3]
22. Brown DL, Emerson DS, Felker RE, et al. Diagnosis of embryonic demise by endovaginal sonography. *J Ultrasound Med.* 1990;9:631–636. [II-3]
23. Goldstein I, Zimmer EA, Tamir A, et al. Evaluation of normal gestational sac growth: Appearance of embryonic heartbeat and embryo body movements using transvaginal technique. *Obstet Gynecol.* 1991;77:885–888. [II-]
24. Westin M, Saltvedt S, Bergman G, et al. Routine ultrasound examination at 12 or 18 gestational weeks for prenatal detection of major congenital heart malformations? A randomised controlled trial comprising 36 299 fetuses. *BJOG.* 2006;113:675–682. [RCT, $n = 39,572$]
25. Wax J, Minkoff H, Johnson A, et al. Consensus report on the detailed fetal anatomic ultrasound examination: Indications, components, and qualifications. *J Ultrasound Med.* 2014 Feb;33(2):189–195. [III]
26. McKenna D, Tharmaratnam S, Mahsud S, et al. A randomized trial using ultrasound to identify the high-risk fetus in a low-risk population. *Obstet Gynecol.* 2003 Apr;101(4):626–632. [RTC, $n = 1,998$]
27. Bricker L, Medley N, Pratt JJ. Routine ultrasound in late pregnancy (after 24 weeks' gestation). *Cochrane Library.* 2015. [meta-analysis; 13 RCTs, $n = 34,980$]
28. Roma E, Arnau A, Berdala R, et al. Ultrasound screening for fetal growth restriction at 36 vs 32 weeks' gestation: A randomized trial (ROUTE). *Ultrasound Obstet Gynecol.* 2015;46:391–397. [RCT, $n = 2,586$]
29. Sovio U, White IR, Dacey A, et al. Screening for fetal growth restriction with universal third trimester ultrasonography in nulliparous women in the Pregnancy Outcome Prediction (POP) study: A prospective cohort study. *Lancet.* 2015 Sept 7. Pii: S0140–6736(15)00131–00132. [II-1]
30. Proud J, Grant AM. Third trimester placental grading by ultrasonography as a test of fetal wellbeing. *BMJ.* 1987;1641–1644. [RCT, n-2,000]
31. Chen KH, Seow KM, Chen LR. The role of preterm placental calcification on assessing risks of stillbirth. *Placenta.* 2015 Sep;36(9):1039–1044. [II-2]
32. Alfirevic Z, Stampalija T, Medley N. Fetal and umbilical Doppler ultrasound in normal pregnancy. *Cochrane Database Syst Rev.* 2015. [meta-analysis, 5 RCTs; $n = 14,185$]
33. Alfirevic Z, Stampalija T, Medley N. Fetal and umbilical Doppler ultrasound in high-risk pregnancies. *Cochrane Database Syst Rev.* 2013. [meta-analysis, 18 RCTs; $n = 10,000+$]
34. Berkley E, Chauhan SP, Abuhamad A. Doppler assessment of the fetus with intrauterine growth restriction. *Am J Obstet Gynecol.* 2012 Apr;206(4):300–308. [Review]
35. Bhide A, Acharya G, Bilardo CM, et al. ISUOG practice guidelines: Use of Doppler ultrasonography in obstetrics. *Ultrasound Obstet Gynecol* 2013 Feb;41(2):233–239. [III]
36. Pretlove SJ, Fox CE, Khan KS, Kilby MD. Noninvasive methods of detecting fetal anaemia: A systematic review and meta-analysis. *BJOG.* 2009;116:1558–1567. [meta-analysis, 9 RCTs; $n = 675$]
37. Mari G, Norton ME, Stone J, et al. Society for Maternal-Fetal Medicine (SMFM) Clinical Guideline #8: The fetus at risk for anemia—Diagnosis and management. *Am J Obstet Gynecol.* 2015;212(6):697–710. [Guideline; III]
38. Mari G, Hanif F, Treadwell MC, Kruger M. Gestational age at delivery and Doppler waveforms in very preterm intrauterine growth-restricted fetuses as predictors of perinatal mortality. *J Ultrasound Med.* 2007 May;26(5):555–559. [II-2]
39. Morris RK, Seiman TJ, Verma M, et al. Systemic review and meta-analysis of the test accuracy of ductus venosus Doppler to predict compromise of fetal/neonatal wellbeing in high risk pregnancies with placental insufficiency. *Eur J Obstet Gynecol Reprod Biol.* 2010;152(1):3–12. [meta-analysis, 16 cohort, 2 cross-sectional; $n = 2,267$]
40. Lees CC, Marlow N, van Wassenaer A, et al. 2 year neurodevelopmental and intermediate perinatal outcomes in infants with very preterm fetal growth restriction (TRUFFLE): A randomized trial. *Lancet.* 2015 May 30:385(9983):2162–2172. [RCT]
41. Stampalija T, Gyte GM, Alfirevic Z. Utero-placental Doppler ultrasound for improving pregnancy outcome. *Cochrane Database of Syst Rev.* 2010;(9). [metaanalysis, 2 RCTs; $n = 4993$]
42. American College of Obstetricians and Gynecologists. Hypertension in pregnancy. Report of the American College of Obstetricians and Gynecologists' Task Force on Hypertension in Pregnancy. *Obstet Gynecol.* 2013;122(5):1122–1131. [Guideline; III]
43. Lalor JG, Fawole B, Alfirevic Z, Devane D. et al. Biophysical profile for fetal assessment in high risk pregnancies. *Cochrane Library.* 2012;(3). [metaanalysis, 5 RCTs, $n = 2974$]
44. Domin CM, Smith EJ, Terplan M. Transvaginal ultrasonographic measurement of cervical length as a predictor of preterm birth. *Ultrasound Q.* 2010 Dec:241–248. [metaanalysis, 23 RCTs, $n = 26,792$]
45. Conde-Agudelo A, Romero R, Hassan SS, Yeo L. Transvaginal sonographic cervical length for the prediction of spontaneous preterm birth in twin pregnancies: A systematic review and metaanalysis. *AJOG.* 2010;203:128.e1–12. [metaanalysis, 21 RCTs, $n = 3523$]
46. Mancuso MS, Szychowski JM, Owen J, et al. Cervical funneling: Effect on gestational length and ultrasound-indicated cerclage in high-risk women. *AJOG.* 2010;203:259.e1–5. [RCT, $n = 301$]
47. Berghella V, Bega G, Tolosa JE, Berghella M. Ultrasound assessment of the cervix. *Clin Obstet Gynecol.* 2003 Dec;46(4):947–962. [Review]
48. American College of Obstetricians and Gynecologists. Prediction and Prevention of Preterm Birth. ACOG Practice Bulletin No. 130. Washington, DC: American College of Obstetricians and Gynecologists; 2012. [review]
49. Parry S, Simhan H, Elovitz M, Iams J. Universal maternal cervical length screening during the second trimester: Pros and cons of a strategy to identify women at risk of spontaneous preterm delivery. *Am J Obstet Gynecol.* 2012 Aug;207(2):101–106. [III]
50. Orzechowski KM, Boelig RC, Baxter JK, Berghella V. A universal transvaginal cervical length screening program for preterm birth prevention. *Obstet Gynecol.* 2014 Sep;124(3):520–525. [II-1]

51. Fonseca EB, Celik, E, Parra M, et al. Progesterone and the risk of preterm birth among women with a short cervix. *N Eng J Med*. 2007 Aug 2:357(5):462–469. [RCT]
52. Hassan SS, Romero R, Vidyadhari D, et al. Vaginal progesterone reduces the rate of preterm birth in women with a sonographic short cervix: A multicenter, randomized, double-blind, placebo-controlled trial. *Ultrasound Obstet Gynecol*. 2011 Jul;38(1):18–31. [RCT]
53. Khalifeh A, Berghella V. Universal cervical length screening in singleton gestations without a prior preterm birth: Ten reasons why it should be implemented. *Am J Obstet Gynecol*. 2015 Dec 18. pii:S0002–9378(15)02517-X. doi: 10.1016/j.ajog.2015.12.017. [Epub ahead of print] [III]
54. Meis PJ, Klebanoff M, Thom E, et al. Prevention of recurrent preterm delivery by 17 alpha-hydroxyprogesterone caproate. *N Engl J Med*. 2003 Jun 12;348(24):2379–2385. [RCT]
55. Berghella V, Mackeen AD. Cervical length screening with ultrasound-indicated cerclage compared with history-indicated cerclage for prevention of preterm birth: A meta-analysis. *Obestet Gynecol*. 2011 Jul;118(1):148–155. [meta-analysis; 4 RCTs, $n = 467$]
56. Ness A, Visintine J, Ricci E, Berghella V. Does knowledge of cervical length and fetal fibronectin affect management of women with threatened preterm labor? A randomized trial. *Am J Obstet Gynecol*. 2007 Oct;197(4):426. [RCT]
57. Abuhamad A (2016). Three-dimension fetal echocardiography: Basic and advanced applications In *A Practical Guide to Fetal Echocardiography: Normal and Abnormal Hearts*. 3rd ed, pp. 215. Philadelphia, PA: Lippincott, Williams & Wilkins. [III]
58. Lapaire O, Alder J, Peukert R, et al. Two versus three dimensional ultrasound in the second and third trimester of pregnancy: Impact on recognition and maternal-fetal bonding. A prospective pilot study. *Arch Gynecol Obstet*. 2007;276:475–479. [RCT, $n = 60$]
59. Leung KY, Ngai CS, Lee A, et al. The effects on maternal anxiety of two-dimensional versus two-plus three-/four-dimensional ultrasound in pregnancies at risk of fetal abnormalities: A randomized study. *Ultrasound Obstet Gynecol*. 2006:28;249–254. [RCT, $n = 124$]
60. Hoffman JI, Kaplan S. The incidence of congenital heart disease. *J Am Coll Cardiol*. 2002 Jun 19;39(12):1890–1900. [II-3]
61. Cuneo BF, Curran LF, Davis N, Elrad H. Trends in prenatal diagnosis of critical cardiac defects in an integrated obstetric and pediatric cardiology imaging center. *J Perinatol*. 2004 Nov;24(11):674–678. [II-3]
62. Abuhamad A. Congenital heart disease: Incidence, risk factors, and prevention. In *A Practical Guide to Fetal Echocardiography: Normal and Abnormal Hearts*. 3rd ed, pp 3. Philadelphia, PA: Lippincott, Williams & Wilkins, 2016. [III]
63. Carvalho JS, Allan LD, Chaoui R, et al. ISUOG Practice Guidelines (updated): Sonographic screening examination of the fetal heart. *Ultrasound Obstet Gynecol*. 2013 Mar;41(3): 348–359 [Guidelines; III]
64. Lee W, Allan L, Carvalho JS, et al. ISUOG consensus statement: What constitutes a fetal echocardiogram? *Ultrasound Obstet Gynecol*. 2008 Aug;32(2):239–242. [Guideline; III]
65. American Institute of Ultrasound in Medicine. AIUM practice guideline for the performance of fetal echocardiography. *J Ultrasound Med*. 2013 Jun;32(6):1067–1082. [Guideline; III]
66. Wiechec M, Knafel A, Nocun A. Prenatal detection of congenital heart defects at the 11- to 13-week scan using a simple color Doppler protocol including the 4-chamber and 3-vessel and trachea views. *J Ultrasound Med*. 2015 Apr;34(4):585–594. [II-2]

Prenatal diagnosis and screening for aneuploidy

Dawnette Lewis

KEY POINTS

- **All women should be offered aneuploidy screening**, ideally starting in the first trimester. Population screening should have **genetic counseling services available** to discuss the different modalities, advantages and disadvantages, and the time frame for each test prior to screening. All women should have counseling available if desired or if an "abnormal" result occurs. The difference between a screening and a diagnostic test should be clearly explained before any testing.
- Issues of **sensitivity, specificity, positive, and negative predictive values** are vital to the interpretation of a screening test. Positive predictive value of a screening test is greatly influenced by **prevalence** rates in the population tested.
- **The performance of a screening test depends on the age of the women** screened (which determines prevalence of trisomies), **women's preference** of screening methods, their **choice of invasive testing**, and their **attitudes toward pregnancy termination**. There is as of now **no definitive noninvasive prenatal diagnostic test. The only diagnostic tests are invasive, i.e., chorion villus sampling (CVS) and amniocentesis.**
- Compared with a Down's screening policy of amniocentesis for age ≥35 years of age and universal ultrasound at 18 weeks, a policy of **nuchal translucency (NT) screening is associated with similar numbers of Down's neonates born and a decrease in invasive tests.**
- **First-trimester screening (FTS)** includes NT, pregnancy associated plasma protein-A (PAPP-A), and human chorionic gonadotropin (B-HCG), and can be performed at 10 3/7 to 13 6/7 weeks, with the best detection rate achieved at 11 weeks. The overall detection rate (sensitivity) is about **84–87%** (false positive rate or FPR, 5%). FTS should be offered only if
  - Appropriate training and ongoing quality monitoring programs are in place for both ultrasound (NT) and laboratory assays of analytes
  - Sufficient information and resources are available to provide comprehensive counseling to women regarding the different options and limitations of these tests
  - Access to an appropriate diagnostic test (i.e., CVS) is available when screening results are positive
- **Compared with management using second-trimester screening (STS), management using FTS is associated with a significant reduction in induction for post-term pregnancy because of better dating with first-trimester ultrasound.**
- **Analyte screening (quadruple marker screen)** can **detect approximately 70%–81% of affected pregnancies (FPR 5%).**
- **Integrative screening** has the **best detection rate for Down's syndrome (95%)**, with a low (1%–4%) FPR, but **results** are available **only in the second trimester.**
- **Stepwise or contingent sequential screening** offer the same 95% detection rate, a reasonable 5% FPR, and availability of results in the first trimester.
- **Cell-free fetal DNA** screens for Trisomy 21, 18, and 13 and can be performed at ≥10 weeks. In a mixed population of low and high risk women the sensitivity of cell free DNA (cfDNA) for trisomy 21 was reported between 99% and 100%, for trisomy 18 between 90% and 99%, and for trisomy 13 greater than 99%, with a very low (usually <1%) FPR. Experts in general currently still recommend first- and second-trimester noninvasive aneuploidy screening over cfDNA in low-risk populations, but this is an area of intense research currently. Indications for cfDNA screening are currently maternal age ≥35 years at delivery; fetal ultrasound findings that indicate an increased risk for aneuploidy, specifically for trisomies 21, 18, 13; previous pregnancy with a trisomy detectable by cfDNA screening; positive screen results for aneuploidy; and parental balanced translocation with increased risk of fetal trisomy 13 or 21.
- **Second-trimester "genetic" ultrasound** has an impact, among other things, on dating, induction rates, and anatomic evaluation of the fetus. As a modality for genetic screening, the data is more limited compared with other available tests. Major anomalies (e.g., congenital cardiac defects and duodenal atresia), and some markers (especially nuchal thickening, short humerus or femur, and echogenic bowel) are associated with a significantly higher risk for Down's syndrome.
- **Second-trimester amniocentesis is safer than transcervical (TC) CVS or early amniocentesis (<15 weeks). Early amniocentesis should never be performed. With expert operators (>400 CVS), CVS by any route may be as safe as second-trimester amniocentesis.**
- If **earlier diagnosis is required, transabdominal (TA) CVS is preferable to early amniocentesis or TC CVS.** In circumstances where TA CVS may be technically difficult, the preferred options are TC CVS in the first trimester with expert operator, or second-trimester amniocentesis, per patients' preference.
- Chromosomal microarray analysis **(CMA) should be recommended as the primary test (replacing conventional karyotype) to patients undergoing prenatal diagnosis in whom a structural abnormality is detected by ultrasound.**
- Trisomy 21 is the most common trisomy at birth. Its incidence increases with increasing maternal age.

DEFINITION

Prenatal diagnosis: Prenatal diagnosis incorporates screening for fetal aneuploidies and anomalies, with many different modalities, including population screening, individual risk assessment, genetic counseling and diagnostic testing.

SCREENING VERSUS DIAGNOSTIC TESTS

Prior to screening a population with an available test, test specifics should be assessed. **Issues of prevalence, sensitivity, specificity, and positive and negative predictive values are vital to the interpretation of a screening test** and are a large part of the problem that exists in interpreting the value of a test by either practitioners or the public. Sensitivity of a screening test can also be called detection rate. Table 5.1 lists the characteristics of an ideal perinatal screening test. High sensitivity and specificity are preferable; however, the prevalence of a condition (based upon the population tested) will ultimately determine the value of a positive or negative result (Figure 5.1). With lower prevalence, the chance of a particular "positive" test to be a true finding is much less. For example, based upon the numbers from Figure 5.1, if all the women with a positive test from group "A" had a chorionic villus sampling (CVS), there would be one positive result for every 55 CVS performed. If all the women in "B" had a CVS, one out of every 2.4 tests would yield a positive result.

The performance of a screening test depends on the age of the women screened (which determines prevalence of trisomies), **women's preference** of screening methods, their **choice of invasive testing,** and their **attitudes toward pregnancy termination. There is as of now no definitive noninvasive prenatal diagnostic test.** The only **diagnostic tests are invasive, i.e., CVS and amniocentesis.**

PRETEST GENERAL COUNSELING

There is no treatment for aneuploidy, so the woman must be aware that the **main aims of screening for aneuploidy** are the **possibility of termination,** and the **knowledge of the diagnosis,** with no definite proof that this knowledge will improve outcome. Similarly, there are usually minimal, experimental, and often no treatments for fetal anomalies, so the woman must be aware that the main aims of screening for anomalies are (similarly) the possibility of termination, and the knowledge of the diagnosis, with no definite proof that this knowledge will improve outcome. Down's syndrome is the most frequent chromosomal disorder among live-born infants, with an expected prevalence of about 1/600–1/800 live births, and the most common identifiable cause of mental retardation, with a life expectancy of almost 50 years (see later in this chapter).

While complicated, discussion of sensitivity (detection rates) at 5% FTR of main screening tests (highlighted in Table 5.2) is necessary. Specific resources (time, expertise, plus the availability of genetic counseling) are paramount. Continuing education of health care providers is necessary. Some couples might prefer a screening approach with earliest detection even with an higher, for example 5%, FPR (e.g., FTS), some highest detection with lowest FPR (e.g., integrative screening). Most women who present in first trimester and opt for aneuploidy screening in centers of excellence choose sequential screening, such as stepwise or contingent screening.

No matter the sensitivity of available tests, for women undergoing screening, particularly those in a higher risk group, **detailed discussions regarding the advantages and disadvantages of screening versus diagnostic testing should occur.** After such counseling, each woman can make the most informed and best choice for their situation. **Since screening tests will never detect 100% of disease, the option of**

Table 5.1 Ideal Perinatal Screening Test

- Identify common or important fetal disorder
- Be cost effective
- High detection rate; low FPR
- Be reliable and reproducible
- Diagnostic test exists
- Be positive early in pregnancy
- Possible intervention if screening test if positive

Abbreviation: FPR, false positive rate.

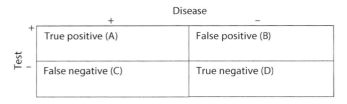

Sensitivity = A/A + C

Specificity = D/B + D

Positive predictive value (PPV) = A/A + B

Negative predictive value (NPV) = D/C + D

Effect of prevalence

N = 100,000

Sensitivity 90%

False positive = 5%

Prevalence = 0.1%		Prevalence = 4%	
90	5,000	3,600	5,000
10	94,900	400	91,000

PPV = 1.8%   PPV = 41.9%

NPV = 99.9%   NPV = 99.5%

Figure 5.1 Screening test concepts and effect of prevalence.

Table 5.2 Screening Tests for Down's Syndrome

Test	FPR (%)	Sensitivity (%)
Age	5	25–30
First trimester (11–14 weeks)		
NT	5	65–80
PAPP-A and β-HCG	5	60–80
Age, NT, PAPP-A, and β-HCG (FTS)	5	85
Age, NT, PAPP-A, and HCG (FTS)	5	80–85
Cell-free DNA	.5	99.9
Second trimester (15–21 weeks)		
Age, MSAFP, HCG, uE$_3$ (TS)	5	60–70
Age, MSAFP, HCG, uE$_3$, inhibin (QS)	5	70–81
Integrative (nondisclosure of FTS)		
Integrated (NT, PAPP-A, QS)	4	95
Serum integrated (PAPP-A, QS)	5	85–90
Sequential (disclosure of FTS)		
Independent	11	95
Stepwise	5	95
Contingent	5	88–94
Genetic ultrasound	5	50–70
Extended ultrasound*	5	80–85

Abbreviations: uE$_3$, unconjugated estriol; TS, triple screen; *, genetic ultrasound and serum screening; QS, quadruple screen; FTS, first trimester screen; FPR, false positive rate.

diagnostic testing in higher risk populations can be offered. Several studies have shown that **most pregnant women prefer early (vs. later) screening** for Down's syndrome.

Many women still believe that the whole purpose behind screening for aneuploidy is so that a couple can terminate a pregnancy prior to viability. While it is true that couples faced with the reality of an aneuploid pregnancy may opt for termination, **the purpose of prenatal diagnosis and screening is to provide information.** If an abnormality is found, depending on the specifics, couples can be provided with specific information regarding their situation. When a couple decides to carry an abnormal pregnancy to term, the antenatal, intrapartum, and postpartum care can be performed under more ideal circumstances, hopefully altering the outcome. Also, one can not underestimate the effect that preparation can have for the individuals involved (Table 5.2).

ANTENATAL NONINVASIVE ANEUPLOIDY SCREENING
History

Langdon Down, in 1866, reported that the skin of individuals with trisomy 21 appears enlarged. In the 1970's data became available on the relationship with maternal age and increased risk for aneuploidy. A statistically relevant difference was seen between the 30- to 34-year-old group, and the 35- to 39-year-old group, so that this difference led to the offering of women 35 years of age diagnostic evaluation for karyotype. Maternal serum alpha-fetoprotein (MSAFP) was originally found to be elevated in women carrying fetuses with neural tube defects (NTDs), then in 1984 a low MSAFP was associated with a higher risk of Down's syndrome. NT first-trimester ultrasound screening was introduced by in the early 1990s [1]. While live births to women >35 years of age continue to increase, due to better, more diffuse screening the number of Down's neonates is decreasing.

Principles

All women should be offered aneuploidy screening, ideally in the first trimester. There is presently a general consensus in the United States that invasive testing for Down's syndrome be offered to those with a second-trimester risk of 1:270 or higher (live-born risk of 1:380). The cut-off level and subsequent public policy was determined over 30 years ago and was based on a maternal age risk of 35 years at delivery. Factors considered in determining this value included the prevalence of disease, a perceived significant increase in the trisomy 21 risk after this age, the risk of invasive testing, the availability of resources, and a cost benefit analysis. Since that time, a number of additional screening tests for Down's syndrome have become available that challenge the validity of maternal age as a single indication for invasive testing. There are a limited amount of randomized control trials (RCTs) for the evaluation of different tests. Most data comes from cohort studies or cross-sectional analysis.

Age

The risk of fetal trisomy 21 increases with maternal age, but decreases with the gestational age (GA) at assessment in determining the risk, secondary to in utero death rates (Table 5.3) [2].

Women greater than 35 years of age have a higher individual risk than younger women; however, the vast majority of Down's syndrome pregnancies are born to the <35-year-old age group. Screening programs have developed to try and detect affected pregnancies in both the "higher" and "lower" risk groups.

Table 5.3 Risk for Down's Syndrome Based on Maternal and Gestational Age

Maternal age	Gestational age (weeks)			
	12	16	20	Live-born
20	1/1068	1/1200	1/1295	1/1527
25	1/946	1/1062	1/1147	1/1352
30	1/626	1/703	1/759	1/895
31	1/543	1/610	1/658	1/776
32	1/461	1/518	1/559	1/659
33	1/383	1/430	1/464	1/547
34	1/312	1/350	1/378	1/446
35	1/249	1/280	1/302	1/356
36	1/196	1/220	1/238	1/280
37	1/152	1/171	1/185	1/218
38	1/117	1/131	1/142	1/167
39	1/89	1/100	1/108	1/128
40	1/68	1/76	1/82	1/97
42	1/38	1/43	1/46	1/55
44	1/21	1/24	1/26	1/30
45	1/16	1/18	1/19	1/23

FIRST-TRIMESTER SCREENING
Nuchal Translucency

NT is elevated in fetuses with Down's syndrome at **10 3/7 to 13 6/7 weeks** (crown-rump length [CRL] about 36–86 mm). The NT measurement is obtained in a mid-sagittal plane with the neck of the fetus in a neutral position. The amnion should be seen separately from the neck. The image should be enlarged >75% of the screen. The measurement is obtained from the inner to inner aspect of the NT, and multiples of the medians are used to calculate the Down's risk via computer software. An increased NT is >70% sensitive for trisomy 21, trisomy 18, and trisomy 13 (Table 5.2) [1]. Rigorous training, certification, and on-going quality control are necessary to achieve the detection rates published in the literature (www.fetalmedicine.com; www.ntqr.org). The optimal time to perform NT for Down's screening is about 11 weeks.

Compared with a Down's screening policy of amniocentesis for age ≥35years of age and ultrasound at 18 weeks, a policy of NT screening is associated with similar numbers of Down's neonates born (a nonsignificant 37.5% decrease) and **a significant 82% decrease in invasive tests** [3]. One explanation for the small nonsignificant difference in Down's neonates born alive may be that NT screening certainly identifies better Down's fetuses, but the majority of these identified Down's fetuses are those that would have miscarried without intervention.

Biochemistry

The maternal serum analytes measured are B-HCG and PAPP-A. **B-HCG** normally decreases in pregnancy, but is **increased** in fetuses affected with trisomy 21. **Free B-HCG** performs better than **total HCG** as an independent marker, but there does not appear to be a clinically significant difference in sensitivity when either is combined with NT and PAPPA-A for FTS [4]. **PAPP-A** normally increases in pregnancy, but is *decreased* in fetuses affected with trisomy 21. HCG discrimination is greatest at 13 weeks, while PAPP-A's is greatest at 10 weeks, making 11 weeks the optimal time for first-trimester analyte screening.

First Trimester Screening

FTS consists of measurement of the **NT** combined with maternal serum screening (**PAPP-A** and **B-HCG**). Over 20 studies in over 200,000 women have been performed to assess the sensitivity of this screening test, making this the best studied screening test in pregnancy [4–7]. The GA for FTS is about **10 3/7 to 13 6/7 weeks** (about 73–98 days; CRL about 36–86 mm). The usual cutoff risk is 1:270. The detection rate (sensitivity) is about **84–87%** (95% CI 80%–90%). **The best detection rate is achieved at 11 weeks.**

FTS should be offered only if the following criteria can be met [4–7]:

1. Appropriate training and ongoing quality monitoring programs are in place for both ultrasound (NT) and laboratory assays of analytes.
2. Sufficient information and resources are available to provide comprehensive counseling to women regarding the different options and limitations of these tests.
3. Access to an appropriate diagnostic test (i.e., CVS) is available when screening results are positive.

The Maternal-Fetal Medicine Foundation (www.mfmf.org) and the Fetal Medicine Foundation (www.fetalmedicine.com) both provide NT education and quality review programs. There is sufficient evidence to support implementing FTS for Down's syndrome provided the above three requirements are met. Almost 85% of women in the United States present for care within 12 weeks and can be offered FTS. FTS can provide high detection, early reassurance, more time / diagnostic options, earlier completion of aneuploidy screening.

Compared with management using STS, management using FTS is associated also with a significant reduction in induction for post-term pregnancy because of better dating with first-trimester ultrasound [8].

Nasal Bone
Over 12 studies in over 18,000 women demonstrated that nasal bone when imaged at 11–14 weeks is absent in approximately 70% of Down's fetuses, and in only 1.5% of unaffected fetuses. When added to FTS (NT, PAPP-A, and B-HCG), it can increase the detection rate to about 95%, decreasing the FPR to 2%. Possibly given to the difficulty of this exam, these data have not been confirmed in all studies. Abnormal ductus venosus Doppler flow and tricuspid regurgitation have also been found to be >70% sensitive for trisomy 21, but there is insufficient prospective data for any increase in accuracy over FTS alone.

SECOND-TRIMESTER SCREENING
Maternal analyte screening had the first reported association with Down syndrome with low **MSAFP** (multiples of the median [MoM] 0.75), followed by the association of high **hCG** (MoM 2.3) and a low **unconjugated estriol** (MoM 0.7) to form the **"triple screen."** The detection rate for women under 35 with a triple screen ranges between 57% and 74%, with a constant 5% FPR [3,5]. For women above 35 (using similar cutoff values), the sensitivity increases to 87%, but the FPR also balloons to 25% [9]. **Inhibin** was added to analyte screening **(quadruple screen)**, but, since levels correlate somewhat with hCG, it is not an independent predictor like the other markers, and the increase in detection is more limited (7–11 percentage points). Approximately 70–81% of cases are detected in the majority of studies, holding the FPR at 5% [4,6]. This screening test can be performed between 15 and 22 weeks, with best results obtained at 16–18 weeks. Values need to be adjusted, as needed, for diabetes, obesity, and other factors.

Other combinations of markers have been assessed; however, with the addition of extra markers, the potential benefit versus the cost must be balanced. With each additional marker, costs to society reach into the millions secondary to the numbers of pregnancies tested each year. The relative cost and value of raising the sensitivity or lowering the false-positive rate a few percentage points is an ongoing debate.

COMBINING BOTH FIRST- AND SECOND-TRIMESTER TESTS
Combined screening programs in the first trimester (using both ultrasound assessments of the NT as well as maternal analytes) and the second trimester (using maternal analytes) have been described. Patterns of testing include sequential testing (results given after each test) and integrated testing (delaying reporting until both tests have been completed).

Integrative Screening
Performance of screening tests at different times during pregnancy with a single result provided to the patient only after all tests have been completed. A protocol for integrated screening for Down syndrome is based upon tests performed during the first and second trimester (NT, PAPP-A, MSAFP, HCG, estriol, and inhibin). Mathematical models calculated that >85% of affected pregnancies would be detected with a FPR of only 0.9%. The FASTER trial (First- And Second-Trimester Evaluation of Risk) performed integrated screening in 33,557 women (84 with Down syndrome) [6]. Cut-off values for the different tests varied (first-trimester combined test cutoff 1:150, second-trimester "quad screen", 1:300). The authors report a sensitivity of 86% with first-trimester screening (FPR 5%), 85% with second-trimester (FPR high at 8.5%), and, when combined, a 94% detection of Down syndrome cases. If results are revealed after second-trimester screening, the FPR is only 4.9%, with the **best sensitivity**. If NT is not available, an "integrated serum screening test" has a detection rate of 85% with 3.9% FPR [4]. Disadvantages of integrative screening include the lack of early diagnosis, the physical and psychological ramifications created if an abnormality is found and the woman opts for termination (compared with the first trimester), the increase in costs (compared with either FTS or STS), the perception of "hiding" abnormal results, as well as the limitations it places on multiple gestations if discordant karyotypes are found.

Sequential Screening
It involves performance of different screening tests at different times during pregnancy with results provided to the patient after each test. There are three approaches to sequential testing: independent, stepwise, and contingent.

Independent
This approach involves the independent interpretation of FTS and STS. While the sensitivity is as exemplary with this approach as with integrative screening (94–95%), combining screening tests and revealing the results after each increases the chance for false-positive results. The FASTER trial's [6] FPR was 10.8% with sequential independent screening, far too high for population-based usage. As a high FPR means higher loss rates due to more invasive testing, independent sequential screening is the least efficient risk assessment strategy, and should NOT be used.

Step-Wise
Both FTS and STS (usually quadruple screen or QS) are performed, with results revealed after FTS: If FTS risk is above a certain cutoff, invasive testing (i.e., CVS) is offered; if FTS is below a certain cutoff, STS is recommended with a final risk revealed at that point. In the FASTER trial, such an approach (low cutoff 1:150; high cutoff 1:300) had a **detection rate of 95% with an FPR of 4.9%** [6]. The advantages of this approach are a very high detection rate (as with integrative screening), with the option of early results in first trimester for the highest risk women. **This is currently the most common way to perform screening for aneuploidy in women presenting in the first trimester** in centers with adequate expertise and facilities. With FTS and such low FPRs, there has also been a decrease in the number of women requesting invasive prenatal diagnosis.

Contingent
Both FTS and STS (usually QS) are performed, with results revealed after FTS: If FTS risk is above a certain cutoff (e.g., 1/150), invasive testing (i.e., CVS) is offered; if FTS is below a certain cutoff (e.g., 1/300), no further screening is necessary; if FTS is in between, STS is recommended with a final risk revealed at that point. Careful determination of risk cutoffs is necessary. This strategy has not been studied prospectively.

CELL-FREE FETAL DNA SCREENING
The discovery of cell free fetal DNA (placental DNA) in maternal plasma opened up new possibilities for noninvasive maternal prenatal screening for fetal chromosomal aneuploidy. The methods utilized for detecting fetal aneuploidy differ based on whether amplified regions throughout the genome, chromosome specific regions or single nucleotide polymorphisms are the targets for sequencing are used [10–14]. In the high-risk population—those who have undergone prenatal diagnosis—the sensitivity of cfDNA for trisomy 21 is greater than 99%, for trisomy 18 greater than 99% and for trisomy 13 greater than 90% [15–19].

In a mixed population of low and high risk women the sensitivity of cfDNA for trisomy 21 was reported between 99% and 100%, for trisomy 18 between 90% and 99% and for trisomy 13 greater than 99% [19–21].

These studies have all shown that fetal fraction increases with GA and that the fetal fraction is decreased in obese patient. These studies also seem to say that an equivocal result or non-result on cfDNA should be cause for concern because this raises this possibility of aneuploidy.

The Society for Maternal-Fetal Medicine regarding prenatal aneuploidy screening using cell-free DNA made the following recommendations [22]:
Indications:

1. Maternal age ≥ 35 years at delivery
2. Fetal ultrasound findings that indicate an increased risk for aneuploidy, specifically for trisomies 21, 18, 13
3. History of a previous pregnancy with a trisomy detectable by cfDNA screening
4. Positive screen results for aneuploidy
5. Parental balanced translocation with increased risk of fetal trisomy 13 or 21

After failed cfDNA test, genetic counseling should be performed that includes offering diagnostic testing [15].

"GENETIC" ULTRASOUND SCREENING FOR DOWN'S SYNDROME
An ultrasound of the fetus performed at **18–24 weeks** is associated with several important benefits (see Chapter 4). One of the benefits is the antenatal detection of anomalies. The identification of a fetus with an issue allows for directed counseling and optimization of antepartum, intrapartum, and postpartum care. Whether routine or targeted anatomic assessment is being performed, it should be done by experienced centers with ongoing quality assessment to increase detection of anomalies and limit false positive results.

The in-utero diagnosis of Down's syndrome can be suspected when anomalies or physical features that occur more frequently in Down's syndrome than in the general population are noted on an ultrasound examination. Certain of these major structural congenital anomalies, such as atrioventricular canal or duodenal atresia, strongly suggest the possibility of Down syndrome and are independent indications to offer invasive testing. Although, when present, there is a high risk of trisomy 21, these anomalies have low sensitivity and, thus, are not useful in screening. For example, when **duodenal atresia** is identified, there is approximately a 40% risk of Down's syndrome, yet it is seen in only 8% of affected fetuses. About 50% of Down's fetuses have **congenital heart defects**.

Physical characteristics that are not structural anomalies but occur more commonly in fetuses with Down's syndrome are called **markers.** By comparing the prevalence of markers in Down's syndrome fetuses to their prevalence in the normal population, a likelihood ratio (LR) can be calculated which can be used to modify risk. This is the basis for ultrasound screening for Down's syndrome. In order for a marker to be useful for Down's syndrome screening, it should be sensitive (i.e., present in a high proportion of Down's syndrome pregnancies), specific (i.e., not commonly seen in normal fetuses), easily imaged in standard sonographic examination, and present early enough in the second trimester that diagnostic testing can be performed so that results are available when pregnancy termination remains an option. A list of presently available markers and LRs are seen in Tables 5.4 and 5.5, respectively [23–25]. Markers commonly sought to assess the risk of Down syndrome are discussed in the following sections.

Table 5.4 Selected Ultrasound Findings Associated with Down's Syndrome

Major anomalies
- Congenital heart defects
- Duodenal atresia

Major markers
- Increased nuchal thickness
- Hyperechoic bowel
- Shortened humerus
- Shortened femur
- Echogenic intracardiac focus
- Renal pyelectasis

Minor markers
- Shortened or absent nasal bone
- Foot length
- "Sandal gap" of the foot
- Widened ischial spine angle
- Hypoplasia of the mid-phalynx of the fifth digit
- Brachycephaly

Table 5.5 LRs and 95% Confidence Limits for Isolated Ultrasound Markers

Isolated Sonographic marker	Nyberg et al. [10] LR (95% CI)	Smith-Bindman et al. [11] LR (95% CI)	Nicolaides et al. [12] LR
Nuchal fold/thickening	11 (5.2–22)	17 (8–38)	9.8
Hyperechoic bowel	6.7 (2.7–16.8)	6.1 (3–12.6)	3.0
Short humerus	5.1 (1.6–16.5)	7.5 (4.7–12)	4.1
Short femur	1.5 (0.8–2.8)	2.7 (1.2–6)	1.6
Echogenic intracardiac focus (EIF)	1.8 (1.0–3)	2.8 (1.5–5.5)	1.1
Pyelectasis	1.5 (0.6–3.6)	1.9 (0.7–5.1)	1.0

Increased Nuchal Fold
About 35% of Down's syndrome fetuses, but only 0.7% of normal fetuses, have a nuchal skin fold measurement ≥6 mm (some studies use ≥5 mm). When an increased nuchal fold is an isolated finding, the LR is strong at 10–17. Thus, the presence of an increased nuchal fold alone is usually an indication to offer invasive testing.

Increased Echogenicity of the Fetal Bowel
When brighter than the surrounding bone, this marker has a Down's syndrome LR of 3.0 to 6.7. This finding can also be seen with fetal cystic fibrosis, congenital cytomegalovirus (CMV) infection, swallowed bloody amniotic fluid, and severe fetal growth restriction (FGR).

Short Humerus, and in a Lesser Degree Short Femur
These markers in the second trimester are associated with Down's syndrome, relative to the length expected from their biparietal diameter. This can be used to identify at-risk pregnancies by calculating a ratio of observed to expected (O/E) femur/humerus length based on the fetus' biparietal diameter (BPD). An O/E ratio for femur length of <0.91 has a reported LR of 1.5–2.7 when present as an isolated finding. A short humerus is more strongly related to Down's syndrome, with reported LRs ranging from 4.1 to 7.5.

Pyelectasis
This marker is defined as a renal anteroposterior (AP) diameter of ≥4–5mm, and has a LR that ranges from 1.1 to 1.9 as an isolated marker. This has been found by some not to be significantly more frequent in Down's syndrome pregnancies than in normals (low specificity) [25].

Echogenic Intracardiac Foci
This marker occurs in up to 5% of normal pregnancies and in approximately 13–18% of Down syndrome gestations. The LR for Down's syndrome when an echogenic focus is present as an isolated marker has ranged from 1.0 to 2.8. This has been found by most investigators not to be significantly more frequent in Down syndrome pregnancies than in normals (low specificity) [12]. The risk does not seem to vary if the focus is in the right or left ventricle or if it is unilateral or bilateral, but may be affected by ethnicity.

Other markers described include a hypoplastic fifth middle phalanx of the hand, short ears, a sandal gap between the first and second toes, an abnormal iliac wing angle, an altered foot to femur ratio, short or absent nasal bone, and others. These markers are inconsistently used because of the time and expertise required to obtain them. Mild ventriculomegaly (10–15 mm) can be an indication for invasive prenatal diagnosis, since it is associated with 1%–2% risk of aneuploidy if isolated. If the karyotype is normal, mild ventriculomegaly is still associated with about 8% structural anomalies, 3% perinatal death, and 10%–20% abnormal neurodevelopment.

Except for major anomalies and increased nuchal thickness, isolated 'genetic ultrasound' markers should in general not be used as the sole indication for invasive testing. As with other screening modalities, "genetic" ultrasound can be used to alter the a priori risk in either direction. A positive LR can be used to increase estimated risk. The magnitude of the increase depends upon the marker(s) or anomalies seen. While most of the clinical prospective data justifying this approach have come from a baseline age-related risk, some have advocated using these LRs to adjust whichever baseline risk, even that derived by other screening tests (e.g., FTS and/or QS, or even integrative or consecutive approaches). A benign second-trimester scan having none of the known markers and no anomalies has been suggested to have a LR of 0.4–0.5, assuming the image quality is satisfactory when the "genetic ultrasound" is normal. It is doubtful that the same sensitivity can be achieved in every center.

Ultrasound Screening for Other Chromosomal Abnormalities
Fetal aneuploidy other than Down's syndrome can be suspected based on ultrasound findings [26]. The rates reported are usually in high-risk populations, and may overestimate the strength of the association when such findings are noted on a screening examination.

Trisomy 18
FTS and STS with MSAFP, HCG, unconjugated estriol and inhibin (QS) have a high detection rate for trisomy 18. Second-trimester ultrasound also has a high detection rate for trisomy 18.

Choroid plexus cysts (CPCs) have a very weak association with trisomy 18, and should not be the sole indication for invasive testing if isolated. The presence of CPCs CPC should be an indication for a detailed second-trimester ultrasound for trisomy 18 major anomalies, such as cardiac, central nervous system (CNS), hands defects, etc.

Positive Screening for Aneuploidy but Normal Karyotype
NT
A NT above the 95% percentile for GA, and especially ≥3.5 mm at 10 3/7–13 6/7 weeks is associated with an increased risk of other anomalies and syndromes, with the risk directly proportional to the increase in NT [27] (Table 5.6). The list of anomalies is long [14], and a detailed second-trimester ultrasound is recommended. The incidence of cardiac anomalies is ≥3.7% for NT ≥3.5 mm, so that a fetal cardiac ultrasound by experienced operator is recommended.

Table 5.6 Risk of Chromosome Abnormalities and (If Normal Karyotype) of Fetal Death or Anomalies According to Nuchal Translucency

NT	Chromosomal defects (%)	Normal karyotype			
		Fetal death (%)	Major fetal anomalies (%)	Alive and well (%)	Cardiac defects (%)
<95th centile	0.2	1.3	1.6	97	0.6
95th–99th centiles	3.7	1.3	2.5	93	0.6
3.5–4.4	21.1	2.7	10.0	70	3.7
4.5–5.4	33	3.4	18.5	50	6.7
5.5–6.4	50	10	24	30	13
≥6.5	65	19	46	15	20

Abbreviation: NT, nuchal translucency.

First Trimester PAPP-A and B-HCG
Low PAPP-A in FTS in the presence of a normal karyotype is associated with several adverse pregnancy outcomes, including fetal loss, PTB, and FGR. Low free HCG is associated with fetal loss. There are no randomized trials assessing any type of intervention or treatment for patients with abnormal serum markers [28].

Second Trimester Screening
High MSAFP is associated with NTDs, as well as abdominal wall defects and several other fetal abnormalities. High MSAFP, negative acetylcholinesterase (AChE) and normal ultrasound can be associated with congenital nephrosis or other syndromes, or normal pregnancy. Unexplained high MSAFP is associated with mild increases in the incidence of preeclampsia, abruption, placental ischemia, preterm birth, fetal demise, low birth weight, and sudden infant death syndrome (SIDS). No trials have assessed specific management to prevent these complications [28].

Low unconjugated estriol is associated with steroid sulfatase deficiency, Smith–Lemli–Opitz or other conditions when very low, usually <0.3 MoM [28].

MSAFP Screening for NTD
Elevated (usually ≥2.5 MoM) MSAFP between 14 and 21 weeks is associated with a ≥90%–95% sensitivity for NTDs (false negative rate 5%). Given that ultrasound is also ≥95% sensitive for NTDs, the routine use of MSAFP screening is most important for pregnancies that will not have a detailed second-trimester ultrasound.

Screening for Aneuploidies in Twins
NT is accurate in estimating Down's risk in dizygotic twins, using each NT separately for each fetus. In monochorionic twins, the average NT is the most effective screening method. Detection rates comparable to singletons can be achieved. Detection rates of FTS or STS tests are usually lower than in singletons, with higher rates of false positive and false negative results. Chorionicity does not seem to affect serum analytes in FTS or STS (see Chapter 44 in *Maternal-Fetal Evidence Based Guidelines*)

DIAGNOSTIC TESTS
CVS and Amniocentesis
Selected common indications for invasive prenatal diagnosis of fetal aneuploidy are listed in Table 5.7. Both CVS and amniocentesis have been performed for many years and can fairly safely diagnose a karyotypic or genetic abnormality.

Table 5.7 Selected Common Indications for Invasive Prenatal Diagnosis

- Abnormal first or second-trimester aneuploidy screen
- Abnormal ultrasound findings
- Parental concern/anxiety

Both procedures have been studied extensively. Differences in technique, as well as timing of the procedure, affect loss rates. To fairly compare procedure-induced loss rates between the two procedures, adjustments must be made for the higher background frequency of pregnancy loss earlier in gestation.

Second Trimester Amniocentesis
One study in a low-risk population (n = 4606) with a background pregnancy loss of around 2% found that a second-trimester amniocentesis increases total pregnancy loss by another 1% compared with no amniocentesis (relative risk [RR] 1.41; 95% confidence interval (CI) 0.99–2.00) [29]. **Compared with no amniocentesis, second-trimester amniocentesis is associated with a 0.8% increase in spontaneous miscarriage** (2.1% versus 1.3%; RR 1.60; 95% CI 1.02–2.52), but similar incidence of perinatal deaths (0.4% vs. 0.7%) [29,30]. In non-RCT data, the procedure-related risk of miscarriage following amniocentesis has been reported to be about **1/1000** [31].

There is insufficient data to assess the effect of PCR testing (fluorescent in situ hybridization [FISH]). In a small trial, reporting karyotype in 3 days with PCR did not affect maternal anxiety level compared with about 3 weeks later in Chinese women with an abnormal screening test for Down's syndrome [32]. Another study compared median trait- and state-anxiety scores and found no difference between the two groups [33]. Therefore, there is insufficient evidence that, while waiting for the full karyotype following amniocentesis, issuing results from a rapid analysis reduces maternal anxiety. The limited evidence from the two trials does not help resolve the dilemma about whether full karyotyping should be abandoned in favor of limited rapid testing for women undergoing Down's syndrome screening. This choice rests on clinical arguments and cost-effectiveness rather than impact on anxiety [34].

Early amniocentesis
Early amniocentesis (<15 weeks) is not a safe early alternative to second-trimester amniocentesis, because it is associated with increased pregnancy loss (7.6% versus 5.9%; RR 1.29; 95% CI 1.03–1.61), and higher incidence of talipes (1.8% versus 0.2%) compared with CVS (RR 4.61; 95% CI 1.82–11.66) [30,35].

CVS

CVS before 10 weeks is associated with an unacceptably high incidence of limb deficiencies, and should not be performed. *The optimal time for CVS is 10–12 weeks,* with trials of safety performed only in this GA. TA CVS can also be performed after 12 weeks (called usually placental biopsy) in cases in which placental karyotype is needed, but there are no trials on this "late" CVS.

Compared with second-trimester amniocentesis, CVS in general (TA and TC combined) is associated with a slight increased incidence of pregnancy losses and a slight increased incidence of spontaneous miscarriages [30].

Compared with second trimester amniocentesis, TC CVS is associated with a higher risk of pregnancy loss (14.5% versus 11%) **and higher** (12.9% versus 9.4%) **risk in spontaneous miscarriage,** although the results are quite heterogeneous and certainly operator-and experience-dependent [30].

Compared with second-trimester amniocentesis, TA CVS is associated with similar risk of pregnancy loss (6.3% versus 7.0%) **and spontaneous miscarriage** (3.0% versus 3.9%) in one study [30,36].

A systemic review of procedure related losses for CVS and amniocentesis revealed pooled loss rates for CVS at 14 days, 30 days and prior to 24 weeks of 0.7%, 1.3%, and 1.3% respectively. The pooled loss rates for amniocentesis for the same time period were 0.6%, 0.8%, and 0.9% [37]. In non-RCT data, the procedure-related risk of miscarriage following CVS has been reported to be about 2/1,000 [31]. Since CVS and amniocentesis are performed at different time periods, it is difficult to compare these procedures due to the higher background loss rate for the time period when CVS is performed. The benefit of earliest diagnosis with CVS compared with amniocentesis should not be underestimated. With the advent of FTS, prenatal diagnosis has moved more to the first trimester. While the total miscarriage rate is higher following first-trimester CVS because of the higher background rate in early pregnancy, for experienced centers, the rates of procedure-induced losses secondary to CVS are similar to those of second-trimester amniocentesis.

The learning curve for TA and TC CVS has been estimated to exceed 400 cases, with post-procedure loss rates for operators having performed less than 100 cases being two to three times higher when compared with more experienced operators. **The importance of operator experience cannot be overemphasized,** particularly for route of CVS, with TC CVS requiring more experience.

TC vs. TA CVS

Compared with TA CVS, TC CVS is associated with similar pregnancy loss rates (9.0% vs. 7.4%) **and similar spontaneous miscarriages** (7.9% vs. 4.5%) [30]. The results related to comparative pregnancy loss between TA and TC CVS are inconclusive, with significant heterogeneity between studies [30].

TC CVS technical instrument

There is some evidence to support the use of **small forceps** compared with cannulas for TC chorionic villus sampling. When different types of cannulae are compared, Portex cannula is more likely to result in an inadequate sample and a difficult or painful procedure when compared with either the silver or aluminum cannula respectively. The evidence is not strong enough to support change in practice for clinicians who have become familiar with aspiration cannulae, and no recent studies have been performed [38].

Microarrays and Other Genetic Tests

Advances in technology have demonstrated many new avenues for **noninvasive** diagnostic testing in utero (i.e., fetal cells from maternal circulation or cervical sampling, free fetal DNA in the maternal circulation, etc.).

Array comparative genomic hybridization (aCGH) is a new technique (based on *invasive* prenatal samples such as CVS and amniocentesis results) which has found clinical use. It can query the entire human genome for copy number changes such as aneuploidy, deletions, duplications, and unbalanced translocations. Unlike traditional cytogenetics which requires dividing cells, aCGH does not [39–44]. Conventional karyotype remains the principal cytogenetic tool for prenatal diagnosis, but the indications for aCGH are

- Abnormal ultrasound findings with normal karyotype
- Intrauterine fetal demise with congenital anomalies and culture failure with conventional karyotype [45]

In a high risk population referred for prenatal diagnosis, chromosomal microarray analysis (CMA) was compared with conventional karyotyping. The indications for prenatal diagnosis were ultrasound abnormalities, advanced maternal age or a positive result on prenatal screening. Microarray was similar to conventional karyotyping in detecting common chromosomal aneuploidy. In addition microarray was able to detect clinically significant aneuploidies not detected by karyotype [46]. Another study demonstrated that microarray was more likely to provide genetic results after stillbirth when compared with conventional karyotype [47]. When structural abnormalities are detected by prenatal ultrasound, chromosomal microarray can identify clinically significant chromosomal abnormalities in approximately 6% of the fetuses that have a normal karyotype [46]. For this reason, **CMA should be recommended as the primary test (replacing conventional karyotype) to patients undergoing prenatal diagnosis in whom a structural abnormality is detected by ultrasound.**

COMMON KARYOTYPE ABNORMALITIES
Trisomy 21 (Down's Syndrome)

Historic Notes

First complete description in 1846 by Seguin. Report by Down in 1866 established the name of the syndrome. In 1959 LeJeune and Jacobs independently described that Down syndrome was caused by trisomy 21.

Definition

Down syndrome is **trisomy 21,** or the presence of an extra chromosome number 21, either as three number 21s, or as a translocation between 21 and another chromosome, usually an acrocentric in a Robertsonian translocation.

Epidemiology/Incidence

About **1 in 800 live births**. This is the most common trisomy at birth. Incidence increases with increasing maternal age.

Embryology

The Down's syndrome critical region on chromosome 21 is being studied extensively to identify the genes involved in the Down's **syndrome phenotype**. However, this region is not one small isolated spot, but most likely several areas on chromosome 21 that are not necessarily side by side.

Genetics/Inheritance
Error in cell division at the time of conception (**nondisjunction**) is responsible for 92% of Down's syndrome resulting in **full trisomy 21**. Approximately 90% of nondisjunction occurs in the eggs. The cause of the nondisjunction error isn't known, but there is definitely a connection with maternal age. The recurrence risk is empirically 1% or the age related risk as a woman gets older. About 3%–4% of all cases of trisomy 21 are due to a **Robertsonian translocation** usually between chromosome #14 and 21. In the balanced state the individual is healthy and has 45 chromosomes with a #21 stuck on #14, or another acrocentric chromosome (15, 21, or 22). An individual with Down's syndrome due to a translocation has 46 chromosomes but one is actually a combination of #21 and another acrocentric like #14. Translocations resulting in trisomy 21 may be inherited, so parental chromosomes must be checked. A female carrier of a balanced Robertsonian translocation has about a 12% risk of recurrence of Down's syndrome in future pregnancies while a male carrier has approximately a 3% risk of recurrence. **Mosaic trisomy 21** occurs when there is a mixture of cell lines, some of which have normal chromosomes and another cell line with trisomy 21. It is impossible to know how the normal and trisomy 21 cells are distributed in the different organs therefore the percentage of mosaic to normal cells in the peripheral blood cannot be used to predict outcome. Another tissue can be examined to help determine the level of mosaicism, usually skin.

Teratology
None.

Classification
Full trisomy 21, translocation trisomy 21, and mosaic trisomy 21.

Risk Factors/Associations
Advanced maternal age. Individuals who are carriers of balanced Robertsonian translocations involving #21 have an increased risk unrelated to age.

Pregnancy Management
Screening (nonultrasound and/or ultrasound) First and second-trimester ultrasound, first-trimester screen, second-trimester multiple marker screening, or combinations are earlier in this chapter.

Ultrasound Findings in Fetus
- Thickened NT at 11–14 weeks (80%) (at times cystic hygroma –10%)
- Thickened nuchal fold (≥6 mm) at 16–23 weeks
- Congenital heart disease (CHD) (40%–50%)
- Duodenal atresia (2%)
- Omphalocele (2%)
- Ventriculomegaly
- Hydrops or some hydropic changes (pleural effusion, ascites, etc.)
- Several "soft markers," such as short humerus and femur, echogenic bowel, renal pyelectasis, cardiac (usually left ventricular) echogenic focus, short middle phalanx 5th digit, "sandal foot," iliac crest >90° angle, short ear length
- Biometry may reveal symmetric FGR by the third trimester
  - Amniotic fluid: Polyhydramnios (if gastrointestinal [GI] obstruction or macroglossia present)
  - Placenta: Normal
- Biometry/measurement data: Symmetric FGR
- When detectable: At 11–14 weeks if increased NT is detected

Ultrasound after 14 weeks only detects ~50% of fetuses with Down syndrome. CPCs do not increase the risk. Screening provides the mother and family with a risk for Down's syndrome, but true diagnosis can only be achieved with CVS or amniocentesis.

Diagnosis
CVS or amniocentesis achieve the diagnosis by a study of the fetal chromosomes, which reveal trisomy 21. In the neonate, usually peripheral blood is cultured and karyotyped.

Counseling
The major abnormalities are increased risk of FGR, congenital heart defects, fetal and postnatal death, and developmental delay, with average IQ 50–75. Congenital heart defects are major contributors to mortality.

Work-Up/Investigations and Consultations
A *fetal echocardiogram* is recommended. Depending on the lesions detected, specific pediatric subspecialty consultation can be offered. Genetic counseling can be offered as well. Care in a tertiary care center is indicated if there are significant associated anomalies, or if they cannot be ruled-out adequately.

Fetal Intervention
None available.

Termination Issues
Termination can be offered as sole intervention as regulated by local law (usually legal <24 weeks)

Fetal Monitoring/Testing
No specific trials. Nonstress tests (NSTs) weekly at ≥32 weeks can be offered. Nonreassuring fetal heart rate (NRFHR) is common.

Delivery/Anesthesia
Mode and management of delivery should not be affected by the diagnosis of Down syndrome. NRFHT is common.

Neonatology Management
Resuscitation
Providing life support as needed as in any other infant is generally appropriate.

Transport
Indicated if counseling, general care, and/or major anomalies cannot be assessed and treated adequately at the birth institution.

Testing and Confirmation
Karyotype is usually confirmed by blood lymphocyte culture.

Nursery Management
Neonatal echocardiogram, and physical exam to assess any anomaly. **Surgery** may need to be scheduled for GI or cardiac anomalies. Down's syndrome presents with a wide variety of features and characteristics. There is a wide range of intellectual disability and developmental delay noted among children

with Down's syndrome. There is a great deal of variability in the presence of other anomalies such as CHD, GI, and hematological problems in these children. Hypothyroidism occurs in a high percentage of individuals with DS and should be monitored closely for their lifetime. **Early intervention** and specialized help with education and home rearing has improved the outcome in children with Down's syndrome. Many young adults with Down syndrome move in to community living arrangements and work regular jobs or in sheltered workshops.

Future Pregnancy Preconception Counseling

With full trisomy 21, the recurrence risk is empirically 1% or the age related risk as a woman gets older. With Robertsonian translocation, parental chromosomes should be checked, with genetic counseling regarding specific future risks. There are other rare translocations leading to DS. One is a Robertsonian translocation between two chromosomes 21, t(21;21); this has a 100% risk for DS when transmitted by a carrier parent. Also rare is a non-Robertsonian translocation formed by the union of two 21s such that the translocation forms a mirror image of the normal 21. There is some literature that suggest in some families where there have been recurrent trisomies, a relationship exists with their MTHFR status. This has not been proven in large studies.

Helpful Websites
General: http://www.ds-health.com/
Health care guidelines for care of individual with DS: http://www.denison.edu/collaborations/dsq/health96.html
Risk and recurrence risk of Down's syndrome: http://www.nas.com/downsyn/benke.html

Trisomy 18 (Edward Syndrome)

Historic Notes
Trisomy 18 was independently described by Edwards et al. and Smith et al. in 1960.

Definition
Edward syndrome is *trisomy 18*, or the presence of an extra chromosome number 18.

Epidemiology/Incidence
Incidence of 1 in 6600 live births in the United States and the United Kingdom. This is the second most common trisomy at birth. Incidence increases with increasing maternal age.

Embryology
Extra number 18 affects development of all organs.

Genetics/Inheritance/Recurrence
Extra chromosome number 18 is usually (95%) secondary to de novo **meiotic nondisjunction** associated with advanced maternal age. In approximately 90% of cases, the extra chromosome is maternal in origin, with meiosis II errors occurring twice as frequently as meiosis I errors. Other human trisomies have a higher frequency of nondisjunction in maternal meiosis I. Approximately 80% of nondisjunctions occurs in females. **Mosaicism** occurs in approximately 10% and is due to post zygotic nondisjunction or anaphase lag. The causes of meiotic and mitotic nondisjunction are unknown. **Translocations** may also result in trisomy or partial trisomy 18 with varying phenotype due to monosomy of another chromosome and variable size of piece of chromosome number 18 involved. The smallest extra region necessary for expression of serious anomalies of trisomy 18 appears to be 18q11–q12.

Teratology
None.

Classification
Trisomy 18 (95%), mosaic trisomy 18, and variable partial trisomy 18 related to translocations.

Risk Factors/Associations
Advanced maternal age and translocation carriers have increased risk. Recurrence risk approximately 1% for full trisomy 18.

Pregnancy Management
Screening NT has a sensitivity of >80%; FTS has a sensitivity of >90%, second-trimester multiple marker screening is typically low alpha-fetoprotein (AFP), low HCG, low estriol with a sensitivity of about >80%. Accurate ultrasound is usually >90% sensitive for trisomy 18.

Ultrasound Findings in Fetus
- Thickened NT at 11–14 weeks (80%) (at times cystic hygroma –15%)
- Thickened nuchal fold (≥6 mm) at 16–23 weeks
- CHD (90%)
- Omphalocele (25%)
- NTDs (20%)
- Clenched hands with overlapping fingers
- Clubbed or rocker-bottom feet
- CPCs (25%) (most commonly isolated and seen in normal fetuses; karyotyping probably not indicated if isolated)
- Enlarged (>1 cm) cisterna magna
- Single umbilical artery
- Micrognathia
- Cleft lip or palate
- Hydrops or some hydropic changes (pleural effusion, ascites, etc.)
- Biometry may reveal FGR by the third trimester
  - Amniotic fluid: Polyhydramnios (25%)
  - Placenta: Normal
  - Biometry/measurement data: Symmetric FGR (>50%) microcephaly in third trimester
  - When detectable: At 11–14 weeks if increased NT is detected

Diagnosis
CVS or amniocentesis

Counseling [48,49]:
Approximately 95% of conceptuses with trisomy 18 die in embryonic or fetal life. Five to ten percent of affected children born alive survive beyond the first year of life. In utero, there are decreased fetal movements. Clinical findings the parents should be informed about include severe psychomotor and growth delay, microcephaly, microphthalmia, malformed ears, micrognathia or retrognathia, microstomia, distinctively clenched fingers, rocker-bottom feet and other congenital malformations. **CHD occurs in 90%,** with ventricular septal defect (VSD) and poly-valvular heart disease (pulmonary and aortic valve defects) common. Renal anomalies, GI and brain malformations are common. Classical dermatoglyphics with digital arch patterns on finger and toe tips and distal palmar triradius with hypoplastic finger tips and small nails. Central apnea is

a frequent cause of death, along with cardiac, CNS and renal malformations.

If diagnosed prenatally, recommend discussion with parents about how to proceed in labor and delivery allowing "nature to take its course" without monitoring, or level of intervention desired by parents including the extent of resuscitation after delivery. Indication for C-section for fetal indications may be futile. **Parents need to be counseled that some children with trisomy 18 do survive and require life-long complete care**, but never achieve any independence. Few milestones are reached. There is an increased incidence Wilms tumor in trisomy 18 children who survive. Cardiac surgery is controversial. In first weeks it may be considered a heroic measure, but if the child is surviving it may make life more comfortable (comfort care). Apnea is a common cause of death, and can happen at home; there is the need to understand "nobody's fault" if this happens.

Work-up/Investigations and Consultations Required
A fetal echocardiogram is recommended. Genetic counseling can be offered. **Neonatal consultation** is extremely important, to help the couple decide regarding neonatal management; usually just comfort care for the baby and psychological support for the parents is most appropriate. Fetal intervention: None available.

Termination Issues
Termination can be offered as sole intervention as regulated by local law (usually legal <24 weeks).

Antepartum Testing
As NRFHT is very common, and prognosis poor, fetal testing is not recommended. Many pregnancies continue without spontaneous labor until post-term (>42 weeks).

Delivery/Anesthesia
Fetal heart monitoring is usually declined, and not indicated. Every attempt should be made to maximize the chances of vaginal delivery to minimize maternal morbidity given frequently fatal neonatal prognosis. Cesarean delivery for fetal indications is not recommended and should be discussed.

Neonatology Management
Resuscitation
Comfort care only. Allow parents to grieve appropriately. Providing life support is usually not appropriate.

Transport
Not indicated.

Testing and confirmation
Karyotype is usually confirmed by blood lymphocyte culture.

Future Pregnancy Preconception Counseling
Test parents if due to translocation.

Helpful Websites
http://www.emedicine.com/ped/topic652.htm

Trisomy 13

Historic Notes
Patau first identified in laboratory in 1960 noting three of the group 13–15 chromosomes.

Definition
Patau syndrome is *trisomy 13*, or the presence of an extra chromosome number 13.

Epidemiology/Incidence
1 in 10,000 live births. Incidence increases with increasing maternal age. Approximately 1% of all first-trimester spontaneous losses are due to trisomy 13.

Embryology
Extra chromosome number 13 affects development of all organs.

Genetics/Inheritance
Extra number 13 chromosome resulting in **full trisomy 13** (80% of cases). This is due to maternal nondisjunction usually in meiosis I. About 15% of cases are due to **translocation**, mostly Robertsonian translocation t(13q14). In 5% translocation is familial with recurrence risk of 5% and risk of spontaneous abortion (SAB) of 20%. The other cases are due to **mosaicism** (5%) with trisomy 13 and a normal cell line. Mosaicism cases may have milder phenotype.

Teratology
None.

Classification
Trisomy 13, mosaic trisomy 13 and translocation trisomy or partial trisomy 13.

Risk Factors/Associations
Advanced maternal age. Individuals who are carriers of balanced Robertsonian translocations involving number 13 have an increased risk.

Pregnancy Management
Screening   First-trimester ultrasound (with NT). First or second-trimester multiple marker screening are not sensitive and clinically useful for detecting trisomy 13. Accurate ultrasound is usually 90% sensitive for trisomy 13.

Ultrasound Findings in Fetus
Thickened NT at 11–14 weeks (>70%) (at times cystic hygroma –20%)
- Thickened nuchal fold (≥6 mm) at 16–23 weeks
- CHD (80%) (atrial septal defect (ASD) and VSD most common, but also often complex CHD)
- Holoprosencephaly (40%)
- Cleft lip and palate (45%)
- Hypotelorism/microphthalmia
- Polydactyly
- Rocker-bottom feet
- Omphalocele (10%)
- Polycystic kidneys (30%)
- Enlarged (>1 cm) cisterna magna (15%)
- NTDs
- Hydrops or some hydropic changes (pleural effusion, ascites, etc.)
- Biometry may reveal symmetric FGR by the third trimester
  - Amniotic fluid: Polyhydramnios or oligohydramnios
  - Placenta: Normal
  - Biometry/measurement data: Symmetric FGR (50%)
  - When detectable: At 11–14 weeks if increased NT is detected

Diagnosis
CVS or amniocentesis achieve the diagnosis by a study of the fetal chromosomes, which reveals trisomy 13. In the neonate, usually peripheral blood is cultured and karyotyped.

Counseling

Most trisomy 13 conceptions result in SABs. Median survival is fewer than 3 days. Mean life expectancy is 130 days with most dying in first month of life, 95% die within 6 months. Apnea is a common cause of death, and can happen at home; there is the need to understand "nobody's fault" if this happens. Family needs to be prepared for intense care needs and possible sudden death. Most common causes of death are cardiopulmonary arrest, 69%; CHD, 13%; and pneumonia, 4% [48,49].

Some infants do survive and those need complete care and achieve few milestones. Survival depends on associated medical problems. Survivors with trisomy 13 have severe intellectual disability and developmental delays. For survivors there are specific growth charts available for monitoring growth. Children with trisomy 13 are irritable, do not achieve milestones beyond smiling and most need to be fed by tube.

If diagnosed prenatally, recommend discussion with parents about how to proceed, usually allowing "nature to take its course" given the grim prognosis. Parents need to be counseled that some children with trisomy 13 do survive and require life-long complete care, never achieve any independence.

Work-up/Investigations and Consultations
A fetal echocardio-gram is recommended. Genetic counseling can be offered. **Neonatal consultation** is extremely important, to help the couple decide regarding neonatal management; usually just comfort care for the baby and psychological support for the parents is most appropriate.

Fetal intervention
None available.

Termination Issues
Termination can be offered as sole intervention as regulated by local law (usually legal <24 weeks).

Antepartum Testing
As NRFHT is very common, and prognosis poor, fetal testing is not recommended. Many pregnancies continue without spontaneous labor until post-term (>42 weeks).

Delivery/Anesthesia
Fetal heart monitoring is usually declined, and not indicated. Every attempt should be made to maximize the chances of vaginal delivery to minimize maternal morbidity given almost universally fatal neonatal prognosis.

Cesarean delivery for fetal indications is not recommended and should be discussed.

Neonatology Management
Resuscitation Comfort care only. Allow parents to grieve appropriately. Providing life support is usually not appropriate.

Transport
Not indicated.

Testing and confirmation
Karyotype is usually confirmed by blood lymphocyte culture.

Long-term care
Feeding issues, gastrostomy; irritability; chronic infections, aspiration pneumonia; heart failure; frequent hospitalizations; seizures; blindness and hearing loss; few milestones achieved (smile, laugh); parental stress.

Future Pregnancy Preconception Counseling
With full trisomy 13, the recurrence risk is empirically 1% or the age related risk as a woman gets older. With Robertsonian translocation, parental chromosomes should be checked, with genetic counseling regarding specific future risks. There are other rare translocations leading to trisomy 13. Rare translocation of t(13q13q) the risk of recurrence or SAB is 100%.

Helpful Website
http://www.emedicine.com/ped/topic1745.htm

Turner Syndrome

Historic Notes
In 1938 Turner described the combination of sexual infantilism, webbed neck and cubitus valgus. Ford showed in 1959 that this combination of findings was associated with a missing X chromosome.

Definition
Turner syndrome is the **presence of single X chromosome,** or **any karyotype with Xp missing** such as isochromosome Xq, ring X or deletion Xp. Also called 45X0 or 45X syndrome.

Epidemiology/Incidence
1/2500 female births (**1/5000** total births). Approximately 98%–99% of Turner fetuses are spontaneously aborted; about 20% of all SABs are due to Turner syndrome.

Embryology
Lymphedema usually due to congenital hypoplasia of lymphatic channels.

Genetics/Inheritance
The **presence of single X chromosome,** or **any karyotype with Xp missing** such as isochromosome Xq, ring X or deletion Xp. The presence of a single X chromosome results from chromosomal nondisjunction. **Mosaicism** is common (40%) and may include a 46,XY karyotype associated with ambiguous genitalia. Since features of Turner syndrome are seen in other syndromes, karyotype is essential to make the diagnosis. Chromosome studies on more than one tissue may be needed to detect mosaicism. Not associated with advanced maternal age.

Teratology
None.

Classification
45,X in 50%. 46,X,i(Xq) in 17%, mosaicism in 40%.

Risk Factors/Associations
Not associated with advanced maternal age. Differentiate from Noonan syndrome by karyotype which is normal in Noonan syndrome.

Pregnancy Management
Screening First-trimester screen with NT measurement. Biochemical screening is usually not sensitive enough for clinical use.

Ultrasound findings in fetus
- Cystic hygroma
- Thickened nuchal fold (≥ 6mm) at 16–23 weeks;
- CHD (20%) (usually left side: coarctation, aortic stenosis, bicuspid aortic valve, left hypoplastic heart)

- Renal anomalies (60%)
- Hydrops or some hydropic changes (pleural effusion, ascites, etc.)
  - Amniotic fluid: Occasionally oligohydramnios
  - Placenta: Normal
  - Biometry/measurement data: Usually normal
  - When detectable: At 10+ weeks if cystic hygroma detected

Diagnosis
CVS or amniocentesis achieve the diagnosis with a study of the fetal chromosomes, which reveals 45,X or missing Xp. In the neonate, usually peripheral blood is cultured and karyotyped.

Counseling
45,X conceptions frequently (>95%) end in SAB. **The presence of a cystic hygroma with the diagnosis of Turner syndrome is >99% fatal.** If cystic hygroma is not present or resolves, and fetus is still alive >20 weeks, many survive until birth. Female infants with Turner syndrome have excess nuchal skin and edema of the hands and feet (80%) due to lymphedema. CHD, if present, usually most affects prognosis, requires surgery and long-term care. In childhood short stature is apparent. Teenagers have delayed puberty and primary amenorrhea (>90%), with infertility (>99%). Other clinical findings include shield-shaped chest with widely spaced nipples, low posterior hair line with webbing or shortness of neck, renal anomalies (60%), cubitus valgus, short 4th metacarpal, narrow, hyper convex and deep set nails, hearing loss and thyroid dysfunction. Some girls with Turner syndrome have learning difficulties including difficulty with math and reading maps related to a deficit in spatial ability. Intelligence and verbal skills are usually within the normal range. Mosaicism with a normal female cell line may result in a milder phenotype and spontaneous puberty with fertility but often early menopause. If there is a deleted X but the X-inactive specific transcript (XIST) locus is intact, normal random X-inactivation may occur and the phenotype may be milder. If XIST is not present in a small X chromosome marker the phenotype may be more severe. In mosaic 45X/46,XY individuals clitoral enlargement may be present and virilization may occur. In these cases there is an increased risk of gonadoblastoma and the gonad should be removed. Psychological impact of short stature, infertility, and learning difficulties needs to be discussed.

Work-up/Investigations and Consultations
A fetal echocardiogram is recommended. Depending on the lesions detected, specific pediatric subspecialty (in particular for cardiac anomalies) consultation can be offered. Genetic counseling can be offered as well. Care in a tertiary care center is indicated if there are significant associated anomalies, or if they cannot be ruled-out adequately. Endocrine follow-up is indicated.

Fetal intervention
None available.

Termination issues
Termination can be offered as sole intervention as regulated by local law (usually legal <24 weeks).

Fetal monitoring/testing
No specific trials. NSTs weekly at ≥32 weeks can be offered.

Delivery/anesthesia
Mode and management of delivery should not be affected by the diagnosis of Turner syndrome.

Neonatology Management
Resuscitation
Providing life support as needed as in any other infant is generally appropriate.

Transport
Indicated if counseling, general care, and/or major anomalies cannot be assessed and treated adequately at the birth institution.

Testing and confirmation
Karyotype is usually confirmed by blood lymphocyte culture.

Nursery Management
Neonatal echocardiogram, renal ultrasound, and physical exam are indicated to assess any anomaly. **Surgery** may need to be scheduled for cardiac anomalies. **Early intervention** and specialized help with education has improved the outcome in children with Turner syndrome.

Long-Term Care
Thyroid studies annually; hearing test if otitis and not done before; speech evaluation, if needed; blood pressure checks routinely (hypertension a complication); annual echocardiogram to measure aortic root; annual urinalysis and culture if renal anomaly; use Turner growth curve after 2 years old; monitor diet (calories and calcium); ophthalmology follow-up as indicated; psychological support; individualized education plan (IEP) at school if indicated; refer to endocrinologist in infancy, discuss growth hormone (GH) and hormone replacement therapy (HRT): GH treatment can improve growth and influence a girl's final adult height. HRT helps the girl with Turner syndrome develop the physical changes of puberty. In vitro fertilization can make it possible for some women with Turner syndrome to become pregnant using a donor egg. It is important to discuss at what age to inform the child of her diagnosis and its implications.

Future Pregnancy Preconception Counseling
Recurrence risk in 45,X is not increased over population risk. There is an increased risk if associated with a translocation.

Klinefelter Syndrome
Historic Notes
In 1942, Dr. Harry Klinefelter described males who had enlarged breasts, sparse facial and body hair, small testes, and azospermia. By the late 1950s these findings were associated initially with an extra Barr body and later the extra X chromosome was identified with the karyotype 47,XXY.

Diagnosis/Definition
Chromosome study 47,XXY. There are no specific phenotypic features to identify Klinefelter syndrome in an infant.

Epidemiology/Incidence
1 in 500 to 1 in 1000 male births.

Genetics/Inheritance/Recurrence/Future Prevention
Advanced maternal age slightly increases the risk for the XXY. Recent studies have shown that half the time, the extra chromosome comes from the father.

Risk Factors/Associations
Advanced maternal age.

Screening
No phenotypic features noted prenatally.

Clinical Features
Occasional breast enlargement, lack of facial and body hair, and a female-type body configuration. Small testes. Taller than others in their family. Delayed speech occurs in >50%. Poor gross motor coordination is present in ~27%. School difficulties are relatively common and many boys with 47,XXY need assistance at school. Many are shy and somewhat passive and easy babies to care for. The average IQ is 90, verbal IQ higher than performance IQ. XXY boys enter puberty normally, without any delay of physical maturity. But as puberty progresses, they fail to keep pace with other males. Most XXY boys benefit from receiving an injection of testosterone every 2 weeks, beginning at puberty.

Counseling
Regular injections of the male hormone testosterone, beginning at puberty, can promote strength and facial hair growth as well as bring about a more muscular body type.

Psychological support and therapy can help with self-esteem issues and interaction with peers. Depression also may be a problem in adults.

Boys with 47, XXY have a slightly increased risk of autoimmune disorders such as type I (insulin dependent) diabetes, autoimmune thyroiditis, and lupus erythematosus. XXY males with enlarged breasts have the same risk of breast cancer as do women-roughly 50 times the risk of XY males. XXY males who do not receive testosterone injections may have an increased risk of developing osteoporosis in later life.

It is unnecessary to share this diagnosis outside of medical providers as diagnosis may be misunderstood.

Rare/Related
Variations include the XY/XXY mosaic who may have enough normally functioning cells in the testes to allow them to father children. Males with two or even three additional X chromosomes have also been reported in the medical literature. In these individuals, the classic features of Klinefelter syndrome may be exaggerated, with low IQ or moderate to severe mental retardation also occurring. Testosterone injections may not be appropriate for all of them.

Helpful Website
http://www.nichd.nih.gov/publications/pubs/klinefelter.htm#xwhat

47,XXX
Diagnosis/Definition
Karyotype shows 47,XXX.

Epidemiology/Incidence
1 in 1000 newborn females.

Genetics/Inheritance/Recurrence
Sporadic, increased by advanced maternal age.

Risk Factors/Associations
Advanced maternal age.

Screening
No identifying physical features. Must have karyotype to make diagnosis.

Clinical Features
Girls with 47,XXX are usually tall. Pubertal development is usually normal and fertility is probably normal but there may be an increased incidence of offspring with chromosome abnormalities.

Counseling
Girls with 47,XXX are shy and may demonstrate immaturity. The support of a loving and understanding family can improve the outcome for these girls. Many have learning difficulties (math and reading) but they are not intellectually disabled. The IQ of a girl with 47,XXX may be a few points lower than that of her siblings. Those diagnosed on amniocentesis or CVS with normal ultrasound, where indication is AMA, have better prognosis than those diagnosed postnatally because a problem has been noted.

SELECTED MICRODELETIONS AND DUPLICATIONS
Di George Syndrome (22q11.2 Deletion Syndrome)
Historic Notes
DiGeorge syndrome, described in 1965 and velo-cardiofacial syndrome described in 1978 are different manifestations of the same deletion of chromosome 22q11.2.

Diagnosis/Definition
FISH study reveals an interstitial deletion of chromosome 22 p11.2. Can be detected on microarray.

Epidemiology/Incidence
1 in 2000–4000 births.

Embryology
Defects occur in the 3rd and 4th pharyngeal pouches, which later develop into the thymus and parathyroid glands. Developmental abnormalities may also occur in the 4th branchial arch.

Genetics/Inheritance/Recurrence/Future Prevention
Autosomal dominant inheritance. In 6% of affected individuals one of the parents is affected. Expression is very variable so both parents of an affected child should be tested for the deletion.

Risk Factors/Associations
Other conditions have been noted to be associated with de 22q11.2 including Conotruncal Anomaly Face syndrome (CAFS) (Japan) and sometimes Opitz G/BBB syndrome, CHARGE Association and Cayler-Cardiofacial syndrome.

Screening
All women with a fetus or neonate with a diagnosis of congenital heart defect, especially if conotruncal, can be offered testing (usually FISH) for this deletion. Testing is available from amniocytes or chorionic villi.

Clinical Features
Characteristic facies, cardiovascular defects in 85%, most are VSD. Cleft of secondary palate, may be submucous cleft or velo-pharyngeal incompetence, nasal reflux in infants, transient neonatal hypocalcemia, hypotonia, immune system dysfunction, postnatal growth delay, developmental delay,

learning disability and psychological problems especially in adolescence, hypernasal speech.

Counseling (Prognosis, Complications, Pregnancy Considerations)
Clinical features should be reviewed. Early death due to congenital heart defects before 6 months of age in 8%. Early intervention for speech and motor delays. Special education for older children. Chance of psychiatric disorders in 10%. Very variable phenotype, not predictable from laboratory result.

5p-(Cri-Du-Chat Syndrome)
Historic Notes
In 1963, Lejeune et al. described a syndrome of multiple congenital anomalies, developmental delay, microcephaly, dysmorphic features, and a high-pitched, cat-like cry in infants with deletion of a B group chromosome (Bp-), later identified as 5p-.

Diagnosis/Definition
5p-Syndrome is characterized at birth by a high pitched cat-like cry, low birth weight, poor muscle tone, microcephaly. The cry is caused by abnormal laryngeal development. The cry disappears by age 2 years in about one-third of children with 5p-.

A karyotype is needed for the diagnosis. The size of the deletion of the short arm of chromosome 5 is variable and a very small deletion may be missed using conventional G-banding. High resolution studies may be needed or a FISH study using a specific probe for the small deleted area of 5p that is essential for this diagnosis. Microarray would identify this deletion.

Epidemiology/Incidence
Estimated prevalence is about 1 in 50,000 live births. Up to 1% of profoundly retarded individuals have 5p-.

Genetics/Inheritance/Recurrence/Future Prevention
May be sporadic (80%–85%) if both parents have normal chromosomes with a recurrence risk of less that 1%. In rare cases gonadal mosaicism in one parent may result in a recurrence. If one parent carries a balanced translocation (10%–15%) involving 5p, the recurrence risk is substantially higher.

Most cases have a terminal deletion of 5p. The cat-like cry maps to 5p15.3 and the Cri-du-chat critical region is 5p15.2, which is associated with all the clinical features of the syndrome. The deletion is paternal in origin in 80% of cases.

Affected females are fertile and have a 50% of passing on the deletion to their offspring although none is documented to have reproduced.

Risk Factors/Associations
Increased risk if translocation carrier involving 5p.

Screening
Amniocentesis, CVS, ultrasound.

Counseling
Early feeding problems are common because of swallowing difficulties; poor suck with resultant failure to thrive. Death occurs in 6%–8% of the overall population with Cri-du-chat due to pneumonia, aspiration pneumonia, and congenital heart defects. Survival to adulthood is possible. Children who are raised at home with early intervention and schooling do better than those described in the early literature. Almost all individuals with 5p- have significant cognitive, speech, and motor delays (IQ rarely above 35). Many children can develop some language and motor skills. They may also become independent in self-care skills. Physical features include microcephaly, growth retardation, hypertelorism, epicanthal folds, down-slanting palpebral fissures, round face with full cheeks, flat nasal bridge, down-turned corners of mouth, micrognathia, low-set ears, and variable cardiac defects. Renal anomalies have been described as have cleft lip and palate, talipes equinovarus and gut malrotation. Treatment is symptomatic.

Helpful Websites
http://www.emedicine.com/ped/topic504.htm

REFERENCES
1. ACOG Practice Bulletin. Screening for fetal chromosome anomalies. *Obstet Gynecol.* 2007;109:217–227. [Review]
2. Hook EB. Rates of chromosome abnormalities at different maternal ages. *Obstet Gynecol.* 1981;58(3):282–285 [II-1]
3. Salvedt A, Almstrom H, Kublickas M, et al. Screening for Down's syndrome based on maternal age or fetal nuchal translucency: A randomized controlled trial in 39,572 pregnancies. *Ultrasound Obstet Gynecol.* 2005;25:537–545. [RCT, $n = 39,572$]
4. Wald NJ, Rodeck C, Hackshaw AK, et al. SURUSS Research Group. First and second trimester antenatal screening for Down's syndrome: The results of the serum, urine and ultrasound screening study. *Health Technol Assess.* 2003;7:1–77. [II-3]
5. Nicolaides KH, spencer K, Avgidou K, et al. Multicenter study of first-trimester screening for trisomy 21 in 75,821 pregnancies: Results and estimation of the potential impact of individual risk-orientated two-stage first-trimester screening. *Ultrasound Obstet Gynecol.* 2005;25:221–226. [II-3]
6. Malone FD, Canick JA, Ball RH, et al. For the First-and-Second Trimester Evaluation of Risk (FASTER) Research Consortium. First-trimester or second-trimester screening, or both, for Down syndrome. *N Engl J Med.* 2005;353:2001–2011. [II-3]
7. Wapner R, Thom E, Simpson JL, et al. For the First Trimester Maternal Serum Biochemistry and Fetal Nuchal Translucency Screening (BUN) Study Group. First-trimester screening for trisomies 21 and 18. *N Engl J Med.* 2003;349:1405–1413. [II-3]
8. Bennett KA, Crane JMC, O'shea P, et al. First trimester ultrasound screening is effective in reducing postterm labor induction rates: A randomized controlled trial. *Am J Obstet Gynecol.* 2004;190:1077–1081. [RCT, $n = 218$]
9. Haddow JE, Palomaki GE, Knight GJ, et al. Reducing the need for amniocentesis in women 35 years of age or older with serum markers for screening. *N Engl J Med.* 1994;330(16): 1114–1118. [II-2]
10. Lo YMD, Lun FMF, Allen Chan KC et al. Digital PCR for molecular detection of fetal chromosome aneuploidy. *PNAS.* 2007;104:13116–13121. [II-2]
11. Fan HC, Blumenfeld YJ, Chitkara U et al. Noninvasive diagnosis of fetal aneuploidy by shotgun sequencing DNA from maternal blood. *PNAS.* 2008;105:16266–16271. [II-2]
12. Chiu RWK, Allen Chan KC, Gao Y, et al. Noninvasive prenatal diagnosis of fetal chromosomal aneuploidy by massively parallel genomic sequencing of DNA in maternal plasma. *PNAS.* 2008;105:20458–20463. [II-2]
13. Palomaki GE, Deciu C, Kloza EM, et al. DNA sequencing of maternal plasma reliably identifies trisomy 18 and trisomy 13 as well as Down syndrome: An international collaborative study. *Genet Med.* 2012;14:296–305. [II-2]
14. Ashoor G, Syngelaki A, Wagner M, et al. Chromosome-selective sequencing of maternal plasma cell-free DNA for first trimester detection of trisomy 21 and trisomy 18. *Am J Obstet Gynecol.* 2012;206:322.e1–5. [II-2]
15. Sparks AB, Struble CA, Wang ET, et al. Noninvasive prenatal detection and analysis of cell-free DNA obtained from maternal blood: Evaluation for trisomy 21 and trisomy 18. *Am J Obstet Gynecol.* 2012;206:319e1–9. [II-2]

16. Norton ME, Brar H, Weiss J, et al. Noninvasive chromosomal evaluation (NICE) study: Results of a multicenter prospective cohort study for detection of fetal trisomy 21 and trisomy 18. *Am J Obstet Gynecol.* 2012;207:137.e1–8. [II-2]
17. Sparks AB, Wang ET, Struble CA, et al. Selective analysis of cell free DNA in maternal blood for evaluation of fetal trisomy. *Prenat Diag.* 2012;32:3–9. [II-2]
18. Zimmerman B, Hill M, Gemelos G, et al. Noninvasive prenatal aneuploidy testing of chromosomes 13, 18, 21, X, and Y, using targeted sequencing of polymotphic loci. *Prenat Diag.* 2012;32:1233–1241. [II-2]
19. Nicolaides KH, Syngelaki A, Ashoor G, et al. Noninvasive prenatal testing for fetal trisomies in a routinely screened first-trimester population. *Am J Obstet Gynecol.* 2012;207:374.e1–6. [II-2]
20. Bianchi DW, Parker RL, Wentworth J, et al. DNA sequencing versus standard prenatal aneuploid screening. *N Engl J Med.* 2014;370:799–808. [II-2]
21. Norton ME, Jacobson B, Swamy GK, et al. Cell-free DNA analysis for noninvasive examination of trisomy. *N Engl J Med.* 2015;372(17):1589–1597 doi: 10.1056/NEJMoa1407349. [II-2]
22. Society for Maternal-Fetal Medicine Publication Committee. Society for Maternal Fetal Medicine (SMFM) consult series #36. Prenatal aneuploidy screening using cell free DNA. *Am J Obstet Gynecol.* 2015;212(6):711–716. [II-2]
23. Nyberg DA, Souter VL, El-Bastawissi A, et al. Isolated sonographic markers for detection of fetal Down syndrome in the second trimester of pregnancy. *J Ultrasound Med.* 2001;20(10):1053–1063. [II-2]
24. Smith-Bindman R, Hosmer W, Feldstein VA, et al. Second-trimester ultrasound to detect fetuses with Down syndrome: A meta-analysis. *JAMA.* 2001;285(8):1044–1055. [II-2]
25. Nicolaides KH, Snijders RJM, Sebire N, eds. *The 11–14 Week Scan: The Diagnosis of Fetal Anomalies.* London: Taylor & Francis. [Review]
26. Snijders R, Nicolaides K. *Ultrasound Markers for Fetal Markers for Chromosomal Defects.* New York, NY: Parthenon Publishing Group, 1996. [II-2]
27. Souka AP, von Kaisenberg CS, Hyett JA, et al. Increased nuchal translucency with normal karyotype. *AJOG.* 2005;192:1005–1021. [Review]
28. Dugoff L, for the Society for Maternal-Fetal Medicine. First- and second-trimester maternal serum markers for aneuploidy and adverse obstetric outcomes. *Obstet Gynecol.* 2010;115:1052–1061. [Review]
29. Tabor A, Madsen M, Obel EB, et al. Randomised controlled trial of genetic amniocentesis in 4606 low-risk women. *Lancet.* 1986;1:1287–1293. [RCT, $n = 4,606$]
30. Alfirevic Z, Mujezinovic F, Sundberg K. Amniocentesis and chorionic villus sampling for prenatal diagnosis. *Cochrane Database of Systematic Reviews.* 2003;3.
31. Akolekar R, beta J, Picciarelli G, et al. Procedure-related risk of miscarriage following amniocentesis and chorionic villus sampling: A systematic review and meta-analysis. *Ultrasound Obstet Gynecol.* 2015;45:16–26. [II-1]
32. Leung WC, Lam YH, Wong Y, et al. The effect of fast reporting by amnio-PCR on anxiety levels in women with positive biochemical screening for Down's syndrome—A randomized controlled trial. *Prenatal Diagnosis.* 2002;22:256–259. [RCT, $n = 60$]
33. Hewison J, Nixon J, Fountain J, et al. A randomised trial of two methods of issuing prenatal test results: The ARIA (Amniocentesis Results: Investigation of Anxiety) trial. *BJOG: An International Journal of Obstetrics and Gynaecology.* 2007;114(4):462–468. [RCT, $n = 226$]
34. Mujezinovic F, Prosnik A, Alfirevic Z. Different communication strategies for disclosing results of diagnostic prenatal testing. *Cochrane Database of Systematic Reviews.* 2010;11. [Meta-Analysis, 2 RCTs, $n = 286$]
35. Collaborative. Randomised trial to assess safety and fetal outcome of early and midtrimester amniocentesis. The Canadian Early and Mid-trimester Amniocentesis Trial (CEMAT) Group. *Lancet.* 1998;351(9098):242–247. [RCT, $n = 4,334$]
36. Smidt-Jensen S, Permin M, Philip J, et al. Randomized comparison of amniocentesis and transabdominal and transcervical chorionic villus sampling. *Lancet.* 1992;340:1237–1244. [RCT, $n = 2,234$]
37. Mujezinovic F, Alfirevic Z. Procedure-related complications of amniocentesis and chorionic villus sampling. A systemic review. *Obstet Gynecol.* 2007;110:687–694. [Meta-Analysis]
38. Alfirevic Z, von Dadelszen P. Instruments for chorionic villus sampling for prenatal diagnosis. *Cochrane Database of Systematic Reviews.* 2003;1. [Meta-Analysis; 5 RCTs, $n = 472$]
39. Schaeffer AJ, Chung J, Heretis K, et al. Comparative genomic hybridization-array analysis enhance the detection of aneuploidies and submicroscopic imbalances in spontaneous miscarriages. *Am J Hum Genet.* 2004;74:1168–1174. [II-3]
40. Oostlander AE, Meijer GA, Yistra B. Microarray-based comparative genomic hybridization and its applications in human genetics. *Clin Genet.* 2004;66:488–495. [II-3]
41. Schaffer LG, Bui TH. Molecular cytogenetic and rapid aneuploidy detection methods in prenatal diagnosis. *Am J Med Genet.* 2007;145C:87–98. [Review]
42. Van den Veyver IB, Patel A, Shaw CA, et al. Clinical use of array comparative genomic hybridization (aCGH) for prenatal diagnosis in 300 cases. *Prenat Diagn.* 2009;29:29–39. [II-3]
43. Fruhman G, Van den Veyver IB. Applications of array comparative genomic hybridization in obstetrics. *Obstet Gynecol Clin N Am.* 2010;37:71–85. [Review]
44. Park JH, Woo JH, Shim SH, et al. Application of a target array comparative genomic hybridization to prenatal diagnosis. *BMC Medical Genetics.* 2010;11:102. [II-3]
45. ACOG Committee Opinion Number 446. Array comparative genomic hybridization in prenatal diagnosis. *Obstet Gynecol.* 2009;114(5):1161–1163. [Review]
46. Wapner RJ, Martin CL, Levy B et al. Chromosomal microarray versus karyotyping for prenatal diagnosis. *N Engl J Med.* 2012;367:2175–2184.
47. Reddy UM, Page GP, Saade GR. Karyotype versus microarray testing for genetic abnormalities after stillbirth. *N Engl J Med.* 2012;367:2185–2193.
48. Baty BJ, Blackburn BL, Carey JC. Natural history of trisomy 18 and trisomy 13: I. Growth, physical assessment, medical histories, survival, and recurrence risk. *Am J Med Genet.* 1994;49(2):175–188. [Review]
49. Baty BJ, Jorde LB, Blackburn BL. Natural history of trisomy 18 and trisomy 13: II. Psychomotor development. *Am J Med Genet.* 1994;49(2):189–194. [Review]

Carrier screening for inherited genetic conditions

Lorraine Dugoff

KEY POINTS
- The primary goals of carrier screening are to identify individuals and couples who are carriers of genetic mutations that place them at increased risk of having a child with a serious medical disorder and provide them with information to optimize pregnancy outcomes based on their personal values and preferences.
- Most inherited genetic conditions are autosomal recessive. Carriers for these conditions are usually asymptomatic, have no significant family history and are unaware of their carrier status.
- **Patients with a positive family history of a genetic condition should be referred for genetic counseling** to review the family history, provide accurate information regarding risk, offer the appropriate genetic testing, and discuss reproductive options.
- **Information regarding genetic carrier screening should be provided to every pregnant woman.**
- **Preconception carrier screening is preferred to prenatal carrier screening** as it enables couples to consider the most complete range of reproductive options. Information regarding the risk of having an affected child may influence a couple's decision to conceive or to consider the use of donor gametes, preimplantation genetic diagnosis, or prenatal genetic testing.
- Professional practice guidelines currently recommend offering **targeted carrier screening** for individual conditions based on race or ethnicity, condition severity, carrier frequency, prevalence, detection rates, and residual risk. This approach is limited due to inaccurate or unavailable information regarding ancestry, increased intermixing between different races/ethnicities and the presence of carriers for genetic conditions in the nontargeted populations.
- Technological advances have made it possible to perform **expanded carrier screening** which involves screening for mutations associated with multiple genetic diseases simultaneously irrespective of ancestry.
- While many practitioners are currently offering expanded carrier screening, professional practice guidelines and recommendations are needed regarding patient and provider education and the conditions that should be included on the screening panels. Future research in expanded carrier screening is needed to assess the impact of this approach on reproductive outcomes.
- Appropriate counseling regarding prognosis, possible complications, long-term issues, and follow-up should be provided to every couple with a pre- or postnatal diagnosis of aneuploidy or other genetic disorders.
- **Cystic fibrosis** (CF) screening should be offered to all women of reproductive age.
- Individuals of African, southeast Asian, and Mediterranean ancestry should have screening for **hemoglobinopathies** with a CBC in combination with a hemoglobin electrophoresis.
- Prenatal testing for **fragile X syndrome** should be offered to known carriers of the fragile X premutation or full mutation. Women with a family history of fragile X-related disorders, unexplained intellectual disability or developmental delay, autism, or premature ovarian insufficiency are candidates for genetic counseling and fragile X premutation carrier screening.
- Preconception and prenatal screening for spinal muscular atrophy (SMA) should be offered to individuals with a family history. Pan-ethnic screening is controversial.
- Carrier screening for Tay–Sachs disease (TSD) (enzyme and DNA), Canavan disease, CF, and familial dysautonomia should be offered to **Ashkenazi Jewish (one Jewish grandparent)** individuals before conception or during early pregnancy. The availability of genetic carrier screening for mucolipidosis IV, Niemann–Pick disease type A, Fanconi anemia group C, Bloom syndrome, and Gaucher disease should be discussed.

BACKGROUND
Ultrasound (see Chapter 4) as well as prenatal diagnosis and screening for aneuploidy (see Chapter 5) have been reviewed in previous chapters. Carrier screening for inherited genetic conditions is an important component of preconception and prenatal care. There are no trials to assess the downstream effects of any intervention for genetic screening and testing in pregnancy, but clearly there are significant effects. For example, the incidence of TSD in the Ashkenazi Jewish population has decreased by 90% since screening was initiated.

GENETIC COUNSELING
All individuals and couples should have a basic screen for family history of genetic disorders, with a pedigree to at least the second prior generation (three-generation pedigree). Questions should also involve history of birth defects, stillbirth, intellectual disability, developmental delay, recurrent spontaneous pregnancy loss and history of a previous fetus or child who was affected by a genetic disorder. Information regarding genetic carrier screening should be provided to **every pregnant woman. Those patients belonging to an ethnic** group at increased risk for a recessive condition (e.g., sickle cell—African-American; TSD and others—Jewish; TSD in Irish, Cajun, and French Canadian; α-thalassemia—southeast Asian; and β-thalassemia—Mediterranean) should be offered specific screening (see Chapters 14 and 15 in *Maternal-Fetal Evidence*

Based Guidelines). Genetic carrier screening should be performed on potential gamete donors. Providers may offer an expanded carrier screening panel. Individuals offered expanded carrier screening should have appropriate pretest counseling. It is **optimal to offer carrier screening preconception** so that women and their partners have the option to consider how much genetic information they would like to have before starting a family. Carrier screening results in the preconception period may influence a couple's decision to conceive or to consider the use of donor gametes, preimplantation genetic diagnosis, or prenatal genetic testing.

Women with a specific indication for genetic testing should be referred for genetic counseling and a discussion of options available for prenatal diagnosis. **Responsibilities of clinicians** (e.g., ob-gyns, family medicine specialists, and nurse midwives) caring for pregnant women regarding genetic screening are shown in Table 6.1 [1]. **Possible indications for genetic consultation** for preconception and prenatal patients are shown in Table 6.2 [2]. Possible indications for genetic consultation for adult patients are shown in Table 6.3 [2].

COMMON GENETIC DISORDERS AND CARRIER SCREENING GUIDELINES
Cystic Fibrosis

CF is an autosomal recessive disorder. The most common mutation is DF508, but >1700 other mutations have been described [3]. The mutation leads to faulty chloride transport, increased sweat chloride levels, and increased thick mucus in lungs, pancreas, biliary tree, and intestines. This is the most common life-limiting genetic disorder in Caucasians (Table 6.4) [3].

CF screening should be offered to all women of reproductive age [3–6]. It is generally more cost effective and practical to initially perform CF carrier screening for the patient only [3]. Nonetheless, screening can be concurrent or sequential, and both strategies are acceptable alternatives.

Concurrent screening:

- Both partners tested simultaneously
- Both partners' results revealed
- Assesses couple's risk
- Identifies couples at risk more rapidly
- More precise

Sequential screening:

- Initial screening of one partner
- Other partner tested if first partner is positive
- Low-risk racial/ethnic groups
- Other partner not available

Interpretation of Results

- Both partners negative (–/–)—prenatal diagnostic testing not indicated
- One partner carrier (–), one not screened:
  - Intermediate risk—prenatal diagnostic testing not indicated
- One partner carrier (+), one carrier (–):
  - Prenatal diagnostic testing not recommended
- One partner carrier (+), one untested:
  - Partner should be tested if possible genetic counseling
  - Availability/limitations of prenatal testing

Table 6.1 Responsibilities of Clinicians Caring for Pregnant Women Regarding Genetic Screening

1. Clinicians should be able to identify patients within their practices who are candidates for genetic testing and should maintain competence in the face of increasing genetic knowledge.
2. Obstetrician–gynecologists should recognize that geneticists and genetic counselors are an important part of the healthcare team and should consult with them and refer as needed.
3. Discussions with patients about the importance of genetic information for their kindred, as well as a recommendation that information be shared with potentially affected family members as appropriate, should be a standard part of genetic counseling.
4. Obstetrician–gynecologists should be aware that genetic information has the potential to lead to discrimination in the workplace and to affect an individual's insurability adversely. In addition to including this information in counseling materials, physicians should recognize that their obligation to professionalism includes a mandate to prevent discrimination.

Source: Modified from American College of Obstetricians and Gynecologists, *Obstet Gynecol*, 111, 1495–1502, 2008.

Table 6.2 Possible Indications for Genetic Consultation for Preconception and Prenatal Patients

Either Member of the Couple with	Reason to Consider Consultation
A positive carrier screening test for a genetic condition such as cystic fibrosis	Discuss additional testing strategies and inheritance, testing of partner and siblings
A personal history of stillbirths, previous child with hydrops, recurrent pregnancy losses, or a child with sudden infant death syndrome (SIDS)	Rule out a chromosomal, metabolic, or syndromic diagnosis associated with an unexplained neonatal death or SIDS
A progressive neurologic condition known to be genetically determined such as progressive ataxia	Discuss a potential diagnosis, the differential diagnosis, inheritance, and testing options
A statin-induced myopathy	Discuss a potential mitochondrial disorder, inheritance, and testing options
A family or personal history of:	Reason to consider consultation
A birth defect such as cleft lip	Discuss recurrence risks and testing options
A chromosomal abnormality such as translocation	Discuss risks to the fetus and testing options
Significant hearing or vision loss thought to be genetically determined	Discuss risks to the fetus and testing options
Intellectual disability, developmental delay, or autism	Discuss risks to the fetus and testing options

Source: Modified from Pletcher BA et al., *Genet Med*, 9, 385–389, 2007.

Table 6.3 Possible Indications for Genetic Consultation for Adult Patients

Personal History of	Reason to Consider Consultation
Abnormal sexual maturation or delayed puberty	Rule out an intersex condition, chromosomal abnormality, or syndromic diagnosis
Recurrent pregnancy losses (more than two)	Rule out a chromosomal rearrangement such as a balanced translocation with karyotype
Tall or short stature for genetic background	Rule out a skeletal dysplasia, chromosomal or syndromic diagnosis
One or more birth defects	Rule out a chromosomal or syndromic diagnosis, and provide genetic counseling
Six or more cafe-au-lait macules >1.5 cm in diameter	Rule out neurofibromatosis Type 1
Statin-induced myopathy	Rule out a mitochondrial disorder
A cancer or cancers known to be associated with specific genes or mutations in the context of a compelling family history: young age at onset, bilateral lesions, and familial clustering of related tumors	Rule out an identifiable mutation in a gene such as BRCA1; rule out a cancer syndrome (MEN2); discuss surveillance, treatment, testing options, and inheritance
Cardiovascular problems known to be associated with genetic factors such as cardiomyopathy	Rule out a mutation in a causative or contributory gene; discuss surveillance, treatment, testing options, and inheritance
Suspected genetic disorder affecting connective tissue	Rule out a syndromic diagnosis (Marfan syndrome); discuss surveillance, treatment, testing options, and inheritance
Hematologic condition associated with excessive bleeding or excessive clotting	Confirm or rule out genetic condition; discuss treatment, testing options, and inheritance
Progressive neurologic condition known to be genetically determined such as unexplained myopathy	Confirm or rule out suspected diagnosis; discuss surveillance, treatment, testing options, and inheritance
Visual loss known to be associated with genetic factors such as retinitis pigmentosa	Rule out a syndromic diagnosis (Stickler syndrome); discuss testing options, if applicable, and inheritance
Early-onset hearing loss	Rule out a syndromic or nonsyndromic genetic form of hearing loss; discuss surveillance, testing options, and inheritance
Recognized genetic disorder including a chromosomal or single-gene disorder	Confirm the diagnosis, discuss prognosis, medical management, and inheritance
Mental illness such as schizophrenia	Rule out a genetic condition associated with this history
A close relative with a sudden, unexplained death, particularly at a young age	Discuss diagnosis, inheritance, recurrence risks, and identify syndromes, when possible

Source: Modified from Pletcher BA et al., *Genet Med*, 9, 385–389, 2007.
Abbreviation: MEN2, type 2 multiple endocrine neoplasia.

Table 6.4 Incidence and Carrier Risk for CF Based on Race or Ethnicity

Racial or Ethnic Group	Detection Rate (%)	Estimated Carrier Risk Before Test	Estimated Carrier Risk After a (−) Test
Ashkenazi Jewish	94	1/24	~1/380
Non-Hispanic white	88	1/25	~1/200
Hispanic white	72	1/58	~1/200
African-American	64	1/61	~1/170
Asian-American	49	1/94	~1/180

Source: Modified from American College of Obstetrics and Gynecology, *Obstet Gynecol*, 117, 1028–1031, 2011.
Abbreviation: CF, cystic fibrosis.

- Both partners carrier (+):
  - 25% Chance of having an affected offspring
  - Genetic counseling
  - Prenatal diagnosis offered (chorionic villus sampling [CVS], amniocentesis)
  - Counseling regarding continuation versus termination of pregnancy for affected pregnancies

Risk of affected offspring depends also on prevalence of carrier status in the specific ethnic group (Table 6.4).

If a patient or the patient's partner has a family history of CF, medical record review should be performed to identify of cystic fibrosis transmembrane conductance regulator (CFTR) mutation analysis in the affected family member is available. If a woman's reproductive partner has apparently isolated congenital bilateral absence of the vas deferens, the couple should be referred for a genetics consultation to discuss potential clinical implications and mutation analysis.

Hemoglobinopathies

Hemoglobinopathies are a diverse group of inherited single-gene disorders that result from variations in the structure and/or function of hemoglobin. The most common hemoglobinopathies, sickle cell disease, β-thalassemia and α-thalassemia, are all autosomal recessive conditions. The American College of Obstetricians and Gynecologists (ACOG) recommends carrier screening for individuals of African, southeast Asian, and Mediterranean ancestry. A complete blood count (CBC) in combination with a hemoglobin electrophoresis is recommended for screening individuals of African ancestry. A CBC with red cell indices is the initial recommended screening test for individuals of southeast Asian, and Mediterranean ancestry. Individuals with a low mean corpuscular volume (MCV) and normal iron status should have a hemoglobin electrophoresis. Southeast Asians with a normal hemoglobin electrophoresis should have molecular testing to rule out α-globin gene deletions characteristic of α-thalassemia. Couples determined to be at increased risk for having a child with sickle cell disease or thalassemia should be referred to a genetic counselor [7]. For additional information regarding hemoglobinopathies, refer to Chapters 14 and 15 in *Maternal-Fetal Medicine Evidence Based Guidelines*.

Fragile X Syndrome

Diagnosis/Definition

Most common inherited cause of intellectual disability; caused by expansion of a repetition of the cytosine–guanine–guanine (CGG) trinucleotide segment of the fragile X mental retardation 1 (FMR-1) gene that is located on the X chromosome at Xq27.3.

The diagnosis is based on molecular genetic analysis. Most laboratories use a combination of two approaches: (1) Southern blot analysis to measure the degree of methylation and (2) polymerase chain reaction (PCR) to discriminate small differences in the intermediate and premutation sizes. Fragile X syndrome occurs when expansion of the CGG repeat occurs.

Epidemiology/Incidence

Both males and females can be affected. The prevalence is 1 in 3600 males and 1 in 4000–6000 females.

Genetics/Inheritance/Recurrence

The FMR-1 gene is typically comprised of a limited number of CGG repeats. This region is usually stable, relatively small (<45 repeats), and passes from one generation to the next. However, during meiosis in oocytes, the region can expand, reaching either intermediate (45–54 repeats) or premutation (55–200 repeats) lengths. As repeat size increases, stability decreases and further increases in the number of repeats become likely. Once the premutation reaches expansion to >90 repeats, the likelihood of expansion to a full mutation is at least 80% (Table 6.5) [8].

Only women with a premutation FMR-1 can pass the full mutation to their offspring. Fathers with premutations usually pass the gene in a stable fashion to all of their daughters and none of their sons and will have affected grandsons. Premutation male and female carriers are at risk for fragile X-associated tremor/ataxia syndrome (FXTAS) usually after age 50 years [9].

Table 6.5 Fragile X: Risk of Full Mutation (and Therefore Affected Child) Based on Number of Maternal CGG Repeats

No. Maternal CGG Repeats	% Risk Expansion to Full Mutation
55–59	4
60–69	5
70–79	31
80–89	58
90–99	80
100–200	98

Source: Modified from Nolin SL et al., *Am J Hum. Genet*, 72, 454–464, 2003.
Abbreviation: CGG, cytosine–guanine–guanine.

Screening

Prenatal testing for fragile X syndrome should be offered to known carriers of the fragile X premutation or full mutation. Women with a family history of fragile X-related disorders, FXTAS, unexplained intellectual disability or developmental delay, autism, or premature ovarian insufficiency are candidates for genetic counseling and fragile X premutation carrier screening [9]. General population screening is not recommended. A careful assessment of the family history for males with cognitive impairment related through females should be performed to identify individuals at sufficient likelihood of premutation or full mutation carrier status to warrant screening.

Women who accept fragile X premutation screening should be offered FMR-1 DNA mutation analysis after genetic counseling about the risks, benefits, and limitations of screening [9]. All identified carriers should be referred for follow-up genetic counseling. Diagnostic modalities for prenatal diagnosis (including CVS and amniocentesis) should be discussed.

Clinical Features

Males: Wide range of behavioral and cognitive manifestations and often subtle physical manifestations, but never asymptomatic. The behavioral phenotype is characterized by autism spectrum behaviors such as attention deficit/hyperactivity, expressive delay, tactile defensiveness, perseverative speech, and echolalia as well as social anxiety and avoidance of eye contact. The cognitive phenotype generally is **moderate to severe mental impairment.** Ten to twenty percent have seizures. Physical characteristics are more readily identifiable around puberty. Findings similar to a connective tissue disorder including hyperextensible joints, soft, smooth skin, flat feet, and mitral valve prolapse may be present. The facial appearance is often described as long and narrow with prognathism and large ears. Macrocephaly may be present. Most develop macroorchidism, and height tends to be below average.

Females: Tend to have fewer and milder abnormalities than males. More likely to have relatively normal cognitive development.

Spinal Muscular Atrophy

Diagnosis/Definition

SMA refers to a group of diseases that affect the motor neurons of the spinal cord and brainstem, which are responsible for supplying electrical and chemical signals to muscle cells. Without proper signals, muscle cells do not function properly and thus become much smaller (atrophy). This leads to muscle weakness. Individuals affected with SMA have progressive muscle degeneration and weakness, eventually leading to death.

Incidence

The incidence is 1/10,000 infants.

Genetics/Classification

There are several forms of SMA, depending on the age of onset and the severity of the disease. Two genes, SMN1 and SMN2, have been linked to SMA types I, II, III, and IV. Type I is the most severe form of SMA and characterized by muscle weakness present from birth, often manifested by difficulties with breathing and swallowing, and death usually by age 2–3 years. Type II has onset of muscle weakness after 6 months of age and can obtain some early physical milestones like sitting without support. Type III is a milder form of SMA, with onset of symptoms after 10 months of age. Individuals with Type III SMA often achieve the ability to walk but may have frequent falls and difficulty with stairs. The weakness is more in the extremities and affects the legs more than the arms. Type IV is the mildest form and is characterized by adult onset of muscle weakness.

SMA is most often caused by a deletion of a segment of DNA, in exon 7 and exon 8, in the SMN1 gene located on chromosome 5. Rarely, SMA is caused by a point mutation in the SMN1 gene.

Screening

The American College of Medical Genetics and Genomics (ACMG) recommends pan-ethnic screening for SMA while the ACOG only recommends screening when a family history is present [10,11]. Approximately 1 in 50 individuals is a carrier for SMA.

Carrier testing for SMA measures the number of copies of the deleted segment in the SMN1 gene. A noncarrier is expected to have two copies present (no deletion), while a carrier will have only one copy present (a deletion of one copy). SMA carriers most commonly have one functional SMN1 gene on one chromosome and an SMN1 gene deletion on the other chromosome. Carriers can also have two functional SMN1 gene copies on one chromosome (in cis) and none on the other chromosome (the '2 + 0' genotype), or one chromosome with a nonfunctional SMN1 gene with a point mutation or a microdeletion. Since carrier testing relies on a PCR-based gene-dose approach to determine SMN1 copy number, this method will not identify carriers with the '2 + 0' genotype. Carrier testing will also not identify point mutations. Approximately 90% of SMA carriers in the Ashkenazi Jewish population can be identified with this PCR-based testing method. A systematic review and meta-analysis including 169,647 SMA carrier tests in 14 studies reported an 87%–95% detection rate of SMA carrier testing in a non-Black population and a 71% sensitivity in the Black population due to a relatively high incidence of the "2 + 0" genotype in the black population. The positive predictive value of carrier testing when one copy of the SMN1 gene is identified is 100%, regardless of the population tested. There is a 5%–13% false-negative rate in non-Black individuals with a two-copy SMN1 result while there is a 29% false-negative rate in Black individuals with this result. Individuals with three SMN1 copies are almost always noncarriers [12].

ASHKENAZI JEWISH ANCESTRY GENETIC SCREENING
Who to Screen

The family history of individuals considering pregnancy, or who are already pregnant, should determine whether either member of the couple is of Eastern European (Ashkenazi) Jewish ancestry (one grandparent is Ashkenazi Jewish) or has a relative with one or more of the following genetic conditions: TSD, Canavan disease, CF, familial dysautonomia, Fanconi anemia group C, Niemann–Pick disease type A, mucolipidosis IV, Bloom syndrome, and Gaucher disease [13].

What to Screen for

The ACOG and the ACMG guidelines differ with respect to the conditions that should be included when performing carrier screening in individuals of Ashkenazi Jewish descent. **The ACOG recommends that carrier screening for TSD, Canavan disease, CF, and familial dysautonomia** should be offered to Ashkenazi Jewish individuals before conception or during early pregnancy so that a couple has an opportunity to consider prenatal diagnostic testing options. If the woman is already pregnant, it may be necessary to screen both partners simultaneously so that the results are obtained in a timely fashion to ensure that prenatal diagnostic testing is an option. ACOG acknowledges that carrier screening is available also for **mucolipidosis IV, Niemann–Pick disease type A, Fanconi anemia group C, Bloom syndrome, and Gaucher disease.** The ACMG recommends screening for these five additional disorders, for a total of nine [14]. ACMG provides criteria for adding new diseases to the panel of Jewish genetic diseases based on significant burden of the disorder, carrier rate >1/100 and/or test sensitivity >90%. Patient education materials can be made available so that interested patients can make an informed decision about having additional screening tests. Some patients may benefit from genetic counseling.

There are currently 19 diseases that are being made available for screening on Jewish genetic disease panels. In addition to those mentioned above, the following diseases are included in the new panels: maple syrup urine disease, glycogen storage disease type 1a, dihyrolipoamide dehydrogenase (DLD) deficiency, familial hyperinsulinism, Joubert syndrome, nemaline myopathy, SMA, Usher syndrome type 1F, Usher syndrome type III, and Walker–Warburg syndrome [15].

How to Screen

All the disorders on the Ashkenazi Jewish genetic disease panel are autosomal recessive. A carrier is unaffected but if two carriers of a mutation in the same gene have a child together, they have a 25% risk with each pregnancy of having an affected child (Figure 6.1).

When only one partner is of Ashkenazi Jewish descent, that individual should be screened first. If it is determined that this individual is a carrier, the other partner should be offered screening for that disorder. However, the couple should be informed that the carrier frequency and

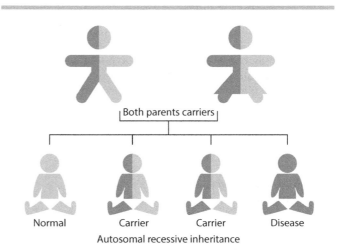

Figure 6.1 Autosomal recessive inheritance: where both parents are carriers, there is a one in four chance a child will be free of disease and not a carrier, a one in two chance a child will be a carrier, and a one in four chance a child will have the disease.

the detection rate in non-Jewish individuals are unknown for many of these disorders. Therefore, it is difficult to accurately predict the couple's risk of having a child with the disorder, and gene sequencing may be necessary to determine whether a non-Jewish partner is a carrier. Referral to a genetic counselor is recommended in these cases.

Individuals with a positive family history of one of these disorders should be offered carrier screening for the specific disorder (and others for this group) and may benefit from genetic counseling.

When both partners are carriers of one of these disorders, they should be referred for genetic counseling and offered prenatal diagnosis. Carrier couples should be informed of the disease manifestations, range of severity, and available treatment options. Prenatal diagnosis by DNA-based testing can be performed on cells obtained by CVS and amniocentesis.

When an individual is found to be a carrier, his or her relatives are at risk for carrying the same mutation. The patient should be encouraged **to inform his or her relatives of the risk and the availability of carrier screening.** The provider should not contact these relatives because there is no provider-patient relationship with the relatives, and confidentiality must be maintained [13].

SELECT DISORDERS

Carrier frequencies apply to the Ashkenazi Jewish population [15].

Tay–Sachs Disease

Carrier frequency is 1 in 30 in the Ashkenazi Jewish population. The carrier frequency is also increased in individuals of French Canadian and Cajun descent.

Clinical Features
The most well-known of these diseases. An apparently healthy child begins to lose skills around 4–6 months of age, and there is a progressive neurological decline leading to blindness, seizures, and unresponsiveness. Death usually occurs by the age of 4–6 years.

Testing
Carrier testing should be performed using DNA-based testing and hexosaminidase enzymatic activity testing [15]. The enzyme assay detects all carriers, regardless of ethnicity. DNA-based testing detects 94% of carriers and hexosaminidase A enzyme testing detects 98% of carriers in the Ashkenazi Jewish population [13]. Enzyme testing in pregnant women and women taking oral contraceptives should be performed using leukocyte testing as serum testing is associated with an increased false-positive rate in these populations.

Familial Dysautonomia

Carrier frequency is 1/32 with disease incidence of 1/3700.

Clinical Features
Causes the autonomic and sensory nervous system to malfunction, affecting the regulation of body temperature, blood pressure, and stress response, and causes decreased sensitivity to pain. Frequent pneumonia and poor growth may occur. Survival into adulthood is possible but with careful medical care.

Testing
Carrier testing for one major mutation and one other mutation accounts for 99.5% of carriers.

Canavan Disease

Carrier frequency is 1 in 40 with a disease incidence of 1 in 3000 to 1 in 6000.

Clinical Features
Appear normal at birth; then progressive loss of skills, hypotonia, macrocephaly, and spasticity. Most die within first year of life but may survive to second decade.

Testing
Carrier testing detects 98% carriers.

Bloom Syndrome

Carrier frequency is 1/100 with a disease incidence of 1/48,000.

Clinical Features
Short stature, a sun-sensitive skin rash, an increased susceptibility to infections and higher incidence of leukemia and other cancers, infertility, and immunodeficiency.

Testing
Carrier testing detects 95%–97% of carriers.

Fanconi Anemia Type C

Carrier frequency is 1/89 with disease incidence of 1/32,000.

Clinical Features
Associated with short stature, bone marrow failure, and a predisposition to leukemia and other cancers. Some children have limb, heart, or kidney abnormalities and learning difficulties.

Treatment
Pancytopenia can be treated with stem cell transplantation.

Testing
Carrier testing detects 99% of carriers.

Gaucher Disease

Carrier rate is 1/15 with disease incidence of 1/900.

Clinical Features
A variable condition both in age of onset and symptoms. It may present with a painful, enlarged spleen, anemia, and low white blood cell count. Bone deterioration is a major cause of pain and disability.

Treatment
Treatment is available.

Carrier Testing
Seven mutations account for >96% mutations.

Mucolipidosis Type IV

Carrier frequency is 1/127.

Clinical Features
A progressive neurological disorder with variable symptoms beginning in infancy. Characteristics include muscle weakness, mental retardation, and eye problems—both corneal clouding and retinal abnormalities develop.

Treatment
No treatment is available [15].

Carrier Testing
95% detection rate.

Glycogen Storage Disease, Type 1a
Carrier frequency is 1 in 64.

Clinical Features
A metabolic disorder that causes poor blood sugar maintenance with sudden drops in blood sugar, growth failure, enlarged liver, and anemia.

Treatment
Disease management involves lifelong diet modification.

Carrier Testing
95% detection rate.

Maple Syrup Urine Disease
Carrier frequency is 1 in 97.

Clinical Features
A variable disorder of amino acid metabolism. Named for the characteristic maple syrup smell of urine in those with the disorder.

Treatment
With careful dietary control, normal growth and development are possible. If untreated, it can lead to poor feeding, lethargy, seizures, and coma.

Carrier Testing
95% detection rate.

Niemann–Pick Disease Type A
Carrier frequency is 1 in 90.

Clinical Features
A progressive neurodegenerative disease characterized by hepatosplenomegaly, leading to death by age 2–4 years.

Carrier Testing
95% detection rate.

DLD Deficiency
Carrier frequency is 1 in 107.

Clinical Features
Presents in early infancy with poor feeding, frequent episodes of vomiting, lethargy, and developmental delay. Affected individuals develop seizures, enlarged liver, blindness, and ultimately suffer an early death.

Carrier Testing
>95% detection rate.

Familial Hyperinsulinism
Carrier frequency is 1 in 68.

Clinical Features
Characterized by hypoglycemia that can vary from mild to severe. It can be present in the immediate newborn period through the first year of life with symptoms such as seizures, poor muscle tone, poor feeding, and sleep disorders.

Carrier Testing
90% detection rate.

Joubert Syndrome
Carrier frequency is 1 in 92.

Clinical Features
Characterized by structural mid- and hindbrain malformations. Affected individuals have mild to severe motor delays, developmental delay, decreased muscle tone, abnormal eye movements, and characteristic facial features.

Carrier Testing
Detection rate is unknown (not enough data).

Nemaline Myopathy
Carrier frequency is 1 in 168.

Clinical Features
Most common congenital myopathy. Infants are born with hypotonia and usually have problems with breathing and feeding. Later some skeletal problems may arise, such as scoliosis. In general, the weakness does not worsen during life but development is delayed.

Carrier Testing
95% detection rate.

Usher Syndrome Type 1F
Carrier frequency is 1 in 147.

Clinical Features
Characterized by profound hearing loss, which is present at birth, and adolescent-onset retinitis pigmentosa, a disorder that significantly impairs vision.

Carrier Testing
≥75% detection rate.

Usher Syndrome Type III
Carrier frequency is 1 in 120.

Clinical Features
Causes progressive hearing loss and vision loss. Hearing is often normal at birth with progressive hearing loss typically beginning during childhood or early adolescence. Often leads to blindness by adulthood.

Carrier Testing
95% detection rate.

Walker–Warburg Syndrome
The carrier frequency in the Ashkenazi population for one Ashkenazi founder mutation is 1 in 149.

Clinical Features

It is a muscle, eye, and brain syndrome. It is a severe condition that presents with muscle weakness, feeding difficulties, seizures, blindness, brain anomalies, and delayed development. Life expectancy is below 3 years.

Carrier Testing

Detection rate is unknown (not enough data).

EXPANDED CARRIER SCREENING

Expanded carrier screening involves **simultaneous screening for multiple genetic conditions regardless of a patient's race/ethnicity.** Technological advances have made it possible to efficiently screen for a large number of conditions simultaneously for the same cost as one or two single-gene carrier tests. Expanded carrier screening has a number of advantages compared with the targeted screening approach. It can overcome the limitations associated with the targeted ethnicity-based screening approach including inaccurate and unavailable information regarding ancestry, increased intermixing between different races/ethnicities and the presence of carriers for genetic conditions in the nontargeted populations. Data from expanded carrier screening on 23,453 individuals from practices in the United States demonstrated that diseases currently recommended for screening only in certain populations, such as Canavan disease and sickle cell disease, are widely distributed outside of their targeted populations. Twenty-four percent of individuals were identified as carriers of at least one mutation [16]. **Future research in expanded carrier screening is needed** to assess the impact of this approach on reproductive outcomes. A 2012 survey of ACOG Fellows indicated that 15% of the responders offered expanded carrier screening to all of their patients and 52% provided this screening upon patient request [17].

Practice guidelines from national societies are needed to recommend conditions that should be included on expanded carrier panels and provide guidance to practitioners regarding pretest counseling. Since expanded carrier screens can include over 100 conditions, it is not feasible to counsel patients regarding the specific conditions on the panel. Table 6.6 lists points to include in the pretest counseling and consent process. If a patient and her partner both test positive as carriers for the same autosomal recessive genetic condition, they should be referred to a certified genetics professional to discuss the implications and reproductive options [19,20].

DIRECT-TO-CONSUMER GENETIC TESTING

Direct-to-consumer (DTC) genetic testing differs from traditional genetic testing in that consumers order tests and receive test results without an independent medical provider serving as an intermediary. Some DTC companies offer genetic counseling (generally by telephone), whereas others do not. These tests are typically advertised and sold over the Internet. DTC is permitted in about half the states in the United States and is subject to little oversight at the federal level. Internationally, several countries have issued reports cautioning against its use, and **several European countries have banned or are considering banning it entirely.** The American Society of Human Genetics has issued guidelines for transparency, provider education, and test and laboratory quality on DTC genetic testing [18]. The ACMG suggests the following regarding DTC genetic testing (www.acmg.net):

- A knowledgeable professional should be involved in the process of ordering and interpreting a genetic test.
- The consumer should be fully informed regarding what the test can and cannot say about his or her health.
- The scientific evidence on which a test is based should be clearly stated.
- The clinical testing laboratory must be accredited by Clinical Laboratory Improvement Amendments (CLIA), the State, and/or other applicable accrediting agencies.
- Privacy concerns must be addressed.

Table 6.6 Discussion Points for Pretest Counseling and Consent Process for Expanded Carrier Screening

1. Carrier screening is voluntary. Patients can choose to participate or decline.
2. Genetic testing results are confidential and protected in employment and health insurance by the Genetic Information Non-Discrimination Act of 2008.
3. Expanded carrier screening panels include conditions that may vary in severity. The panels include many conditions that are associated with significant adverse outcomes including decreased life expectancy, cognitive impairment and the need for medical and/or surgical intervention.
4. Accurate knowledge of paternity is necessary to provide accurate information regarding risk. DNA (or blood) from the biological father is necessary in order to provide risk assessments for autosomal recessive conditions.
5. There is a residual risk for having an affected offspring even if both partners screen negative. This risk may vary depending on ethnicity, the specific condition and the laboratory performing the testing.
6. It is common to identify carriers for one or more conditions when using expanded screening panels. In most cases, being a carrier has no significant medical consequences for the individual. If two partners are carriers of different autosomal recessive conditions, offspring are not likely to be affected.
7. It is possible that carrier screening will determine that an individual has two pathogenic variants for a condition and thus has an autosomal recessive condition that might affect their health. Expanded carrier screening panels that include autosomal dominant and X-linked conditions may detect individuals affected with one of these conditions. In these situations, individuals should be referred for genetic counseling and appropriate medical management.

Source: Modified from Edwards JG et al., *Obstet Gynecol*, 125, 653–662, 2015.

REFERENCES

1. American College of Obstetricians and Gynecologists. ACOG Committee Opinion No. 410: Ethical issues in genetic testing. *Obstet Gynecol.* 2008;111:1495–1502. [III]
2. Pletcher BA, Toriello HV, Noblin SJ, et al. Indications for genetic referral: A guide for healthcare providers. *Genet Med.* 2007;9:385–389. [III]
3. American College of Obstetrics and Gynecology. Update on carrier screening for cystic fibrosis. Committee Opinion No. 486. American College of Obstetrics and Gynecology. *Obstet Gynecol.* 2011;117:1028–1031. [III]
4. Edwards JG, Feldman G, Goldberg J, et al. Expanded carrier screening in reproductive medicine-Points to consider. A joint statement of the American College of Medical Genetics and Genomics, American College of Obstetrics and Gynecologists, National Society of Genetic Counselors, Perinatal Quality Foundation, and Society for Maternal-Fetal Medicine. *Obstet Gynecol.* 2015;125:653–662. [III]
5. Watson MS, Cutting GR, Desnick RJ, et al. Cystic fibrosis population carrier screening: 2004 Revision of American College of Medical Genetics mutation panel. *Genet Med.* 2004;6:387–391. [III]
6. Lanfelder-Schwind E, Karczeki B, Strecker MN, et al. Molecular testing for cystic fibrosis carrier status practice guidelines: Recommendations of the National Society of Genetic Counselors. *J Genet Couns.* 2014;23:5–15. [III]
7. American College of Obstetrics and Gynecology. Hemoglobinopathies in pregnancy. ACOG Practice Bulletin No. 78. American College of Obstetricians and Gynecologists. *Obstet Gynecol.* 2007;109:229–237. [III]
8. Nolin SL, Brown WT, Glicksman A, et al. Expansion of the Fragile X CGG repeat in females with permutation or intermediate alleles. *Am J Hum Genet.* 2003;72:454–464. [II]
9. American College of Obstetrics and Gynecology. ACOG Committee Opinion No. 469: Carrier screening for fragile X syndrome. *Obstet Gynecol.* 2010;116:1008–1010. [III]
10. Prior TW. Professional Practice and Guidelines Committee. Carrier screening for spinal muscular atrophy. *Genet Med.* 2008;10:840–842. [III]
11. American College of Obstetrics and Gynecology. Spinal muscular atrophy. ACOG Committee Opinion No. 432. American College of Obstetrics and Gynecology. *Obstet Gynecol.* 2009;113:1194–1196. [III]
12. MacDonald WK, Hamilton D, Kuhle S. SMA carrier testing: A meta-analysis of differences in test performance by ethnic group. *Prenat Diagn.* 2014;34:1219–1226. [II]
13. American College of Obstetricians and Gynecologists. ACOG Committee Opinion No. 442: Preconception and prenatal carrier screening for genetic disease in individuals of Eastern European Jewish descent. *Obstet Gynecol.* 2009;114:950–953. [III]
14. Gross SJ, Pletcher BA, Monaghan KG for the Professional Practice and Guidelines Committee. Carrier screening in individuals of Ashkenazi Jewish descent. *Genet Med.* 2008;10(1):54–56. Available at: www.acmg.net. [III]
15. Carlos J, Ferreira P, Schreiber-Agus N, et al. Carrier testing for Ashkenazi Jewish disorders in the prenatal setting: Navigating the genetic maze. *Am J Obstet Gynecol.* 2014;197–201. [III]
16. Lazarin GA, Haque IS, Nazareth S, et al. An empirical estimate of carrier frequencies for 400+ causal Mendelian variants: Results from an ethnically diverse clinical sample of 23,453 individuals. *Genet Med.* 2013;15:178–186. [II-2]
17. Benn P, Chapman AR, Erickson K, et al. Obstetricians and gynecologists' practice and opinions of expanded carrier testing and noninvasive prenatal testing. *Prenat Diagn.* 2014;34:145–152. [III]
18. American Society of Human Genetics. ASHG statement on direct-to-consumer genetic testing in the United States. *AM J Hum Genet. 2007;145–152.*
19. Langlois S, Benn P, Wilkins-Haug L. Current controversies in prenatal diagnosis 4: Pre-conception expanded carrier screening should replace all current prenatal screening for specific single gene disorders. *Prenat Diagn.* 2015;35:23–28. [III]
20. Rose NC. Expanded carrier screening: Too much of a good thing? *Prenat Diagn.* 2015;10:936–937. [III]

Before labor and first stage of labor

Serena Xodo

KEY POINTS

- **Before labor**
  - Prediction of spontaneous labor is imprecise, with best evidence for transvaginal ultrasound (TVU) cervical length (CL) having good predictive accuracy for spontaneous labor within 7 days.
  - If nonvertex presentation, perform **cesarean delivery (CD) at 39 0/7–39 6/7 weeks**. For timing and indications of other planned cesarean or vaginal deliveries, see Chapters 13 and 56 in *Maternal-Fetal Evidence Based Guidelines*.
  - If woman is candidate for vaginal delivery and ≥41 **weeks,** start **induction** (see Chapter 21).
  - **Maternal antenatal training to prepare for** labor and delivery **(L&D) is associated with arriving to L&D ward more often in active labor, less visits to the labor suite,** and **using less epidural analgesia.**
  - **X-ray pelvimetry should not be performed** as it is associated with no benefits, and it increases incidence of CDs. There is insufficient data regarding MRI or clinical pelvimetry.
- **There is limited evidence to assess the safety and efficacy of planned home birth for low-risk pregnant women.** Compared with planned hospital birth, **planned home birth is associated with a higher risk of neonatal deaths (0.2% vs. 0.09%), low Apgar scores, and neonatal seizures. The hospital is the safest setting for L&D.**
- A birth center in the hospital is a safe location for birth. The trend for a 67% higher perinatal mortality should be weighted during counseling against the significant 4% increase in spontaneous vaginal delivery (SVD) and 96% higher satisfaction.
- **Most women (those without risk factors) should be offered midwife-led models of care,** as midwife-led care is associated with a lower incidence of preterm birth, regional analgesia, instrumental vaginal birth, and fetal/neonatal death, and with shorter labor and a higher incidence of spontaneous vaginal birth. **So women should be encouraged to ask for this option.**
- **Training of traditional birth assistants in middle- and low-income countries is associated with a trend for less maternal mortality and significantly less perinatal mortality.**
- **Delayed hospital admission until** active labor (regular painful contractions and cervical dilatation >3 cm) **is associated with less time in the labor ward, less intrapartum oxytocics, and less analgesia.**
- Admission tests such as fetal heart rate (FHR) tracing and amniotic fluid assessment have not been associated with any benefit.
- Routine enema is not recommended.
- Perineal shaving is not recommended.
- Vaginal chlorhexidine irrigation is not recommended.
- **Universal prenatal maternal screening with anovaginal specimen at 35–37 weeks and intrapartum antibiotic treatment** are the most efficacious of the current strategies for prevention of neonatal early-onset group B streptococcus (GBS) disease.
- **All women should have continuous, one-on-one support throughout labor and birth (e.g., doula),** as it is associated with less intrapartum analgesia, cesarean birth, operative birth, and dissatisfaction with the childbirth experiences, and more spontaneous vaginal birth.
- There is insufficient evidence for providing nutritional recommendations for women in labor. **There is little justification for the restriction of fluids and food in labor for women at low risk of complications.**
- **Intravenous (IV) fluids at 250 mL/hour are associated with shorter duration of labor and less cesarean deliveries compared with 125 mL/hour.**
- **Upright positions** (either standing, sitting, kneeling, or walking around) in the first stage of labor **reduce the length of labor** by approximately **over 1 hour** and are associated with **less epidural analgesia.** Since walking does not seem to have a beneficial or detrimental effect on **L&D,** women can choose freely to walk or lay in bed, preferably upright, during labor, whichever is more comfortable for them.
- **Water immersion** during the **first stage** of labor **reduces the use of analgesia and by about 30 minutes the duration of the first stage of labor,** without adverse maternal or neonatal outcomes.
- Routine early (or even late) **amniotomy cannot be recommended as part of standard labor management and care.**
- **The use of the partogram cannot be recommended as a routine intervention in labor.**
- There is insufficient evidence to recommend any particular frequency of vaginal cervical examinations in labor. Most studies, including those with active management, perform cervical examinations every 2 hours in active labor, but the risk of chorioamnionitis increases with increasing number of examinations.
- **For women making slow progress in the first stage of spontaneous labor,** the use of **oxytocin augmentation** is associated with a **reduction in the time to delivery of approximately 2 hours.**
- The individual interventions that are part of **active management of labor** should be studied separately, and only those that are beneficial (e.g., support by doula) implemented.
- **Dystocia cannot be diagnosed unless rupture of membranes (ROM) has occurred,** and adequate oxytocin to

achieve at least three to five adequate contractions per hour has been instituted. Dystocia also **cannot be diagnosed reliably before the first stage of labor has entered the active phase, which has been defined, especially in nulliparous with epidurals in place, as at least 6 cm of cervical dilatation. Before performing a CD for active phase labor arrest, labor should be arrested for a minimum of 4 hours (if uterine activity is greater than 200 Montevideo units as documented with intrauterine pressure catheter [IUPC]) or 6 hours (if greater than 200 Montevideo units could not be sustained).**

INTRODUCTION

For management of induction, meconium, oligo/polyhydramnios, intrapartum monitoring (including amnioinfusion for variables), operative vaginal delivery, shoulder dystocia, trial of labor after cesarean (TOLAC), intrauterine growth restriction (IUGR), macrosomia, abnormal third stage, etc., **see appropriate distinct guidelines in this book and its companion,** *Maternal-Fetal Evidence Based Guidelines.* This chapter discusses prediction of the onset of spontaneous labor, and especially interventions before labor and in the first stage of labor that can influence L&D outcomes.

PREDICTION OF THE ONSET OF SPONTANEOUS LABOR
Weather Effects

There is no strong association between changes in barometric pressure and onset of labor [1].

Time of Day

Diurnal rhythms seem to show a higher rate of starting labor in the evening and night hours [2].

Cervical Status

Both the Bishop score and CL measure usually by TVU have been evaluated for their predictive accuracy for the onset of spontaneous labor. TVU CL is associated with very good prediction of onset of spontaneous labor: for example, the chance of labor within 7 days is about 10% for a woman with a TVU CL of 40–45 mm at about 37–39 weeks, and about 90% if TVU CL is about 10 mm at about 37–39 weeks [3].

BEFORE LABOR
Antenatal Classes

Antenatal classes to improve the birth process have been studied in at least three randomized controlled trials (RCTs).

Compared with no such training, 9 hours of antenatal training to prepare for L&D are associated with **arriving to L&D ward more often in active labor** (relative risk [RR] 1.45, 95% confidence interval [CI] 1.26–1.65) and **using less epidural analgesia** (RR 0.84, 95% CI 0.73–0.97) [4].

Compared with no such education, antenatal education focusing on natural childbirth preparation with training in breathing and relaxation techniques is not associated with any effects on maternal or perinatal outcomes, including similar incidences of epidural analgesia, childbirth, or parental stress, in nulliparous women and their partners [5].

In a small RCT, **specific antenatal education program is associated with a reduction in the mean number of visits to the labor suite before the onset of labor** [6]. It is unclear whether this results in fewer women being sent home because they are not in labor.

Fear of Childbirth

Fear of childbirth is associated with a 47 minutes longer duration of labor, compared with no fear of childbirth [7]. Intensive counseling in women with fear of childbirth reduces anxiety and concerns related to pregnancy and birth, and is associated with shorter labors [8].

Nonvertex Presentation

If **nonvertex presentation** is detected, CD at 39 0/7–39 6/7 weeks is recommended (see Chapter 24). For timing and indications of other planned cesarean or vaginal deliveries, see Chapters 13, and 56 in *Maternal-Fetal Evidence Based Guidelines.*

Late-Term Gestation

Induction advised at ≥**41 weeks** (see Chapter 27).

Pelvimetry

There is not enough evidence to support the use of X-ray pelvimetry in women whose fetuses have a cephalic or noncephalic presentation. **Women undergoing X-ray pelvimetry are more likely to be delivered by cesarean section** [9]. No significant impact is detected on perinatal outcome, but numbers are small, insufficient for meaningful evaluation (e.g., perinatal mortality 1% vs. 2%). The results are similar for women with or without a prior CD.

There is insufficient data regarding MRI or clinical pelvimetry.

Interventions to Expedite the Onset of Labor

For acupuncture, breast stimulation, castor oil, enemas and baths, homeopathy, sexual intercourse, as well as other nonpharmacologic and pharmacologic techniques to expedite the onset of labor, or for induction, see Chapter 21.

SITE OF LABOR MANAGEMENT
Planned Home Birth

There is limited evidence to assess the safety and efficacy of planned home birth for low-risk pregnant women as there is only one RCT with only 11 women ever published [10,11]. In healthy low-risk women, compared with planned hospital birth, **planned home birth is associated with a higher risk of neonatal deaths (0.2% vs. 0.09%)** in a meta-analysis of nonrandomized studies including over 500,000 births [12]. In a large (>79,000 women with singletons, term, cephalic, nonanomalous pregnancies) retrospective cohort study, planned out-of-hospital births were associated with a higher rate or **perinatal deaths** (3.9 vs. 1.8 deaths per 1000 deliveries; OR 1.52, 95% CI 0.51–2.54) than planned in-hospital deliveries, as well as more neonatal seizures [13]. Data from U.S. births showed a significantly increased risk of **neonatal deaths, low Apgar scores, and neonatal seizures** associated with home births or births in free standing birth centers, compared with hospital births [14,15]. Some of these studies included freestanding birth centers with home births. This means, therefore, that the **hospital is the safest setting for L&D** [16]. A home birth service ought to be backed up by a modern hospital system. There are diverging opinions even in Western countries, with about 30% of Dutch births occurring at home, versus <1% of U.S. births. In the United States, about 75% of home births are delivered by **noncertified** midwives. In the Netherlands, travel time of >20 minutes from home to hospital is associated with increased risk of perinatal mortality and other adverse outcomes [17]. **Women with risk factors for abnormal outcome should deliver in a hospital setting.** All women should be aware of possible maternal and fetal risks, including severe morbidity and mortality, associated with L&D even in low-risk women, and should be aware of the **absence of intensive care and operative capabilities in the home setting** [10]. Inference from results of "home-like" versus conventional ward setting (see below) should warn against home birth.

Ethical experts agree that hospital birth is safer. Some medical ethics experts emphasize that physicians should counsel strongly against home birth [18]. Some other medical ethics experts argue instead that, given the increased risk of perinatal mortality is about 1–2/1000 in home compared with hospital birth, women should be counseled on these absolute numbers and allowed a choice based on autonomy [19].

Freestanding Birth Center
There are no RCTs of freestanding birth centers, and therefore the evidence is insufficient to recommend this setting [20]. For non-RCT evidence, see above, under "Planned home births."

Planned Hospital Birth: Alternative Setting (Home-Like, e.g., Hospital Birth Center) versus Conventional Hospital Ward Setting
Several RCTs have evaluated the option of "alternative setting" versus conventional hospital ward setting for L&D. For alternative setting, most trials included care by midwives in a location in the hospital, close to the regular L&D ward, that did not look like a usual L&D setting. There are no RCTs of freestanding birth centers or Snoezelen rooms. Some RCTs randomized women in labor, while others at the beginning of pregnancy. So continuity of care was usually higher in the alternative setting group. **Usually about 40%–50% of patients randomized to alternative setting** (often about 60% for nulliparous women, 20%–30% for multiparous women) **need to be moved in labor to the conventional L&D ward.**

Compared with conventional hospital ward, allocation to an alternative hospital setting **increased the likelihood of the following: no intrapartum analgesia/anesthesia** (RR 1.18, 95% CI 1.05–1.33); **SVD** (RR 1.03, 95% CI 1.01–1.05); **breast-feeding at 6–8 weeks** (RR 1.04, 95% CI 1.02–1.06); and **very positive views of care** (RR 1.96, 95% CI 1.78–2.15). Allocation to an alternative setting **decreased the likelihood of epidural analgesia** (RR 0.80, 95% CI 0.74–0.87); **oxytocin augmentation** of labor (RR 0.77, 95% CI 0.67–0.88); and **episiotomy** (RR 0.83, 95% CI 0.77–0.90) [13]. There was no apparent effect on maternal morbidity and mortality, serious perinatal morbidity/mortality (RR 1.17, 95% CI 0.51–2.67), perinatal mortality (RR 1.67, 95% CI 0.93–3.00), other adverse neonatal outcomes, or postpartum hemorrhage. The 4% increase in SVD may be secondary to less epidural anesthesia, which may in turn be secondary to less availability in home-like settings, and/or to less intrapartum monitoring. **The trend for a 67% higher perinatal mortality should be weighted against the significant 4% increase in SVD and 96% higher satisfaction, during counseling.** Episiotomy should be avoided in general (see Chapter 8). No firm conclusions can be drawn regarding the effects of variations in staffing, organizational models, or architectural characteristics of the alternative settings [20]. **A birth center in the hospital is a safe location for birth** [16].

PROVIDER
Midwife-Led Care
In many parts of the world, midwives are the primary providers of care for childbearing women. Elsewhere it may be medical doctors or family physicians who have the main responsibility for care, or the responsibility may be shared. The underpinning philosophy of midwife-led care is normality, continuity of care, and being cared for by a known and trusted midwife during labor. There is an emphasis on the natural ability of women to experience birth with minimum intervention [21].

The effect of midwife-lead care compared with physician-led care or to other provider-led care has been evaluated mostly for the whole pregnancy, including together both antepartum care and care during L&D (see also Chapter 2). Therefore, it is difficult to assess the effect of midwife-led care just on L&D.

A systematic review compared the midwife-led continuity model versus other models, including 15 RCTs, for a total of 17,674 women. Women who midwife-led continuity models of care were **less likely to experience regional analgesia** (RR 0.85, 95% CI 0.78–0.92), **instrumental vaginal birth** (RR 0.90, 95% CI 0.83–0.97), **preterm birth less than 37 weeks** (RR 0.76, 95% CI 0.64–0.91), and **less overall fetal/neonatal death** (RR 0.84, 95% CI 0.71–0.99) [21]. Women who had midwife-led continuity models of care were **more likely to experience spontaneous vaginal birth** (RR 1.05, 95% CI 1.03–1.07). There were no differences between groups for cesarean births or intact perineum. In addition, women assisted by midwives were **less likely to receive** some medical interventions, such as **amniotomy** (RR 0.80, 95% CI 0.66–0.98), **episiotomy** (RR 0.84, 95% CI 0.77–0.92), and **intrapartum analgesia/anesthesia** (RR 1.21, 95% CI 1.06–1.37). Women who had midwife-led continuity models of care were **less likely to experience longer mean length of labor** (hours) (mean difference [MD] 0.50, 95% CI 0.27–0.74), to be **attended at birth by a known midwife** (RR 7.04, 95% CI 4.48–11.08), and had **less fetal loss/neonatal death before 24 weeks** (RR 0.81, 95% CI 0.67–0.98). There were no differences between groups for fetal loss or neonatal death more than or equal to 24 weeks, induction of labor, antenatal hospitalization, antepartum hemorrhage, augmentation/artificial oxytocin during labor, opiate analgesia, perineal laceration requiring suturing, postpartum hemorrhage, breast-feeding initiation, low birth weight infant, 5-minute Apgar score ≤ 7, neonatal convulsions, admission of infant to special care or neonatal intensive care unit(s), or mean length of neonatal hospital stay (days). The majority of included studies reported a **higher rate of maternal satisfaction** in midwife-led continuity models of care [21] (see also section "Continuous Support in Labor").

Training of Birth Assistants
Training of traditional birth assistants **in middle- and low-income countries is associated with a trend for less maternal mortality and significantly less perinatal mortality** [22]. There are no trials in high-income countries.

Teamwork Training
There is **insufficient evidence** to assess the effects of training and teamwork education for L&D personnel. Quality and safety initiatives are probably beneficial but have not been sufficiently studied in RCTs. Compared with no such training, a standardized teamwork training curriculum based on crew resource management that emphasized communication and team structure was not associated with significant effect on adverse maternal and perinatal outcomes in one RCT [23].

ADMISSION
Delayed versus Early Hospital Admission
Labor assessment programs, which aim to **delay hospital admission until active labor,** may benefit women with term pregnancies. Active labor was defined as regular painful contractions and cervical dilatation >3 cm. In one RCT, compared with direct admission to hospital, delayed admission until active labor is associated with **less time in the labor ward, less intrapartum oxytocics, and less analgesia** [24]. Women in the labor assessment and delayed admission group report **higher levels of control during labor. CD rates are similar, with a nonsignificant 30% decrease.** A 30%–40% decrease in CD has been reported in retrospective studies with delayed versus direct admission. There is insufficient evidence (a larger trial needed) to assess true effects on rate of CD and other important measures of maternal and neonatal outcome. Potential risks of delayed admission include unplanned out-of-hospital births and the potentially harmful effects of withholding caregiver support and attention to women in early or latent phase labor.

In another RCT, compared with no use of algorithm, use of an algorithm by midwives to assist in their diagnosis of active labor (painful, regular contractions with at least one of the following: 3 cm dilated, ROM, or "show") was associated with more women being discharged after their first labor ward assessment, and no effect of oxytocin augmentation and other medical interventions in labor [25].

Suggested criteria for admission based on these studies are a cervix of at least 3–4 cm dilatation and regular painful contractions. Pregnant women should be informed of these data during prenatal care.

Fetal Assessment Tests upon Admission
FHR Tracing for 20 Minutes
Women allocated to admission cardiotocography (CTG) have an increase in incidence of cesarean section than women allocated to intermittent auscultation (RR 1.20, 95% CI 1.00–1.44). There is no significant difference in instrumental vaginal birth (RR 1.10, 95% CI 0.95–1.27) and fetal and neonatal deaths (RR 1.01, 95% CI 0.30–3.47) [26].

Amniotic Fluid Volume Index
Obtaining an amniotic fluid volume index (AFI) in early labor is associated with a higher incidence of CD, and similar neonatal outcomes, compared with no AFI [27].

Neither a 2 × 1 pocket (abnormal in 8%) nor an AFI (abnormal in 25%) upon admission for labor identifies a pregnancy at risk for adverse outcome such as nonreassuring fetal heart rate tracing (NRFHT) or CD for NRFHT [28].

Other Tests
There is insufficient evidence to support the use of vibroacoustic stimulation or Doppler ultrasound as fetal admission tests, as there are no RCTs on these interventions.

Enemas
Enemas do not have a significant beneficial effect on infection rates such as perineal wound infection or other neonatal infections and women's satisfaction. Compared with no enema, enema in labor is associated with no significant differences for infection rates in puerperal women (RR 0.66, 95% CI 0.42–1.04) and no significant differences in neonatal umbilical infection rates (RR 3.16, 95% CI 0.50–19.82). No significant differences are found in the incidence of neonatal lower or upper respiratory tract infections [29].

One RCT described labor to be significantly shorter (50 minutes) with enema versus no enema. A second RCT found labor to be significantly longer (112 minutes) with enema compared with no enema. No significant differences in the duration of labor were found in the third RCT that scored as having a low risk of bias and was adjusted for parity. One RCT that researched women's views found no significant differences in satisfaction between groups. **The routine use of enemas during labor should be discouraged** [29]. This intervention (enema) generates discomfort in women and increases the costs of delivery.

Perineal Shaving
There is **no support for routine perineal shaving** (shaving with a razor) for women prior to or in labor. In a very old trial, 389 women were alternately allocated to receive either skin preparation and perineal shaving or clipping of vulvar hair only. In the second old trial, which included 150 participants, perineal shaving was compared with the cutting of long hairs for procedures only. In the third trial, 500 women were randomly allocated to shaving of perineal area or cutting of perineal hair. Compared with no shaving, shaving was associated with a similar incidence of maternal febrile morbidity (RR 1.14, 95% CI 0.73–1.76), perineal wound infection (RR 1.47, 95% CI 0.80–2.70), and perineal wound dehiscence (RR 0.33, 95% CI 0.01–8.00). In the smaller trial, fewer women who had not been shaved had Gram-negative bacterial colonization compared with women who had been shaved (OR 0.43, 95% CI 0.20–0.92). There were no differences in maternal satisfaction immediately after birth [30]. The potential for complications (redness, multiple superficial scratches and burning and itching of the vulva, and embarrassment and discomfort afterward when the hair grows back), which often occur later, suggests that **shaving should not be part of routine clinical practice.** The first two trials are old (1922 and 1965) and included the clipping of long hairs in their control groups to aid in operative procedures, which is itself usually unnecessary and can lead to complications.

Morphine Sleep
Morphine sleep, also called therapeutic rest, given usually in the latent phase of the first stage of labor, has never been evaluated with an RCT [31].

FIRST STAGE
Chlorhexidine
There is **no evidence to support the use of vaginal chlorhexidine by either irrigation or vaginal wipes during labor** in order to prevent maternal and neonatal infections. The effect on the incidence of postpartum endometritis is not statistically significant (RR 0.83; 95% CI 0.61–1.13) [32]. Chlorhexidine solution is safe, not expensive, and vaginal irrigation is easy to perform, but apparently not beneficial.

GBS Prophylaxis
In the United States and some European countries **universal prenatal maternal GBS screening** is performed, with **anovaginal specimen collected at 35–37 weeks and antibiotic (ampicillin first line) treatment** administered intrapartum to GBS colonized women [33]. **Women with GBS bacteriuria** in the

current pregnancy or who had a **prior infant with GBS sepsis are candidates for intrapartum antibiotics prophylaxis and should be the only two groups not screened. Intrapartum treatment for chorioamnionitis is recommended regardless of GBS maternal status** (see Chapter 22 and Chapter 37 in *Maternal-Fetal Evidence Based Guidelines*). Other European countries use a risk-based strategy, which means to offer intrapartum antibiotic treatment to all women with recognized risk factors: previous infant affected by GBS sepsis, GBS bacteriuria during current pregnancy, preterm labor < 37 weeks, prelabor ROM ≥18 hours and/or fever in labor ≥38°C. **Support for the universal screening strategy is based on a large retrospective study**, which concluded that this policy was more than 50% effective in preventing early GBS sepsis [33]. However, no RCTs are available on this issue. There is no intervention shown to be efficacious for prevention of late-onset GBS sepsis.

Continuous Support in Labor

Definition
For support, it is generally intended emotional support (continuous presence, reassurance, and praise), information about labor progress and advice regarding coping techniques, comfort measures (comforting touch, massage, warm baths/showers, promoting adequate fluid intake and output), and advocacy (helping the woman articulate her wishes to others) [34].

Mechanism of Action
Anxiety during labor is associated with high levels of the stress hormone epinephrine in the blood, which may in turn lead to abnormal FHR patterns in labor, decreased uterine contractility, a longer active labor phase with regular well-established contractions, and low Apgar scores. One example of possible mechanisms of action for support to reduce complications of L&D is decreased anxiety [34]. This in turn can lead to a beneficial "chain-reaction": for example, if continuous support leads to reduced use of epidural analgesia, then several complications associated with regional anesthesia (see Chapter 11) can be prevented.

Types of Support
Family member or friend (not part of hospital staff) or hospital-based (part of hospital staff). Doula (a Greek word for "handmaiden") is a support person with the sole job of providing support to the laboring woman. They are usually not part of the hospital staff. This member of the caregiver team may also be called a labor companion, birth companion, labor support specialist, labor assistant, or birth assistant.

Effectiveness
Continuous support during labor has clinically meaningful benefits for women and infants and no known harm. **All women should have support throughout labor and birth.** Women allocated to continuous support are more likely to have a **spontaneous vaginal birth** (RR 1.08, 95% CI 1.04–1.12) and **less likely to have intrapartum analgesia** (RR 0.90, 95% CI 0.84–0.96) **or to report dissatisfaction** (RR 0.69, 95% CI 0.59–0.79). In addition, their labors are about 1-hour shorter (MD −0.58 hours, 95% CI −0.86 to −0.30) (MD −0.58 hours, 95% CI −0.85 to −0.31), they are **less likely to have a cesarean** (RR 0.78, 95% CI 0.67–0.91) or **instrumental vaginal birth** (RR 0.90, 95% CI 0.85–0.96), or regional analgesia (RR 0.93, 95% CI 0.88–0.99) **or a baby with a low 5-minute Apgar score** (RR 0.69, 95% CI 0.50–0.95). There is no apparent impact on other intrapartum interventions, maternal or neonatal complications, or on breast-feeding. **Continuous support is most effective when provided by a woman who is neither part of the hospital staff nor the woman's social network, and in settings in which epidural analgesia is not routinely available.** No conclusions could be drawn about the timing of onset of continuous support. **Hospitals should permit and encourage women to have a companion of their choice during labor and birth, and administrators and policymakers should ensure that these services are available to every pregnant woman** [34] (see also the section "Midwife-Led Care").

It may be possible to increase access to one-to-one continuous labor support worldwide by encouraging women to invite a family member or friend to commit to being present at the birth and assuming this role. The mother selects her doula during pregnancy; they establish a relationship (which is likely to involve the woman's partner, if any) and discuss the mother's and partner's preferences and concerns before labor. The doula brings her experience and training (often to the level of certification) to the labor support role during childbirth, and the mother and doula frequently have telephone and/or face-to-face contact in the early postpartum period. Other models of support, for which there are little or no data, include support by a female family member and support by the husband/partner [34].

Aromatherapy

There **is insufficient evidence** to assess the effects of aromatherapy in labor. Compared with no such intervention, administration of selected essential oils during labor is not associated with significant effects on CD, instrumental delivery, or use of oxytocin. While maternal pain perception in nulliparous women was decreased in one RCT on this intervention, this RCT was also not blind [35].

Nutrition in Labor

Since the evidence shows no benefits or harms, **there is little justification for the restriction of fluids and food in labor for women at low risk of complications.** All studies looked at women in active labor and at low risk of potentially requiring a general anesthetic. One study looked at complete restriction versus giving women the freedom to eat and drink at will; two studies looked at water only versus giving women specific fluids and foods; and two studies looked at water only versus giving women carbohydrate drinks.

When comparing any restriction of fluids and food versus **women given some nutrition in labor** (three RCTs), the meta-analysis was dominated by one study undertaken in a highly medicalized environment. There were no statistically significant differences identified in the following: cesarean section (RR 0.89, 95% CI 0.63–1.25), operative vaginal births (RR 0.98, 95% CI 0.88–1.10), and Apgar scores <7 at 5 minutes (RR 1.43, 95% CI 0.77–2.68), nor in any of the other outcomes assessed. Women's views were not assessed. The pooled data were insufficient to assess the incidence of Mendelson syndrome (bronchopulmonary reaction following aspiration of gastric contents during anesthesia), an extremely rare outcome [36].

Oral carbohydrate intake, equivalent to about 10 teaspoons of sugar, in labor is not associated with any effect on labor outcomes, like length of labor or mode of delivery [37]. Some umbilical cord studies revealed lactate transport to the fetal circulation with potential (but not observed) fetal academia [38,39].

No studies looked specifically at women at increased risk of complications; hence, there is no evidence to support restrictions in this group of women [36].

Ice chips to moisten the mouth and sips of clear liquids are the only oral intake recommended by U.S. authorities [40]. Some experts also allow sport drinks, yogurt, or sherbet. In the Netherlands women in labor are allowed to eat and drink. The reason for avoiding solid food is risk of aspiration ("Mendelson syndrome"), which is rare (about 15/10,000 CDs) [41]. When there is increased gastric volume, there is increased risk of vomiting and therefore aspiration. Airway precautions in L&D are paramount to avoid aspiration.

Acid Prophylaxis Drugs

There is **no good evidence to support** the routine administration of acid prophylaxis drugs in normal labor to prevent gastric aspiration and its consequences [42]. Giving such drugs to women once a decision to give general anesthesia is made is discussed in Chapter 11.

IV Fluids

Two RCTs compared **IV fluids** (up to 250 mL/hour + oral intake) versus oral intake only. There was a **reduction in the duration of labor** in IV fluids + oral intake of **29 minutes** (MD −28.86, 95% CI −47.41 to −10.30, two studies, 241 women). There was no statistically significant reduction in the number of cesarean deliveries. There was no evidence of a statistically significant difference in admission to the neonatal unit and in low Apgar score at five minutes [43].

Four RCTs compared **250 mL/hour** with 125 mL/hour IV fluids in labor in women with **restricted oral intake**. There was a significant **reduction of over one and an half hour in the duration of labor** in women who received 250 mL/hour (MD 105.61 minutes, 95% CI 53.19–158.02 ($P < 0.0001$). There was a **significant reduction in the cesarean section rate** in women receiving a higher rate of IV fluid infusion (RR 1.56, 95% CI 1.10–2.21; ($P = 0.01$) [36].

Three RCTs compared women who received **250 mL/hour** versus 125 mL/hour of IV fluids with **free oral fluids** in both groups. Women receiving 250 mL/hour had **shorter labors** than those receiving 125 mL/hour (MD **23.87 minutes**, 95% CI 3.72–44.02, 256 women). There was no statistically significant reduction in the number of cesarean deliveries in the 250 mL IV fluid group (RR 1.00, 95% CI 0.54–1.87). In one study the number of assisted vaginal deliveries was lower in the group receiving 125 mL/hour (RR 0.47, 95% CI 0.27–0.81).

The benefits are substantiated by the fact that several trials in nonpregnant adults demonstrate that increased fluid intake improves exercise performance.

Compared with normal saline without dextrose, normal saline with **5% dextrose,** both given IV at 125 mL/hour in early labor (3–5 cm), is associated with a **shorter (by about 70 minutes) duration of labor** from initiation of IV infusion to delivery. The incidence of labor lasting >12 hours was decreased from 22% to about 10% [44]. Five percent dextrose has also been associated with less umbilical cord acidemia compared with lactated Ringer's solution [45].

In summary, **IV fluids at 250 mL/hour are associated with shorter duration of labor and less cesarean deliveries compared with 125 mL/hour and should be preferred.** There is insufficient evidence for which type of IV fluids to use, with possibly some benefit for those containing 5% dextrose.

Maternal Position

Upright and mobile positions (either standing, sitting, kneeling, or walking around) **in the first stage of labor reduce the length of labor** and do not seem to be associated with increased intervention or negative effects on mothers' and babies' well-being. Compared with recumbent positions, the first stage of labor is approximately **1 hour and 22 minutes shorter for** women randomized to upright and mobile positions. Women randomized to upright positions are **less likely to have epidural analgesia** (RR 0.81, 95% CI 0.66–0.99), **and cesarean section** (RR 0.71, 95% CI 0.54–0.94) [46]. There are no differences between groups for other outcomes including length of the second stage of labor, or other outcomes related to the well-being of mothers and babies, except for a **lower incidence of neonatal intensive care unit admission** in the upright group. For women who had epidural analgesia there were no differences between those randomized to upright and recumbent positions for any of the outcomes examined in the review. Little information on maternal satisfaction was collected, and none of the studies compared different upright or recumbent positions. A woman semireclining or lying down on the side or back during the first stage of labor may be more convenient for staff and can make it easier to monitor progression and check the baby. Fetal monitoring, epidurals for pain relief, and use of IV infusions also limit movement. **Women should be encouraged to take up whatever position they find most comfortable in the first stage of labor** [46].

Ambulation

Compared with remaining in bed, walking in labor is associated with similar length of first stage of labor, use of oxytocin, use of analgesia, need for forceps vaginal delivery, or CD, and also similar neonatal outcomes in women at term with cephalic presentation starting at 3–5 cm of dilatation [47] or in other groups of women [46,48–51]. Since walking does not seem to have a beneficial or detrimental effect on L&D, **women can choose freely to walk or stay upright** (see the section "Maternal Position") **in bed during labor, whichever is more comfortable for them.** See also the section "Maternal Position," as upright position *and* mobility have been associated with shorter labors.

Immersion in Water

Compared with controls (labor not in water), water immersion **during the first stage of labor reduces by 10% the use of epidural/spinal analgesia** (RR 0.90, 95% CI 0.82–0.99) **and by about 30 minutes the duration of the first stage of labor.** There is **no difference in other outcomes:** assisted vaginal deliveries (RR 0.86, 95% CI 0.71–1.05), cesarean sections (RR 1.21, 95% CI 0.87–1.68), use of oxytocin infusion (RR 0.64, 95% CI 0.32–1.28), perineal trauma or maternal infection, Apgar score <7 at 5 minutes (RR 1.58, 95% CI 0.63–3.93), neonatal unit admissions (RR 1.06, 95% CI 0.71–1.57), or neonatal infection rates (RR 2.00, 95% CI 0.50–7.94) [52]. There is limited information for other outcomes related to water use during the first and second stages of labor, due to intervention and outcome variability. There is no evidence of increased adverse effects to the fetus/neonate or woman from laboring in water. Laboring in water is usually linked to midwifery care, which is associated with its own benefits (see the section "Midwife-Led Care"). There are no trials evaluating different baths/pools, immersion in water during pregnancy, or during the third stage of labor. For water birth and immersion in water in the second stage, see Chapter 8.

Stripping in Labor
There are no trials to evaluate stripping during spontaneous labor (see also Chapter 21 for stripping before labor).

Early Artificial Rupture of Membranes (AROM) (aka Amniotomy)
Compared with no amniotomy, amniotomy is not associated with significant differences in length of the first stage of labor (MD −20.43 minutes, 95% CI −95.93–55.06), cesarean section (RR 1.27, 95% CI 0.99–1.63), maternal satisfaction with childbirth experience, or low Apgar score <7 at 5 minutes (RR 0.53, 95% CI 0.28–1.00). Other maternal and perinatal outcomes are also not different. There is no consistency between RCTs regarding the timing of amniotomy during labor in terms of cervical dilatation. An association between early amniotomy and CD for NRFHT is noted in one large trial [53]. Therefore, routine early (or even late) **amniotomy cannot be recommended as part of standard labor management and care.** Women should be counseled regarding these results, and make an informed decision regarding the option of this intervention [53]. Early amniotomy may be possibly reserved for women with slow labor progress.

Use of Partogram
A partogram is a preprinted form, the aim of which is to provide a pictorial overview of labor to plot progress in labor and to alert health professionals to any problems with the mother or baby. The general intervention with the partogram is early use of oxytocin as soon as the cervical dilatation falls to the right of the partogram, usually on the 2-hour cervical examinations.

The use of the partogram cannot be recommended as a routine intervention in labor. Compared with no partogram, the use of the partogram is **not associated with significant effects** on cesarean section (RR 0.64, 95% CI 0.24–1.70), instrumental vaginal delivery (RR 1.00, 95% CI 0.85–1.17), or Apgar score <7 at 5 minutes (RR 0.77, 95% CI 0.29–2.06), in two RCTs including 1590 women [54].

Compared with a 4-hour action line, women in the 2-hour action line group are more likely to require oxytocin augmentation (RR 1.14, 95% CI 1.05–1.22). When the 3- and 4-hour action lines are compared, cesarean section rate is lowest in the 4-hour action line group (RR 1.70, 95% CI 1.07–2.70) [53–56]. When a partogram with a latent phase (composite) and one without (modified) were compared, the cesarean section rate was lower in the partogram without a latent phase [54].

Frequency of Cervical Examinations
Only one RCT assessed different frequencies of cervical assessment in labor. Comparing two-hourly with four-hourly vaginal examinations in labor, there was no difference in length of labour (MD in minutes −6.00, 95% CI −88.70 to 76.70; one RCT, $n = 109$). There were no data on maternal or neonatal infections requiring antibiotics, and women's overall views of labor. There were no differences in augmentation, epidural for pain relief, cesarean section, spontaneous vaginal birth and operative vaginal birth [57].

The only other RCT on cervical assessment in labor compared routine vaginal examinations with routine rectal examinations to assess the progress of labor. There was no difference in neonatal infections requiring antibiotics (RR 0.33, 95% CI 0.01–8.07; one RCT, $n = 307$). There were no data on length of labor, maternal infections requiring antibiotics, and women's overall views of labor. The study did show that significantly fewer women reported that vaginal examination was very uncomfortable compared with rectal examinations (RR 0.42, 95% CI 0.25–0.70). There were no differences in augmentation, cesarean section, spontaneous vaginal birth, operative vaginal birth, perinatal mortality, and admission to neonatal intensive care.

In summary, cervical assessment should be done by cervical and not rectal examination, as per patient's safety and comfort. **There is insufficient evidence to recommend any particular frequency of vaginal cervical examinations in labor.** Most studies, including those regarding active management, perform cervical examinations every 2 hours in labor. The risk of chorioamnionitis though increases with increasing number of examinations [58].

Oxytocin Augmentation
There are **no trials to evaluate the timing and dosing of oxytocin in labor in women making normal progress in labor.**

For women making slow progress in the first stage of spontaneous labor, treatment with oxytocin as compared with no treatment or delayed oxytocin treatment does not result in any discernable difference in the number of cesarean sections performed, in one meta-analysis. In addition there are no detectable adverse effects for mother or baby [59]. The meta-analysis included eight appropriate studies, for a total of 1338 women with low risk singleton pregnancies at term in the active stage of labor. **IV oxytocin versus placebo or no treatment** (three trials; 138 women) showed **no difference** as for cesarean section rates; only three small trials were considered so that the comparison was clearly underpowered to make any firm conclusions. **Early use of IV oxytocin versus delayed use** (five trials; 1200 women), however, was much larger and also showed **no effect on cesarean section rates.** The early use of oxytocin did significantly increase uterine hyperstimulation with FHR changes; however, this did not translate into serious neonatal morbidity or perinatal death. The early use of oxytocin, as opposed to its delayed use, did significantly **shorten the time to delivery by approximately two hours,** which might be important to some women.

In a different meta-analysis, early oxytocin was associated with a 9% significant increase in the probability of SVD, but also a tripling of the rate of hyperstimulation, without apparent perinatal consequences [60].

In summary, **oxytocin augmentation in women making slow progress in the first stage seems to be associated with a 2-hour shortening of labor,** with apparent effect on mode of delivery or other maternal and perinatal outcomes.

There is insufficient evidence to assess how to best use (i.e., dosing issues) oxytocin for augmentation of labor. There are four variables to assess: (1) type of dilution, (2) initial dose, (3) incremental increase, and (4) maximum dose [61]. In a meta-analysis, a higher initial dose (e.g., 2 mU/minute) of oxytocin and incremental dose (e.g., 4 mU/minute or more) was associated with a significant reduction in length of labor reported from one trial (MD −3.50 hours, 95% CI −6.38 to −0.62, one RCT, $n = 40$). There was a decrease in rate of cesarean section (RR 0.62; 95% CI 0.44–0.86) and an increase in the rate of spontaneous vaginal birth (RR 1.35; 95% CI 1.13–1.62). There were no significant differences for neonatal mortality, hyperstimulation, chorioamnionitis, epidural analgesia; or neonatal outcomes of Apgar scores, umbilical cord pH, or admission to special care baby unit. Many outcomes were not evaluated, such as perinatal mortality, women's satisfaction, instrumental vaginal birth, uterine rupture, postpartum hemorrhage, abnormal cardiotocography, women's pyrexia, dystocia, and neonatal neurological morbidity [62]. Based mostly on physiologic studies, an oxytocin dilution of 10 mU/mL, and initial dose of 2 mU/minute (12 mL/hour), incremental increase of 2 mU (12 mL) every 30–45 minutes until adequate labor, and maximum dose of 16 mU/minute (up to 24 mU) have been proposed [61].

Stopping oxytocin, instead of continuing it, once the active phase of labor is reached in women in spontaneous labor is **not associated in maternal or perinatal benefits.** Stopping oxytocin is associated with **longer (by about 30 minutes) time to delivery** [63].

For use of oxytocin in induction, see Chapter 21.

Active Management of Labor

Active management of labor was originally devised to shorten labor, and therefore prevent prolonged labor. Its components have varied somewhat in the literature but generally include antenatal classes, admission not before premature rupture of membranes (PROM) or 2 cm dilatation and full effacement (active labor), early amniotomy, support by doula, use of partogram, and vaginal examinations every 2 hours, with oxytocin started for rate of progress off the partogram or < 1 cm/hour. Oxytocin rate is started at 4–6 mU/minute, increased by 4–6 mU every 15 minutes to reach contractions every 2–3 minutes (but not more than 7/15 minutes) or 40 mU/minutes. Early amniotomy and early use of high-dose oxytocin are the two most characteristic interventions of active management of labor.

Compared with "routine" care (no active management), active management of labor is associated with a trend for a slightly lower incidence of CD (RR 0.88, 95% CI 0.77–1.01). However, in one study there were a large number of postrandomization exclusions. On excluding this study, **CD rates in the active management group were statistically significantly lower than in the routine care group** (RR 0.77, 95% CI 0.63–0.94). **More women in the active management group had labors lasting less than 12 hours,** but there was wide variation in length of labor within and between trials. The **reduced duration of labor** is about 50–100 minutes, mostly in the first stage. There were no differences between groups in use of analgesia, rates of assisted vaginal deliveries, or maternal or neonatal complications. Only one RCT examined maternal satisfaction; the majority of women (over 75%) in both groups were very satisfied with care [64–68]. The shorter labor is probably due to the early amniotomy (see the section "Early Artificial Rupture of Membranes (AROM) [(aka Amniotomy]"). The effects on incidence of CD may be due to the fact that some aspects of active managements (e.g., support by doula) decrease CD rate, but some others (e.g., early amniotomy) may increase it. It is recommended that **the individual interventions that are part of active management of labor should be studied separately, and only those that are beneficial (e.g., support by doula) implemented.**

Use of Continuous versus Intermittent Monitoring, Amnioinfusion for Variables, Scalp Sampling, etc.
See Chapter 10.

Bladder Catheterization
There are *no trials* to evaluate the necessity, timing, and frequency of bladder catheterization in labor per se.

Epidural or Other Anesthesia
See Chapter 11.

Use of Ultrasound During Labor
There is growing evidence, including RCTs, to assess the effect of using ultrasound during L&D. There are several potential uses, including as an aid to the diagnosis of malposition, dystocia, etc. [69]. Performing routine ultrasound to assess fetal head position in singleton pregnancies in labor ≥8 cm, compared with digital vaginal assessment alone, is associated with an increase in operative vaginal delivery, with no other effects on maternal or perinatal outcomes [70].

Use of Intrauterine Pressure Catheter
The IUPC can measure more objectively than external tocomonitor the intensity of uterine contractions. It necessitates ROM. Intensity is usually calculated by Montevideo units, that is, sum of peak pressures above baseline of all contractions in 10 minutes.

Several RCTs have assessed the effect of IUPC on labor outcomes. In the largest RCT, compared with no IUPC, IUPC use is associated with **no effect** in rate of operative deliveries, maternal or fetal infection, or other maternal or perinatal recorded outcome [71]. In the meta-analysis, the neonatal outcome was not statistically different between groups: Apgar score < 7 at 5 minutes (RR 1.78, 95% CI 0.83–3.83); umbilical artery pH < 7.15 (RR 1.31, 95% CI 0.95–1.79); admission to the neonatal intensive care unit (RR 0.34, 95% CI 0.07–1.67); and more than 48 hours hospitalization (RR 0.92, 95% CI 0.71–1.20). The pooled risk for instrumental delivery (including cesarean section, vacuum and forceps extraction) was not statistically significantly different (RR 1.05, 95% CI 0.91–1.21). Hyperstimulation was similar between groups (RR 1.21, 95% CI 0.78–1.88). **No serious complications** were reported in the trials and **no neonatal or maternal deaths occurred** [72]. See also section "Criteria for Diagnosis of Failure to Progress in First Stage."

CRITERIA FOR DIAGNOSIS OF FAILURE TO PROGRESS IN FIRST STAGE

According to studies now >60 years old in women without regional anesthesia by Friedman, the active phase began at 2.5 cm and ended at complete dilatation, with an average duration of 4.6–4.9 hours, a mean rate of cervical dilation of 3 cm/hour and the slowest acceptable rate (95th percentile) of 1.2 cm/hour [73,74]. More recently investigators found that the active phase labor in nulliparous women lasts longer than previously thought. According to a systematic review, which included 18 studies (for a total of 7009 women), the active phase of labor among healthy, low risk, nulliparous women at term with a spontaneous labor onset, lasts 6 hours on average, and the average cervical dilation rate is 1.2 cm/hour. This means that rates of cervical dilatation during active labor from 4 cm forward are much slower than those reported by Friedman. According to recent evidence it seems that the slowest acceptable rate of cervical dilation is 0.6 cm/hour. In term women in labor necessitating oxytocin and with epidural, the fifth percentile rate for dilatation is about 0.5 cm/hour for both nulliparous and parous women [75]. In term women with epidural, **labor may take more than 6 hours to progress from 4 to 5 cm, and more than 3 hours to progress from 5 to 6 cm of dilation** [76]. Moreover, cervical dilation during active phase labor is often conceptualized linearly, however recent evidence suggest that cervical dilation rates accelerate throughout the majority of labor. So, in common practice, the likelihood of accelerative intervention is much greater in earlier active labor. It must be kept in mind that progression in the earlier part of "active labor" will typically be slower than 0.6 cm/hour, while progression in more advanced active labor will typically be more rapid [77].

Abnormal progression of labor, including terms such as dystocia, dysfunctional labor, failure to progress, cephalopelvic disproportion, and others, is the most common problem in labor, and the **reason for the majority of CDs** [78]. Risk factors for dystocia are, among others, as follows: obesity, induction, Bishop <5 at start of labor, station higher than −2, persistent occiput posterior, macrosomia, epidural anesthesia, etc. There are no RCTs on interventions for asynclitism [79] (see also Chapter 24). For malposition, see Chapter 24. **Dystocia cannot be diagnosed unless ROM has occurred, and adequate oxytocin** to achieve at least three to five adequate contractions per hour has been instituted. Dystocia also **cannot be diagnosed reliably before the first stage of labor has entered the active phase, which has been defined, especially in nulliparous with epidurals in place, as at least 6 cm of cervical dilatation** [76]. The majority (>60%) of women who experience 2 hours of labor arrest despite a sustained uterine contraction pattern of at least 200 Montevideo units in the first stage of labor will achieve a vaginal delivery if oxytocin is continued [80]. **Before performing a CD for active phase labor arrest, labor should be arrested for a minimum of 4 hours (if uterine activity is greater than 200 Montevideo units as documented with IUPC) or 6 hours (if greater than 200 Montevideo units could not be sustained)** [80,81]. These data are not from an RCT, and there was a significant higher risk of shoulder dystocia among parturient who had arrest for 4 hours or more. Vaginal birth after cesarean (VBAC) and diabetics were not included in this study. Please see Chapter 8 for additional evidence on dystocia.

In women at term with singleton gestations and requiring oxytocin by obstetrician because of "dystocia" at 4–6 cm, **meperidine 100 mg IV does not affect operative delivery rates and worsens neonatal outcomes compared with placebo** [82] (see also Chapter 8).

REFERENCES

1. Noller KL, Resseguie LL, Voss V. The effect of changes in atmospheric pressure on the occurrence of the spontaneous onset of labor in term pregnancies. *Am J Obstet Gynecol*. 1996;174:1192–1199. [II-2]
2. Cagnacci A, Soldani R, Melis GB, et al. Diurnal rhythms of labor and delivery in women: Modulation by parity and seasons. *AJOG*. 1998;178:140–145. [II-2]
3. Saccone G, Simonetti B, Berghella V. Transvaginal ultrasound cervical length for prediction of spontaneous labour at term: A systematic review and meta-analysis. *BJOG*. 2016;123:16–22. [Meta-analysis]
4. Maimburg RD, Vaeth M, Durr J, et al. Randomized trial of structured antenatal training sessions to improve the birth process. *BJOG*. 2010;117:921–928. [RCT, n = 1193]
5. Bergstrom M, Kieler H, Waldenstrom U. Effects of natural childbirth preparation versus standard antenatal education on epidural rates, experience of childbirth and parental stress in mothers and fathers: A randomized controlled trial. *BJOG*. 2009;116:1167–1176. [RCT, n = 1087]
6. Bonovich L. Recognizing the onset of labour. *J Obstet Gynecol Neonatal Nurs*. 1990;19(2):141–145. [RCT, n = 245;208 analyzed]
7. Adams SS, Eberhard-Gran M, Eskild A. Fear of childbirth and duration of labour: A study of 2206 women with intended vaginal delivery. *BJOG*. 2012;119:1238–1246. [II-1]
8. Saisto T, Salmela-Aro K, Nurmi JE, et al. A randomized controlled trial of intervention in fear of childbirth. *Obstet Gynecol*. 2001;98(5):820–826. [RCT, n = 176].
9. Pattinson RC, Farrell E. Pelvimetry for fetal cephalic presentations at or near term. *Cochrane Database Syst Rev*. 2005;(4):CD003514. [Meta-analysis: 4 RCTs (all used X-ray pelvimetry; all not of good quality), n = 895]
10. Dowswell T, Thornton JG, Hewison J, et al. Should there be a trial of home versus hospital delivery in the United Kingdom? Measuring outcomes other than safety is feasible. *BMJ*. 1996;312:753. [RCT, n = 11]
11. Olsen O, Clausen JA. Planned hospital birth versus planned home birth. *Cochrane Database Syst Rev*. 2012;(9):CD000352. [Meta-analysis: 1 RCT, n = 11]
12. Wax JR, Lucas FL, Lamont M, et al. Maternal and newborn outcomes in planned home birth vs planned hospital births: A meta-analysis. *Am J Obstet Gynecol*. 2010;203:243.e1–243.e8. [Meta-analysis on non-RCTs]
13. Snowden JM, Tolden EL, Snyder J, et al. Planned out-of-hospital birth and birth outcomes. *NEJM*. 2015;373:2642–2653. [II-1]
14. Grunebaum A, McCullough LB, Sapra KJ, et al. Early and total mortality in relation to birth setting in the United States, 2006–2009. *AJOG*. 2014;211:390.e1–7. [II-1]
15. Grunebaum A, McCullough LB, Sapra KJ, et al. Apgar score of 0 at 5 minutes and neonatal seizures or serious neurologic dysfunction in relation to birth setting. *Am J Obstet Gynecol*. 2013;209:323.e1–6. [II-1]
16. American College of Obstetricians and Gynecologists. ACOG Committee Opinion No. 476: Planned home birth. *Obstet Gynecol*. 2011;117:425–427. [Review]
17. Ravelli ACJ, Jager KJ, de Groot MH, et al. Travel time from home to hospital and adverse perinatal outcomes in women at term in the Netherlands. *BJOG*. 2010;118(4):457–465. [II-2]
18. Chervenak FA, McCullough LB, Arabin B. Obstetric ethics: An essential dimension of planned home birth. *Obstet Gynecol*. 2011;117(5):1183–1187. [Review]
19. Ecker J, Minkoff H. Home birth. What are physicians' ethical obligations when patient choices may carry increased risk? *Obstet Gynecol*. 2011;117:1179–1182. [Review]
20. Hodnett ED, Downe S, Walsh D, et al. Alternative versus conventional institutional settings for birth. *Cochrane Database Syst Rev*. 2012;(8):CD000012. [Meta-analysis: 10 RCTs, n = 11,795]
21. Sandall J, Soltani H, Gates S, et al. Midwife-led versus other models of care for childbearing women. *Cochrane Database Syst Rev*. 2015;(9):CD004667. [15 RCTs, n = 17674]
22. Jokhio AH, Winter HR, Cheng KK. An intervention involving traditional birth attendants and perinatal and maternal mortality in Pakistan. *NEJM*. 2005;352:2091–2099. [1 RCT, n = 20,557]
23. Nielsen PE, Goldman MB, Mann S, et al. Effects of teamwork training on adverse outcomes and process of care in labor and delivery: A randomized controlled trial. *Obstet Gynecol*. 2007;109:48–55. [RCT, n = 1307 personnel, 28,536 deliveries]
24. McNiven PS, Williams, JI, Hodnett E, et al. An early labour assessment program: A randomised, controlled trial. *Birth*. 1998;25(1):5–10. [RCT, n = 209]
25. Cheyne H, Hundley V, Dowding D, et al. Effects of algorithm for diagnosis of active labour: Cluster randomized trial. *BMJ*. 2008;337:a2396. [RCT, n = 4503]
26. Devane D, Lalor JG, Daly S, et al. Cardiotocography versus intermittent auscultation of fetal heart on admission to labour ward for assessment of fetal wellbeing. *Cochrane Database of Systematic Reviews*. 2012;(2):CD005122. DOI: 10.1002/14651858. CD005122.pub4. [Meta-analysis; 4 RCTs, n = 13,000]
27. Chauhan SP, Washburne JF, Magann EF, et al. A randomized study to assess the efficacy of the amniotic fluid index as a fetal admission test. *Obstet Gynecol*. 1995;86:9–13. [RCT, n = 883]

28. Moses J, Doherty DA, Magann EF, et al. A randomized clinical trial of the intrapartum assessment of amniotic fluid volume: Amniotic fluid index versus the single deepest pocket technique. *Am J Obstet Gynecol.* 2004;190:1564–1570. [RCT, n = 499]
29. Reveiz L, Gaitán HG, Cuervo LG. Enemas during labour. *Cochrane Database Syst Rev.* 2013; (7):CD000330. [Meta-analysis; 4 RCTs, n = 1917]
30. Basevi V, Lavender T. Routine perineal shaving on admission in labour. *Cochrane Database Syst Rev.* 2014; CD001236. [Meta-analysis, 3 RCTs]
31. Mackeen AD, Fehnel E, Berghella V, Klein T. Morphine sleep in pregnancy. *Am J Perinatol.* 2014;31:85–90. [II-3]
32. Lumbiganon P, Thinkhamrop J, Thinkhamrop B, et al. Vaginal chlorhexidine during labour for preventing maternal and neonatal infections (excluding Group B Streptococcal and HIV). *Cochrane Database Syst Rev.* 2014;(9):CD004070. [3 RCTs, n = 3012]
33. Schrag S, Gorwitz R, Fultz-Butts K, et al. Prevention of perinatal group B streptococcal disease. *MMWR Recomm Rep.* 2002;51(RR-11):1–24. [Review/Guideline; www.cdc.gov/groupbstrep]
34. Hodnett ED, Gates S, Hofmeyr GJ, Sakala C. Continuous support for women during childbirth. *Cochrane Database Syst Rev.* 2013;(7):CD003766. [Meta-analysis:22 RCTs; n = 15,288]
35. Burns E, Zobbi V, Panzeri D, et al. Aromatherapy in childbirth: A pilot randomized controlled trial. *BJOG.* 2007;114:838–844. [RCT, n = 513]
36. Singata M, Tranmer J, Gyte GML. Restricting oral fluid and food intake during labour. *Cochrane Database Syst Rev.* 2013;(8):CD003930. [Meta-analysis: 5 RCTs, n = 3130]
37. Malin GL, Bugg GJ, Thornton J, et al. Does oral carbohydrate supplementation improve labour outcomes? A systematic review and individual patient data meta-analysis. *BJOG.* 2016;123:510–517. [Meta-analysis, 8 RCTs, n = 691]
38. Scheepers HCJ, Thans MCJ, de Jong PA, et al. A double-blind, placebo controlled study on the influence of carbohydrate solution intake during labor. *BJOG.* 2002;109:178–181. [RCT, n = 201]
39. Scheepers HCJ, de Jong PA, Essed GGM, et al. Carbohydrate solution intake during labour just before the start of the second stage: A double-blind study on metabolic effects and clinical outcome. *BJOG.* 2004;111:1382–1387. [RCT, n = 2021]
40. Practice guidelines for obstetrical anesthesia. A report by the American Society of Anesthesiologist Task Force on Obstetrical Anesthesia. *Anesthesiology.* 1999;90:600–611. [Review]
41. Olsson GL, Hallen B, Hambreas-Jonzon K. Aspiration during anaesthesia: A computer aided study of 185358 anaesthetics. *Acta Anaesthesiol Scand.* 1986;30:84–92. [II-2]
42. Gyte GML, Richens Y. Routine prophylactic drugs in normal labour for reducing gastric aspiration and its effects. *Cochrane Database Syst Rev.* 2006;(3):CD005298. [Meta-analysis; 3 RCTs, n = 2465]
43. Dawood F, Dowswell T, Quenby S. Intravenous fluids for reducing the duration of labour in low risk nulliparous women. *Cochrane Database Syst Rev.* 2013;(6):CD007715. [Meta-analysis; 9 RCTs, n = 1617]
44. Shrivastava VK, Garite TJ, Jenkins SM, et al. A randomized, double-blinded controlled trial comparing parenteral normal saline with and without dextrose on the course of labor in nulliparas. *Am J Obstet Gynecol.* 2009;200:379.e1–379.e6. [RCT, n = 300]
45. Fisher AJ, Huddleston JF. Intrapartum maternal glucose infusion reduces umbilical cord acidemia. *Am J Obstet Gynecol.* 1997;177:765–769. [RCT, n = 106]
46. Lawrence A, Lewis L, Hofmeyr GJ, et al. Maternal positions and mobility during first stage labour. *Cochrane Database Syst Rev.* 2013;(10):CD003934. [Meta-analysis: 25 RCTs, n = 5128]
47. Bloom SL, McIntire DD, Kelly MA, et al. Lack of effect of walking on labor and delivery. *NEJM.* 1998;339:76–79. [RCT, n = 1067]
48. McManus TJ, Calder AA. Upright posture and the efficiency of labour. *Lancet.* 1978;1:72–74. [RCT, n = 40]
49. Flynn AM, Kelly J, Hollins G, et al. Ambulation in labour. *BMJ.* 1978;2:591–593. [RCT, n = 68].
50. Read JA, Miller FC, Paul RH. Randomized trial of ambulation versus oxytocin for labor enhancement: A preliminary report. *Am J Obstet Gynecol.* 1981;139:669–672. [RCT, n = 14]
51. Hemminki E, Saarikoski S. Ambulation and delayed amniotomy in the first stage of labor. *Eur J Obstet Gynecol Reprod Biol.* 1983;15:129–139. [RCT, n = 630]
52. Cluett ER, Burns E Immersion in water in labour and birth. *Cochrane Database Syst Rev.* 2009;(2):CD000111. [Meta-analysis: 12 RCTs, n = 3243]
53. Smyth RM, Markham C, Dowswell T. Amniotomy for shortening spontaneous labour. *Cochrane Database Syst Rev.* 2013;(6): CD006167. [Meta-analysis: 15 RCTs, n = 5583]
54. Lavender T, Hart A, Smyth RM. Effect of partogram use on outcomes for women in spontaneous labour at term. *Cochrane Database Syst Rev.* 2013;(7):CD005461. [Meta-analysis: 6 RCTs, n = 7706; of which 2 RCTs partogram vs no partogram; 4 RCTs assessed different partogram designs]
55. Pattison RC, Howarth GR, Mdluli W, et al. Aggressive or expectant management of labour: A randomized clinical trial. *BJOG.* 2003;110:457–461. [RCT, n = 694]
56. World Health Organization Maternal Health and Safe Motherhood Programme. World Health Organization partograph in the management of labour. *Lancet.* 1994;343:1399–1404. [RCT, n = 35,484]
57. Downe S, Gyte GML, Dhalen HG, Singata M. Routine vaginal examinations for assessing progress of labour to improve outcomes for women and babies at term. *Cochrane Database Syst Rev.* 2013. [Meta-analysis; 2 RCTs, one n = 109; the other n = 307]
58. Soper DE, Mayhall CG, Dalton HP. Risk factors for intraamniotic infection: A prospective epidemiologic study. *Am J Obstet Gynecol* 1989;161:562–566; discussion 566–568. [II-2]
59. Bugg GJ, Siddiqui F, Thornton JG. Oxytocin versus no treatment or delayed treatment for slow progress in the first stage of spontaneous labour. *Cochrane Database Syst Rev.* 2013;(6):CD007123. [Meta-analysis: 8 RCTs, n = 1338]
60. Wei S-Q, Luo Z-C, Xu H, et al. The effect of early oxytocin augmentation in labor—A meta-analysis. *Obstet Gynecol.* 2009;114:641–649. [Meta-analysis: 9 RCTs, n = 1983]
61. Hayes EJ, Weinstein L. Improving patient safety and uniformity of care by a standardized regimen for the use of oxytocin. *Am J Obstet Gynecol.* 2008;198(6):622.e1–622.e7. [Review]
62. Kenyon S, Tokumasu H, Dowswell T, et al. High-dose versus low-dose oxytocin for augmentation of delayed labour. *Cochrane Database Syst Rev.* 2013;(7):CD007201. [Meta-analysis: 4 RCTs, n = 660]
63. Ozturk FH, Yilmaz SS, Yalvac S, et al. Effect of oxytocin discontinuation during the active phase of labor. *JMFNM.* 2015;28:196–198. [RCT, n = 140]
64. Brown HC, Paranjothy S, Dowswell T, Thomas J. Package of care for active management in labour for reducing caesarean section rates in low-risk women. *Cochrane Database Syst Rev.* 2013;(9):CD004907. [Meta-analysis: 7 RCTs, n = 5390]
65. Lopex-Leno JA, Peaceman AM, Adashek JA, et al. A controlled trial of a program for the active management of labor. *NEJM.* 1992;326:450–454. [RCT, n = 705]
66. Frigoletto FD, Leiberman E, Lang JM, et al. A clinical trial of active management of labor. *NEJM.* 1995;333:745–750. [RCT, n = 1915]
67. Rogers R, Gilson GJ, Miller AC, et al. Active management of labor: Does it make a difference? *AJOG.* 1997;599–605. [RCT, n = 405]
68. Sadler LC, Davison T, McCowan LME. A randomized controlled trial and meta-analysis of active management of labour. *BJOG.* 2000;107:909–915. [RCT, n = 651]
69. Vintzileos AM, Chavez M, Kinzler WL. Use of ultrasound in labor and delivery. *J Matern Fet Neo Med.* 2010;23:469–475. [Review]
70. Popowski T, Porcher R, Fort J, et al. Influence of ultrasound determination of fetal position on mode of delivery: A pragmatic

randomized trial. *Ultrasound Obstet Gynecol.* 2015;46:520–525. [RCT, $n = 1903$]
71. Bakker JJH, Verhoeven MS, Janssen PF, et al. Outcomes after internal versus external tocodynamometry for monitoring labor. *NEJM.* 2010;362:306–313. [RCT, $n = 1456$]
72. Bakker JJH, Janssen PF, van Halem K, et al. Internal versus external tocodynamometry during induced or augmented labor. *Cochrane Databsase Syst Rev.* 2012;(12):CD006947. [Meta-analysis, 3 RCTs, $n = 1945$]
73. Friedman EA. Primigravid labor: A graphicostatistical analysis. *Obstet Gynecol.* 1955;6:567–589. [II-3]
74. Friedman EA. *Labour: Clinical Evaluation and Management.* 2nd ed. New York, NY: Appleton-Century-Croft, 1978. [II-3]
75. Rouse DJ, Owen JO, Hauth JC. Active-phase labor arrest: Oxytocin augmentation for at least 4 hours. *Obstet Gynecol.* 1999;93:323–328. [II-3]
76. Zhang J, Landy HJ, Branch DW, et al. Contemporary patterns of spontaneous labor with normal neonatal outcomes. *Obstet Gynecol.* 2010;116(6):1281–1287. [II-1]
77. Neal JL, Lowe NK, Ahijevych KL, et al. "Active labor" duration and dilation rates among low-risk, nulliparous women with spontaneous labor onset: A systematic review. *J Midwifery Womens Health.* 2010;55(4):308–318.
78. Ness A, Goldberg J, Berghella V. Abnormalities of the first and second stages of labor. *Obstet Gynecol Clin N Am.* 2005;32:201–220. [Review]
79. Malvasi A, Barbera A, Di Vagno G, et al. Asynclitism: A literature review of an often forgotten clinical condition. *JMFNM.* 2015;28:1890–1894. [Review]
80. Rouse DJ, Owen JO, Savage KG, et al. Active-phase labor arrest: Revisiting the 2-hour minimum. *Obstet Gynecol.* 2001;98:550–554. [II-3]
81. American College of Obstetricians and Gynecologists (College); Society for Maternal-Fetal Medicine, Caughey AB, et al. Safe prevention of the primary cesarean delivery. *Am J Obstet Gynecol.* 2014;210(3):179–193. [Guideline]
82. Sosa CG, Balaguer E, Alonso JG, et al. Meperidine for dystocia during the first stage of labor: A randomized controlled trial. *AJOG.* 2004;191:1212–1218. [RCT, $n = 407$]

Second stage of labor

Alexis Gimovsky

KEY POINTS

- Prophylactic intrapartum maternal oxygen should not be used in the second stage of normal labor, since it is associated with more frequent low cord blood pH values (<7.20) than the control group.
- Prophylactic intrapartum betamimetics should not be used in the second stage of normal labor, since their usage is associated with an increase in forceps deliveries.
- Women should be encouraged to give birth in the position they find most comfortable, which is usually upright. Use of any **upright or lateral position,** compared with supine or lithotomy positions, is associated, **in women without epidural analgesia,** with reduction in duration of second stage of labor, reduction in assisted deliveries, reduction in episiotomies, increase in second-degree perineal tears, increase in estimated blood loss >500 mL, reduction in reporting of severe pain during second stage of labor and reduction in abnormal fetal heart rate patterns. In women with epidural anesthesia, the evidence is limited and insufficient to make a recommendation.
- There is insufficient evidence to recommend for or against maternal stirrup use in the second stage of labor.
- There is insufficient evidence to recommend water immersion in second stage of labor, and the risks have not been adequately assessed.
- In women at term with **epidural** analgesia and a singleton, cephalic fetus, **delayed pushing** (waiting 1–3 hours or until "urge to push") is associated with similar rate of operative vaginal delivery and cesarean delivery (CD), and a **higher incidence of spontaneous vaginal delivery** compared with early (immediate upon entering second stage) pushing. Additionally, the duration of the second stage is **longer by about 60 minutes,** the duration of pushing is similar, as are all other studied maternal and perinatal outcomes. **Careful monitoring of mother and fetus is necessary** to allow labor to continue safely.
- In women without epidural anesthesia, compared with encouraging a woman's own urge to push (open glottis), **pushing using the Valsalva maneuver (closed glottis) is associated with shorter (by 19 minutes) duration of labor,** similar incidences of operative vaginal deliveries, need for perineal repair, postpartum hemorrhage, and similar neonatal outcomes. Labor attendant should counsel women in labor regarding these data and **support the parturient in her own choice of pushing technique.**
- Coaching during pushing in the second stage of labor may shorten the second stage of labor, but lack of available coaching support does not adversely affect labor outcomes.
- Use of a dental support device/mouthguard has been associated with a shorter second stage of labor and reduction in the number of failures to descend requiring operative intervention.
- Both **manual and belt fundal pressure** to aid in vaginal delivery have not been associated with effect on maternal and perinatal outcomes, except for **decreased maternal satisfaction.**
- **Perineal massage and stretching of the perineum with a water-soluble lubricant** in the second stage of labor is associated with **similar rates of intact perineum** compared with the control group. The incidence of **third-degree lacerations is decreased**.
- Use of **perineal warm packs in the second stage of labor is associated with a reduction in third- and fourth-degree tears, as well as a reduction in pain on postpartum days 1 and 2.**
- Routine use of the Ritgen's maneuver does not appear to be associated with any benefits.
- "Hands-poised" is preferred to the "hands-on" method, since they are associated with similar incidences of perineal and vaginal tears, but the hands-on method is associated with a higher incidence of episiotomies.
- **Routine episiotomy should not be performed during the second stage of labor,** as restricting episiotomy use is associated with less posterior perineal trauma, less suturing, and fewer healing complications.
- **Nulliparous women with epidurals should be allowed to labor for at least one additional hour after prolonged (3 hours) second stage of labor,** since this results in a lower chance of CD (by 55%) without increasing maternal or neonatal morbidities. Apart from this trial, there is insufficient evidence to determine exactly when the second stage is considered to be prolonged and associated with enough complications as to justify either operative vaginal delivery or CD.

PROPHYLACTIC INTERVENTIONS
Maternal Oxygen
Prophylactic intrapartum maternal oxygen in the second stage of normal labor is associated with more frequent low (<7.20) cord blood pH values than the control group [1]. There are no other statistically significant differences between the groups. There is a tendency toward reduced cord arterial blood oxygen content and oxygen saturation in mothers treated with oxygen compared with controls. Therefore, **routine maternal oxygenation throughout the second stage should not be performed.** Short-term oxygenation may be beneficial and long-term oxygenation harmful.

Prophylactic Tocolysis
There is no evidence to support the prophylactic use of betamimetics to prevent nonreassuring fetal heart rate tracing (NRFHT) during the second stage of labor. Compared with placebo, prophylactic betamimetic therapy is associated with

an increase in forceps deliveries. The trial protocol required forceps to be used if the second stage of labor exceeded 30 minutes in both groups. There are no clear effects on postpartum hemorrhage, neonatal irritability, feeding slowness, umbilical arterial pH values, or Apgar scores at 2 minutes [2].

Therefore, **routine prophylactic tocolysis should not be performed in the second stage of labor.**

Prophylactic Positioning to Prevent Shoulder Dystocia
See Chapter 25.

MANAGEMENT
Maternal Position
There are several benefits for **upright posture**: sitting (obstetric chair/stool); semirecumbent (trunk tilted backward 30° to the vertical), kneeling, squatting (unaided or using squatting bars) and squatting (aided with Birth cushion) during the second stage of labor.

Use of any **upright or lateral position,** compared with supine or lithotomy positions, is associated, **in women without epidural analgesia,** with a **small (4 minutes) reduction in duration of second stage of labor,** a **20% reduction in assisted deliveries,** a **17% reduction in episiotomies,** a **23% increase in second-degree perineal tears,** a **63% increase in estimated blood loss >500 mL,** a **23% reduction in reporting of severe pain during second stage of labor,** and a **69% reduction in abnormal fetal heart rate patterns** [3]. Use of the birth stool showed no effect and results with the birth chair were variable. Estimation of blood loss in the upright group may be influenced by the fact that blood loss in the birth chair is collected in a receptacle. Physiological advantages for upright labor may include lessened risk of aortocaval compression, improved acid–base outcomes in the neonates, stronger and more efficient uterine contractions, improved alignment of the fetus for passage through the pelvis ("drive angle") and larger anteroposterior and transverse pelvic outlet diameters, resulting in an increase in the total outlet area in the squatting and kneeling positions [3].

In women with epidural anesthesia, the evidence is limited and insufficient to make a recommendation. In a small randomized controlled trial (RCT), compared with a supported sitting position, lateral position was associated with a lower chance of an operative vaginal delivery [4]. Kneeling and sitting upright are associated with similar duration of second stage and other outcomes, except for a more favorable maternal experience and less pain associated with kneeling [5]. In a Cochrane review of five RCTs, it was concluded that there was no significant difference in operative vaginal delivery, CD, lacerations or neonatal outcomes when comparing women with analgesia during labor in the upright or recumbent positions [6].

In summary, **women** without epidural anesthesia **should be encouraged to give birth in the upright position,** which is also the position they usually find most comfortable [3]. The evidence is insufficient for a recommendation on women with epidural anesthesia.

Maternal Stirrup Use
Routine use of stirrups during labor has had limited **study insufficient to make a recommendation.** In one small RCT, women who delivered in bed with stirrups versus those who delivered without stirrups had similar perineal lacerations, incidence of prolonged second stage, operative vaginal delivery and CD incidence [7].

Epidural or Other Anesthesia
See Chapter 11.

Water Immersion
Although there is some evidence that water immersion in the first stage of labor may reduce the need for epidural/spinal anesthesia and the length of first stage of labor (see Chapter 7), **immersion during the second stage has been insufficiently studied** and may be best avoided given lack of sufficient safety data. Of the three trials that compared water immersion during the second stage with no immersion, only one trial showed a significantly higher level of satisfaction with the birth experience (relative risk [RR] 0.24, 95% confidence interval [CI] 0.07–0.70). There are reports of neonatal water aspirations from birth (end of second stage) in water [8,9]. American College of Obstetricians and Gynecologists (ACOG) Committee Opinion concludes that, as safety has not been well established, water immersion in the second stage of labor should be **considered experimental** [10]. **In summary, there is insufficient evidence to recommend water immersion in second stage of labor, and risks have not been adequately assessed.**

Pushing
Delayed versus Early Pushing
In women at term with **epidural** analgesia and a singleton, cephalic fetus, **delayed pushing** (waiting 1–3 hours or until urge to push) is associated with **a similar rate of operative vaginal delivery and of CD,** and a **higher incidence of spontaneous vaginal delivery** compared with early (immediate upon entering second stage) pushing (RR 1.22, 95% CI 1.05–1.42) [11]. The duration of the second stage is **longer by about 60 minutes,** the duration of pushing is similar, as are all other studied maternal outcomes. The neonatal outcomes are also similar, including incidence of admission to neonatal intensive care unit (NICU). In a meta-analysis of 12 RCTs, similar results were noted. Second stage is longer in the delayed pushing group by 57 minutes, while there is a **shortened duration of active pushing** (by 22 minutes). Delayed pushing increases spontaneous vaginal delivery rate compared to immediate pushing, while operative vaginal delivery rates are not different [12]. The longer duration of second stage with delayed pushing has not been associated with detrimental effects on the fetus, but **careful monitoring of both mother and fetus is necessary to allow labor to continue safely** (see also section "Criteria for Diagnosis of Prolonged Second Stage"). There is no evidence available regarding **how long to delay pushing.** The 2012 International Federation of Gynecology and Obstetrics (FIGO) guideline for management of the second stage of labor recommends allowing nulliparous women to wait up to four hours before pushing and multiparous women up to one hour before pushing [13].

Pushing Method: Valsalva versus Spontaneous
Most women spontaneously choose to Valsalva during the second stage of labor. In women without epidural anesthesia, compared with encouraging a woman's own urge to push (open glottis), **pushing using the Valsalva maneuver (closed glottis:** taking a deep breath, holding it and pushing for as long and hard as possible, two to three times during each contractions) is **associated with shorter (by 19 minutes) duration of labor, similar incidences of operative vaginal deliveries, need for perineal repair, postpartum hemorrhage, and**

neonatal outcomes [14]. Urodynamics 3 months after delivery are worse in the closed glottis group, but long-term outcome has not been studied [14]. Labor attendants should counsel women in labor regarding these data and **support the parturient in her own choice of pushing technique.**

Coached Pushing
Although **coached pushing confers the benefit of a slightly shorter second stage,** coached maternal pushing confers no other advantages and withholding such coaching is not detrimental to maternal or fetal outcomes [15].

Use of a Dental Support Device
Wearing a dental support device (mouthguard) is associated with a shorter second stage (19 minutes) in one RCT. In addition, less operative intervention was used in the dental support group. Further research into optimizing maternal expulsive efforts is needed to evaluate the overall benefit of dental devices [16].

Fundal Pressure
In the second stage of labor, fundal pressure has been evaluated either as just manual pressure or with an obstetric belt wrapped around the woman's abdomen above the level of the uterine fundus.

Compared with no manual fundal pressure, **manual fundal pressure (Kristeller maneuver) concomitant with each contraction while patient has the urge to push during the second stage is not associated with any significant changes in duration of labor or with other maternal and perinatal outcomes** in one RCT [17].

The fundal pressure belt inflates with each contraction to a maximum of 200 mmHg for 30 seconds. Compared with no belt, the **inflatable obstetric belt is associated with similar incidence of spontaneous vaginal delivery** in nulliparous women with singleton term pregnancies and an epidural at term. All other maternal and neonatal outcomes are similar, but **women with no belt have greater satisfaction** [18].

In summary, **neither manual nor belt fundal pressures** to aid in vaginal delivery have been associated with effect on maternal and perinatal outcomes, except for **decreased maternal satisfaction.**

Perineal Massage
Perineal massage has been evaluated for decrease in perineal lacerations. Perineal massage has not been associated with complications. For perineal massage during pregnancy and before labor, see Chapter 2. Perineal massage and stretching of the perineum with a water-soluble lubricant in the second stage of labor are associated with similar rates of intact perineum compared with the control group. The incidence of third-degree lacerations is decreased [19]. In another RCT, perineal massage with lubricant was associated with similar incidence of genital tract trauma compared to no massage or to warm compresses [20]. A meta-analysis favored perineal massage versus hands off for a **reduction in third or fourth degree lacerations** (RR 0.52, 95% CI 0.29–0.94) [21]. The most recent double-blinded RCT comparing perineal oil with liquid wax (jojoba oil) showed no significant difference in perineal lacerations [22].

Perineal Warm Packs
Although no difference was seen in minor perineal trauma or requirement for suturing, **application of perineal warm packs during the second stage of labor was associated with less severe (third- or fourth-degree) tears** than was standard management. In addition, **pain scores were less** on postpartum days 1 and 2 in the intervention group. After 3 months, a trend toward decreased symptoms of urinary incontinence was seen in the intervention group [23]. In another RCT, warm compresses were associated with similar incidence of genital tract trauma compared to the presence or absence of a "no touch" technique or to perineal massage [20]. The decrease in third or fourth degree lacerations with perineal warm packs in the second stage of labor is also supported by a Cochrane review (RR 0.48, 95% CI 0.28–0.84) [21].

Manual Rotation
Persistent fetal occiput posterior position is a risk factor for prolonged labor and higher rate of CD. **Malposition includes usually occiput transverse or posterior positions.** These are often associated with asynclitism, defined often as the "oblique malpresentation of the fetal head in labor" [24]. **There is insufficient evidence (no trials) to evaluate the efficacy of manual rotation in labor.** In a retrospective cohort study of women with a fetus in persistent occiput posterior or transverse position in the second stage of labor, manual rotation was associated with lower rates of CD, perineal lacerations, postpartum hemorrhage and chorioamnionitis, but with a higher rate of cervical lacerations [25]. Another prospective study (but not randomized) of singletons with occiput posterior position reported an increase in fetuses delivered in occiput anterior position (93% vs. 15%) and in spontaneous vaginal delivery (77% vs. 27%) compared with no manual rotation, using historic controls [26] (see also Chapter 24).

Ritgen's Maneuver
Ritgen's maneuver (originally described by Ritgen in 1855) involves reaching for the fetal chin when it reaches the plane between the maternal anus and the coccyx and pulling it anteriorly, while using the fingers of the other hand on the fetal occiput to control speed of delivery and keep flexion of the fetal neck. Its aim is usually to protect the perineum from lacerations. Compared with no Ritgen's maneuver, Ritgen's maneuver performed for delivery of fetal head during uterine contractions is **not associated with any effect** on the incidence of perineal tears or other reported maternal or perinatal outcomes. The length of second stage and several perinatal outcomes were not reported in this RCT [27]. **In summary, Ritgen's maneuver does not appear to be associated with any benefits.**

"Hands-On" versus "Hands-Poised"
The hands-on method (also described by Ritgen) involves employing pressure on the infant's head upon crowning and supporting the perineum with the other hand. The aim is to protect against lacerations. In the hands-poised method, the fetal head and perineum are not touched or supported by the delivering personnel. These two methods are associated with **similar incidences of perineal and vaginal tears, but the hands-on method is associated with higher incidence of episiotomies** (RR 0.69, 95% CI 0.50–0.96) [21,28]. A policy of hands-poised has also been supported by a quasi-randomized study, reporting less third-degree tears compared with hands-on [29]. In a meta-analysis of five RCTs, the hands-on method **does not protect against** obstetric and anal sphincter injuries (RR 1.03, 95% CI 0.32–3.36) [30]. Therefore, **the hands-on method should not be routinely employed in labor.**

Episiotomy

Routine episiotomy should not be performed, as restrictive episiotomy policies have a number of benefits compared with routine episiotomy policies. In the most recent meta-analysis of RCTs, 75% of women had episiotomies in the routine episiotomy group, while the rate in the restrictive episiotomy group was 28%. Compared with routine use, **restrictive episiotomy is associated with less severe perineal trauma** (RR 0.67, 95% CI 0.49–0.91), *less suturing* (RR 0.71, 95% CI 0.61–0.81), **and fewer healing complications** (RR 0.69, 95% CI 0.56–0.85) [22]. Restrictive episiotomy is associated with **more anterior perineal trauma** (RR 1.84, 95% CI 1.61–2.10). There was no difference in severe vaginal/perineal trauma (RR 0.92, 95% CI 0.72–1.18), dyspareunia (RR 1.02, 95% CI 0.90–1.16), urinary incontinence (RR 0.98, 95% CI 0.79–1.20), or several pain measures. Results for restrictive versus routine mediolateral versus midline episiotomy were similar to the overall comparison [31]. There is insufficient evidence to evaluate if there are indications for any use of episiotomy, such as in operative vaginal delivery, preterm delivery, breech delivery, predicted macrosomia or presumed imminent tears. **Episiotomy should be avoided if at all possible;** but, if used, it is unknown which episiotomy technique (mediolateral or midline) provides the best outcome.

CRITERIA FOR DIAGNOSIS OF PROLONGED SECOND STAGE

There is insufficient evidence to determine when the second stage is prolonged, and associated with enough complications with continuing labor so as to justify either operative vaginal delivery or CD. Some have proposed the criteria in Table 8.1 for the diagnosis of prolonged second stage (or criteria for dystocia or failure to progress), but these are not based on level 1 evidence [32–35]. Clinically, the start of the second stage is imprecise and begins when the subjectively timed cervical examination reveals complete (10 cm) cervical dilation. It is also important to realize that, based on data above, women often do not begin to push until 1 hour or more after complete dilation has been ascertained.

American guidelines discuss the concepts of passive and active second stage [36]. Passive second stage is defined as full dilation of the cervix without voluntary or involuntary pushing. Active second stage is defined as when the fetus is visible or once pushing has started with or without contractions. These guidelines suggest that the passive phase in a nulliparous women be up to 2 hours regardless of anesthesia. In a multiparous woman, passive phase is suggested to be 1 hour without an epidural and 2 hours with an epidural. The active phase of the second stage of labor is suggested in nulliparous women to have a time limit of 1 hour without an epidural and 2 hours with an epidural. In a multiparous woman, active phase is suggested as 1 hour regardless of anesthesia [36]. The suggestions regarding length of the active second stage are not supported by level 1 data, and we allow longer second stages (see Table 8.1).

Several non-level-1 studies have compared maternal and perinatal outcomes between women with shorter versus "prolonged" second stage. In a review of all studies up to 2004, a strong **association between prolonged second stage and operative vaginal delivery** was noted [37]. The definition of prolonged second stage was inconsistent across studies. In addition, significant associations with maternal outcomes such as **postpartum hemorrhage, infection, and severe obstetric lacerations** were reported, but methods varied widely. From other data, urinary incontinence may also be increased with prolonged second stage [34]. Anal incontinence does not seem to be affected [38]. **No clear associations between prolonged second stage and adverse neonatal outcomes were reported** [26]. The length of the second stage is not associated with poor neonatal outcome as long as reassuring fetal testing is present. A recent large retrospective study suggested that neonatal sepsis (odds ratio [OR] 2.08, 95% CI 1.60–2.70), asphyxia (OR 2.39, 95% CI 1.28–4.27), and mortality (OR 5.92, 95% CI 1.43–24.51) were increased in nulliparous women with prolonged second stage of labor [39]. Nevertheless, these data are limited by their retrospective nature.

The problem with the evidence above is that these maternal detriments of prolonged second stage occur when these women are compared with women without prolonged second stage. It is evident that a planned CD before labor might decrease some of these complications (e.g., bleeding, infection, lacerations, and incontinence). **The clinical issue is different, though. Once a woman has prolonged second stage, should she be delivered operatively or should she continue labor?** CD performed after prolonged second stage has been associated with longer surgery time, increased postoperative fevers, maternal intraoperative trauma including higher risk of extensions of the uterine incision and higher composite maternal morbidity, but similar perinatal outcomes, compared with CD performed before prolonged second stage [40].

In a recent RCT, extending the second stage of labor beyond 3 hours by at least one additional hour in nulliparous women with epidural anesthesia decreased the CD incidence by 55% without incurring any additional increase in neonatal or perinatal morbidity (RR 0.45, 95% CI 0.22–0.93) [41]. Operative intervention is not warranted based solely on the time elapsed in the second stage. **If there are no signs of infection (maternal or fetal), no maternal exhaustion and reassuring fetal testing, labor can be allowed to continue beyond current limits** (Table 8.1) **as long as some progress has been made.** Nevertheless, if contractions are adequate, the chance of vaginal delivery decreases progressively after 3–5 hours of pushing in the second stage [42].

Mandatory second opinion is associated with 22 fewer intrapartum CDs per 1000 deliveries, without affecting maternal or perinatal outcomes [43] (see Chapter 13).

Table 8.1 Proposed Criteria for Prolonged Second Stage

Maternal Characteristics	Suggested Upper Limit of Length of Second Stage (Hours)
Nulliparous, epidural	4
Nulliparous, no epidural	3
Multiparous, epidural	3
Multiparous, no epidural	2

Source: Spong CY et al., *Obstet. Gynecol.*, 120, 1181–1193, 2012.

REFERENCES

1. Fawole B, Hofmeyr GJ. Maternal oxygen administration for fetal distress. *Cochrane Database Syst Rev.* 2005;(4) :CD000136. [2 RCTs, *n* = 245]
2. Campbell J, Anderson I, Chang A, et al. The use of ritodrine in the management of the fetus during the second stage of labour. *Aust N Z J Obstet Gynaecol.* 1978;18:110–113. [RCT, *n* = 100. Normal obstetric women selected during the first stage of labor. Infusion of ritodrine 5 mg/kg/min starting when the second stage of labor is diagnosed, compared with placebo infusion (dextrose water)]

3. Gupta JK, Hofmeyr GJ. Position in the second stage of labour for women without epidural anaesthesia. *Cochrane Database Syst Rev.* 2005;(3):CD002006. [Meta-Analysis: 20 RCTs; n = 6135. Variable trial quality, inconsistencies within trials, and heterogeneity of subjects]
4. Downe S, Gerrett D, Renfrew MJ. A prospective randomized trial on the effect of position in the passive second stage of labour on birth outcome in nulliparous women using epidural anesthesia. *Midwifery.* 2004;20:157–168. [RCT, n = 107]
5. Ragnat I, Altman D, Tyden T, et al. Comparison of the maternal experience and duration of labour in two upright delivery positions—A randomized controlled trial. *BJOG.* 2006;113:165–170. [RCT, n = 271]
6. Kemp E, Cj K, Kibuka M, et al. Position in the second stage of labour for women with epidural anaesthesia (Review). *Cochrane Database Syst Rev.* 2013;(1):CD008070. doi: 10.1002/14651858. CD008070.pub2. [Meta-Analysis of 5 RCTs, n = 879, I]
7. Corton MM, Lankford JC, Ames R, et al. A randomized trial of birthing with and without stirrups. *Am J Obstet Gynecol.* 2012; 207:133.e1–133.e5. [RCT, n = 108, I]
8. Cluett ER, Burns E. Immersion in water in labour and birth. *Cochrane Database Syst Rev.* 2009;(2):CD000111. [Meta-Analysis: 12 RCTs, n = 3243]
9. Mammas IN, Thiagarajan P. Water aspiration at birth: Report of 2 cases. *J Matern Fetal Neonatal Med.* 2009;22:365–367. [Case Report]
10. American College of Obstetrics and Gynecology. ACOG Committee Opinion no. 594: Immersion in water during labor and delivery. *Obstet Gynecol.* [Internet]. 2014;123(4):912–915. Available at: http://www.ncbi.nlm.nih.gov/pubmed/24785637.
11. Roberts CL, Torvaldsen S, Cameron CA, et al. Delayed versus early pushing in women with epidural analgesia: A systematic review and meta-analysis. *BJOG.* 2004;111:1333–1340. [Meta-Analysis: 9 RCTs; n = 2953]
12. Tuuli MG, Frey HA, Odibo AO, et al. Immediate compared with delayed pushing in the second stage of labor: A systematic review and meta-analysis. *Obstet Gynecol.* 2012;120:660–668. [Meta-Analysis of 12 RCTs, n = 3115, I]
13. FIGO Safe Motherhood and Newborn Health (SMNH) Committee. Management of the second stage of labor. *Int J Gynaecol Obstet.* 2012;119:111–116. [FIGO Guideline, III]
14. Prins M, Boxem J, Lucas C, Hutton E. Effect of spontaneous pushing versus valsalva pushing in the second stage of labour on mother and fetus: A systematic review of randomized trials. *BJOG.* 2011;118(6):662–670. [Meta-Analysis: 3 RCTs, n = 425]
15. Bloom SL, Casey BM, Schaffer JI, et al. A randomized trial of coached versus uncoached maternal pushing during the second stage of labor. *Am J Obstet Gynecol.* 2006;194:10–13. [RCT, n = 320]
16. Matsuo K, Mudd JV, Kopelman JN, Atlas RO. Duration of the second stage in labor while wearing a dental support device: A pilot study. *J Obstet Gynaecol Res.* 35(4):672–678. [RCT, n = 64]
17. Api O, Blacin ME, Ugurel V, et al. The effect of uterine fundal pressure on the duration of the second stage of labor: A randomized controlled trial. *Acta Obstet Gynecol.* 2009;88:320–324. [RCT, n = 197]
18. Cox J, Cotzias CS, Siakpere O, et al. Does an inflatable obstetric belt facilitate spontaneous vaginal delivery in nulliparae with epidural analgesia? *BJOG.* 1999;106:1280–1286. [RCT, n = 500]
19. Stamp G, Kruzins G, Crowther C. Perineal massage in labour and prevention of perineal trauma: Randomized controlled trial. *BMJ.* 2001;322:1277–1280. [RCT, n = 1340]
20. Albers LL, Sedler KD, Bedrock EJ, et al. Midwifery care measures in the second stage of labor and reduction of genital tract trauma at birth: A randomized trial. *J Midwifery Women Health.* 2005;50:365–372. [RCT, n = 1211]
21. Aasheim V, Nilsen AB, Lukasse M, Reinar LM. Perineal techniques during the second stage of labour for reducing perineal trauma. *Cochrane Database Syst Rev.* 2011;(12):CD006672. doi: 10.1002/14651858.CD006672.pub2. [Meta-Analysis of 8 RCTs, n = 11,651, I]
22. Harlev A, Pariente G, Kessous R, et al. Can we find the perfect oil to protect the perineum? A randomized-controlled double-blind trial. *J Matern Fetal Neonatal Med.* 2013;26:1328–1331. [RCT, n = 164, I]
23. Dahlen HG, Homer CS, Cooke M, et al. Perineal outcomes and maternal comfort related to the application of perineal warm packs in the second stage of labor: A randomized controlled study. *Obstet Gynecol Surv.* 2008;63(5):286–287. [RCT, n = 717]
24. Malvasi A, Barbera A, Di Vagno G, et al. Asynclitism: A literature review of an often forgotten clinical condition. *J Matern Fetal Neonatal Med.* 2015;28(16):1890–1894. [III; Review]
25. Shaffer BL, Cheng YW, Vargas JE, et al. Manual rotation to reduce caesarean delivery in persistent occiput posterior position. *J Matern Fetal Neonatal Med.* 2010;24:65–72. [II-2]
26. Reichman O, Gdanski E, Latinsky B, et al. Digital rotation from occipito-posterior to occipito-anterior decreases the need for cesarean section. *Eur J Obstet Gynecol Reprod Biol.* 2008;136:25–28. [II-2]
27. Jonsson ER, Elfaghi I, Rydhstrom H, Herbst A. Modified Ritgen's maneuver for anal sphincter injury at delivery. *Obstet Gynecol.* 2008;112:212–217. [RCT, n = 1623]
28. McCandlish R, Bowler U, Van Asten, et al. A randomized controlled trial of care of the perineum during second stage of normal labor. *BJOG.* 1998;105:1262–1272. [RCT, n = 5471]
29. Mayerhofer K, Bodner-Adler B, Bodner K, et al. Traditional care of the perineum during birth: A prospective, randomized, multicenter study of 1,076 women. *J Reprod Med.* 2002;47:477–482. [Quasi-RCT, n = 1076]
30. Bulchandani S, Watts E, Sucharitha A, et al. Manual perineal support at the time of childbirth: A systematic review and meta-analysis. *BJOG.* 2015;122:1157–1165. [Meta-Analysis of 5 RCTs n = 6816) and 7 non-randomized studies, (n = 108,156) I, and II-1]
31. Carroli G, Mignini L. Episiotomy for vaginal birth. *Cochrane Database Syst Rev.* 2014;(1):CD000081. [Meta-Analysis: 8 RCTs, n = 5541]
32. American College of Obstetricians and Gynecologists. *ACOG Practice Bulletin No. 17: Operative vaginal delivery.* Washington, DC: American College of Obstetricians and Gynecologists, 2000. [Review]
33. Royal College of Obstetricians and Gynaecologists. *NICE Guideline No. 26: Operative vaginal delivery.* London, UK: RCOG Press, Revised 2005. [Review]
34. Brown SJ, Gartland D, Donath S, et al. Effects of prolonged second stage, method of birth, timing of cesarean section and other obstetric risk factors on postnatal urinary incontinence: An Australian nulliparous cohort study. *BJOG.* 2011;118:991–1000. [II-2]
35. Spong CY, Berghella V, Wenstrom KD, et al. Preventing the first cesarean delivery: summary of a joint Eunice Kennedy Shriver National Institute of Child Health and Human Development, Society for Maternal-Fetal Medicine, and American College of Obstetricians and Gynecologists Workshop. *Obstet Gynecol.* 2012;120:1181–1193. [Review, III]
36. AHRQ Agency for Healthcare Research and Quality National Guideline Clearinghouse (US). Clinical practice guideline on care in normal childbirth [Internet]. Available at: http://www.guideline.gov/content.aspx?id=47076&;search=Obstetric+Labor+Complications+. Accessed October 11, 2015. [National Guideline, III]
37. Altman MR, Lydon-Rochelle MT. Prolonged second stage of labor and risk of adverse maternal and perinatal outcomes: A systematic review. *Birth.* 2006;33(4):315–322. [Systematic review of PubMed, Cochrane Library, and CINAHL from 1980 until 2005]
38. Badiou W, Bousquet PJ, Prat-Pradal D, et al. Short vs long second stage of labour: Is there a difference in terms of postpartum anal incontinence? *Eur J Obstet Gynecol Reprod Biol.* 2010;152:168–171. [II-2]

39. Laughon SK, Berghella V, Reddy UM, et al. Neonatal and maternal outcomes with prolonged second stage of labor. *Obstet Gynecol.* [Internet] 2014;124(1):57–67. Available at: http://www.pubmedcentral.nih.gov/articlerender.fcgi?artid=4065200&tool=pmcentrez&rendertype=abstract. Accessed September 4, 2015. [Retrospective cohort, n = 43,810 nulliparous women, II-2]
40. Sung JF, Daniels KI, Brodzinsky L, et al. Cesarean delivery outcomes after a prolonged second stage of labor. *Am J Obstet Gynecol.* 2007;197:306. [II-1]
41. Gimovsky AC, Berghella V. Randomized controlled trial of prolonged second stage: Extending the time limit vs usual guidelines. *AJOG.* 2016;214(3):361.e1–6. [RCT, n = 78, I]
42. Menticoglou SM, Manning F, Harman C, Morrison I. Perinatal outcome in relation to second stage duration. *Am J Obstet Gynecol.* 1995;173:906–912. [Retrospective, n = 6041, II-2]
43. Althabe F, Belizan JM, Villar J, et al. Mandatory second opinion to reduce rates of unnecessary caesarean sections in Latin America: A cluster randomized controlled trial. *Lancet.* 2004;363:1934–1940. [RCT, n = 149,276]

Third stage of labor

Jennifer Salati and Jorge E. Tolosa

PART 1—NORMAL THIRD STAGE OF LABOR
Key Points
- **Oxytocin is the prophylactic uterotonic of choice at delivery** as it reduces blood loss and has fewer side effects compared with other agents such as ergot alkaloids and prostaglandins, including misoprostol. Oxytocin **10 IU intramuscular (IM), preferably to 5 IU IM, or 20 IU (10–40 IU) intravenous (IV)** in 500 cc normal saline (NS) or lactated Ringer's (LR) infused over 1 hour should be routinely **administered following vaginal delivery,** either after delivery of the anterior shoulder or immediately after delivery of the neonate and before delivery of the placenta.
- Active management of the third stage of labor (AMTSL), including routine, prophylactic use of an **oxytocic agent, early cord clamping (ECC) and cutting, and cord traction, shortens the third stage and reduces blood loss and postpartum hemorrhage (PPH),** compared with expectant management.
- **Tranexamic acid (TA), (in addition to oxytocin administered after delivery),** *before skin incision at cesarean section could be given,* as current data suggest it can significantly decrease blood loss > 1000 cc. It reduces the risk of blood loss >400 or >500 cc but not >1000 cc after vaginal delivery.
- **Carbetocin, (not currently available in the United States)** has been shown to reduce the need for therapeutic uterotonics compared with oxytocin in women who underwent cesarean section, but not for vaginal delivery. Carbetocin is associated with **less blood loss and fewer side effects** when used prophylactically compared with syntometrine.
- For cesarean, **misoprostol combined with oxytocin appears to be more effective than oxytocin alone** in reducing intraoperative and postoperative hemorrhage.
- **Delayed cord clamping (DCC) in preterm neonates** by 30–120 (maximum 180) seconds is associated with fewer transfusions and lower risk of intraventricular hemorrhage (IVH).
- DCC in term neonates is associated with higher hematocrit and lower risk of iron deficiency at less than a year of age, but with an increased risk of hyperbilirubinemia requiring phototherapy.
- Vaginal and perineal **lacerations should be repaired with one continuous absorbable synthetic suture,** including continuous subcuticular skin repair.
- Rectal nonsteroidal anti-inflammatory drugs (NSAIDs), topical anesthetics, and therapeutic ultrasound can each decrease perineal pain and need for additional pain therapy.

Definitions
Third stage of labor is defined as the **interval between delivery of the neonate and expulsion of the placenta.** Mean length of time of the third stage is about 6 minutes. An interval of **greater than 30 minutes** is the 97th percentile, and represents the definition of a **prolonged third stage.**

Pathophysiology
The third stage involves separation of the placenta with capillary hemorrhage and shearing of the placental surface when the uterus contracts after delivery of the infant. Signs of separation include a gush of blood, cord lengthening, and the uterine fundus becoming more globular and firm.

Complications (Chapter 26)
- PPH—classically defined as an estimated blood loss (EBL) >500 cc after vaginal delivery or >1000 cc after cesarean delivery
- Retained placenta—placenta not expelled ≥30 minutes after infant delivery
- Uterine inversion—collapse of uterine fundus into the uterine cavity

Management
An algorithm including uterotonics use and active management of placental delivery is shown in Figure 9.1.

Uterotonics

Oxytocin (Syntocinon®). Oxytocin binds to specific uterine receptors with immediate action causing increasing strength and frequency of contractions (Table 9.1). The mean **half-life is 3 minutes** with the plateau reached after 30 minutes. It can either be given as IV or IM, though IM injection has time of onset of 3–7 minutes and clinical effect is longer, lasting 30–60 minutes. It is metabolized by the liver and kidneys with a known 5% antidiuretic effect of vasopressin. If given in large volumes, greater than 40–50 cc/minute, and high concentration, or when given without dilution, it may result in hyponatremia and syndrome of inappropriate antidiuretic hormone hypersecretion (SIADH) with symptoms of headache, vomiting, drowsiness, and convulsions.

Many different ways of administering oxytocin for prophylaxis in the third stage of labor following vaginal delivery have been used, including IM, IV (either undiluted or as a diluted infusion), and intraumbilical. The **IM dose is 5–10 IU,** administered at the delivery of the anterior shoulder, or soon after, before delivery of the placenta. Oxytocin can also be given as an undiluted IV bolus, or a **diluted IV infusion consisting of 10–40 IU diluted in 500–1000 cc of NS or LR.** A recent randomized controlled trial (RCT) compared various oxytocin doses (10 IU, 40 IU, and 80 IU IV in 500 mL) given over 1 hour after placental delivery for primary PPH prophylaxis at vaginal delivery, and showed no differences overall in incidence of PPH. However, **the 80 IU dose was associated with** less need for additional uterotonics, and less risk of decline in hematocrit ≤6% [1]. The comparative effectiveness and safety of these various approaches have not been well quantified in high-quality RCTs so **there is insufficient evidence to recommend a specific route or dosage** [2]. The IM route is favored in some institutions, particularly in resource-poor settings, as it can be administered rapidly by providers with minimal training. **Undiluted IV boluses are generally not recommended** as they are associated with transient hypotension and tachycardia. Intraumbilical injection is not superior to IV administration and has not been shown to be effective in reducing blood loss or manual placental removal [3].

Oxytocin is the prophylactic uterotonic of choice in the third stage of labor. Compared with no uterotonics, prophylactic oxytocin reduces blood loss of >500 cc after vaginal delivery and the need for therapeutic uterotonics [4]. There are similar incidences of manual removal of the placenta and rates of blood transfusions with the use of oxytocin compared with no uterotonic.

Compared with ergot alkaloids (methergine or ergometrine [ergonovine]), oxytocin is associated with **fewer side effects** including nausea and vomiting, with no difference in length of the third stage or need for manual placental removal [4]. There is no clear evidence that oxytocin is superior to ergot alkaloids in blood loss prevention, however the side effect profile makes oxytocin a better first-line option [4].

Compared with oxytocin alone, ergometrine in addition to oxytocin is associated with increased side effects with only modest benefits. Benefits include a statistically significant reduction in the risk of PPH when compared with oxytocin alone for blood loss of 500 ml or more. There is no difference in PPH for blood loss >1000 cc. In addition, there are no differences in blood transfusion, retained placenta, or other neonatal outcomes. Unfortunately, adverse side effects are significant including nausea, vomiting, and hypertension, from the ergometrine added to oxytocin [5]. When compared with ergot alkaloids alone, oxytocin in addition to ergot alkaloids was not beneficial in PPH prevention [4].

As part of AMTSL, oxytocin is routinely administered after delivery of the anterior shoulder or immediately after delivery of the neonate and before delivery of the placenta. Timing

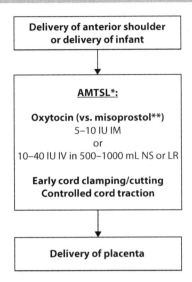

Figure 9.1 Algorithm for active management of the third stage of labor (AMSTL). IM, intramuscular; IU, international units; LR, lactated Ringer's solution; NS, normal saline; RCT, randomized controlled trial. *There is heterogeneity in the literature regarding different definitions for AMTSL. We have used the one utilized for evaluation of the existing RCTs of AMTSL by the Cochrane collaboration. **Misoprostol is an equally-effective alternative to oxytocin if oxytocin is not available. (From Giacalone PL et al., *BJOG*, 107, 396, 2000.)

Table 9.1 Commonly Used Uterotonic Agents

	Route/Dose	Maximum Dose	Side Effects	Contraindications
Oxytocin	5–10 IM *or* 10–80 IU IV infusion in 500–1000 mL NS/LR	80–100 IU	Hypotension Hyponatremia Fluid overload Flushing Nausea/emesis	None
Ergometrine/methergine	0.2 mg IM *or* 0.2 mg PO, every 15 minutes ×2 doses then every 2–4 hours	1 mg (five doses)	Nausea/emesis Vasoconstriction Hypertension	Hypertension Cardiac disease[a] Peripheral vascular disease[a]
Prostaglandin F2α/hemabate	0.25 mg IM, every 15–90 minutes	2 mg (eight doses)	Bronchoconstriction Hypertension Nausea/emesis Diarrhea	Asthma Active cardiac, pulmonary, renal, or hepatic disease[a]
Misoprostol	200–1000 μg PO, PR, or PV	Unknown	Pyrexia Shivering Nausea/emesis Diarrhea	None
Carbetocin	100 μg IV (single dose)	100 μg	Hypotension Flushing Pruritus Headache Nausea/emesis	None

Abbreviations: IM, intramuscular; IU, international units; IV, intravenous; LR, lactated Ringer's solution; NS, normal saline; PO, per os; PR, per rectum; PV, per vagina.
[a] Relative contraindication.

of oxytocin administration before or after placental delivery, did not show differences in rates of blood loss, length of third stage of labor and rates of retained placenta [6,7]. Nonsignificant trends for less PPH but more retained placenta are associated with oxytocin given before compared with after placental separation [6].

Oxytocin prophylaxis with 20–80 IU in 500 cc over 30 minutes after cord clamping is recommended following delivery by cesarean section [8]. However, the optimal route and dosing in this situation has not been established (see Chapter 13).

Oxytocin Agonists
Carbetocin (not currently available in the United States) is a synthetic analogue of oxytocin; 100 µg IV has been shown to **reduce the need for therapeutic uterotonics compared with oxytocin, for those women who underwent cesarean section,** but not for vaginal delivery; and **reduced need for uterine massage following any mode of delivery** [9]. There is limited comparative evidence on adverse events [9,10]. Compared with syntometrine (oxytocin plus ergometrine), carbetocin is associated with less blood loss and fewer side effects when used prophylactically following vaginal delivery; however the risk of PPH is not decreased [9]. The World Health Organization (WHO) together with pharmaceutical companies is conducting a multicountry trial, in low, middle and high income countries, expecting to enroll 29,000 women to test effectiveness of a proprietary formulation of carbetocin compared with oxytocin to reduce PPH.

Ergot Alkaloids (Methergine® or Ergometrine). Methylergonovine and its parent compound ergometrine result in sustained tonic contraction of uterine smooth muscle by stimulation of α-adrenergic myometrial receptors. The dose is **0.2 mg IM injection or per os (PO)** with a mean elimination half-life of 3.39 hours (range 1.5–12.7 hours). Intravenous administration is not recommended as it is associated with more severe side effects. Nausea and vomiting are common side effects, although the most concerning side effect is vasoconstriction of the vascular smooth muscle. This results in elevation of central venous pressure and systemic blood pressure increasing the risk of pulmonary edema, stroke, or myocardial infarction. Contraindications include cardiac disease, autoimmune diseases associated with Raynaud's phenomena, peripheral vascular disease, arteriovenous shunts, hypertension, preeclampsia, and eclampsia.

Compared with oxytocin, ergot alkaloids used as a prophylactic uterotonic have similar benefits, but **worse side effects,** making oxytocin preferable as the first-line prophylactic agent [11]. Methergine can instead be used as a second-line agent for treatment of PPH (see Chapter 26).

Syntometrine (Oxytocin Plus Ergometrine). Syntometrine is a combination drug containing oxytocin 5 IU and ergometrine 0.5 mg, and is administered intramuscularly. Side effects are significant, including nausea, vomiting, and hypertension. This combination is not recommended over oxytocin for PPH prophylaxis [4].

Prostaglandins
Misoprostol is a synthetic analog of prostaglandin E1 and is metabolized in the liver. The tablet can be given by oral or sublingual route at 400–600 µg, or by vaginal or rectal route at 400–1000 µg. It does not require sterile needles and syringes for administration. It is inexpensive, heat and light stable, and has a long shelf life, making it more accessible and beneficial in low-resource settings. Side effects include shivering, elevated body temperature >38°C, and gastrointestinal (GI) upset with nausea, vomiting, and diarrhea. Studies suggest that these side effects are dose dependent, particularly with doses exceeding 600 µg [12].

Compared with placebo, prophylactic oral or sublingual misoprostol reduces the risk of severe PPH and need for blood transfusion. When compared with conventional injectable uterotonics (oxytocin, oxytocin–ergometrine, or ergometrine) the risk of PPH is comparable, and possibly even increased [13–15]. One recent double-blind RCT though showed that sublingual misoprostol 400 µg was associated with less PPH compared with oxytocin 10 IU IM given within 1 minute of cord clamping at vaginal delivery [16]. Moreover, for cesarean, misoprostol combined with oxytocin appears to be more effective than oxytocin alone in reducing intraoperative and postoperative hemorrhage [17]. There is a limited but growing role for prophylactic use of misoprostol in the routine management of the third stage of labor, or can be used as an agent for treatment of PPH in certain circumstances, when rectal misoprostol may be a useful "first-line" therapy for the treatment of PPH. It may be a more appropriate first-line agent in the setting of no IV access, patients with contraindications to other uterotonics, **or in resource-poor settings** (see Chapter 26).

Prostaglandin F2α (hemabate/carboprost) causes contraction of uterine smooth muscle cells. Administration is either 0.25 mg IM or as a direct injection into the myometrium, which may be repeated every 15–20 minutes for a maximum of 8 doses or 2 mg. Side effects are secondary to smooth muscle constriction and include bronchoconstriction, venoconstriction, and constriction of GI smooth muscle. Common side effects are nausea, vomiting, diarrhea, pyrexia, bronchospasm, and case reports of hypotension and intrapulmonary shunting with arterial oxygen desaturation. It is contraindicated in patients with cardiac and pulmonary disease. There is **no high-quality evidence to support the use of carboprost for PPH prophylaxis, but it can be used as a second-line agent for treatment of PPH** (see Chapter 26).

Tranexamic Acid. TA is a synthetic derivative of the amino acid lysine that is metabolized in the kidney and functions as an antifibrinolytic. For prophylaxis, it is administered intravenously at a dose of 10 mg/kg (usually maximum of 1 g), before skin incision (e.g., 30 minutes prior), with rapid onset of action and a mean elimination half-life of 2–10 hours. Side effects include nausea, vomiting and dizziness [18].

TA given **in combination with routine prophylactic uterotonics** appears to decrease the risk of postpartum blood loss >400 cc, >500 cc, and >1000 cc, need for blood transfusion in women at low risk for PPH following a cesarean delivery with data from clinical trials of mixed quality and meta-analysis from such data [18,19]. For vaginal delivery, there is insufficient evidence to recommend the routine use of TA alone for PPH prophylaxis, as well as its use in a population at high risk for PPH. It has been reported it reduces the risk of blood loss >400 or >500 cc but not >1000 cc after vaginal delivery. There is variability amongst available studies, which are too small to assess rare outcomes of venous thromboembolism or maternal mortality. Therefore, **we recommend it be considered for routine prophylactic use at cesarean section in addition to prophylactic oxytocin.** Currently a large multi-country RCT "The Woman Trial" is testing the use of 1 g of TA initially, followed by 1 g if bleeding continues, **in women diagnosed with PPH,** compared with placebo. It is expected 20,000 women will be recruited and that this RCT will provide definitive data on use of TA for treatment of PPH (Chapter 13).

Summary
Oxytocin (5–10 IU IM or 10–40 IU IV in 500–1000 cc NS or LR bolus) should be routinely administered with delivery of the anterior shoulder or before delivery of the neonate, in all pregnancies as prophylaxis to prevent PPH. **At cesarean, TA before skin incision should be given, in addition to oxytocin after delivery of the fetus.** Methergine, syntometrine, and prostaglandin F2α should generally not be used for prophylaxis in normal third stage of labor, unless oxytocin is unavailable. Methergine, prostaglandin F2α, and misoprostol are often used for treatment of PPH (see Chapter 26).

Umbilical Cord

Cord Gases
Cord gases are stable in a clamped segment of cord for up to 60 minutes and in a heparinized syringe for up to 60 minutes. Umbilical artery pH, pCO2, and base deficit may be helpful in indicating timing of insult and can be collected in cases of nonreassuring fetal heart rate tracings (NRFHTs), meconium, low Apgar scores (defined as below 7 at 5 minutes), growth restriction, preterm birth, or any sentinel event including cord prolapse, uterine rupture, or placental abruption. Umbilical vein pH may be helpful in cases of uteroplacental problems like growth restriction, placental abruption, asthma, and hypertension. While there are **no RCTs on this issue, routine sending of umbilical cord gases** is usually not necessary or recommended for normal labor, delivery, and Apgar scores, without risk factors.

Cord Blood Collection
Cord blood is routinely sent for Rh status of the infant, especially in Rh-negative women. Cord blood collection for stem cells has increased in popularity in recent years. Obstetricians should support public banking of cord blood [20]. **Public banking is recommended over private banks** secondary to more stringent U.S. Food and Drug Administration (FDA) guidelines, given its increased legal responsibilities, cost-effectiveness, and greater access to cord blood by the general population. The chance of a child requiring an autologous transplant from privately banked cord blood is about 1/2700. Directed donation of cord blood when there is a disease in the family amenable to stem cell transplantation can be arranged through many public banks with other applications not yet proven.

Timing of Cord Clamping
In preterm neonates <37 weeks, **DCC by about 30–120 seconds** (180 maximum) **is associated with fewer transfusions for anemia, less IVH and lower risk for necrotizing enterocolitis** than ECC at <30 seconds [21]. This intervention also benefits very preterm neonates <32 weeks, with decreased mortality, risk of blood transfusion and IVH [22]. In addition, DCC has been shown to be safe and does not compromise the preterm infant [23]. There are no clear differences in other outcomes including respiratory distress, death, initial adaptation phase, or long-term outcomes. There is **no current recommendation on positioning of the preterm infant during DCC secondary to insufficient data.** One RCT showed no differences in neonatal outcomes during a 120 second DCC after vaginal delivery with the neonate held either at the level of the vagina, or the level of the abdomen or chest, concluding that mothers can safely be allowed to hold their baby on their abdomen or chest for skin-to-skin and breastfeeding [24].

Milking of the cord following preterm delivery has been examined in a few RCTs with benefits similar to DCC. Compared with no milking, milking of the cord has been associated with higher hematocrit, lower transfusion rates and less need for circulatory and respiratory support [25–27]. One study examined the effect of DCC in addition to cord milking versus cord milking only, and found no differences [28].

In **term neonates**, DCC has also been shown to have some benefits, but also some risks. Compared with early clamping, DCC is associated with higher hematocrit and a lower risk of iron deficiency at less than a year of age. There was no increased risk of PPH, however, there was an increased risk of the neonate needing phototherapy for hyperbilirubinemia. The possible **increased risk of neonatal jaundice requiring phototherapy must be weighed against the physiological benefit of greater hemoglobin and iron levels** conferred by DCC in term infants, which may be of clinical value particularly in infants where access to good nutrition is poor [29].

Placenta

Cord Drainage with or without Traction
Immediate cord drainage and traction is associated with a **shorter duration of the third stage of labor and a smaller decrease in hemoglobin** compared with no drainage or traction [30]. Cord drainage with traction reduces the length of the third stage of labor and decreases blood loss compared with traction and no cord drainage [31].

Cord Traction
As mentioned above, the combination of cord drainage with traction appears to shorten the third stage of labor and leads to a smaller decrease in hemoglobin compared with no drainage or traction [30]. **Cord traction alone has been associated with lower mean blood loss and decreased risk of PPH, shorter third stage of labor, and lower risk of needing manual placental removal compared with no cord traction** [32].

Massage of the Uterus
There is limited evidence to evaluate the effect of massage of the uterus alone. Three trials have examined the use of massage in addition to oxytocin. In one small trial, use of uterine massage resulted in decreased mean blood loss and need for additional uterotonics. A larger trial did not demonstrate benefit when uterine massage was added to oxytocin treatment [33]. A more recent RCT from China also did not show a significant decrease in blood loss with addition of uterine massage to 10 IU oxytocin IM prophylaxis [34]. However, uterine massage has been evaluated as a component of AMTSL and found to be beneficial in prevention of a prolonged third stage and PPH. Therefore, uterine massage after delivery of the placenta is recommended.

Injection of Oxytocin in Umbilical Cord
Injection of oxytocin into the umbilical cord is not recommended. Compared with IV/IM oxytocin or to injection of saline alone, the umbilical vein injection of oxytocin does not have a significant effect on postpartum blood loss, need for transfusion, length of the third stage of labor or need for manual placental removal [3].

Active Management of the Third Stage of Labor
AMTSL usually consists of

- Prophylactic oxytocin at delivery of the anterior shoulder or immediately after delivery of the baby
- ECC and cutting
- Controlled cord traction

Expectant management usually consists of:
- No uterotonics
- No ECC, cutting, or traction
- Use of gravity and maternal expulsive efforts for placenta delivery

There is heterogeneity in the literature regarding different definitions for AMTSL. We have used the one utilized for evaluation of the existing RCTs of AMTSL by the Cochrane collaboration [35]. AMTSL has been used mostly in pregnancies at term after vaginal births, so recommendations are limited to this population. AMTSL reduces the risk of PPH and should be offered and recommended to all women, including women following preterm birth. Compared with expectant management, active management is associated with reduced risk of maternal primary hemorrhage of blood loss >1000 cc and >500 cc, and of maternal hemoglobin <9 g/dL following birth [35]. Adverse effects were identified including increases in vomiting after birth, increased maternal diastolic blood pressure, increased use of analgesia and pain, more women returning to the hospital with bleeding, and decrease in infant birth weight, possibly reflecting some degree of lower blood volume from placental transfusion if ECC is performed. There was no effect on risk of infant admission to the neonatal unit or incidence of jaundice requiring treatment. Each element of AMTSL should be assessed separately, as we have done in the preceding sections "*Umbilical cord*" and "*Placenta*."

Repair of Laceration
Closure and Repair
Compared with nonclosure, closure of first- and second-degree perineal lacerations after vaginal delivery is associated with **better healing seen at 10 days and 6 weeks** and similar pain scores [36–38]. The **continuous suturing** techniques, compared with the interrupted, are associated with less short-term pain in second-degree and episiotomy repairs [39]. Furthermore, approximation (end-to-end) and overlap technique for third- and fourth-degree laceration repair are associated with similar outcomes in two RCTs [40,41], while in the most recent RCT end-to-end repair was associated with significantly lower rates of anal incontinence, with no difference in long-term outcomes [42]. One small randomized trial showed that use of **antibiotics** at the time of third- and fourth-degree repairs decreased perineal wound complications (wound disruption and purulent discharge) [43] (see also Chapter 30).

Suture
Absorbable synthetic materials should be used for all layers of the repair. Compared with catgut (plain or chromic), **absorbable synthetic sutures (e.g., Vicryl)** used for perineal repair decreased women's experience of short-term (3-day) pain, less need for analgesia, reduced rate of suture dehiscence up to day 10, and less need for resuturing at <3 months. There is no significant difference in long-term pain or dyspareunia experienced by women [44]. More women with catgut sutures required resuturing compared with synthetic sutures, while more women in the standard synthetic suture group required suture removal compared with the rapidly absorbed group. Clinical experience has shown **suture removal is necessary <5% of the time when using 3–0 or finer sutures and performing subcuticular skin closures** [44]. Polyglactin (Vicryl) and polydioxanone (PDS) have similar outcomes [45].

Anal Ultrasound
Anal endosonography with clinical examination immediately after delivery in nulliparous women with second-degree lacerations detected more sphincter tears than clinical examination. Anal endosonography with immediate repair of these tears is associated with less severe fecal incontinence at 1 year compared with clinical examination only [46].

Perineal Pain Control
Nonsteroidal Anti-Inflammatory Drugs
There are no RCTs to accurately assess the effectiveness of oral NSAIDs for perineal pain control. However, clinical experience shows a reduction in perineal pain. Rectally administrated NSAIDs appear to provide effective pain relief in postpartum women. Rectal indomethacin or diclofenac are associated with less pain up to 24 hours after birth and less requirement for additional analgesia in the first 24 hours and 48 hours postpartum [47]. No information is available on pain experienced >72 hours after birth or other outcomes of importance such as the impact on daily activities, resumption of sexual intercourse, and the impact on the mother-baby relationship. More studies are needed to assess the acceptability of this route of administration and comparison to oral NSAIDs.

Topical Anesthetics
Compared with placebo, topical anesthetics applied to the perineum are associated with similar pain relief up to 24 hours to 72 hours postpartum, but women are more satisfied after administration of an anesthetic [48]. Epifoam (1% hydrocortisone acetate and 1% pramaxine hydrochloride in the mucoadhesive foam base) use is associated with less additional analgesia, while lignocaine/lidocaine showed no difference with regard to additional analgesia use compared with placebo [48]. A lidocaine/prilocaine cream appears to be as effective as local mepivacaine injection for pain relief during repair [49]. Compared with indomethacin vaginal suppositories, topical anesthetics have similar mean pain scores.

Therapeutic Ultrasound for Perineal Pain
There is insufficient evidence to evaluate the use of ultrasound in treating perineal pain and/or dyspareunia following vaginal delivery. Women treated with active ultrasound for acute perineal pain are more likely to report improvement in pain, less pain at 10 days and 3 months, but more likely to have bruising at 10 days compared with placebo [50]. Additionally, women with persistent perineal pain or dyspareunia treated with ultrasound are less likely to report pain with sexual intercourse.

Anesthesia
Epidural is commonly used during labor for pain control. Spinal, epidural, paracervical block, or general anesthesia may be used if complications arise in the management of retained placenta, intractable PPH, uterine inversion, or assisted vaginal deliveries (Chapter 11).

Breast-Feeding
Hypertension and headache are associated with misoprostol and ergotamine use. There are no other known complications with breastfeeding after use of other uterotonics. There are no differences in breastfeeding or onset of jaundice with AMTSL.

Delivery Note
If a complicated delivery occurs with possible fetal compromise, a detailed note should address the pertinent and immediate neonatal status, including Apgar scores, umbilical cord pH, and base deficit (if obtained), and assessment of fetal heart testing prior to delivery.

PART 2—CARE OF THE JEHOVAH'S WITNESS PREGNANT WOMAN

Key Points

- Members of the Jehovah's Witness faith refuse blood transfusions due to their beliefs that accepting them violates God's law, and would lead to excommunication and eternal damnation.
- Refusal of blood can lead to an increased risk of maternal (and at times therefore fetal) death, especially in cases of obstetric hemorrhage.
- All obstetrical providers are responsible to ask *each* woman at her first prenatal visit (or preconception) if she has any objection to receiving any blood product in case of necessity.
- The woman's wishes should be respected, following the principle of autonomy.
- After counseling, the patient should be asked to sign the consent for blood products, as well as the Health Care Power of Attorney.
- The third stage should be managed actively, and PPH prevented as much as possible. The use of cell saver is safe and effective in pregnancy.

Historic

"That is why I have said to the sons of Israel: 'No soul of you must eat blood and no alien resident who is residing as an alien in your midst should eat blood.'" (Holy Bible: Leviticus 17:12). Charles Russell started the Jehovah's Witness Christian sect in Pennsylvania in 1872.

Members of the Jehovah's Witness faith refuse blood transfusions due to their beliefs that prohibit use of blood products, because they believe that accepting them violates God's law, and would lead to excommunication and eternal damnation, as they take literally the statement reported in the Bible.

Complications

The risk of obstetric hemorrhage is approximately 6% in Jehovah's Witness women [51]. The risk of maternal death is about 0.5%, a 44-fold increase compared with non-Jehovah's Witness controls [51].

Management

There are **no trials to assess the efficacy of interventions specifically in women who are Jehovah's witnesses.** Refer to the guidelines of third stage and abnormal third stage for general recommendations.

Preconception Counseling
Counsel regarding complications, and management in pregnancy.

Prenatal Care
All obstetrical providers are responsible to ask *each* woman at her first prenatal visit (or preconception visit) if she has any objection to receiving any blood product in case of necessity. The woman who states she would decline blood transfusion even if medically necessary and/or is a Jehovah's Witness should be managed as follows:

- Counsel the woman and any family member present regarding the reasons and the risks of blood product refusal, including the possibility of maternal and fetal

I hereby consent to the blood products marked below:

- ___Whole blood
- ___Fresh frozen plasma
- ___Cryoprecipitate
- ___Albumin
- ___Erythropoietin
- ___Immune globulins (blood fraction, Rh immunoglobulin)
- ___Clotting factors
- ___PolyHeme (human hemoglobin), hemopure products (bovine hemoglobin)
- ___Recombinant factors
- ___Platelet cell fractions (platelet gel)
- ___Other surgical procedures, medical tests, or current therapy
- ___Using my own blood, i.e., tagged red cells, white cells, blood patching
- ___Hemodialysis equipment (nonblood primed)
- ___Intraoperative blood salvage (cell saver)
- ___Intraoperative hemodilution

Patient's Name _____

Patient's Signature _____

Date _____

Figure 9.2 Blood product consent for Jehovah's Witness patients.

death. **The counseling should be documented on the medical record.** The patient might want to consult with the "elders" before **signing informed refusal.** Her wishes should be respected, following the principle of autonomy. A physician has the right of refusing to provide care for a Jehovah's Witness only if an alternative caregiver agrees to accept and care for the patient [52].
- After counseling, the patient should be asked to sign the **consent for blood products** (Figure 9.2), as well as the **Health Care Power of Attorney** [52]. These two consents should be kept in the medical record chart and available at labor and delivery. Approximately 39% of Jehovah's Witness pregnant women accept a variety of donated blood products, and 55% accept either intraoperative normovolemic hemodilution or transfusion of their own blood obtained by a cell saver [53].
- Consider including a copy of this guideline in the medical record, for reference.
- Selected high-risk patients, for example, those with hemoglobin <9 mg/dL, may be considered for appropriate replacement of iron, folic acid, and erythropoietin, which can be coordinated by a maternal-fetal medicine and/or a hematologist specialist.
- A routine consult with the Maternal-Fetal Medicine service is not required, but can be considered.
- A routine ethics consult is not indicated, but can be considered in specific cases.

Antepartum Testing

No specific antepartum testing is indicated.

Delivery

- Consents: Upon admission and prior to the surgery/delivery, all Jehovah's Witness patients should have signed a consent form (Figure 9.2) and the previously mentioned healthcare power of attorney. If consents have not been previously signed or are not available, the patient should be recounseled and consents signed.
- The third stage should be managed actively with the goal of PPH prevention. Oxytocin, methylergonovine, 15-methylprostaglandin F2a, misoprostol, and other medical and, if necessary, surgical therapies should be employed [54].
- If an operative delivery or bleeding disorder is anticipated, if the patient has a history of a low-lying placenta or a placenta previa, or if an operative delivery is to occur, a **cell saver** can be on standby in labor and delivery throughout the patient's labor and delivery. Use of the cell saver is safe in obstetrics [55].

Anesthesia

An anesthesiology consult should be obtained. The anesthesiologist will review the patient's medical record and consents, including consent or refusal for blood products.

REFERENCES

1. Tita ATN, Szychovski JM, Rouse DJ, et al. Higher dose oxytocin and hemorrhage after vaginal delivery. A randomized controlled trial. *Obstet Gynecol.* 2012;119:293–300. [RCT, $n = 1,798$] [I]
2. Oladapo OT, Okusanya BO, Abalos E. Intramuscular versus intravenous prophylactic oxytocin for the third stage of labour. *Cochrane Database Syst Rev.* 2012;(2):CD009332. [Meta-analysis: 0 RCTs] [I]
3. Mori R, Nardin JM, Yamamoto N, et al. Umbilical vein injection for the routine management of third stage of labour. *Cochrane Database Syst Rev.* 2012;(3):CD006176. [Meta-analysis: 9 RCTs, $n = 1118$] [I]
4. Westhoff G, Cotter AM, Tolosa JE. Prophylactic oxytocin for the third stage of labour to prevent postpartum hemorrhage. *Cochrane Database Syst Rev.* 2013;(10):CD001808. [Meta-analysis: 20 RCTs, $n = 10,806$] [I]
5. McDonald SJ, Abbott JM, Higgins SP. Prophylactic ergometrine-oxytocin versus oxytocin for the third stage of labour. *Cochrane Database Syst Rev.* 2009;(3):CD000201. [Meta-analysis: 6 RCTs; $n = 9332$] [I].
6. Soltani H, Hutchon DR, Poulose TA. Timing of prophylactic uterotonics for the third stage of labour after vaginal birth. *Cochrane Database Syst Rev.* 2010;(8):CD006173. [Meta-analysis: 3 RCTs, $n = 1671$] [I]
7. Jackson KW Jr., Allbert JR, Schemmer GK, et al. A randomized controlled trial comparing oxytocin administration before and after placental delivery in the prevention of postpartum hemorrhage. *Am J Obstet Gynecol.* 2001;185:873. [RCT, $n = 1486$] [I]
8. Roach MK, Abramovici A, Tita AT. Dose and duration of oxytocin to prevent postpartum hemorrhage: A review. *Am J Perinatol.* 2013;30(7):523–528. doi: 10.1055/s-0032-1329184 [Review]
9. Su LL, Chong YS, Samuel M. Carbetocin for preventing postpartum haemorrhage. *Cochrane Database Syst Rev.* 2012;(4):CD005457. [Meta-analysis: 11 RCTs, $n = 2635$] [I]
10. Leung SW, Ng PS, Wong WY, et al. A randomized trial of carbetocin versus syntometrine in the management of the third stage of labor. *BJOG.* 2006;113:1459–1464. [RCT, $n = 329$] [I]
11. Liabsuetrakul T, Choobun T, Peeyananjarassri K, et al. Prophylactic use of ergot alkaloids in the third stage of labour. *Cochrane Database Syst Rev.* 2007;(2):CD005456. [Meta-analysis: 6 RCTs, $n = 3941$] [I]
12. Hofmeyr GJ, Gülmezoglu AM, Novikova N, Lawrie TA. Postpartum misoprostol for preventing maternal mortality and morbidity. *Cochrane Database Syst Rev.* 2013;(7):CD008982. [Meta-analysis: 78 RCTs, $n = 59,216$] [I]
13. Chaudhuri P, Biswas J, Mandal A. Sublingual misoprostol versus intramuscular oxytocin for prevention of postpartum hemorrhage in low-risk women. *Int J Gynaecol Obstet.* 2012;116(2):138–142. [RCT, $n = 530$] [I]
14. Atukunda EC, Siedner MJ, Obua C, et al. Sublingual misoprostol versus intramuscular oxytocin for prevention of postpartum hemorrhage in Uganda: A double-blind randomized non-inferiority trial. *PLoS Med.* 2014;11(11):e1001752. doi:10.1371/journal.pmed.1001752. [I]
15. Tuncalp O, Hofmeyr GJ, Gullmezoglu AM. Prostaglandins for preventing postpartum hemorrhage. *Cochrane Database Sys Rev.* 2012;(8):CD000494. [Meta-analysis: 72 RCTs, $n = 52,678$] [I]
16. Bellad MB, Tara D, Ganachari MS, et al. Prevention of postpartum haemorrhage with sublingual misoprostol or oxytocin: A double-blind randomized controlled trial. *BJOG.* 2012;119:975–986 [RCT, n=652] [I]
17. Conde-Agudelo A, Nieto A, Rosas-Bermudez A, Romero R. Misoprostol to reduce intraoperative and postoperative hemorrhage during cesarean delivery: A systematic review and metaanalysis. *Am J Obstet Gynecol.* 2013;209(1):40.e1–40. [Meta-analysis; 17 RCTs, $n = 3,174$] [I]
18. Novikova N, Hofmeyr GJ, Cluver C. Tranexamic acid for preventing post-partum haemorrhage. *Cochrane Database Syst Rev.* 2015;(6):CD007872. [Meta-analysis: 12 RCTs, $n = 3285$] [I]
19. Simonazzi G, Bisulli M, Saccone G, et al. Tranexamic acid for preventing postpartum blood loss after cesarean delivery: A systematic review and meta-analysis of randomized controlled trials. *Acta Obstet Gynecol Scand.* 2015; DOI: 10.1111/aogs.12798. [meta-analysis, 9 RCTs, $n = 2365$] [I]
20. Moise KJ. Umbilical cord stem cells. *Obstet Gynecol.* 2005;106:1393–1407. [Review]
21. Rabe H, Diaz-Rossello J, Duley L, Dowswell T. Effect of timing of umbilical cord clamping and other strategies to influence placental transfusion at preterm birth on maternal and infant outcomes. *Cochrane Database of Syst Rev.* 2012;(8):CD003248. [15 RCTs, $n = 738$] [I]
22. Backes CH, Rivera BK, Haque U, et al. Placental transfusion strategies in very preterm neonates. *Obstet Gynecol.* 2014;(124):47–56. [Meta-analysis: 12 RCTs, $n = 531$] [I]
23. Rabe H, Reynolds G, Diaz-Rossello J. A systemic review and meta-analysis of a brief delay in clamping the umbilical cord of preterm infants. *Neonatology.* 2007;93:138–144. [Meta-analysis: 10 RCTs, $n = 454$] [I]
24. Vain NE, Satragno DS, Gorenstein AN, et al. Effect of gravity on volume of placental transfusion: A multicenter, randomized, non-inferiority trial. *Lancet.* 2014;384(9939):235–240. [RCT, $n = 546$] [I]
25. Hosono S, Mugishima H, Fijita H, et al. Umbilical cord milking reduces the need for red blood cell transfusions and improves neonatal adaptation in infants born at less than 29 weeks' gestation: A randomized controlled trial. *Arch Dis Child Fetal Neo Ed.* 2008;93:F14–F19. [RCT, $n = 40$] [I]
26. Rabe H, Jewison A, Fernadez Alvarez R, et al. Milking compared to delayed cord clamping to increase placental transfusion in preterm neonates. *Obstet Gynecol.* 2011;117:205–211. [RCT, $n = 58$]
27. Patel S, Clark EAS, Rodriguez CE, et al. Effect of umbilical cord milking on morbidity and survival in extremely low gestational age neonates. *Am J Obstet Gynecol.* 2014;211(5):519.e1–7. [Retrospective cohort, $n = 318$] [I]
28. Krueger MS, Eyal FG, Peevy KJ, et al. Delayed cord clamping with and without cord stripping: A prospective randomized trial of preterm neonates. *Am J Obstet Gynecol.* 2015;212(3):394.e1–5. [RCT, $n = 67$] [I]
29. McDonald SJ, Middleton P. Effect of timing of umbilical cord clamping of term infants on maternal and neonatal outcomes. *Cochrane Database Syst Rev.* 2013;(7):CD004074. [Meta-analysis: 15 RCTs, $n = 3911$] [I]

30. Giacalone PL, Vignal J, Daures JP, et al. A randomized evaluation of two techniques of management of the third stage of labor in women at low risk of postpartum hemorrhage. *BJOG*. 2000;107:396. [RCT, *n* = 477] [I]
31. Soltani H, Dickinson F, Symonds IM. Placental cord drainage after spontaneous vaginal delivery as part of the management of the third stage of labour. *Cochrane Database Syst Rev*. 2011;(4):CD004665. [Meta-analysis: 3 RCTs, *n* = 1257] [I]
32. Hofmeyr GJ, Mshweshwe NT, Gulmezoglu AM. Controlled cord traction for the third stage of labour. *Cochrane Database Syst Rev*. 2015;(1):CD008020. [3 RCTs, *n* = 27,873] [I]
33. Hofmeyr GJ, Abdel-Aleem H, Abdel-Aleem MA. Uterine massage for preventing postpartum haemorrhage. *Cochrane Database of Syst Rev*. 2013;(7):CD006431 [Meta-analysis: 2 RCTs, *n* = 2164] [I]
34. Chen M, Chang Q, Duan T, et al. Uterine massage to reduce blood loss after vaginal delivery: A randomized controlled trial. *Obstet Gynecol*. 2013;122:290–295. [RCT, 2,340] [I]
35. Begley CM, Gyte GML, Murphy DJ, et al. Active versus expectant management for women in the third stage of labour. *Cochrane Database Syst Rev*. 2015;(3):CD007412. [Meta-analysis: 7 RCTs; *n* = 8247] [I]
36. Fleming VEM, Hagen S, Niven C. Does perineal suturing make a difference? The SUNS trial. *BJOG*. 2003;110:684–689. [RCT, *n* = 74]
37. Lunquist M, Olsson A, Nissen E, et al. Is it necessary to suture all lacerations after vaginal delivery? *Birth*. 2000;27:79–85. [RCT, *n* = 78] [I]
38. Gordon B, Mackrodt C, Fern E, et al. The Ipswich childbirth study: 1. A randomized evaluation of two stage postpartum perineal repair leaving the skin unsutured. *BJOG*. 1998;105:435–440. [RCT, *n* = 1780] [I]
39. Kettle C, Hills RK, Ismail KMK. Continuous versus interrupted sutures for repair of episiotomy or second degree tears. *Cochrane Database Syst Rev*. 2009;(1):CD00947. [Meta-analysis: 7 RCTs, *n* = 3822] [I]
40. Fitzpatrick M, Behan M, O'Connell PR, et al. A randomized clinical trial comparing primary overlap with approximation repair of third degree obstetric tears. *Am J Obstet Gynecol*. 2000;183:1220–1224. [RCT, *n* = 112] [I]
41. Williams A, Adams EJ, Tincello DG, et al. How to repair an anal sphincter injury after vaginal delivery: Results of a randomized controlled trial. *BJOG*. 2006;113:201–207. [RCT, *n* = 112] [I]
42. Farrell SA, Flowerdew G, Gilmour D, et al. Overlapping compared with end-to-end repair of complete third-degree or fourth-degree obstetric tears. Three year follow-up of a randomized controlled trial. *Obstet Gynecol*. 2012;120:803–808. [RCT, *n* = 174] [I]
43. Buppasira P, Lumbiganon P, Thinkhamrop J, et al. Antibiotic prophylaxis for third and fourth degree perineal tear during vaginal birth. *Cochrane Database of Syst Rev*. 2014;(10):CD005125 [1 RCT, *n* = 147] [I]
44. Kettle C, Dowswell T, Ismail KMK. Absorbable suture materials for primary repair of episiotomy and second degree tears. *Cochrane Database Syst Rev*. 2010;(6):CD000006. [18 RCTs, *n* = 10,171] [I]
45. Dencker A, Lundgren I, Sporrong T. Suturing after childbirth—A randomized controlled study testing a new monofilament material. *BJOG*. 2006;113:114–116. [RCT, *n* = 1139] [I]
46. Flatin DL, Boulvain M, Floris LA, Irion O. Diagnosis of anal sphincter tears to prevent fecal incontinence. *Obstet Gynecol*. 2005;106:6–13. [RCT, *n* = 752] [I]
47. Hedayati H, Parsons J, Crowther CA. Rectal analgesia for pain from perineal trauma following childbirth. *Cochrane Database Syst Rev*. 2009;(4):CD003931. [Meta-analysis: 3 RCTs, *n* = 249] [I]
48. Hedayati H, Parsons J, Crowther CA. Topically applied anaesthetics for treating perineal pain after childbirth. *Cochrane Database Syst Rev*. 2009;(4):CD004223. [Meta-analysis: 8 RCTs, *n* = 976] [I]
49. Franchi M, Cromi A, Scarperi S, et al. Comparison between lidocaine-prilocaine (EMLA) and mepivacaine infiltration for pain relief during perineal repair after childbirth: A randomized trial. *Am J Obstet Gynecol*. 2009;(201):186.e1–5. [RCT, n = 61] [I]
50. Hay-Smith, EJC. Therapeutic ultrasound for postpartum perineal pain and dyspareunia. *Cochrane Database Syst Rev*. 2009;(4):CD00495. [Meta-analysis: 4 RCTs, *n* = 459] [I]
51. Singla AK, Lapinski RH, Berkowitz RL, et al. Are women who are Jehovah's witnessess at risk of maternal death? *Am J Obstet Gynecol*. 2001;185:893–895. [II-2; *n* = 332]
52. Gyamfi C, Gyamfi MM, Berkowitz RL. Ethical and medicolegal considerations in the obstetric care of a Jehovah's Witness. *Obstet Gynecol*. 2003;102:173–180. [Review]
53. Gyamfi C, Berkowitz RL. Responses by pregnant Jehovah's Witnesses on health care proxies. *Obstet Gynecol*. 2004;104:541–544. [II-3]
54. Singla AK, Berkowitz RL, Saphier CJ. Obstetric hemorrhage in Jehovah's witnesses. *Conteporary Obstet Gynecol*. 2002; 4:32–43. [Review]
55. Catling S, Joels L. Cell salvage in obstetrics: The time has come. *BJOG*. 2005;112:131–132. [Review]

Intrapartum fetal monitoring

Serena Xodo and Suneet P. Chauhan

KEY POINTS
- Compared with intermittent auscultation (IA), the **use of continuous electronic fetal heart rate (FHR) monitoring significantly increases the rate of operative interventions** (vacuum, forceps, and cesarean delivery [CD]) for nonreassuring patterns, **but it does decrease the likelihood of neonatal seizures.**
- With some persistent category II or III patterns, limited evidence (one randomized controlled trial [RCT]) **showed that intrauterine resuscitation with maternal oxygen, change in maternal position, discontinuation of labor stimulation and/or tocolytics, or amnioinfusion (if variable decelerations) reduce the need to proceed with emergent CD but do not reduce the likelihood of injury from intrapartum hypoxia.** The use of maternal oxygen has been also associated with possible harm, but the evidence is still insufficient for a recommendation. The labor of **women at risk** for poor peripartum outcomes **should be monitored with continuous electronic FHR tracing.**
- Reinterpretation of the FHR tracing, especially knowing the neonatal outcome, should be avoided.
- There is **insufficient evidence** to assess **computerized FHR monitoring,** but the limited evidence so far is promising.
- For singletons at 36 weeks or more, **fetal electrocardiogram (ECG) ST-segment analysis (STAN)** used as an adjunct to conventional intrapartum electronic fetal heart-rate monitoring **does not improve perinatal outcomes.**
- *Fetal pulse oximetry (FPO) is not associated with significant maternal or neonatal benefits* compared with continuous FHR monitoring alone, **except for a significant decrease in CD for nonreassuring FHR (NRFHR).**

BACKGROUND
Electronic FHR monitoring during labor is the most common obstetric procedure in the United States [1]. Between 1997 and 2003 in the United States, monitoring was utilized in 84% (23,273,458) of the over 27 million births [1]. For admission tests at the beginning of labor, see Chapter 7. For meconium, see Chapter 23.

FHR DEFINITIONS
Intrapartum fetal monitoring usually refers to monitoring of the FHR. Outside the United States, this monitoring is often referred to as **cardiotocography (CTG),** while the term **intrapartum FHR monitoring** is more commonly used in the United States. Adapted from the 2008 National Institute of Child Health and Human Development Workshop [2], the definitions of FHR pattern are described in Table 10.1 and depicted in Figures 10.1 through 10.3. The definitions were developed for intrapartum monitoring but may be applicable to antepartum monitoring. No distinction is made between short- and long-term variability [2]. Accelerations, decelerations, bradycardia, and tachycardia can be quantified by describing the nadir/zenith and the duration in minutes and seconds of the FHR change. A **recurrent deceleration** occurs with >50% of uterine contractions in any 20-minute period.

A **three-tier system for categorization of FHR patterns** has been recommended [2]. According to this classification, **category I** tracings are predictive of normal fetal acid–base status at the time of observation and may be followed in a routine manner. **Category II** tracings are indeterminate and not predictive of abnormal fetal acid–base status but require evaluation and continued surveillance and reevaluation. **Category III** tracings are abnormal and predictive of abnormal fetal acid–base status (Table 10.2; Figures 10.4 through 10.6). These tracings require prompt evaluation and should include efforts to expeditiously resolve the abnormal pattern. It is noteworthy that a full description of an electronic fetal monitoring (EFM) tracing requires a qualitative and quantitative description of the following: (1) uterine contractions, (2) baseline FHR, (3) baseline FHR variability, (4) presence of accelerations, (5) periodic or episodic decelerations, and (6) changes or trends of FHR patterns over time [2].

In relation to uterine activity, *tachysystole* is defined as >5 contractions in 10 minutes averaged over 30 minutes, whether the contractions are spontaneous or stimulated. The terms hyperstimulation and hypercontractility should be abandoned. Terms such as "asphyxia," "hypoxia," and "fetal distress" should not be used in the interpretation of FHR tracing.

pH DEFINITIONS
- *Acidemia:* increased concentration of hydrogen ions in blood.
- *Acidosis:* a pathologic condition marked by increased concentration of hydrogen ions in tissue.
- *Hypoxemia:* decreased oxygen content in blood.
- *Hypoxia:* a pathologic condition marked by decreased level of oxygen in tissue.
- *Asphyxia:* acidemia, hypoxia, and metabolic acidosis; must have all of the following: (1) umbilical arterial pH <7.00; (2) Apgar ≤3 at >5 minutes; and (3) neonatal neurologic sequelae (e.g., seizures, coma, and hypotonia) [3]. This term should be used with caution and never before birth (see also Chapter 31).

INCIDENCE
The prevalence of CD for nonreassuring FHR (NRFHR) tracing is about 3% or more, and it is increasing [4]. NRFHR is usually the second most common reason for CD, after arrest of labor [5].

Table 10.1 Definitions of FHR Patterns

	Definitions
Baseline FHR	The mean FHR rounded to increments of 5 bpm during a 10-minute period (excluding accelerations, decelerations, and periods of marked variability). The baseline must be for a minimum of 2 minutes. May need to compare the previous 10-minute segment to determine the baseline. Bradycardia—baseline FHR <110 bpm Tachycardia—baseline FHR >160 bpm Sinusoidal pattern—visually apparent, smooth, sine-wave-like undulating FHR baseline pattern with cycle frequency 3–5/minute, persisting ≥20 minutes
Baseline FHR variability	Fluctuations in the baseline FHR that are irregular in amplitude and frequency (excluding accelerations and decelerations). Variability is quantitated as the amplitude of peak-to-trough in bpm. Absent—amplitude range undetectable Minimal—amplitude range ≤5 bpm Moderate (normal)—amplitude range 6–25 bpm Marked—amplitude range >25 bpm
Acceleration	An abrupt (peak within 30 seconds) increase in the FHR from baseline. Acme is ≥15 bpm above baseline, lasting for 15 seconds or more and <2 minutes from the onset to return to baseline Before 32 weeks, acceleration is acme ≥10 bpm over the baseline and lasting at least 10 seconds but <2 minutes. Prolonged acceleration if it lasts >2 minutes but <10 minutes If the acceleration is >10 minutes, then it is a baseline change.
Deceleration	An abrupt or gradual decrease in FHR as characterized below: Recurrent—occur with ≥50% contractions in 20 minutes Intermittent—occur with <50% contractions in 20 minutes Prolonged—visually apparent decrease in FHR ≥15 bpm, lasting ≥2 minutes but <10 minutes
Early deceleration (Figure 10.1)	In association with a uterine contraction, a visually apparent, usually symmetrical and gradual (onset to nadir ≥30 seconds) decrease in FHR with return to baseline. Onset, nadir, and recovery of deceleration occur at same time as beginning, peak, and ending of contraction, respectively.
Late deceleration (Figure 10.2)	In association with a uterine contraction, a visually apparent, gradual (onset to nadir ≥30 seconds) decrease in FHR Onset, nadir, and recovery of deceleration occur after the beginning, peak, and end of the contraction, respectively.
Variable deceleration (Figure 10.3)	An abrupt (onset to nadir <30 seconds) decrease in FHR The decrease in FHR is at least 15 bpm, lasting ≥15 seconds but <2 minutes. Onset, depth, and duration vary with contractions.

Source: Adapted from Macones GA et al., *Obstet Gynecol*, 112, 661–666, 2008.
Abbreviations: bpm, beats per minute; FHR, fetal heart rate.

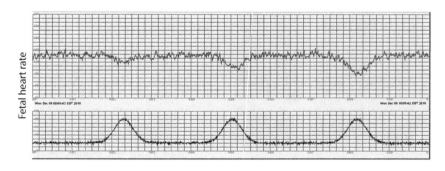

Figure 10.1 Early decelerations of 15, 30, and 45 beats per minute (bpm), respectively.

RISK FACTORS AND PREDICTORS OF ABNORMAL FHR

The risk of CD for NRFHR is >20% in patients with **moderate/severe asthma, severe hypothyroidism, severe preeclampsia, postterm, or fetal growth restriction (FGR) with abnormal Doppler studies** [4].

Use of likelihood ratio suggests that fetal movement count, abnormal FHR on admission, vibroacoustic stimulation, amniotic fluid index, contraction stress test, and modified and completed biophysical profile are poor diagnostic tests to identify which patients will require emergent CD for NRFHR [4]. **Umbilical artery systolic/diastolic**

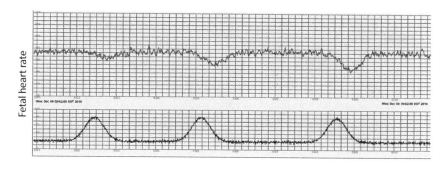

Figure 10.2 Late decelerations of 15, 30, and 45 bpm, respectively.

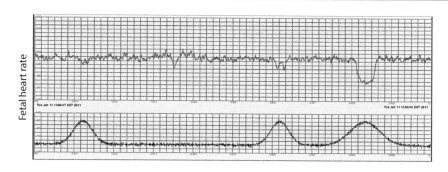

Figure 10.3 Variable decelerations of 15, 40, 30, and 60 bpm, respectively.

Table 10.2 Three-Tier FHR Interpretation System

	Baseline	Variability	Acceleration	Deceleration
Category I (Figure 10.4A–C)	110–160 bpm	Moderate	Possible, not necessary	Possible early; no variable or late
Category II (includes those not in category I or III; Figure 10.5A–I)	1. Bradycardia without absent variability 2. Tachycardia	1. Minimal 2. Absent without recurrent decelerations 3. Marked	After fetal stimulation	1. Recurrent variable with minimal to moderate variability 2. Prolonged 3. Recurrent late with moderate variability 4. Variable with other characteristics (i.e., slow return to baseline, overshoots, or shoulders)
Category III (Figure 10.6A–C)	1. Bradycardia 2. Sinusoidal	Absent		1. Recurrent late 2. Recurrent variable

Source: Adapted from Macones GA et al., *Obstet Gynecol*, 112, 661–666, 2008.

ratio, however, is a reliable test to predict the need for CD for NRFHR.

FETAL HEART MONITORING CONTINUOUS ELECTRONIC FHR MONITORING VERSUS INTERMITTENT AUSCULTATION

Despite the ubiquitous use, there are concerns about the efficacy of EFM. As noted by the American College of Obstetricians and Gynecologists (ACOG) practice bulletin [6], the efficacy of monitoring is adjudicated by comparing the neonatal and infant morbidity, including seizure and cerebral palsy, or mortality averted versus the unnecessary interventions (operative vaginal delivery or CD) undertaken. Since all the randomized clinical trials (RCTs) with EFM compare it to IA, the efficacy is determined by calculating the relative risks (RR) of interventions, neonatal seizures, cerebral palsy, or death.

Compared with IA, continuous EFM (CTG) shows **no significant improvement in overall perinatal death rate** (RR 0.86, 95% confidence interval [CI] 0.59–1.23), but was associated with a **halving of neonatal seizures** (RR 0.50, 95% CI 0.31–0.80). There was no significant difference in cerebral palsy rates (RR 1.75,

114 OBSTETRIC EVIDENCE BASED GUIDELINES

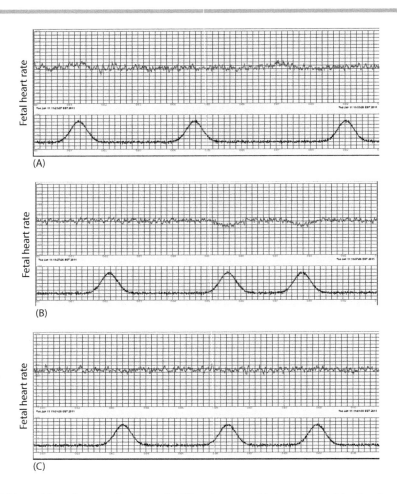

Figure 10.4 Category I. (**A**) Normal baseline, moderate variability, absence of late and variable decelerations, accelerations present. (**B**) Normal baseline, moderate variability, absence of late and variable decelerations, early decelerations present. (**C**) Normal baseline, moderate variability, absence of late and variable decelerations.

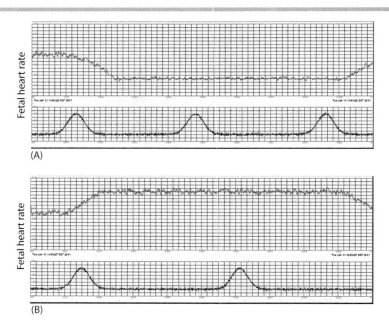

Figure 10.5 Category II. (**A**) Bradycardia with moderate variability. (**B**) Tachycardia. (**C**) Minimal variability. (**D**) Absent variability. (**E**) Marked variability. (**F**) Recurrent variable decelerations, minimal variability. (**G**) Prolonged deceleration. (**H**) Recurrent late decelerations, moderate variability. (**I**) Variable decelerations.

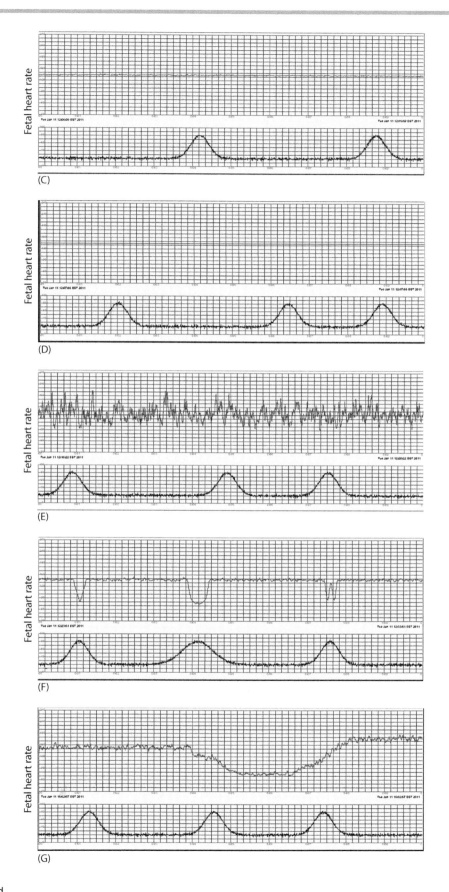

Figure 10.5 Continued

116 OBSTETRIC EVIDENCE BASED GUIDELINES

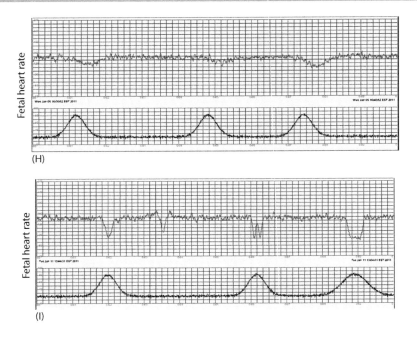

Figure 10.5 Continued

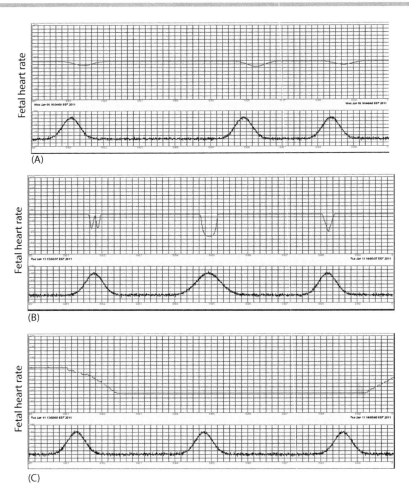

Figure 10.6 Category III. (**A**) Recurrent late decelerations, absent fetal heart rate (FHR) variability. (**B**) Recurrent variable decelerations, absent FHR variability. (**C**) Bradycardia, absent FHR variability.

95% CI 0.84–3.63). There was a **significant increase in cesarean sections** associated with continuous CTG (RR 1.63, 95% CI 1.29–2.07). Women were also **more likely to have an instrumental vaginal birth** (RR 1.15, 95% CI 1.01–1.33). Data for subgroups of low-risk, high-risk, preterm pregnancies and high-quality trials were consistent with overall results [6,7]. EFM is associated with 1 additional CD for every 58 women monitored continuously; 661 women need to have EFM during labor to prevent one neonatal seizure [7].

While the efficacy of EFM is debated, it is noteworthy that there are concerns regarding the 13 RCTs, which are sampled over 37,000 women, on continuous FHR monitoring versus IA [7]. Only two of these trials were of high quality [8,9], and only three trials reported data in low-risk women [8–10]. The authors of the meta-analysis on this subject [7] noted that to test the hypothesis that continuous monitoring can prevent 1 death in 1,000 births, more than 50,000 women would have to be randomized. Additionally, there are concerns that the meta-analysis combines results from RCTs published prior to the introduction of the Consolidated Standards of Reporting Trials (CONSORT) guidelines [11], and that inadequate study size may not reflect the outcomes in contemporary obstetrical practice [12].

Thus, if IA is available on the labor and delivery, it is reasonable to discuss the options with the patients [13]. Admittedly both patients and clinicians prefer continuous FHR monitoring as the method to evaluate the fetus during labor [14]. The explanations for the preference include the ease of use, the reassurance women derive from hearing the heart beat during labor, and the different value patients and clinicians place on the route of delivery and neonatal outcomes. Compared with pregnant patients and mothers, obstetricians overestimate the burden posed by cesarean, and, contrary to obstetricians, women value a newborn with permanent neurologic handicap over neonatal death [14].

Clinicians choosing to utilize IA should be aware of some of the problems associated with its use. **Continuous electronic FHR monitoring has a significantly better ability to detect acidemia** (umbilical arterial pH < 7.15 in this study) than IA: a sensitivity of 97% versus 34% and a higher positive predictive value of 37% versus 22%, respectively [15]. Continuous tracing of the FHR was not only superior with detection of respiratory and mixed acidosis but metabolic as well. It is possible that the ominous FHR patterns are poorly assessed by IA. Logistically **it may not be feasible to adhere to guidelines of how frequently the heart rate should be auscultated with IA.** One prospective study noted that the protocol for IA was successfully completed with only 3% of the cases [16].

Even though the use of continuous electronic monitoring of the FHR does not decrease the prevalence of cerebral palsy, it assists in determining if the injury occurred during the ante- or intrapartum periods. Review of the FHR tracing of neurologically injured newborns indicates that the majority of them had an abnormal pattern consistent with asphyxial injury *prior* to the onset of labor [17]. Moreover, a pregnancy with chronic fetal distress may develop superimposed acute asphyxia, in which case the impairment may be more severe than if the sentinel event and injury occurred during labor.

Not all pregnancies should be monitored with IA because **those at risk for adverse outcomes like cerebral palsy, neonatal encephalopathy, and perinatal death should be monitored with continuous FHR tracing during labor** [18]. Thus, high-risk pregnancies that underwent antepartum surveillance should not be evaluated with IA, nor should those who are likely to have CD for an NRFHR pattern [4]. These include FGR, oligohydramnios, polyhydramnios, placenta previa, postterm (≥42 weeks), multiple gestation, isoimmunized pregnancy, prior intrauterine fetal demise (IUFD), or maternal renal disease, diabetes, preeclampsia, collagen disorders, hemoglobinopathies, and cardiovascular disease. Additionally, parturients should be monitored with continuous tracing of the FHR if they have been induced or augmented, or have dysfunctional labor, tocolytics administered more than once an hour, suspected FHR abnormalities with auscultation, abnormal fetal presentation, regional anesthesia, abruption, infection, preterm labor, prior CD (vaginal birth after cesarean [VBAC] attempt), hypertonic uterus, and meconium staining of the amniotic fluid [19].

FHR monitoring should be continued until delivery. If CD is performed, internal scalp monitoring can be continued until delivery, while external monitoring can be discontinued when the abdominal preparation begins.

REVIEWING ELECTRONIC FHR MONITORING

When EFM is utilized during labor, the nurses or physicians should review it frequently. If the patient is at low-risk pregnancy, the FHR tracing should be reviewed at least every 30 minutes in the first stage of labor and at least every 15 minutes during the second stage. The corresponding frequency for high-risk parturients is 15 and 5 minutes, respectively. The maternal pulse should be taken to make sure the FHR is indeed fetal, and not maternal. **Healthcare providers should document** that they have reviewed the tracing by a narrative note or use of comprehensive flow sheets or by placing one's initials on the monitor strip, if it is reassuring [19]. Among low-risk patients, it is more feasible to confirm that the strips are reviewed according to the guidelines, whereas among high-risk patients, compliance during active phase, and especially during second stage of labor, is more demanding and difficult. The FHR tracing, as a part of the medical chart, should be labeled and available for review if the need arises. Alternatives like computer storage of the FHR tracing that do not permit overwriting or revisions are reasonable, as are microfilm recordings [19].

Due to the **inter- and intraobserver variability**, FHR tracing should be interpreted cautiously and preferably without knowing the neonatal outcome [20–22]. When four obstetricians, for example, examined 50 cardiotocograms, they agreed in only 22% of the cases. Two months later, during the second review of the same 50 tracings, the clinicians interpreted 21% of the tracings differently than they did during the first evaluation [21]. Factors that influence the interpretation of cardiotocograms include the clinician's experience, whether the tracing is normal versus equivocal or ominous with greater agreement if the tracing is reassuring, and the time of the day, with possibly greater error at night. With retrospective reviews, the foreknowledge of neonatal outcome alters the impressions of the tracing. Given the same intrapartum tracing but opposite neonatal outcomes, the reviewer is more likely to find evidence of fetal hypoxia and criticize the obstetrician's management if the outcome was supposedly poor versus good [22].

The positive predictive value of NRFHR for cerebral palsy is about 0.1% [8]. The **false-positive rate is extremely high** (99%) for FHR tracing and abnormal neonatal outcome, especially cerebral palsy [23].

EXTERNAL VERSUS INTERNAL FHR MONITORING

External FHR monitoring is accomplished via a Doppler ultrasound device applied to the maternal abdomen. Internal scalp electrode (scalp lead) for FHR monitoring measures the R-R interval between consecutive beats. This provides an accurate representation of FHR variability. There are **no RCTs comparing these two monitoring techniques.** Internal monitoring is used, in general, for an FHR that cannot be consistently assessed by external monitoring. Contraindications to internal monitoring include maternal infections such as human immunodeficiency virus (HIV), active hepatitis B or C, and fetal thrombocytopenia. Otherwise internal fetal monitoring is safe.

COMPUTERIZED FHR MONITORING (EXPERT SYSTEMS)

Measured by interobserver agreement, the reliability of electronic FHR monitoring is not very good. Computerized evaluation of the intrapartum FHT, also called Expert Systems (ES), has been evaluated to try to improve the sensitivity for perinatal morbidity and mortality of FHR monitoring (CTG), and also try to decrease false positives associated with FH monitoring.

Two RCTs comparing CTG monitoring during labor with an ES versus CTG without an ES have been published, but only one trial ($n = 220$) provides data for quantitative analysis. There is **no strong evidence that CTG with an ES has an effect on the incidence of CD** (RR 0.61; 95% CI 0.35–1.04) when compared with CTG with fetal scalp blood sampling (FSBS). There is **no strong evidence supporting a reduction in the incidence of neonatal seizures** (RR 0.33; 95% CI 0.01–8.09) or *fetal acidemia* (RR 0.50; 95% CI 0.09–2.67) in women monitored using a CTG with an ES versus a CTG without an ES. Perinatal mortality was not reported. No fetal deaths occurred. There was no strong evidence supporting a reduction in the incidence of forceps-assisted vaginal birth (RR 0.50; 95% CI 0.05–5.43), hypoxic ischemic encephalopathy (RR 0.33; 95% CI 0.01–8.09), admission to the neonatal intensive care unit (RR 0.40; 95% CI 0.08–2.02) or an Apgar less than seven at 5 minutes (RR 0.50; 95% CI 0.13–1.95) [24].

Another RCT evaluated computer analysis by the Omniview-SisPorto 3.5 system of intrapartum CTG tracings to standard clinician analysis of *prerecorded cases*. Prediction of abnormal umbilical artery pH was more reproducible and accurate when clinicians had access to the computerized analysis of the CTGs [25].

Therefore, while limited results look promising, **there is insufficient evidence to assess if computerized evaluation of electronic FHR monitoring improves perinatal outcomes.**

OTHER FETAL MONITORING TESTS
Digital Scalp or Vibroacoustic Stimulation

The presence of acceleration usually assures that the fetus is not acidotic (pH < 7.20). If spontaneous acceleration is not present, and/or NRFHR is present, **digital scalp or vibroacoustic stimulation** should be done to elicit an acceleration (see definition in Table 10.1). Allis clamp and scalp puncture have been used to elicit an acceleration but are less safe. Digital scalp stimulation (gentle stroking of the fetal scalp for 15 seconds) is the test with the best predictive accuracy among these four [26]. There are currently **no RCTs that address the safety and efficacy of digital scalp or vibroacoustic stimulation used to assess fetal well-being in labor in the presence of NRFHR.** If the FHR increases, then labor should continue since an acceleration following fetal stimulation indicates that the likelihood of low scalp pH is 2% [26]. In the absence of an acceleration, the likelihood is 38%.

Fetal Scalp Blood Sampling

FSBS to measure scalp pH and lactate was introduced in 1962 by Saling in Berlin, Germany, as a stand-alone fetal status test, before the commercialization of EFM machines in 1968 [27].

It is important to understand fetal intrapartum physiology to assess FSBS. The fetus reacts to intrapartum decreased supply in oxygen by using anaerobic glycolysis, which leads to metabolic acidosis through conversion of pyruvate to lactate. Low pH is a combined measure of both metabolic acidosis (including base deficit) and the more labile component, respiratory acidosis [28].

At FSBS, a pH value >7.25 is considered to be normal, demonstrating a well oxygenated fetus. Values between 7.25 and 7.20 are considered subnormal, thus indicating the need to repeat the sampling within 20–30 minutes. Values of pH < 7.20 (or <7.15 in the second stage of labor) require intervention, such as intrauterine resuscitation or operative delivery. As for lactate concentration, normal values have been described as being <4.2 mmol/L. Values between 4.2 and 4.8 are defined intermediate, and values >4.8 mmol require intervention [29]. If the results are scalp pH < 7.20 or lactate >4.8 mm/L, then delivery should be accomplished expeditiously, usually by CD [30].

The technical aspects of FSBS require ruptured membranes and a cervical dilatation greater than or equal to 3 cm. An amnioscope is then placed vaginally to allow adequate visualization of the fetal head. A small blood sample is then taken from the fetal scalp. Usually 30–50 µL of blood are sufficient to perform the test. For testing lactate a much smaller amount of blood is required [28]. To be beneficial, the scalp pH machine needs to be reliable and readily available with prompt results.

There is no RCT that compares specifically FSBS versus no FSBS as primary, or even secondary, intervention for fetal monitoring intrapartum. Examining then indirect data, the latest Cochrane Review reports, in the meta-analysis on continuous CTG monitoring (with or without FSBS), that FSBS is associated with an increase in instrumental deliveries ($P = 0.04$ and a decrease in neonatal acidosis ($P = 0.04$) [31]. Retrospective studies have also failed to show a positive effect of FSBS on neonatal outcome [32,33].

The only level 1 evidence available on FSBS is that comparing pH or lactate measurement for FSBS [28]. The two RCTs [34,35], enrolled a total of 3348 women in labor having a NRFHR pattern. and investigated maternal and fetal/neonatal/infant outcomes following FSBS for pH or lactate measurement. The Cochrane Review noted that lactate sampling is more likely to be successful than pH sampling; but there were no differences between the two techniques (lactate versus pH analysis of FSBS) in terms of mode of birth, or neonatal outcomes evaluated by umbilical cord blood gases, Apgar score, encephalopathy, or admission to the neonatal intensive care unit (NICU) [29].

Given these data, as well as the several risks of FSBS [27], the ACOG has recommended **against the use of FSBS** [33,36]. Others have also cautioned against its use [27,30]. However, this procedure is still frequently performed in some Northern European countries (e.g., Sweden).

Fetal Electrocardiogram for Fetal Monitoring in Labor

The use of the fetal ECG has been evaluated **as an adjunct to continuous electronic FHR monitoring during labor** [36–43]. The use of internal monitoring with a scalp lead is mandatory to obtain ECG. In most labors, technically satisfactory cardiotocographic traces can be obtained by external ultrasound monitors, which are less invasive than internal scalp electrodes. One study assessed PR intervals and is insufficient to make recommendations [41]. Six RCTs assessed the ST segment [34–40].

A meta-analysis of six RCTs including 26,529 laboring singletons with cephalic presentation at 34 weeks or more reported that, compared with standard CTG only, ST analysis (STAN) plus CTG was associated with similar perinatal composite outcome (1.5% vs. 1.6%; RR 0.90, 95% CI 0.74–1.10), neonatal metabolic acidosis (0.5% vs. 0.7%; RR 0.74, 95% CI 0.54–1.02;), admission to the neonatal intensive care unit (5.4% vs. 5.5%; RR 0.99, 95% CI 0.90–1.10), perinatal death (0.1% vs. 0.1%; RR 1.71, 95% CI 0.67–4.33), neonatal encephalopathy (0.1% vs. 0.2%; RR 0.62, 95% CI 0.25–1.52), CD (13.8% vs. 14.0%; RR 0.96, 95% CI 0.85–1.08), and operative delivery (either cesarean or operative vaginal delivery) (23.9% vs. 25.1%; RR 0.93, 95% CI 0.86–1.01) [42]. The Cochrane review confirms these findings, and found an 8% decrease in operative vaginal deliveries associated with STAN [36].

As there is no difference in perinatal outcomes between STAN with CTG compared with CTG alone, this modality cannot be yet recommended for routine clinical care. Nonetheless, given heterogeneity in inclusion criteria among RCTs, issues regarding learning curve for STAN, Hawthorne effect in RCTs, different (3 vs. 4) tier classification used in RCTs, and sample size and power issues given abnormal perinatal outcomes (e.g., metabolic acidosis) are uncommon, more research is needed before the STAN technology can be deemed of no value for fetal monitoring in labor [43].

Fetal Pulse Oximetry

A normal fetal oxygen saturation ($FSpO_2$) in labor is 35%–65%. Fetal pulse oximetry (FPO) showing $FSpO_2$ <30% for at least >2 minutes is associated with a higher risk for declining fetal arterial pH and metabolic acidosis. The fetal oxygen sensor lies against the fetal cheek. The use of the FPO has been evaluated **as an adjunct to continuous electronic FHR monitoring during labor** [44–49].

RCTs on FPO are at high risk of bias because the impractical nature of blinding participants and clinicians. In RCTs not requiring FSBS prior to study entry, there was **no evidence of differences in the overall cesarean section rate** between those monitored with FPO and those not monitored with FPO or for whom the FPO results were masked (RR 0.99, 95% CI 0.86–1.13). There was evidence of a higher risk of cesarean section in the group with FPO plus CTG than in the group with fetal ECG plus CTG (one study only, n = 180, RR 1.56, 95% CI 1.06–2.29). No studies reported details of long-term disability [44].

There was evidence of a **decrease in cesarean section for nonreassuring fetal heart rate tracing (NRFHT) in the FPO plus CTG group compared with the CTG group** (RR 0.65, 95% CI 0.46–0.90) in women ≥34weeks without use of FSBS. There was no evidence of differences between groups in cesarean section for dystocia, although the overall incidence rates varied between the RCTs [44]. No differences are seen for endometritis, intrapartum or postpartum hemorrhage, uterine rupture, low Apgar scores, umbilical arterial pH or base excess, admission to the NICU, or fetal/neonatal death [44,45].

Given the above evidence, **routine use of FPO in labor is not recommended,** but can be considered in venues that do not use FSBS, to reduce rates of cesarean for NRFHT.

MANAGEMENT OF ABNORMAL FHR

The best time to evaluate the FHR tracing is after a contraction. The frequency with which the FHR should be evaluated depends on the risk status of pregnancy (see above). To correctly interpret the FHR pattern, the clinician must be cognizant of the gestational age, medications (Table 10.3) [50], prior fetal assessment, and obstetric and medical conditions. There is no evidence to support the prophylactic use of betamimetics during the second stage of labor. Compared with placebo, prophylactic betamimetic therapy is associated with an increase in forceps deliveries in one trial (Figure 10.7) [51].

Amnioinfusion

Amnioinfusion means, as the word says, infusing fluid (usually saline solution) in the amniotic cavity. Amnioinfusion has been proposed in order to prevent or relieve possible umbilical cord compression during labor either after rupture of membranes (ROM), or in cases of oligohydramnios with intact membranes. This technique consists of introducing into the uterine cavity saline or ringers lactate transcervically through a catheter in women with ROM, or transabdominally through a spinal needle when membranes are intact. Amnioinfusion can be used prophylactically (e.g., in cases of oligohydramnios), or therapeutically (e.g., when repetitive variable decelerations occur during labor). This type of decelerations is typically caused by umbilical cord compression, which occurs more frequently in case of oligohydramnios [52]. For prophylactic amnioinfusion for oligohydramnios before labor, see Chapter 19.

In the Cochrane review, therapeutic **transcervical amnioinfusion for** potential and suspected umbilical cord compression (mostly associated with **variable decelerations**) was found to significantly **reduce the following outcomes: cesarean section** (13 trials, 1493 participants, RR 0.62, 95% CI 0.46–0.83); **FHR decelerations** (seven trials, 1006 participants, RR 0.53, 95% CI 0.38–0.74); **Apgar score less than seven at 5 minutes** (12 trials, 1804 participants; RR 0.47, 95% CI 0.30–0.72); **meconium below the vocal cords** (three trials, 767 participants; RR 0.45, 95% CI 0.25–0.81); and **maternal stay longer than 3 days** (four trials, 1051 participants, RR 0.45, 95% CI 0.25–0.78) [53].

Transcervical amnioinfusion can be done by bolus or continuous infusion technique, with similar ability to relieve recurrent variable decelerations. Neither pumps nor warmers are necessary with amnioinfusion. In fact, the use of infusion pump during amnioinfusion significantly increases the risk of NRFHR. Either lactated Ringer's solution or normal saline can be used to place a crystalloid solution into the uterus without altering the neonatal electrolyte balance [53].

Transabdominal amnioinfusion showed similar results, though a fewer sample of patients was involved in the trials. Mean cord umbilical artery pH was higher in the amnioinfusion group (seven trials, 855 participants; average mean difference 0.03, 95% CI 0.00–0.06) and there was a trend toward fewer neonates with a low cord arterial pH (less than 7.2 or as defined by trial authors) in the amnioinfusion group (8 trials, 972 participants, RR 0.58, 95% CI 0.29–1.14) [53]. ACOG recommends *amnioinfusion for management of recurrent variable decelerations* [54].

Table 10.3 Effect of Medications and FHR Patterns

Medications	Study Design	Effect on FHR
Butorphanol	Case : control	Transient sinusoidal FHR pattern
Cocaine	Case : control	No characteristic changes in FHR pattern
Corticosteroid	RCT	Decrease in FHR variability with betamethasone but not dexamethasone
Magnesium sulfate	RCT and retrospective	A significant decrease in the FHR baseline and variability; inhibits the increase in accelerations with advancing gestational age
Meperidine	RCT	No characteristic changes in FHR pattern
Morphine	Case : control	Decreased number of accelerations
Nalbuphine	RCT	Decreased the number of accelerations, long- and short-term variations
Terbutaline	Retrospective	Abolishment or decrease in frequency of late and variable decelerations
Zidovudine	Case : control	No difference in the FHR baseline, variability, number of accelerations or decelerations

Source: Adapted from Chauhan SP and Macones GA, *Obstet Gynecol*, 105(5 Pt 1), 1161–1169, 2005.
Abbreviation: RCT, randomized clinical trial.

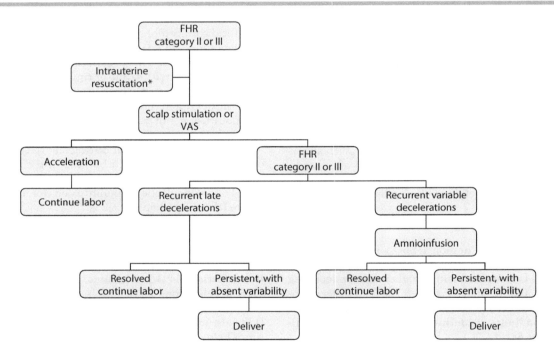

Figure 10.7 Algorithm for the management of abnormal FHR in labor. VAS, vibroacoustic stimulation. *Discontinue labor stimulant, change maternal position, hydration, and oxygenation.

Tocolysis

Tocolysis is a possible tool in the management of intrapartum NRFHR tracing. The rationale behind using intrapartum tocolysis is that uterine relaxation improves uteroplacental blood flow and therefore fetal oxygenation. The most commonly studied tocolytics for intrapartum fetal resuscitation are betamimetic drugs (terbutaline 0.25 mg intravenous [iv], hexoprenalne 10 mg iv, or ritodrine 10 mg in 9 mL saline administered iv over a 1-minute period).

There are some important safety concerns regarding using these drugs. The most serious reported side effects associated with administration of beta-agonists are pulmonary edema and myocardial ischemia [55]. Six RCTs have been performed with the aim to evaluate the use of betamimetics as tocolytics for acute intrapartum fetal resuscitation [56–61]. When betamimetic administration was compared with no treatment, neonatal outcome seemed to improve [57,58]. Four RCTs assessed the efficacy of betamimetics by comparing these drugs with either magnesium sulfate (4.0 g iv magnesium sulfate) [59], or atosiban (6.75 mg in 4.9 mL saline administered iv over a 1-minute period) [56,60], or nitroglycerin (0.4 mg iv) [61]. Betamimetics provided a more effective tocolysis, with similar successful resuscitation rates. The tocolytic potency of a single bolus of atosiban for tocolysis in term labor, especially for spontaneous contractions, needs further research [56].

ACOG recommends the **administration of tocolytic medications (e.g., terbutaline) when tachysystole is associated with FHR abnormalities** [54]. The time gained with this intervention may be useful for preparing for cesarean section or operative delivery, setting up regional analgesia, transferring a woman at home or in a unit without the necessary surgical or neonatal facilities to an appropriate hospital, or reviewing the need for urgent delivery.

Intrauterine Resuscitation

In the presence of NRFHR, concomitantly with performing scalp stimulation and/or scalp pH, intrauterine resuscitation can be attempted with maternal position change, hydration, oxygenation, and/or stopping labor stimulants (i.e., oxytocin) (Figure 10.7). **Intravenous fluid (IVF) bolus of 1000 mL, lateral positioning, and oxygen administration at 10 L/minute via nonbreather face mask have been studies together in one RCT, and are effective resuscitative measures to improve fetal oxygen saturation (FSpO$_2$) during labor** [62]. The evidence is from patients with normal FHR, and at present it is a reasonable assumption that the findings are applicable to NRFHR pattern.

- **Maternal position change**
  Maternal position change to improve fetal status in cases of intrapartum NRFHT **has not been studied separately in an RCT**, but only together with IVF and oxygenations (see above) [62]. Indirect evidence for position change comes from studies on maternal positioning during normal labor. There have been two reports comparing the effects of right lateral, left lateral, and supine maternal positions on fetal oxygen status, each suggesting that lateral positioning is more favorable than a supine position [63,64]. In 2013, a Cochrane review was published on the impact of maternal positions during the first stage of labor on different important outcomes for the mother and the baby. A total of 25 trials were included, with 5218 women considered. It was found that women should be encouraged and supported to use upright and mobile positions, as it seems that they benefit in terms of: a shorter duration of first stage of labor, a reduction in the risk of cesarean birth, a less use of epidural as a method of pain relief, and a lower chance of babies being admitted to the neonatal unit [65]. However, this review does not answer directly the question whether changing maternal position could be considered as a therapeutic measure in case of NRFHT in labor.
- **Hydration**
  There is **insufficient evidence (no trial) to assess by itself the effect of intrapartum maternal hydration on fetal status**. Maternal hydration has been studied in RCTs only together with IVF and oxygenations (see above) [62] Except for the situation where maternal hydration is necessary to correct either maternal hypotension or hypovolemia, the impact of IVFs intrapartum on NRFHT has not been established. Little is known about the effects of additional IVF volume on maternal transfer of oxygen to the fetus [62].
- **Oxygenation**
  Oxygen is frequently given to improve fetal status, though evidence of fetal benefits is lacking. Oxygen can be used either prophylactically, i.e., to prevent NRFHT, or therapeutically, i.e., to improve NRFHR which is already present.

  Only two RCTs have been done on the effects of maternal oxygen therapy for prophylaxis [66]. **The evidence available does not support the use of prophylactic maternal oxygen therapy during labor;** in fact, abnormal cord blood pH values (less than 7.2) were recorded significantly more frequently in the oxygenation group than the control group (RR 3.51, 95% CI 1.34–9.19) [66]. Evidence from animal studies suggests that giving oxygen to the mother raises the markers of free radical activity, which leads to edema and hemorrhage in vital organs for the fetus, such as brain and lungs [67].

  No RCTs on the therapeutic use of maternal oxygen for NRFHT exist. Unfortunately, the limited data available on women in labor does not clarify whether oxygen in labor is beneficial or harmful for the fetus. Oxygen has been associated with decreased umbilical cord pH [68], increased need for neonatal resuscitation [69], and raised level of markers of free radical activity [70]. Moreover neonatal resuscitation with 100% oxygen is no longer recommended [71]. In two FPO studies, maternal administration of oxygen by simple face mask was associated with a 5% increase in fetal oxygen saturation in normally oxygenated fetuses, and 20% in hypoxemic fetuses, returning abnormal to normal level of oxygenation [72,73].
- **Labor stimulant**
  There is **insufficient evidence (no trial) to assess by itself the effect of labor stimulant discontinuation on fetal status.** Nonetheless, **labor stimulants such as oxytocin should be discontinued in cases of NRFHT**, as it is well known that contraction can be associated with decreased fetal oxygenation, especially is too frequent.

Other Interventions

Additional steps with the management of NRFHR tracing might include (no trials available) the following:

- **Tocomonitoring**
  Uterine contraction assessment can be considered especially for suspected for tachysystole.
- **Cervical examination**
  Assessment of cervical status can be helpful to assess rapid dilation or descent, and to ensure that the umbilical cord has not prolapsed.
- **Maternal blood pressure**
  Maternal blood pressure monitoring may be helpful, especially among those who have received regional anesthesia. If hypotension is present in conjunction with NRFHR pattern, ephedrine or phenylephrine may be utilized [6].
- **Piracetam for NRFHR in labor**
  Piracetam, a derivative of γ-aminobenzoic acid, is thought to promote the metabolism of the brain cells when they are hypoxic. There is not enough evidence to evaluate the use of piracetam for NRFHR in labor. Compared with placebo, piracetam is associated with a nonsignificant trend to reduced need for cesarean section, and similar incidences of low Apgar scores, or neonatal respiratory problems and signs of hypoxia [74].
- **Operative delivery for NRFHR in labor**
  There are no contemporary trials of operative delivery versus conservative management of suspected NRFHR. In the only old (1959) trial, there is no difference in perinatal mortality [75].

REFERENCES

1. Chen HY, Chauhan SP, Ananth CV, et al. Electronic fetal heart rate monitoring and infant mortality: A population-based study in the United States. *Am J Obstet Gynecol*. 2011;204:491.e1–10. [II-3]
2. Macones GA, Hankins GDV, Spong CY, et al. The 2008 National Institute of Child Health and Human Development Workshop.

Electronic fetal heart rate monitoring: Update on definitions, interpretation, and research guidelines. *Obstet Gynecol.* 2008;112:661–666. [Review]
3. American College of Obstetricians and Gynecologists. ACOG Committee Opinion No. 197. Inappropriate use of the terms fetal distress and birth asphyxia. Washington, DC: ACOG, 1998. [Review]
4. Chauhan SP, Magann EF, Scott JR, et al. Cesarean delivery for fetal distress: Rate and risk factors. *Obstet Gynecol Surv.* 2003;58:337–350. [Review of 392 articles published in English from 1990 to 2000]
5. American College of Obstetricians and Gynecologists; Society for Maternal-Fetal Medicine. Obstetric care consensus no. 1: Safe prevention of the primary cesarean delivery. *Obstet Gynecol.* 2014;123(3):693–711. [Guideline]
6. American College of Obstetricians and Gynecologists. ACOG Practice Bulletin No. 106. Intrapartum fetal heart rate monitoring: Nomenclature, interpretation, and general management principles. Washington, DC: ACOG, 2009. [Review]
7. Alfirevic Z, Devane D, Gyte GM. Continuous cardiotocography (CTG) as a form of electronic fetal monitoring (EFM) for fetal assessment during labour. *Cochrane Database Syst Rev.* 2013;(3):CD006066. [Meta-Analysis; 13 RCTs, $n = >37,000$]
8. Renou P, Chang A, Anderson I, et al. Controlled trial of fetal intensive care. *Am J Obstet Gynecol.* 1976;126:470–476. [Level I]
9. Macdonald D, Grant A, Sheridan-Pereira M, et al. The Dublin randomized controlled trial of intrapartum fetal heart rate monitoring. *Am J Obstet Gynecol.* 1985;152:524–539. [Level I]
10. Leveno KJ, Cunningham FG, Nelson S, et al. A prospective comparison of selective and universal electronic fetal monitoring in 34,995 pregnancies. *N Engl J Med.* 1986;315:615–619. [Level I, $n = 34,995$]
11. Begg C, Cho M, Eastwood S, et al. Improving the quality of reporting of randomized controlled trials. The CONSORT statement. *JAMA.* 1996;276:637–639. [Level III]
12. Vintzileos AM. Evidence-based compared with reality-based medicine in obstetrics. *Obstet Gynecol.* 2009;113:1335–1340. [Level III]
13. Hundley V, Ryan M, Graham W. Assessing women's preferences for antepartum care. *Birth.* 2001;28:254–263. [Level II-3]
14. Vandenbussche FPHA, De Jong-Potjer LC, Stiggelbout AM, et al. Difference in the valuation of birth outcomes among pregnant women, mothers, and obstetricians. *Birth.* 1999;28:178–183. [Level II-3]
15. Vintzileos AM, Nochimson DJ, Antsaklis A, et al. Comparison of continuous electronic fetal heart rate monitoring versus intermittent auscultation in detecting fetal acidemia at birth. *Am J Obstet Gynecol.* 1995;173:1021–1024. [Level I-1]
16. Morrison JC, Chez BF, Davis ID, et al. Intrapartum fetal heart rate assessment: Monitoring by auscultation or electronic means. *Am J Obstet Gynecol.* 1993;168:63–66. [Level II-1]
17. Phelan JP, Ahn MO. Perinatal observations in forty-eight neurologically impaired term infants. *Am J Obstet Gynecol.* 1994;171:424–431. [Level II-3]
18. Society of Obstetricians and Gynaecologists of Canada Policy Statement. Fetal health surveillance in labour. *J Soc Obstet Gynaecol Can.* 1995;17:865–901. [Review]
19. Royal College of Obstetricians and Gynaecologists. The use of electronic fetal monitoring. The use and interpretation of cardiotocography in intrapartum surveillance. Evidence-Based Clinical Guidelines No. 8. London, UK: RCOG Press, 2001:136. [Review]
20. Chauhan SP, Klauser CK, Woodring TC, et al. Intrapartum nonreassuring fetal heart rate tracing and prediction of adverse outcomes: Interobserver variability. *Am J Obstet Gynecol.* 2008;199:623.e1–623.e5. [II-3]
21. Nielsen PV, Stigsby B, Nickelsen C, et al. Intra- and inter-observer variability in the assessment of intrapartum cardiotocograms. *Acta Obstet Gynecol Scand.* 1987;66:421–424. [Level II-3]
22. Zain HA, Wright JW, Parrish GE, et al. Interpreting the fetal heart rate tracing: Effect of knowledge of neonatal outcome. *J Repro Med.* 1998;43:367–370. [Level II-3]
23. Nelson KB, Dambrosia JM, Ting TY, et al. Uncertain value of electronic fetal monitoring in predicting cerebral palsy. *NEJM.* 1996;324:613–618. [II-2]
24. Lutomski JE, Meaney S, Greene RA, et al. Expert systems for fetal assessment in labour. *Cochrane Database Syst Rev.* 2015;(4):CD010708. doi: 10.1002/14651858.CD010708.pub2. [Meta-Analysis; 2 RCTs]
25. Costa A, Santos C, Ayeres-de-Campos D, et al. Access to computerized analysis of intrapartum cardiotocographs improves clinicians' prediction of newborn umbilical artery blood pH. *BJOG.* 2010;117:1288–1293. [RCT, $n = 204$]
26. Skupski DW, Rosenberg CR, Eglinton GS. Intrapartum fetal stimulation tests: A meta-analysis. *Obstet Gynecol.* 2002;99:129–134. [Meta-Analysis: 11 studies (not RCTs)]
27. Chandraharan E. Fetal scalp blood sampling during labour: Is it a useful diagnostic test or a historical test that no longer has a place in modern clinical obstetrics? *BJOG.* 2014;121(9):1056–1060. [Review]
28. East CE, Leader LR, Sheehan P, et al. Intrapartum fetal scalp lactate sampling for fetal assessment in the presence of a non-reassuring fetal heart rate trace. *Cochrane Database Syst Rev.* 2015;5:CD006174. doi: 10.1002/14651858.CD006174.pub3. [Meta-Analysis; 2 RCTs, $n = 3348$]
29. Jørgensen JS, Weber T. Fetal scalp blood sampling in labor--a review. *Acta Obstet Gynecol Scand.* 2014;93(6):548–555. doi: 10.1111/aogs.12421. [Review; III]
30. Berghella V. Research needed before FSBS can be used as a safe and effective screening test. *BJOG.* 2014;121(9):1061–1062. [Commentary].
31. Alfirevic Z, Devane D, Gyte GM. Continuous cardiotocography (CTG) as a form of electronic fetal monitoring (EFM) for fetal assessment during labour. *Cochrane Database Syst Rev.* 2013;5:CD006066. doi: 10.1002/14651858.CD006066.pub2. [Meta-Analysis]
32. Perkins RP. Requiem for a heavyweight: The demise of scalp blood pH sampling. *J Matern Fetal Med.* 1997;6(5):298–300. [Review; III]
33. Perkins RP. Perinatal observations in a high-risk population managed without intrapartum fetal pH studies. *Am J Obstet Gynecol.* 1984;149(3):327–336. [II-2]
34. Westgate J, Harris M, Curnow JSH, et al. Plymouth randomized trial of cardiotocogram only vs ST waveform plus cardiotocogram for intrapartum monitoring in 2400 cases. *Am J Obstet Gynecol.* 1993;169:1151–1160. [RCT, $n = 2434$]
35. Amer-Wahlin I, Hellsten C, Noren H, et al. Cardiotocography only versus cardiotocography plus ST analysis of fetal electrocardiogram for intrapartum fetal monitoring: A Swedish randomised controlled trial. *Lancet.* 2001;358:534–538. [RCT, $n = 4966$. CTG plus ST analysis of fetal ECG (2519 women) versus CTG alone (2477). The monitoring device was the STAN S21 (Neoventa Medical, Gothenburg) that incorporates an "expert system" to provide advice to clinical staff. In this, it constitutes a technically more advanced system than used in the Westgate 1993 trial.]
36. Neilson JP. Fetal electrocardiogram (ECG) for fetal monitoring during labour. *Cochrane Database Syst Rev.* 2006;(3):CD000116. Updated 2015;(3). [Meta-Analysis; 7 RCTs, $n = 27,403$]
37. Ojala K, Vaarasmaki M, Makikallio K, et al. A comparison of intrapartum automated fetal electrocardiography and conventional cardiography—A randomized controlled study. *Br J Obstet Gynecol.* 2006;113:419–423. [RCT, $n = 1483$]
38. Vayssiere C, David E, Meyer N, et al. A French randomized controlled trial of ST-segment analysis in a population with abnormal cardiotocograms during labor. *Am J Obstet Gynecol.* 2007;197(3):299.e1–299.e6. [RCT, $n = 799$]
39. Westerhuis ME, Visser GH, Moons KG, et al. Cardiotocography plus ST analysis of fetal electrocardiogram compared with cardiotocography only for intrapartum monitoring: A randomized

controlled trial. *Obstet Gynecol.* 2010;115(6):1173–1180. [RCT, n = 5681]
40. Belfort MA, Saade GR, Thom E, et al. A randomized trial of intrapartum fetal ECG ST-segment analysis. *N Engl J Med.* 2015;373(7):632–641. [RCT]
41. Strachan BK, van Wijngaarden WJ, Sahota D, et al. for the FECG Study Group. Cardiotocography only versus cardiotocography plus PR-interval analysis in intrapartum surveillance: A randomised, multicentre trial. *Lancet.* 2000; 55:456–459. [RCT, n = 957]
42. Saccone G, Schuit E, Amer-Wåhlin I, et al. Electrocardiogram ST analysis during labor: A systematic review and meta-analysis of randomized controlled trials. *Obstet Gynecol.* 2016;127:127–135. [6 RCT; n = 26,529]
43. Xodo S, Saccone G, Schuit E, et al. Why STAN might not be dead. *J Matern Fetal Neonatal Med.* 2016 Oct 13:1–10. [Review; III]
44. East CE, Begg L, Colditz PB, Lau R. Fetal pulse oximetry for fetal assessment in labour. *Cochrane Database Syst Rev.* 2007;(2):CD004075. [Meta-Analysis: 7 RCTs, n = 8,013]
45. Garite TJ, Dildy GA, McNamara H, et al. A multicenter controlled trial of fetal pulse oximetry in the intrapartum management of nonreassuring fetal heart rate patterns. *Am J Obstet Gynecol.* 2000;183(5):1049–1058. [RCT, n = 1010. Control group: Fetal heart rate monitoring (CTG) (Doppler/fetal scalp electrode). Study group: CTG plus fetal pulse oximetry. Protocol for action with reassuring and nonreassuring fetal oximetry values]
46. Kuhnert M, Schmidt S. Intrapartum management of nonreassuring fetal heart rate patterns: A randomized controlled trial of fetal pulse oximetry. *Am J Obstet Gynecol.* 2004;191:1989–1995. [RCT, n = 146]
47. Klauser CK, Christensen EE, Chauhan SP, et al. Use of fetal pulse oximetry among high-risk women in labor: A randomized clinical trial. *Am J Obstet Gynecol.* 2005;192:1810–1819. [RCT, n = 360]
48. East CE, Brennecke SP, King JK, et al. The effect of intrapartum fetal pulse oximetry, in the presence of nonreassuring fetal heart pattern, on operative delivery rates: A multicenter, randomized, controlled trial (the FOREMOST trial). *Am J Obstet Gynecol.* 2006;194:606–616. [RCT, n = 600]
49. Bloom SL, Spong CY, Thom E, et al.; National Institute of Child Health and Human Development Maternal-Fetal Medicine Units Network. Fetal pulse oximetry and cesarean delivery. *N Engl J Med.* 2006;355(21):2195–2120. [RCT, n = 5341].
50. Chauhan SP, Macones GA. ACOG Practice Bulletin No. 62. Intrapartum fetal heart rate monitoring. *Obstet Gynecol.* 2005;105(5 pt 1):1161–1169. [Review]
51. Hofmeyr GJ, Kulier R. Tocolysis for preventing fetal distress in second stage of labour. *Cochrane Database Syst Rev.* 1996;(1):CD000037. [Meta-Analysis: 2 RCTs, n = 164]
52. Gabbe SG, Ettinger BB, Freeman RK, Martin CB. Umbilical cord compression associated with amniotomy: Laboratory observations. *Am J Obstet Gynecol.* 1976 Oct 1;126(3):353–355.
53. Hofmeyr GJ, Lawrie TA. Amnioinfusion for potential or suspected umbilical cord compression in labour. *Cochrane Database Syst Rev.* 2012 Jan 18;1:CD000013. doi: 10.1002/14651858. CD000013.pub2. [Meta-Analysis; 19 RCTs]
54. American College of Obstetricians and Gynecologists. Practice Bulletin No. 116. Management of intraprtum fetal heart rate tracings. *Obstet Gynecol.* 2010;116(5):1232–1240. doi: 10.1097/AOG.0b013e3182004fa9. [Guideline; III]
55. Kulier R, Hofmeyr GJ. Tocolytics for suspected intrapartum fetal distress. *Cochrane Database Syst Rev.* 2000;(2):CD000035. [Meta-Analysis]
56. de Heus R, Mulder EJ, Derks JB, et al. A prospective randomized trial of acute tocolysis in term labour with atosiban or ritodrine. *Eur J Obstet Gynecol Reprod Biol.* 2008;139(2):139–145. doi: 10.1016/j.ejogrb.2008.01.001. Epub 2008 Mar 7. [RCT]
57. Patriarco MS, Viechnicki BM, Hutchinson TA, et al. A study on intrauterine fetal resuscitation with terbutaline. *Am J Obstet Gynecol.* 1987;157(2):384–387. [RCT]
58. Kulier R, Gülmezoğlu AM, Hofmeyr GJ, Van Gelderen CJ. Betamimetics in fetal distress: Randomised controlled trial. *J Perinat Med.* 1997;25(1):97–100. [RCT]
59. Magann EF, Cleveland RS, Dockery JR, et al. Acute tocolysis for fetal distress: Terbutaline versus magnesium sulphate. *Aust N Z J Obstet Gynaecol.* 1993;33(4):362–364. [RCT]
60. Afschar P, Schöll W, Bader A, et al. A prospective randomised trial of atosiban versus hexoprenaline for acute tocolysis and intrauterine resuscitation. *BJOG.* 2004;111(4):316–318. [RCT]
61. Pullen KM, Riley ET, Waller SA, et al. Randomized comparison of intravenous terbutaline vs nitroglycerin for acute intrapartum fetal resuscitation. *Am J Obstet Gynecol.* 2007;197(4):414.e1–6. [RCT]
62. Simpson KR, James DC. Efficacy of intrauterine resuscitation techniques in improving fetal oxygen status during labor. *Obstet Gynecol.* 2005;105(6):1362–1368. [RCT]
63. Carbonne B, Benachi A, Lévêque ML, et al. Maternal position during labor: Effects on fetal oxygen saturation measured by pulse oximetry. *Obstet Gynecol.* 1996;88(5):797–800. [RCT]
64. Aldrich CJ, D'Antona D, Spencer JA, et al. The effect of maternal posture on fetal cerebral oxygenation during labour. *Br J Obstet Gynaecol.* 1995;102(1):14–19.
65. Lawrence A, Lewis L, Hofmeyr GJ, Styles C. Maternal positions and mobility during first stage labour. *Cochrane Database Syst Rev.* 2013;(10):CD003934. doi: 10.1002/14651858.CD003934. pub4. [Meta-Analysis]
66. Fawole B, Hofmeyr GJ. Maternal oxygen administration for fetal distress. *Cochrane Database Syst Rev.* 2012;(12):CD000136. doi: 10.1002/14651858.CD000136.pub2. [Meta-Analysis; 2 RCTs]
67. Hamel MS, Andreson BL, Rouse DJ. Oxygen for intrauterine resuscitation: Of unproved benefit and potentially harmful. *Am J Obstet Gynecol.* 2014;211(2):124–127. doi: 10.1016/j.ajog.2014.01.004. Epub 2014 Jan 8. [Review; III]
68. Thorp JA, Trobough T, Evans R, et al. The effect of maternal oxygen administration during the second stage of labor on umbilical cord blood gas values: A randomized controlled prospective trial. *Am J Obstet Gynecol.* 1995;172(2 Pt 1):465–474. [RCT]
69. Nesterenko TH, Acun C, Mohamed MA, et al. Is it a safe practice to administer oxygen during uncomplicated delivery: A randomized controlled trial? *Early Hum Dev.* 2012;88(8):677–681. doi: 10.1016/j.earlhumdev.2012.02.007. Epub 2012 Mar 23. [RCT]
70. Khaw KS, Wang CC, Ngan Kee WD, et al. Effects of high inspired oxygen fraction during elective caesarean section underspinal anaesthesia on maternal and fetal oxygenation and lipid peroxidation. *Br J Anaesth.* 2002;88:18–23. [RCT]
71. Kattwinkel J, Perlman JM, Aziz K, et al. Part 15: Neonatal resuscitation: 2010 American Heart Association Guidelines for Cardiopulmonary Resuscitation and Emergency Cardiovascular Care. *Circulation.* 2010;122(18 Suppl 3):S909–S919. doi: 10.1161/CIRCULATIONAHA.110.971119. [Guideline; III]
72. Haydon ML, Gorenberg DM, Nageotte MP, et al. The effect of maternal oxygen administration of fetal pulse oximetry during labor in fetuses with nonreassuring fetal heart rate patterns. *AJOG.* 2006;195:735–738. [II-3]
73. Simpson KR, James DC. Efficacy of intrauterine resuscitation techniques in improving fetal oxygen status during labor. *Obstet Gynecol.* 2005;105:1362–1368. [II-2]
74. Huaman EJ, Hassoun R, Itahashi CM, et al. Results obtained with piracetam in foetal distress during labour. *J Int Med Res.* 1983;11:129–136. [RCT, n = 96. Peru L. [Fetal distress: Meconium-stained amniotic fluid and/or pathological fetal heart rate pattern. Piracetam (n = 48) vs. placebo (n = 48), intravenously 6 ampoules at once and 2 ampoules hourly]
75. Walker N. A case for conservatism in management of foetal distress. *BMJ.* 1959;2:1221–1226. [RCT, n = 350. Fetal distress: Meconium-stained liquor; fetal heart rate below 110/minute, above 160/minute, or irregular. Drawn envelop from drum for either operative delivery or expectant management]

Analgesia and anesthesia

Kyle Jespersen and Michele Mele

KEY POINTS
- In every hospital providing labor and delivery services, **anesthesia personnel must be available on a 24-hour basis,** with the ability to perform a cesarean delivery (CD) within 30 minutes from decision.
- **Intravenous (IV) pain relief is inferior to neuraxial analgesia,** minimally effective, and associated with several maternal and fetal/neonatal side effects.
- **Neuraxial analgesia provides the best pain relief in labor, and should be available to all laboring women upon request.**
- **Airway complications can occur during induction and emergence of general anesthesia as well as the postoperative period and constitute the most common cause of anesthesia related death.**
- In the absence of a medical condition associated with coagulopathy, it is not necessary to obtain a platelet count before neuraxial techniques. In general, women with platelet counts of ≥75,000/μL can safely receive neuraxial analgesia.
- As there is no benefit to obstetric outcome from delaying neuraxial analgesia until an arbitrary cervical dilation has been reached, **the decision of when to initiate neuraxial analgesia should be made individually with each woman.**
- Patients should be counseled regarding the benefits and risks of neuraxial analgesia in labor. These include the following:
  - **Neuraxial anesthesia is associated with much better pain relief** compared with any other intervention for pain relief, and with lower risk of umbilical cord pH < 7.20 compared with systemic opioids.
  - **Neuraxial analgesia is associated with an increased incidence of hypotension, pruritus, urinary retention, and maternal fever; increased need for oxytocin administration; increased duration of the second stage (by about 15 minutes); and increased risk of instrumental vaginal birth.**
  - Rare complications of neuraxial analgesia include postdural puncture headache (PDPH), respiratory depression from opioid use, epidural or spinal hematoma or abscess.
- Discontinuation of neuraxial analgesia in the second stage does not impact obstetric outcome.
- Use of **low doses of anesthetic medications, prophylactic prehydration,** and **phenylephrine or ephedrine** can **decrease** the incidence of **maternal hypotension and associated** nonreassuring fetal heart rate **(NRFHR).**
- Compared with the standard epidural approach, combined spinal epidural **(CSE)** has been shown to **produce a quicker** (by about 6 minutes) **onset of analgesia,** result in a **lower total dose of local anesthetic** over the course of the labor, achieve a **lower median visual analog pain** score earlier in labor, increase the incidence of **maternal satisfaction,** have a **lower incidence of incomplete block,** but is associated with an increased likelihood of maternal pruritus.
- **For CD, neuraxial anesthesia is the anesthetic technique of choice. Spinal (intrathecal) anesthesia has advantages over epidural anesthesia including quicker onset of surgical anesthesia, simplicity, lower total drug dose, and superior abdominal muscle relaxation.** Compared with epidural anesthesia, the spinal technique is associated with a similar failure rate, need for supplemental intraoperative analgesia, need for conversion to general anesthesia intraoperatively, maternal satisfaction, need for postoperative pain relief and neonatal intervention.
- **Hypotension** following spinal analgesia for CD can **be decreased by crystalloid or colloid administration, phenylephrine, ephedrine, and lower limb compression.**
- **General anesthesia for CD should be avoided if at all possible** as it is associated with a threefold risk of maternal death compared with neuraxial analgesia. Risks include inability to intubate or ventilate the patient at the induction of general anesthesia as well as airway complications at emergence from anesthesia. There are no evident advantages to general anesthesia in the absence of a contraindication to a neuraxial approach.

HISTORIC NOTES
Three months after the first successful public demonstration of the anesthetic properties of ether, on January 19, 1847, Dr. James Simpson Young of the University of Edinburgh used diethyl ether as anesthesia for childbirth to a woman with a deformed pelvis [1]. Before this time, pain during labor and childbirth were seen by both medical professionals and the lay community as a necessary and indeed inseparable part of pregnancy. By 1860 anesthesia for parturition had become common practice thanks to a majority of women demanding it be a part of their medical care. The practice of obstetric anesthesia has changed markedly since. Women in labor now receive analgesia, rather than anesthesia, with the goal of enabling maternal mobility during labor. Refined anesthetic techniques for women requiring CD have substantially decreased the number of maternal deaths directly related to anesthesia.

DEFINITIONS
Pain: an unpleasant sensory and emotional experience associated with actual or potential tissue damage

Analgesia (from the Greek: "no pain"): loss of the ability to feel pain without the loss of consciousness

Anesthesia (from the Greek: "no sensation"): an induced, temporary state of analgesia, paralysis, amnesia, and unconsciousness

GENERAL COMMENTS

In 2008, 60% of women in the United States chose to receive epidural or spinal anesthesia during labor [2]. **While not all laboring women desire the services of an anesthesiologist, maternal request is a sufficient medical indication for pain relief in labor** [3]. Hospitals providing labor and delivery services must have **anesthesia personnel available on a 24-hour basis**, with the ability to perform a CD within 30 minutes from decision [4]. Availability of licensed practitioners to administer anesthetics and support vital functions in emergencies is recommended [3,4].

PHYSIOLOGY OF LABOR PAIN

Labor is associated with two sources of pain: visceral pain at T10 through L1 from uterine contractions and cervical dilatation during the first stage of labor and somatic pain transmitted by the pudendal nerve at S2 through S4 from descent and consequent pressure of the fetal head on the pelvic floor, vagina, and perineum during the second stage of labor [5]. This pain is amenable to safe intervention as the anesthesiologist can interrupt the transmission of peripheral afferents from the cervix, lower uterine segment and perineum by use of neuraxial techniques that block spinal cord transmission of labor pain.

MATERNAL PHYSIOLOGIC CHANGES

Pregnancy is associated with **unique physiologic changes**. As a result of these changes, after the first trimester, parturients are at increased risk for aspiration of gastric contents, have decreased oxygen reserve, and are much more likely to be difficult to intubate than a nonpregnant woman (see also Chapter 3). Maternal mortality associated with general anesthesia is estimated at approximately 32/1,000,000 live births versus 1.9/1,000,000 live births for neuraxial analgesia [5].

Pregnant patients should be positioned with **left uterine displacement** when supine after 20 weeks of gestational age. Left uterine displacement prevents aortocaval compression, which can result in a marked decrease in venous return and a subsequent drop in cardiac output. The ability to compensate for aortocaval compression is compromised in the presence of neuraxial analgesia or anesthesia.

When considering anesthesia or analgesia, one must take into account that pregnant women are **more sensitive to sedative hypnotics, local anesthetics, and the inhaled anesthetic agents** than nonpregnant women. In addition the pregnant patient should be considered *two patients* and occasionally the needs of one must be prioritized over the other. Informed consent should be attempted in case of an emergency, and the patient's wishes for an unmedicated birth always respected. Successful initiation of breast-feeding is not affected by neuraxial analgesia.

NONPHARMACOLOGIC ANALGESIC TECHNIQUES

Increasingly, many pregnant women are seeking alternative approaches to labor pain relief such as water immersion, acupuncture and aromatherapy. While these techniques may not provide complete pain relief, they may diminish labor pain helping parturients delay or even avoid the use of pain relief medications if that is their goal.

Acupuncture and Acupressure

Acupuncture and acupressure are therapeutic techniques based on the concept that energy flows throughout the body and strategic placement of needles or pressure can restore its balance and provide pain relief. Theories on its mechanism of action suggest it stimulates the release of endorphins in the muscles, brain, and spinal cord.

Compared with no intervention or placebo, **acupuncture** for labor pain is associated with **less intense pain, increased satisfaction with pain relief, and reduced use of pharmacological analgesia,** in small trials. Compared with no intervention or placebo, *acupressure* has been associated with *less pain intensity,* in small trials [6]. Therefore, acupuncture and acupressure may have a role with reducing pain, increasing satisfaction with pain management and reduced use of pharmacological management.

Water Immersion

Water immersion is a form of hydrotherapy in which water is used to relieve pain during labor. A Cochrane review suggests that immersion during the first stage of labor was associated with a **reduction in the use of neuraxial anesthesia** compared with controls [7]. There were no difference in perineal trauma, need for assisted vaginal deliveries or cesarean deliveries. There is no evidence that immersion improves perinatal outcome, however, there are case reports of rare but serious adverse effects in the newborn including respiratory distress when practiced during the second stage of labor. Given these rare but serious risks to the newborn, it is the opinion of The American College of Obstetricians and Gynecologists and the American Academy of Pediatrics that the practice of immersion in the second stage of labor (underwater delivery) should be avoided in routine obstetrical care [8]. See also Chapters 7 and 8.

Biofeedback

Biofeedback is a therapy that alloys women to gain control over their body's physiologic response to pain by controlling heart rate, blood pressure and muscle tension. Despite some positive results shown in some very small trials, there is insufficient evidence that biofeedback is effective for the management of pain during labor [9].

Aromatherapy

Aromatherapy is the use of plant derived aromatic essential oils to promote the sense of physical and psychological well-being. The limited evidence available does not show benefit, or harm, from aromatherapy for labor pain relief compared with no aromatherapy [10].

Hypnosis

Hypnotherapy is the use of hypnosis to deeply relax the body through focused concentration. For childbirth hypnosis is often used to focus attention on feelings of comfort or numbness as well as to enhance women's feelings of relaxation and sense of safety. In a review of six studies (1032 women) there was no significant difference between women receiving hypnosis versus controls in the use of pharmacologic pain relief [11].

Massage

There is insufficient evidence to assess the effect of massage therapy on labor pain. However a meta-analysis involving 326 women found that women who used massage felt **less pain** when compared with women given usual care during first stage of labor [12].

Relaxation

A review of eleven randomized controlled trials, with data reported on 1374 women, found that **relaxation techniques and yoga may help manage labor pain** [13].

Transcutaneous Nerve Stimulation

Transcutaneous electrical nerve stimulation (TENS) units emit low voltage electrical impulses and may be used to stimulate acupressure points. A systemic review of nine trials including more than 1000 women concluded that TENS did not reduce labor pain and did not reduce the use of additional analgesic agents [14].

SYSTEMIC ANALGESIA
Parenteral Opioids

Opioids are the most widely used of the systemic medications for labor analgesia. Opioids are low cost, easy to use, and do not require specialized personnel or equipment to be delivered safely. There are a variety of opioid agonist–antagonists in clinical use such as buprenorphine (Buprenex), butorphanol (Stadol), or nalbuphine (Nubain), or pure opioid agonists such as meperidine, fentanyl, morphine, hydromorphone, or their derivatives. Characteristics of some of these drugs are shown in Table 11.1. All provide moderate pain relief with respect to one another. Opioids may be delivered intramuscularly (IM) or IV. IM administration is easy for the healthcare provider, but painful for the patient. IV administration does require an IV line be placed, but allows faster onset of analgesia, predictable magnitude of peak plasma concentration, and titrating of dose to effect. IV opioids may be delivered as intermittent boluses or via patient-controlled analgesia (PCA) technology.

Efficacy

These drugs are similarly efficacious in relief of maternal labor pain. In one small study, **compared with placebo, meperidine** (Demerol, pethidine) **100 mg IM in early labor is associated with a very modest** (17 mm) **reduction in** the visual analog scale (VAS) **pain score at 30 minutes** [15,16]. Request for epidural analgesia is delayed to 232 minutes compared with 75 minutes for parturients receiving placebo, with no further requests for analgesia in 32% versus 4% of women receiving meperidine or placebo, respectively [16].

There is not enough evidence to definitively evaluate the comparative efficacy of the various systemic opioids used to provide labor analgesia. There are problems with the methodological quality of some trials, and lack of consistency in the way various outcomes are reported. Nonetheless, using a variety of measures, including pain relief, maternal satisfaction with analgesia, interval to delivery, and obstetric outcome, there is no evidence of significant differences between **meperidine, tramadol** (Ultram, Meptazinol), or **pentazocine** (Talwin) [15].

Maternal Safety

There is not enough evidence to definitively evaluate the comparative safety of the various systemic opioids used to provide labor analgesia. Maternal side effects are largely dose dependent rather than drug dependent. Across all opioids there exists the potential for maternal nausea, histamine release and pruritus, delayed gastric emptying, constipation, urinary retention, dysphoria, drowsiness, hypoventilation and hypotension. There is weak evidence of more frequent adverse effects such as maternal nausea, vomiting, and drowsiness with meptazinol compared with meperidine. However, both **tramadol and pentazocine** have fewer maternal side effects when compared with meperidine [15], making these two agents the ones with the best evidence of **both moderate efficacy and lowest incidence of side effects among the opioid analgesic agents.** Respiratory and neurobehavioral depression can be reversed with the use of the pure opioid antagonist naloxone. Meperidine, the first synthetic opioid to be used for labor analgesia, is metabolized to normeperidine in the liver, which can cause respiratory depression and convulsions, neither of which can be reversed by naloxone.

Fetal Safety

IV opioids cross the placenta owing to their low molecular weight and lipid soluability and as a result can affect the neonate. When compared with neuraxial analgesia, IV opioids are associated with **increased incidence of NRFHR, lower fetal base excess, and decreased fetal respirations and tone at birth.** Drugs with active metabolites, such as meperidine (active metabolite normeperidine), are associated with more prolonged neonatal sedation. Agonist/antagonists such as nalbuphine can result in both neonatal cardiac and respiratory depression although there is no data that demonstrates adverse outcomes. Naloxone is a pure opioid antagonist and is the drug of choice in treatment of neonatal respiratory and neurobehavioral depression secondary to opioid agonist agents. Repeated doses might be necessary, but excess use can be associated with neonatal withdrawal seizures. **Compared with neuraxial analgesic techniques, systemic medications are much less effective at decreasing visual analog pain scores** (see Efficacy and Advantages in the section "Epidural Analgesia").

Table 11.1 IV or IM Opioid Agents for Maternal Pain Relief in Labor

Agent	Usual Dose (mg)	Frequency (Every Hour)	Onset (Minutes)	Neonatal Half-Life (Hours)
Tramadol	50–100 mg	4		
Pentazocine	30 mg IV or IM	3–4		
Meperidine	25–50 IV	1–2	5	13–22
	50–100 IM	2–4	30–45	>60
Fentanyl	50–100 μg IV	1	1	5
Nalbuphine	10 IV or IM	3	2–3 (IV)	4
			15 (IM)	
Butorphanol	1–2 IV or IM	4	1–2 (IV)	Not known
			10–30 (IM)	
Morphine	2–5 IV	4	5 (IV)	7
	10 IM		30–40 (IM)	

Source: Adapted from American College of Obstetricians and Gynecologists, *ACOG Practice Bulletin No. 36. Obstetric Analgesia and Anesthesia*, Washington, DC, American College of Obstetricians and Gynecologists, 2002.
Abbreviations: IV, intravenous; IM, intramuscular.

PERIPHERAL NERVE BLOCKS
Paracervical Block
During the first stage of labor, pain from cervical dilation (but not uterine contractions) can be blocked by a **paracervical block.** There are **no trials** to assess the effectiveness of paracervical block in labor. Risks include maternal local anesthetic toxicity from IV injection, fetal local anesthetic toxicity from inadvertent fetal injection, and a strong association with fetal bradycardia.

Pudendal Block
During the second stage of labor, perineal pain can be blocked with a **pudendal block.** There are *no trials* to assess the effectiveness of pudendal block in labor. There is a small risk of maternal local anesthetic toxicity in the event of accidental intravascular injection.

Lumbo-Sacral Sterile Water Injection
For patients that desire nonpharmacologic analgesic techniques, back pain during the first stage of labor can be reduced with lumbo-sacral sterile water injection. In a randomized controlled trial studying 128 term parturients, women receiving sterile water injection versus acupuncture reported greater pain relief and higher degrees of relaxation during labor [17]. In another study, women with severe lower back pain, four **injections of sterile water,** either 0.1 mL intracutaneously or 0.5 mL subcutaneously **in the lumbar–sacral region,** has been shown to be effective in reducing severe back pain [18].

NEURAXIAL (REGIONAL) LABOR ANALGESIA (EPIDURAL, SPINAL, OR CSE)
Background
Epidural, spinal, and combined spinal–epidural analgesia techniques are the most effective methods of providing pain relief to the laboring parturient. A large meta-analysis looking at over 300 studies comparing neuraxial analgesic techniques to a variety of other techniques including systemic opioids, inhaled anesthetics, and nonpharmacologic concluded that neuraxial techniques are superior to all other methods in terms of parturient pain relief [19]. In a jointly published opinion, both the American College of Obstetricians and Gynecologists and the American Society of Anesthesiologists (ASA) state: "in the absence of a medical contraindication, maternal request is a sufficient medical indication for pain relief during labor" [20]. As labor results in severe pain for many women, neuraxial anesthesia, when available, should be offered to all women in labor, assuming no medical contraindication.

Overview of Techniques
Neuraxial labor analgesia is also commonly called regional analgesia. It can be provided via the epidural space, the intrathecal (spinal) space, or both.

Medications injected into the epidural space have a relatively slow analgesic onset of 8–15 minutes. Block height is determined by the volume of medication injected into the epidural space. Injecting low concentration local anesthetic produces analgesia and injecting high-concentration local anesthetic produces anesthesia.

By contrast, medication injected into the intrathecal space has a quick onset of 2–5 minutes. Block height is determined primarily by the baricity (density relative to cerebrospinal fluid [CSF]) of the injectate and, to some extent the total volume of drug.

Epidural Analgesia
Technique
The epidural space (Figure 11.1) is located using a loss of resistance (to air or saline) technique [21]. A small catheter is placed into the epidural space through which local anesthetics and opioids can be intermittently injected (bolus) or given as a continuous infusion.

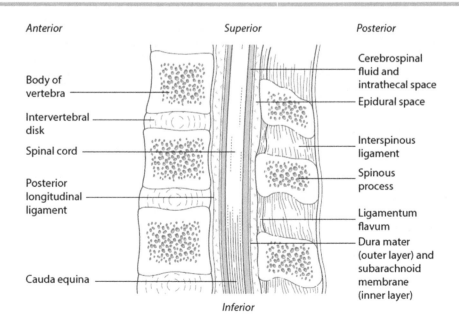

Figure 11.1 The epidural space. (From Macintyre PE and Schug SA, *Acute Pain Management: A Practical Guide*, Fourth Edition, Boca Raton, FL: CRC Press, 2014. With permission.)

The most common local anesthetic choices include low-concentration, long-acting amides such as bupivacaine and ropivicaine in combination with a lipid soluble opioid such as fentanyl and sufentanil. The addition of opioids to local anesthetics produces an additive effect that results in a lower concentration of local anesthetic being required to produce adequate labor analgesia. A lower concentration of local anesthetic increases maternal mobility and decreases the potential for maternal systemic toxicity. There is insufficient evidence comparing concentrations, type of anesthetic used, and several other technical aspects of epidural anesthesia in labor to recommend one specific drug combination [22,23].

The epidural infusion rate can be controlled either by the anesthesiologist or by the patient. **Patient-controlled epidural analgesia** (PCEA) typically employs a background infusion of local anesthetic and opioid together with enabling the parturient to augment the infusion with a bolus dose every 10–15 minutes. This technique can also be used with a spinal catheter with appropriately reduced doses.

Indications
The primary indication for neuraxial analgesia is maternal request during labor [5]. However there are numerous maternal conditions that make neuraxial anesthesia the prudent choice. Examples of such conditions include anticipated difficult intubation, history of malignant hyperthermia, high risk for CD, the presence of a comorbidity that would benefit from the reduced catecholamine levels that result from adequate labor analgesia (e.g., selected respiratory or cardiac disease) and prophylaxis against autonomic hyperreflexia in the woman with a high spinal cord lesion. Functioning epidural catheters can also be used to provide anesthesia for instrumented delivery and extraction of a retained placenta.

In some cases, an epidural catheter can be intentionally inserted into the intrathecal space to provide continuous spinal analgesia. However, the resulting PDPH incidence may be high. Nonetheless, this risk may be acceptable in certain situations such as the presence of certain maternal comorbidities (typically cardiac), the morbidly obese parturient with an airway that appears extremely difficult or impossible to intubate, or following an inadvertent dural puncture during a difficult epidural placement.

Efficacy and Advantages
Compared with nonpharmacologic techniques or to IV opioids, epidural analgesia provides **significantly better pain relief** [24]. In >85% of cases, the pain relief is optimal. **As labor results in severe pain for many women, and neuraxial analgesia is the most effective intervention to decrease or eliminate this pain, neuraxial analgesia should be offered, when available, to all women in labor (assuming no medical contraindication).**

Compared with systemic opioids, **epidural anesthesia is associated with superior pain relief and lower risk of umbilical cord pH <7.20.** There is no evidence of a significant difference in the risk of CD (relative risk [RR] 1.10, 95% confidence interval [CI] 0.97–1.25 27 trials, 8417 women) [24]. In addition there is no evidence of a significant difference in the risk of long-term backache, low neonatal Apgar scores at 5 minutes, and other maternal and neonatal outcomes. No studies reported on rare but potentially serious adverse effects of epidural analgesia [15]. Neuraxial analgesia is the least depressant method of analgesia for the fetus/neonate.

There is no reason to delay epidural placement until an arbitrary cervical dilation has been reached. Data suggest that neuraxial analgesia can be offered as early as 2 cm or less without adversely affecting labor outcome or incidence of CD. Epidural placement at ≤2–5 cm is associated with similar maternal (instrumental delivery, CD, etc.) and neonatal outcomes compared with epidural placement at ≥3–5 cm in women in spontaneous labor or receiving oxytocin [25–29]. Therefore, **the decision of when to place epidural analgesia should be made individually with each woman** [5].

PCEA gives the patient control over her analgesia. Patients receive less local anesthetic overall (and therefore have less motor blockade) and receive fewer manual boluses from the anesthesiologist ("top offs") [22,30]. As patient satisfaction is high with epidural analgesia, PCEA is not associated with additional improvement in maternal satisfaction.

There is insufficient evidence to support the hypothesis that discontinuing epidural analgesia late in labor (e.g., at the beginning of the second stage) reduces the rate of instrumental delivery. There is evidence that it increases the rate of inadequate pain relief in the second stage of labor [31].

Safety, Disadvantages, and Complications
Compared with systemic analgesia, epidural analgesia is associated with an increased need for oxytocin administration, increased duration of the second stage by an average of 15 minutes, **increased risk of operative vaginal birth (forceps or vacuum-assist), and increased risk of mild maternal fever, hypotension, and urinary retention.** (RR 1.42, 95% CI 1.28–1.57) [24]. A recent noninferiority trial assessed the effects of routine epidural analgesia during labor versus epidural upon maternal request suggests that routine epidural analgesia was associated with a statistically significant increase the rate of operative deliveries (difference 8.1%, 95% CI −0.01 to 16.3) [32].

The etiology of the occasional **increase in maternal temperature** associated with epidural use is uncertain. This effect can lead to increased maternal and neonatal antibiotic treatments, as well as neonatal sepsis evaluations, but with no difference in the corresponding rate of neonatal infection or sepsis [33]. In centers with structured protocols for neonatal sepsis workups, there are no increases in the incidence of neonatal sepsis workups in babies born to mothers with epidural analgesia.

The incidence of maternal **hypotension** following neuraxial analgesia during labor is approximately 14%. Hypotension is associated with an increased incidence of NRFHT that **rarely (1%–2%) necessitates** CD. Left uterine displacement should be maintained whenever possible as it will increase maternal preload and increase uterine perfusion. Measures such as fluid preloading and concurrent administration of phenylephrine or ephedrine can mitigate or prevent maternal hypotension.

Although the risk of long-term **backache** in women who utilize epidural analgesia is similar to controls (IM meperidine), it is quite common for a woman to experience soreness or tenderness at the site of epidural insertion for 2–3 days [34].

Disadvantages of epidural analgesia include a slower onset compared with intrathecal (spinal) injection, incomplete blockade of pain (in about 10%–15% of patients), and inadvertent intrathecal or intravascular catheter placement. While the PCEA gives the patient more control and requires less intervention from anesthesiologists, this can lead to underdosing and therefore inadequate analgesia: for example, if the patient does not self-administer a bolus (if she is asleep), or if there is a pump malfunction.

Other complications include a 1%–2% chance of **PDPH** following accidental lumbar puncture, and rarely, epidural **hematoma, respiratory arrest** due to the unrecognized injection of an epidural dose of opioid into the intrathecal space, systemic local anesthetic toxicity due to unrecognized IV injection, or total spinal anesthesia from an unrecognized intrathecal injection of a dose of local anesthetic meant for the epidural space. See sections "Spinal Analgesia" and "Anesthetic Emergencies" for further details on these complications and strategies for their prevention and treatment. **Women should be counseled about these risks before labor** [33].

Interventions to Avoid Some Disadvantages and Complications of Epidural Analgesia
Preloading with IV fluids to prevent hypotension: Preloading with IV fluids (500–1000 mL, or weight-based formula 10–20 mL/kg) prior to traditional high-dose local anesthetic blocks may have some beneficial fetal and maternal effects in healthy women [35]. Using **low concentration** analgesic solutions for epidural techniques, preloading with IV fluids is associated with **no significant difference in maternal hypotension**, although only a very large effect was excluded. There is, however, a **trend toward less frequent FHR** abnormalities [35], therefore some fluid preloading may be beneficial.

Prophylactic ephedrine to prevent NRFHR: Compared with no ephedrine, ephedrine 10 mg IV bolus, followed by a 20 mg continuous infusion over 60 minutes, started in the first minutes after the epidural test dose, significantly **decreases the incidence of NRFHT** from 15% to 3% [36]. This evidence though is insufficient to make a recommendation.

Spinal Analgesia
Technique
Using a small-bore spinal needle (typically a pencil point design that minimizes trauma to the dura thereby reducing the incidence of PDPH), a dural puncture is made and proper location confirmed by CSF aspiration (Figure 11.1). A single injection of an analgesic dose of an opioid such as fentanyl, or sufentanil, with or without a local anesthetic such as bupivacaine or ropivacaine, is administered.

Indications
Indications for single injection spinals include advanced labor where delivery is imminent, forceps deliveries in women without epidurals, and for patients with retained placentas.

Advantages
Advantages for single injection spinals include ease and speed of onset, completeness of block, and lower incidence of PDPH compared with epidural analgesia.

Disadvantages and complications
Disadvantages for single injection spinals are inability to redose.

Postdural puncture headache. PDPH occurs with a frequency of approximately 1%–2% after either spinal or CSE analgesia when administered using a small-gauge pencil-point needle. PDPH is thought to be caused by leak of CSF through the punctured dura. The leak of CSF and subsequent decreased spinal fluid pressure leads to downward traction or stretch on the meninges with resulting symptoms. PDPH is characterized by a positional frontal-occipital headache that is exacerbated by the upright position (gravity worsening stretch on the meninges), with improvement in symptoms when the patient is supine. Diplopia, tinnitus, nausea, and vomiting caused by stretch on the cranial nerves are also common symptoms. Although **pencil-point design spinal needles have significantly reduced the incidence of PDPH following spinal analgesia,** there are no proven interventions to prevent PDPH following inadvertent dural puncture with an epidural needle. Conservative early interventions include **analgesics, supine positioning, caffeine, and hydration.** In about 1/3 of cases, the headache persists and is severe enough to require an epidural blood patch procedure. An epidural **blood patch** is performed by injecting 10–25 mL of autologous blood into the patient's epidural space at the level of the dural puncture using meticulous sterile technique. If the level of the dural puncture is unknown, a more caudad interspace should be chosen. After the procedure, the patient should rest in the supine position for 1–2 hours. Resolution of symptoms with blood patch occurs in 70%–85% of women. Expected side effects following epidural blood patch include backache and leg pain [37].

Respiratory depression or arrest. Respiratory depression or arrest due to intrathecal opioids occurs rarely (1 in 5,000–10,000 patients). Naloxone reverses this complication and should be readily available, along with airway management equipment when administering labor analgesia.

Hematoma. Hematoma after epidural or spinal analgesia is an extremely rare complication of neuraxial anesthesia (1/150,000–250,000). Symptoms include bilateral leg weakness, urinary incontinence and back pain. Prolonged motor paralysis without regression of block should raise suspicion. If suspected the patient should undergo prompt definitive imaging (MRI) of her neuraxis, followed by surgical decompression after diagnosis. Surgical decompression within 6 hours following the onset of symptoms often prevents permanent neurologic injury. The risk of persistent neurologic injury from epidural is about 1/240,000 [21].

Combined Spinal Epidural
Technique
The epidural space is identified with loss of resistance technique (Figure 11.1). A spinal needle is then introduced into the intrathecal space. An intrathecal dose of local anesthetic and opioid is injected through the spinal needle, which is then removed, leaving the epidural needle in place. An epidural catheter is inserted and an epidural local anesthetic and opioid infusion is started. The intrathecal dose generally lasts about 2 hours, after which the epidural catheter will provide continuous analgesia.

Indications
A CSE technique provides the benefit of immediate onset of spinal analgesia coupled with the indefinite duration of an epidural catheter technique. The CSE technique is particularly useful for women in advanced labor requesting pain relief. There are data that associate CSE with an increased rate of cervical dilatation and shorter length of labor compared with both IV opioid and epidural analgesia [38–40]. Indications for a CSE are the same as those for both epidural and spinal techniques.

Advantages
Both CSE and epidural techniques provide effective pain relief in labor. The type of opioid and concentration of local anesthetic used in the CSE or epidural technique impact maternal mobilization and other outcomes more than the technique itself [41]. **There appears to be little basis for offering CSE over epidurals in labor, with no difference in overall maternal satisfaction despite a slightly faster onset (about 6 minutes) with CSE, and less pruritus with epidurals.** There is some evidence that CSE compared with an epidural is associated with a faster

rate of cervical dilatation in nulliparous women less than 5 cm [39], and women close to imminent birth may benefit from the speed of onset a CSE offers. There is no difference in ability to mobilize, obstetric outcome, or neonatal outcome [41]. A recent review revealed however there is a statistically significant difference in risk of instrumental delivery between CSE and epidural analgesia with CSE having decreased rates of instrumentation (RR 0.81; 95% CI 0.67–0.97) [41].

Disadvantages
Disadvantages of CSE are similar to epidural and spinal techniques. Although data is limited, no differences are reported between IV preloading and no preloading to prevent hypotension [35]. Women who receive intrathecal opioids experience **more pruritus** than with a standard epidural [41]. However, pruritus is very common after both spinal and epidural opioids and results from µ-opioid receptor stimulation in the brainstem. Naloxone or nalbuphine are effective interventions. Diphenhydramine and other antihistamines are not effective in treating opioid-induced pruritus because opioids administered via the intrathecal or epidural route do not cause histamine release. **The significantly higher incidence of urinary retention, instrumental deliveries and rescue analgesia interventions with traditional high concentration epidurals would favor the use of low-dose epidurals** [41]. It is not possible to draw any meaningful conclusions as to possible differences between CSE and epidural in producing rare complications such as nerve injury and meningitis.

Contraindications to Regional Anesthesia
Coagulopathy
A routine platelet count is not necessary before administering neuraxial analgesia in the healthy parturient. Indications for platelet count may include hypertensive disorders of pregnancy, idiopathic thrombocytopenia purpura (ITP), abruption and disorders of coagulation. In the absence of DIC, a platelet count of ≥100,000/mL is considered safe. Several studies have also confirmed that platelets levels of 50,000–99,000/mL are not associated with higher risk of complications [3]. Women receiving low-dose aspirin are not at increased risk for complications from neuraxial blocks. Women receiving prophylactic unfractionated heparin, regardless of dosing schedule, should have the medication held for at least 4 hours, ideally 6 hours, before placing a neuraxial block or removing an epidural catheter. Women receiving therapeutic unfractionated heparin are candidates for regional analgesia if the activated partial thromboplastin time (PTT) is normal. If the PTT is elevated, protamine may be used to reverse the heparin effect. Women receiving low–molecular weight heparin are not candidates for regional analgesia for 12–24 hours from last dose, given a higher rate of epidural hematoma with placement during this period. Therefore, consideration should be given to converting women who require anticoagulation from low molecular to unfractionated heparin as they approach term.

The coagulation status of parturients with medical conditions associated with coagulopathy such as the HELLP (hemolysis, elevated liver enzyme levels, and low platelet levels) syndrome should be thoroughly evaluated before initiating a neuraxial block. Patients with platelets less than 75,000/µL should be examined for stigmata of coagulopathy (easy bruising, bleeding from the IV site, and so on) before instrumentation. A prothrombin time, a partial thrombin time, and a platelet count should all be reviewed before proceeding. A fibrinogen level and a d-dimer level are useful to assess the presence of DIC if suspected. A bleeding time is not indicated. Patients with known platelet dysfunction including those on antiplatelet medication (e.g., clopidogrel) should not receive neuraxial analgesia. Aspirin therapy is considered an acceptable risk [42].

Infection
    Systemic. Patients with suspected meningitis (bacterial or viral), sepsis, or viremia should not receive neuraxial blockade. Patients with suspected chorioamnionitis can receive neuraxial analgesia/anesthesia following the administration of appropriate IV antibiotics. Chronic herpes simplex virus (HSV) outbreak is not a contraindication to neuraxial techniques. However a primary outbreak places the parturient at risk for herpetic viremia and the theoretical risk for central nervous system (CNS) infection and should be weighed against the risk of alternative methods of analgesia. Human immunodeficiency virus (HIV)/acquired immunodeficiency syndrome (AIDS) is not a contraindication to spinal or epidural anesthesia, or epidural blood patch.
    Localized. Patients with localized skin or soft tissue infections should not be instrumented at those sites.

ANESTHESIA AND MATERNAL COMORBIDITIES
Hypertensive Disorders
Advantages of Neuraxial Analgesia
Pregnant women with hypertension may benefit from neuraxial analgesia, as it may improve uterine perfusion through several pathways (localized neuraxial vasodilatory effect, reduced catecholamine release). **Neuraxial analgesia is the analgesia of choice in hypertensive pregnant women as it allows clinicians to avoid the possibility of difficult intubation and the severe hypertension that accompanies endotracheal intubation.**

Disadvantages
Patients with gestational hypertension, preeclampsia, and eclampsia are at increased risk for hemodynamic instability during both labor and surgical anesthesia. Neuraxial techniques can be used safely with increased vigilance for maternal hypotension. In one focused review, marked hypotension after spinal in women with preeclampsia did not occur, lending support to the safety of spinal anesthesia in these women [43].

Women with preeclampsia may have thrombocytopenia, which increases the risk of neuraxial hematoma formation. Most anesthesia providers consider a platelet count above 75,000/mm^3 to be adequate for the administration of neuraxial anesthesia.

Cautions
Caution must be taken in fluid management in this patient population as there is altered vascular leaking, decreased oncotic pressure, and a higher incidence of pulmonary edema. Also, there can be an exaggerated hypertensive response to ephedrine and phenylephrine. The prevention, rather than treatment, of hypotension has been associated with better outcomes for the fetus. Women with severe preeclampsia who must undergo general anesthesia are at risk for an exaggerated hypertensive response to intubation and often benefit from pretreatment with an antihypertensive such as labetalol immediately prior to induction. Treatment with magnesium sulfate for preeclampsia/eclampsia can potentiate neuromuscular blockade in patients receiving general anesthesia, so care must be taken when using nondepolarizing muscle relaxants.

Maternal Cardiac Disease

Heart disease in the parturient is the leading cause of maternal mortality outside of obstetric complications. Understandably, the risk increases with severity of maternal disease. The normal changes in maternal cardiac physiology resulting from pregnancy can either unmask subclinical or worsen clinical cardiac disease. Every effort should be made to care for these patients in facilities equipped to provide the multidisciplinary approach that is required to ensure the best possible outcome for mother and neonate. Goals of anesthetic management for parturients with heart disease are: (1) maintain a normal heart rate, sinus rhythm, and adequate SVR; (2) maintenance of intravascular volume and venous return; (3) avoidance of aortocaval compression; and (4) avoidance of myocardial depression during general anesthesia.

Valvular Heart Disease
Patients with acquired valvular disease (rheumatic fever, mitral valve prolapse, artificial valves, and endocarditis) are at increased risk for arrhythmias, pulmonary edema, and cardiac ischemia from the increased heart rate, cardiac output, metabolic demand, and decreased oxygen reserve associated with pregnancy and the pain of labor. Patients with arrhythmias or artificial valves may also be on heparin or low–molecular weight heparin.

Advantages of neuraxial analgesia. Epidurals and CSE block the pain and stress of contractions therefore reducing tachycardia and increased cardiac output. Ablation of the bearing down reflex can be advantageous in patients with aortic or mitral regurgitation.

Disadvantages. Hypotension is the largest disadvantage with neuraxial analgesia; even transient hypotension can lead to coronary hypoperfusion, ischemia, arrhythmias, or arrest. This is especially dangerous in patients with moderate to severe aortic stenosis. However, parturients with aortic stenosis have safely undergone both neuraxial labor analgesia and anesthesia for CD. Meticulous anesthetic technique and allowing adequate time to slowly administer the requisite medication is the key to safe provision of neuraxial anesthesia in these patients. Inadvertent IV injection of local anesthetics is also a significant risk in patients with underlying arrhythmias due to impairment of cardiac automaticity and conduction (especially, with bupivacaine).

Congenital Heart Disease
Women with congenital heart disease (e.g., tetralogy of Fallot, hypoplastic left ventricle, transposition of the great vessels, and septal defects) are now surviving to childbearing years. Depending on the adequacy of their surgical repair, pregnancy may or may not severely impact these patients with underlying cyanotic heart disease. The increased cardiac output, oxygen consumption, changes in systemic and pulmonary resistance, and aortocaval compression can exacerbate preexisting right to left shunts increasing the risk of maternal cyanosis and death.

Advantages of epidural analgesia. Although the hypotension of large-dose spinal anesthesia can be associated with risk of shunting and cyanosis, slowly administered epidural, low-dose spinal, or continuous spinal analgesia are advantageous to these patients by reducing catecholamine levels and preventing maternal expulsive reflexes. Additionally, if an instrumented delivery or CD is required, a surgical anesthetic level can be slowly produced, avoiding the risks of general anesthesia in these patients.

Disadvantages. The largest disadvantage of neuraxial analgesia is the risk of hypotension. Hemodynamic management of these patients should be aggressive and tailored to the underlying cardiac defect.

Previous Lumbar Surgery

Previous lumbar surgery (e.g., discectomy, placement of Harrington rods) is not a contraindication for lumbar epidural or spinal analgesia or anesthesia. One case series found that successful block can be achieved, although at a lower rate (55%) than in the control population. There were no cases of spine infection, low back pain, or headaches [44].

Maternal Obesity

The incidence of maternal obesity has been rapidly increasing worldwide. Obese parturients have higher rates of hypertension, diabetes, preeclampsia, chorioamnionitis and cesarean section compared with normal weight women. Obese patients are also more at risk for hypoventilation and apnea after administration of opioids, complicating postpartum and postoperative pain control. Relative immobility also increases the risk of thromboembolic events [45]. Most importantly, obesity increases the risk for death during pregnancy. The report of *Confidential Enquiries into Maternal Deaths in the United Kingdom* for the 2006–2008 triennium showed that 49% of maternal deaths were overweight or obese [46]. The risks of low Apgar scores, neonatal intensive care unit admission, fetal death, and perinatal death are increased [47]. Respiratory, gastrointestinal, and anatomical changes of pregnancy significantly increase the **risk of a failed intubation and aspiration, which is as high as 15%–33% in obese pregnant women.** Venous access can be difficult increasing the need for central venous access. Bony landmarks and increased adipose and soft tissue can complicate placement of neuraxial analgesia and anesthesia with initial **epidural failure as high as 42%**. Despite this increase in technical difficulty, neuraxial anesthesia is the technique of choice in the obese parturient.

ANESTHESIA FOR CESAREAN DELIVERY

Current guidelines recommend a fasting period for solids of 6–8 hours prior to scheduled CD. Parturients without complications may drink clear liquids for up to 2 hours before induction of anesthesia for planned CD [3].

Epidural

Epidural anesthesia can be used for CD, and for most urgent or emergent deliveries if a functioning catheter is in place. Patients with existing labor epidurals can have their block extended to an adequate level for surgery using a large volume of high-concentration local anesthetic solution containing opioids and epinephrine (which is thought to produce analgesia via α2 receptors in the spinal cord).

Advantages
There are numerous advantages to using epidural anesthesia for CD, including avoiding instrumentation of the maternal airway, the ability to redose the epidural in the event of a delayed or prolonged surgery, the ability to administer long-acting epidural opioids to augment postoperative pain control and the avoidance of a dural puncture. Opioids administered via neuraxial approach are associated with a 35%–55% incidence of maternal pruritus severe enough to require treatment [48]. An additional advantage is that the patient is awake and can experience the birth. The epidural catheter should be

removed after 24 hours to reduce urinary retention, pruritus, and infection risks.

Disadvantages
Disadvantages of epidural for CD include longer onset time for surgical block compared with spinal anesthesia and the possibility of incomplete or patchy block, making epidural anesthesia a less attractive option than spinal anesthesia in emergent situations (when an epidural catheter is not already in place). The higher doses of local anesthetics used in epidural blocks (compared with spinal) increase the risk of maternal systemic toxicity.

Spinal
Spinal anesthesia can be used for both planned cesarean deliveries and in most emergencies. Intrathecal opioids can be added to augment postoperative pain control.

Advantages
Spinal anesthesia is a reliable form of anesthesia that is technically easier to perform and produces adequate anesthesia significantly faster than epidural anesthesia [49]. Other advantages are its simplicity, lower drug doses, and superior abdominal muscle relaxation. **Compared with epidural, spinal technique is associated with similar failure rate, need for additional intraoperative analgesia, need for conversion to general anesthesia intraoperatively, maternal satisfaction, need for postoperative pain relief, and neonatal intervention** [49]. Compared with epidural, spinal anesthesia for cesarean section is associated with reduced time, by about 8 minutes, from start of the anesthetic to start of the operation.

Compared with general anesthesia, women with neuraxial anesthesia have less intraoperative blood loss but significantly more nausea. In a review of randomized clinical trails, no differences in umbilical cord arterial blood pH were found among general and neuraxial anesthetic techniques [50].

Disadvantages
Hypotension, possibly profound, is increased in incidence 23% with spinal versus epidural anesthesia [49]. A number of strategies can be used to mitigate hypotension. No intervention reliably prevents hypotension due to spinal anesthesia for CD, but five interventions have been found to reduce the incidence of hypotension: (1) **crystalloid preload,** (2) **preemptive colloid administration,** (3) **ephedrine,** (4) **phenylephrine,** and (5) **lower limb compression** [35,51,52]. No differences were detected for different doses, rates or methods of administering colloids or crystalloids. High doses of ephedrine may increase the incidence of hypertension and tachycardia and is associated with fetal acidosis of uncertain clinical significance. Patients who receive intrathecal bupivacaine with prophylactic IV phenylephrine infusion have less hypotension than those without phenylephrine [51]. Newer studies have shown that **phenylephrine** is as safe as ephedrine; in fact, fetal pH is higher and the incidence of maternal nausea is lower with phenylephrine [53]. Given the efficacy of phenylephrine and better umbilical cord pH many anesthesia providers now use phenylephrine as a first line agent for the treatment and prevention of maternal hypotension. Different methods of compression appeared to vary in their effectiveness. In summary, **interventions such as crystalloids, colloids, ephedrine, phenylephrine, or lower-leg compression can reduce the incidence of hypotension,** but none have been shown to eliminate maternal hypotension during spinal anesthesia for CD.

Limited duration is another disadvantage of spinal anesthesia. CSEs and spinal catheters combine the advantages of the rapid onset of spinal anesthesia with the ability to redose in the case of prolonged surgical time.

The rate of **PDPH** after spinal anesthesia ranges between 1.5% and 11.2%. To reduce this risk, this technique should be performed using a small-gauge (24 g or smaller), pencil point spinal needle when possible.

In summary, both spinal and epidural techniques are shown to provide effective anesthesia for cesarean section. Both techniques are associated with moderate degrees of maternal satisfaction. Spinal anesthesia has a shorter onset time, but treatment for hypotension is more likely if spinal anesthesia is used. Because of its safety and effectiveness, **spinal anesthesia has evolved as the regional technique of choice for CD** due in particular to rapidity of anesthetic onset, quality of anesthesia, and ease of performance of block.

General Anesthesia
While neuraxial techniques are clearly the preferred anesthetic for CD, general anesthesia is indicated in the case of failed regional anesthesia, an obstetric emergency preventing placement of a neuraxial technique, a contraindication for regional anesthesia, or objection by the patient to regional anesthesia.

Precautions
If a general anesthetic is chosen, patients must receive aspiration prophylaxis that may include a nonparticulate oral antacid within 30 minutes of surgery and/or metoclopramide. Time permitting, an H2 blocker can be given 30–50 minutes before induction of anesthesia, to confer additional protection. Airway protection with **endotracheal intubation** is mandatory.

There is insufficient evidence to assess prevention of aspiration during general anesthesia. When compared with no treatment or placebo, there is a significant reduction in the risk of intragastric pH < 2.5 with antacids, H2 antagonists, and proton pump antagonists [54]. H_2 antagonists are associated with a reduced risk of intragastric pH < 2.5 at intubation when compared with proton pump antagonists, but compared with antacids the findings were unclear. The combined use of antacids plus H2 antagonists is associated with a significant reduction in the risk of intragastric pH < 2.5 at intubation when compared with placebo or compared with antacids alone (RR 0.12, 95% CI 0.02–0.92, 1 trial, 119 women). In general, the quality of the evidence is insufficient to make a recommendation. None of the studies assessed potential adverse effects or substantive clinical outcomes [54].

Advantages
There are *few advantages* to general anesthesia in the absence of a contraindication to a neuraxial approach. One possible advantage is the relaxation properties halogenated anesthetics have on uterine muscle. This property can be useful in the management of uterine inversion, fetal entrapment, or retained placenta. IV nitroglycerine and terbutaline are other options in these situations.

Disadvantages
Compared with neuraxial anesthesia, general anesthesia is associated with a threefold risk of maternal death [55]. The **greatest risk is from the inability to intubate or ventilate the patient.** Parturients have increased upper airway edema, decreased pulmonary functional residual capacity, increased metabolic oxygen consumption, decreased lower esophageal

sphincter tone, and delayed gastric emptying. These conditions increase the risk of both hypoxemia and aspiration. Airway edema can also make anesthetizing the airway for awake fiberoptic intubation more difficult. The incidence of failed intubation in obstetric population is approximately 1 in 300, nearly eight times that of the general population [55,56].

CD is considered a high-risk procedure for intraoperative recall. Concern about neonatal depression and uterine atony has led to minimal use of benzodiazepines and low dose intraoperative halogenated anesthetics intraoperatively. **Compared with nonobstetric surgery, the risk of maternal awareness under general anesthesia is increased (0.4% vs. 0.2% for nonobstetric surgery)** [57]. Although benzodiazepines and opioids can depress the fetus, they are pharmacologically reversible and administration should be considered if their use would benefit the mother. For instance, the judicious use of preintubation opioids can be considered to blunt the sympathetic response to direct laryngoscopy in the hypertensive parturient. The ultra-short-acting synthetic opioid remifentanil can provide this benefit with minimal effect on the neonate.

General anesthesia is also associated with **higher incidence of postoperative nausea and vomiting, maternal sedation, and increased time to breast-feeding.**

General anesthesia's **effect on the fetus** depends on the length of time from induction to umbilical cord clamp; length of time from hysterotomy to cord clamp is also important. Fetal exposure to inhaled anesthetics of >5–8 minutes is associated with **neonatal depression.** General anesthesia compared with neuraxial anesthesia has been shown to increase the incidence of **fetal acidosis, drug exposure, and lower Apgar scores.** IV induction agents, opioids, and hypnotics readily cross the placenta while neuromuscular blocking agents do not [58].

Post-Cesarean Delivery Analgesia
First 24 Hours
There are several safe and effective options for providing post-cesarean analgesia. Preservative-free **morphine** hydrochloride administered **at the time of spinal** anesthesia **or** following cord clamp when using **epidural** anesthesia provides effective pain relief in the first 12–24 hours [5]. An alternative is **PCEA**, which can be associated with increased maternal motor weakness. However, following major surgery, such as cesarean hysterectomy, the effectiveness of continuous epidural analgesia may justify the potential for increased maternal motor weakness.

IV patient-controlled opioids are another reasonable alternative, using morphine, hydromorphone hydrochloride, or fentanyl.

Oral analgesia with oxycodone-acetaminophen 5/325 mg two tablets every 3 hours for 12 hours and then one or two tablets every 4 hours as needed is associated with superior pain control and fewer side effects compared with morphine patient-controlled IV analgesia in one trial [59].

The transversus abdominis plane (TAP) block is performed by injection of local anesthetic between the internal oblique and transversus abdominis muscles to block the plexus of nerves supplying the anterior abdominal wall. In a randomized controlled trial comparing intrathecal opioid to TAP block after CD, intrathecal opioid was superior and patients receiving TAP block had increased opioid consumption in the immediate postoperative period [60]. The TAP block is a reasonable alternative in a patient with a contraindication to a neuraxial block [61].

After 24 Hours
Nonsteroidal anti-inflammatory drugs reduce maternal opioid consumption after CD, even in the first 24 hours, and should be the main intervention for pain control after the first 24 hours. Use of oral narcotics should be quickly weaned.

ANESTHETIC EMERGENCIES
An anesthetic emergency in the obstetric patient necessitates clear and precise communication and cooperation between the anesthesia and obstetric teams. The goal is to stabilize the mother while, if necessary, safely and quickly delivering the neonate.

Total Spinal
A total spinal occurs with cephalad spread of local anesthetic to the breathing centers of the brainstem. This can result from unintentional intrathecal placement of an epidural dose of local anesthetic or from subdural catheter placement with subsequent migration of the catheter. Agitation, difficulty speaking, and profound hypotension are signs of a total spinal. Control of the airway with endotracheal intubation, blood pressure support with fluid, vasopressors and left uterine displacement should be performed immediately. Once the airway has been secured, assessment of the fetus should be facilitated. If the fetus is stable, delivery can safely await maternal recovery.

Local Anesthetic Systemic Toxicity (LAST)
IV injection of local anesthetics can lead to systemic toxicity including seizures and cardiovascular collapse. The mother's airway should be controlled immediately and delivery of the fetus is often indicated because of maternal instability. Seizures can be quickly terminated with administration of diazepam. The pharmacologic treatment of LAST is different from other cardiac arrest scenarios. Management of cardiac arrest includes treatment accordings to the American Heart Association (AHA)/Advanced Cardiac Life Support (ACLS) guidelines with adjustment of medications and possibly prolonged effort as per American Society of Regional Anesthesia and Pain Medicine (ASRA) guidelines [62]. Administration of intralipid, a 20% fat emulsion, has been shown to increase the survival rate of patients who experience cardiac arrest secondary to local anesthetic system toxicity [63].

Failed Intubation
The risk of failed intubation is increased in the parturient at approximately 1 in 300 nearly 8 times that of the general population (1:2330) [55,56]. Increased edema in the upper airway, increased breast size, and increased friability of the mucosa increase chance of failure. In addition, parturients have decreased functional residual capacity that decreases their apneic oxygen reserve and are at higher risk for aspiration secondary to decreased gastric emptying and increased abdominal pressure. In patients where intubation was difficult, it is important to note that emergence is an equally high-risk event. This is emphasized by the number of anesthetic deaths in parturients involving loss of airway, the majority of which occurred during emergence from anesthesia or in the postanesthesia period [64]. Open communication between the obstetric team and anesthesia team is crucial and all decisions should incorporate multidisciplinary communication and cooperation.

Maternal Hemorrhage, Resuscitation, and Massive Transfusion

Maternal hemorrhage can lead to exsanguination and the need for massive transfusion, defined as the need for 10 or more units of packed red blood cells (PRBC) in 24 hours. Volume resuscitation with crystalloid, nonbiologically active colloid, and PRBCs can lead to a dilutional coagulopathy necessitating the transfusion of clotting factors and platelets. Recent retrospective studies from both military and civilian trauma have shown improved outcomes using an empiric ratio of FFP:RBC (fresh frozen plasma:red blood cells) 1:1 in settings that require massive transfusion. Cryoprecipitate may also be needed in patients with low fibrinogen levels. Parturients may acquire a dilutional thrombocytopenia, thus transfusion of platelets may also be warranted; however, the optimal ratio of platelet units to other factors is not known. Risks of massive transfusion include transfusion reactions, viral infection, fluid overload, pulmonary edema, and transfusion related acute lung injury (TRALI) [65]. Intraoperative cell salvage is an addition to the above armamentarium and is gaining acceptance. The ASA Practice Guidelines on Obstetric Anesthesia recommend "in case of intractable hemorrhage when banked blood is not available or the patient refuses banked blood, intraoperative cell salvage should be considered if available" [3].

Cardiopulmonary Resuscitation in the Pregnant Patient

Cardiac arrest during late pregnancy occurs in approximately 1 in 30,000 pregnancies. ACLS protocols apply to pregnant women with a few important adjustments. Pregnant women should be intubated promptly to facilitate oxygenation and protect the airway from aspiration. Left uterine displacement is essential to relieve aortocaval compression. The AHA states the resuscitation team leader should consider delivery of the fetus after 4 minutes to improve cardiopulmonary resuscitation of the mother by relieving aortocaval compression [66]. The AHA further notes improved survival for infants occurs when the delivery occurs no more than 5 minutes after maternal cardiac arrest [66].

REFERENCES

1. Shepherd JA. *Simpson and Syme of Edinburgh*. Edinburgh, Scotland: E&S Livingstone, 1969.
2. Osterman M, Martin J. Epidural and spinal anesthesia use during labor: 27 State reporting area, 2008. *Natl Vital Stat Rep*. 2011;59(5):1–13. [Review]
3. American Society of Anesthesiologists Task Force on Obstetric Anesthesia. Practice Guidelines for Obstetric Anesthesia: An update report by the American Society of Anesthesiologists Task Force on Obstetric Anesthesia. *Anesthesiology*. 2007:106:843–863. [III]
4. American College of Obstetrician and Gynecologists. *ACOG Committee Opinion 433: Optimal Goals for Anesthesia Care in Obstetrics*. Washington, DC: American College of Obstetricians and Gynecologists, 2008. [III]
5. American College of Obstetricians and Gynecologists. *ACOG Practice Bulletin No. 36: Obstetric Analgesia and Anesthesia*. Washington, DC: American College of Obstetricians and Gynecologists, 2002. [III]
6. Smith CA, Collins CT, Crowther CA, et al. Acupuncture or acupressure for pain management in labor. *Cochrane Database Syst Rev*. 2011;(7):CD009232. [Meta-Analysis: 13 RCTs, $n = 1986$]
7. Cluett ER, Burns E. Immersion in water in labour and birth. *Cochrane Database Syst Rev*. 2009;(1):CD000111. [Meta-Analysis: 12 RCTs, $n = 3243$]
8. American College of Obstetricians and Gynecologists. *ACOG Committee Opinion No. 594: Immersion in Water during Labor and Delivery*. Washington, DC: American College of Obstetricians and Gynecologists, 2014. [III]
9. Barragán Loayza IM, Solà I, Juandó Prats C. Biofeedback for pain management during labour. *Cochrane Database Syst Rev*. 2011;(6):CD006168. [Meta-Analysis: 4 RCTs, $n = 186$]
10. Smith CA, Collins CT, Crowther CA. Aromatherapy for pain management in labour. *Cochrane Database Syst Rev*. 2011;(7):CD009215. [Meta-Analysis: 2 RCTs, $n = 535$]
11. Madden K, Middelton P, Cyna AM, et al. Hypnosis for pain management during labour and childbirth. *Cochrane Database Syst Rev*. 2012;(11):CD009356. [Meta-Analysis: 7 RCTs, $n = 1213$]
12. Smith CA, Levett KM, Collins CT, et al. Message, reflexology and other manual methods for pain management in labor. *Cochrane Database Syst Rev*. 2012;(2):CD009290. [Meta-Analysis: 6 RCTs, $n = 326$]
13. Smith CA, Levett KM, Collins CT, et al. Relaxation techniques for pain management in labour. *Cochrane Database Syst Rev*. 2011;(12):CD009514. [Meta-Analysis: 11RCTs, $n = 1374$]
14. Mello LF, Nobrega LF, Lemos A. Transcutaneous electrical stimulation for pain relief during labor: A systemic review and meta-analysis. *Rev Bras Fisioter*. 2011;15:175–184. [Meta-Analysis: 9 RCTs, $n = 1076$]
15. Elbourne D, Wiseman RA. Types of intra-muscular opioids for maternal pain relief in labour. *Cochrane Database Syst Rev*. 2005;(3):CD001237. [Meta-Analysis: 16 RCTs; $n = >5000$]
16. Tsui MHY, Ngan Kee WD, Ng FF, et al. A double blinded randomized placebo-controlled study of intramuscular pethidine for pain relief in the first stage of labour. *Br J Obstet Gynecol*. 2004;111:648–655. [RCT, $n = 112$]
17. Martensson L, Stener-Victorian E, Wallen G. Accupuncture versus subcutaneous injections of sterile water as treatment for labour pain. *Acta Obstetricia et Gynecologica*. 2008;87:171–177. [RCT, $n = 128$]
18. Martensson L, Wallin G. Labour pain treated with cutaneous injections of sterile water: A randomized controlled trial. *Br J Obstet Gynecol*. 1999;106:633–637. [RCT, $n = 99$]
19. Jones L, Othman M, Dowsell T, et al. Pain management for women in labour: An overview of systemic reviews. *Cochrane Database Syst Rev*. 2012;(3):CD009234. [Meta-Analysis 310 RCTs]
20. American College of Obstetricians and Gynecologists. *ACOG Committee Opinion No. 295: Pain Relief during Labor*. Washington, DC: ACOG. July 2004 (Reaffirmed 2015). [Review]
21. Hawkins JL. Epidural analgesia for labor and delivery. *N Engl J Med*. 2010;362:1503–1510. [Review]
22. Anim-Somuah M, Smyth R, Howell C. Epidural versus nonepidural or no analgesia in labour. *Cochrane Database Syst Rev*. 2005;(4):CD000331. [Meta-Analysis: 21 RCTs, $n = 6664$; 20/21 compared epidural analgesia with opiates]
23. Beilin Y, Hapern S. Focused review: Ropivicaine versus bupivicaine for epidural labor analgesia. *Anesth Analg*. 2010;111:482–487. [Review]
24. Amin-Somuah M, Smyth R, Jones L. Epidural versus nonepidural or no analgesia in labour. *Cochrane Database Syst Rev*. 2011;(12):CD000331. [Meta-Analysis: 38 RCTs, $n = 9{,}658$]
25. Chestnut DH, McGrath JM, Vincent RD, et al. Does early administration of epidural analgesia affect obstetric outcome in nulliparous women who are spontaneous labor? *Anesthesiology*. 1994;80:1201–1208. [RCT, $n = 344$]
26. Chestnut DH, Vincent RD, McGrath JM, et al. Does early administration of epidural analgesia affect obstetric outcome in nulliparous women who are receiving intravenous oxytocin? *Anesthesiology*. 1994;80:1193–1200. [RCT, $n = 150$]
27. Luxman D, Wolman I, Groutz A, et al. The effect of early epidural block administration on the progression and outcome of labor. *Int J Obstet Anesth*. 1998;7:161–164. [RCT, $n = 60$]
28. Ohel G, Gonen R, Vaida S, et al. Early versus late initiation of epidural analgesia in labor: Does it increase the risk of cesarean

section? A randomized trial. *Am J Obstet Gynecol*. 2006;194:600–605. [RCT, n = 449]
29. Wassen MMLH, Zuijlen J, Roumen LJM, et al. Early versus late epidural analgesia and risk on instrumental delivery in nulliparous women: A systematic review. *Br J Obstet Gynecol*. 2011;118(6):655–661. [Meta-Analysis: 6 RCTs, 1 cohort, n = 15,399]
30. Usha Kiran TS, Thakur MB, Bethel JA, et al. Comparison of continuous infusion versus midwife administered top-ups of epidural bupivicaine for labour analgesia: Effect on second stage of labour mode of delivery. *Int J Obstet Anesth*. 2003;12:9–11. [RCT]
31. Torvaldsen S, Roberts CL, Bell JC, et al. Discontinuation of epidural analgesia late in labour for reducing the adverse delivery outcomes associated with epidural analgesia. *Cochrane Database Syst Rev*. 2005;(3). [5 RCTs, n = 462]
32. Wassen MMMLH, Smits LJM, Scheepers HCJ, et al. Routine labour epidural analgesia versus labour analgesia on request: A randomized non-inferiority trail. *BJOG*. 2015;122:344–350. [RCT, n = 488]
33. Segal S. Labor epidural analgesia and maternal fever. *Anesth Analg*. 2010;111:1467–1475. [Review]
34. Koughnan F, Crli M, Romney M, et al. Epidural analgesia and backache: A randomized controlled comparison with intramuscular meperidine for analgesia during labor. *Br J Anaesth*. 2002;89(3):466–472. [RCT]
35. Hofmeyr GJ, Cyna AM, Middleton P. Prophylactic intravenous preloading for regional analgesia in labour. *Cochrane Database Syst Rev*. 2005;(3). [6 RCTs, n = 473]
36. Kreiser D, Katorza E, Seidmen DS, et al. The effect of ephedrine on intrapartum fetal heart rate after epidural analgesia. *Obstet Gynecol*. 2004;104:1277–1281. [RCT, n = 145]
37. Harrington BE. Postdural puncture headache and the development of the epidural blood patch. *Reg Anesth Pain Med*. 2004;29:136–163. [II-2]
38. Rawal N, Van Zundert A, Holmstrom B, et al. Combined-spinal technique. *Reg Anesth*. 1997;22:406–423. [Review]
39. Tsen LC, Brad T, Datta S, et al. Is combined spinal-epidural analagesia associated with more rapid cervical dilatation in nulliparous patients when compared with conventional epidural analgesia. *Anesthesiology*. 1999;91:920–925. [RCT; n = 100]
40. Wong CA, Scavone BM, Peaceman AM, et al. The risk of cesarean delivery with neuraxial analgesia given early versus late in labor. *N Engl J Med*. 2005;352:655–665. [RCT, n = 750]
41. Simmons SW, Taghizadeh HN, Dennis A, et al. Combined spinal epidural versus epidural analgesia in labor. *Cochrane Database Syst Rev*. 2012;(10):CD003401 [Meta-Analysis: 27 RCT's n = 3274]
42. Horlocker TT, Wedel DJ, Rowlingson JC, et al. Regional anesthesia in the patient receiving antithrombotic or thrombolytic therapy: American Society of Regional Anesthesia and Pain Medicine Evidence-Based Guidelines (Third Edition). *Reg Anesth Pain Med*. 2010;35(1):64–101. [Review]
43. Henke VG, Bateman BT, Leffert LR. Focused review: Spinal anesthesia in severe preeclampsia. *Anesth Analg*. 2012:117(3): 686–693. [Review]
44. Ho AM, Kee WD, Chung DC. Should laboring parturients with Harrington rods receive lumbar epidural analgesia? *Int J Gynaecol Obstet*. 1999;67(1):41–43. [II-3]
45. Saravanakumar K, Rao SG, Cooper GM. Obesity and obstetric anaesthesia. *Anaesthesia*. 2006;61:36–48. [II-3]
46. Cantwell R, Clutton-Brock T, Cooper G et al. Saving mothers lives: Reviewing maternal deaths to make motherhood safer: 2006–2008: The eight report of the confidential enquiries into maternal deaths in the United Kingdom. *Br J Obstet Gynecol*. 2011;118 (Suppl 1):1–203. [Review]
47. Raatikainen K, Heiskanen N, Heinon S. Transition from overweight to obesity worsens pregnancy outcome in a BMI-dependent manner. *Obesity*. 2006;14:165–171. [II-3]
48. Dahl JB, Jeppesen IS, Jorgensen H, et al. Intraoperative and postoperative analgesic efficacy and adverse effects of intrathecal opioids in patients undergoing cesarean section with spinal anesthesia: A qualitative and quantitative systematic review of randomized controlled trials. *Anesthesiology*. 1999;91:1919–1927. [Meta-Analysis: 11 RCTs]
49. Ng K, Parsons J, Cyna AM, et al. Spinal versus epidural anaesthesia for caesarean section. *Cochrane Database Syst Rev*. 2005; (4). [Meta-Analysis: 10 RCTs, n = 751]
50. Afolabi BB, Lesi AFE, Merah NA. Regional versus general anaesthesia for caesarean section. *Cochrane Database Syst Rev*. 2006;(4):CD004350. [Meta-Analysis: 16 RCTs, n = 1586]
51. Langesaeter E, Rosseland LA, Stubhaug A. Continuous invasive blood pressure and cardiac output monitoring during cesarean delivery: A randomized, double-blind comparison of low-dose versus high-dose spinal anesthesia with intravenous phenylephrine or placebo infusion a randomized, double-blind comparison of low-dose vs. high-dose spinal anesthesia with intravenous phenylephrine or placebo infusion. *Anesthesiology*. 2008;109:856–863. [RCT, n = 80]
52. Emmett RS, Cyna AM, Andrew M, et al. Techniques for preventing hypotension during spinal anaesthesia for caesarean section. *Cochrane Database Syst Rev*. 2005;(4). [Meta-Analysis: 25 RCTs, n = 1477]
53. Lee A, Ngan Kee WD, Gin T. A quantitative, systematic review of randomized controlled trials of ephedrine versus phenylephrine for the management of hypotension during spinal anesthesia for cesarean delivery. *Anesth Anal*. 2002;94:920–926. [Meta-Analysis: 7 RCTs, n = 292]
54. Paranjothy S, Griffiths JD, Broughton HK, et al. Interventions at caesarean section for reducing the risk of aspiration pneumonitis. *Cochrane Database Syst Rev*. 2010;(1):CD004943. [Meta-Analysis: 22 RCTs, 2658]
55. Russell R. Failed intubation in obstetrics: A self-fulfilling prophecy? *International Journal of Obstetric Anesthesia*. 2006;16:1–3. [III]
56. Samsoon GL, Young JR. Difficulty tracheal intubation: A retrospective study. *Anesthesia*. 1987;42:487–490. [II-3]
57. Lyons G, MacDonald R. Awareness during caesarean section. *Anesthesia*. 1991;46:62–64. [II-2]
58. Littleford J. Effects on the fetus and newborn of maternal analgesia and anesthesia: A review. *Can J Anesth*. 2004;51:585–609. [Review]
59. Davis KM, Esposito MA, Meyer BA. Oral analgesia compared to intravenous patient-controlled analgesia for pain after cesarean delivery: A randomized controlled trial. *Am J Obstet Gynecol*. 2006;194:967–971. [RCT, n = 93]
60. Loan H, Preston R, Douglas MJ, et al. A randomized controlled trial comparing intrathecal morphine and transversus abdominus plane block for post-cesarean delivery analgesia. *Int J Obstet Anesthe*. 2012;21:112–118. [RCT, n = 69]
61. Mukhtar K. Transversus abdominis plane (TAP) block. *J N Y School Reg Anesth*. 2009;12:28–33. [II-3]
62. Neal J, Mulroy F, Weinberg G. American Society of Regional Anesthesia and Pain Medicine. Checklist for managing local anesthetic systemic toxicity: 2012 version. *Reg Anesth Pain Med*. 2012;37:16–18. [III]
63. Rosenblatt MA, Abel M, Fischer GW, et al. Successful use of a 20% lipid emulsion to resuscitate a patient after a presumed bupivicaine-related cardiac arrest. *Anesthesiology*. 2006;105:217–218. [III, case report]
64. Mhyre JM, Riesner MN, Polley LS, et al. A series of anesthesia related maternal deaths in Michigan, 1985–2003. *Anesthesiology*. 2007;106:1096–1104. [Review]
65. Bolliger D, Gorlinger K, Tanaka KA. Pathophysiology and treatment of coagulopathy in massive hemorrhage and hemodilution. *Anesthesiology*. 2010;113:1205–1219. [Review]
66. American Heart Association Guidelines for Cardiopulmonary Resuscitation and Emergency Cardiovascular Care. Part 12: Cardiac arrest in special situation. *Circulation*. 2010;122:829–861. [III]

Operative vaginal delivery

Adeeb Khalifeh

KEY POINTS
- Vacuum- and forceps-assisted deliveries have the same indications. There are **no circumstances where operative vaginal delivery (OVD) is definitely indicated.** Alternatives, including allowing the patient to labor longer, oxytocin augmentation, and cesarean delivery (CD), should always be considered.
- **When used by experienced operators, OVD is safe for both mother and baby** and effective in obtaining vaginal delivery, with **forceps having slightly higher success rates.**
- Forceps achieve a vaginal delivery more often than vacuum, 91% versus 86%, respectively. Complication rates differ between vacuum and forceps, with the predominant differences being that **maternal third- and fourth-degree perineal (14% vs. 7.5%) and vaginal wall (26% vs. 8%) injuries are more common with forceps-assisted delivery. Neonatal facial injury is uncommon with operative delivery, 1.7% with forceps, and 0.2% with vacuum.** The choice of instrument is decided after appropriate counseling and depends also on operator experience.
- There is insufficient evidence to compare different types of forceps.
- **Soft vacuum cups fail at attaining vaginal delivery more often than by rigid cups** but have a lower rate of significant fetal scalp trauma. Rigid cups may be better for occiput posterior and other more difficult deliveries, while soft cups may be better suited for less complicated, routine deliveries.
- If attempted, **delivery with a vacuum should ideally be achieved within 5 minutes from vacuum application** and, in general, should be **discontinued if the vacuum cup pops off the fetal head three times.**
- Attempting to use a different extraction instrument after failing with one should be avoided due to increased incidence of fetal injury.

HISTORICAL PERSPECTIVES
OVD has been practiced for centuries. Its initial function was fetal extraction during prolonged dysfunctional labor in an attempt to preserve the life of the laboring women. The invention of modern forceps can be traced back to the Chamberlain family in Europe during the sixteenth century. Vacuum extraction was first described by Dr James Yonge in 1705. The modern evolution of vacuum delivery (also called ventouse) can be attributed to Malmström's metal cup vacuum system developed in 1954. OVD has evolved significantly and today implies a mechanism for facilitating vaginal delivery of a healthy infant while minimizing maternal risk.

In modern obstetrics, OVD, whether forceps or vacuum, is used to expedite safe vaginal delivery for maternal or fetal indications. Despite wide variations in different countries [1], in appropriate circumstances, OVD has a crucial role in safely avoiding primary CD. Emphasis should be placed on indications, contraindications and prerequisites for an OVD with instrument choice based on clinical circumstances and operator skill to minimize maternal and neonatal morbidity.

INCIDENCE
Rates of OVD (forceps and vacuum) have been declining in the United States. The rate of OVD decreased from 9.01% in 1992 to 3.30% in 2013. In 2013, forceps-assisted deliveries accounted for only 0.59% of live births [2].

INDICATIONS
Both **forceps and vacuum have the same indications.** Use should depend mostly on proper evaluation of the patient's labor, risk factors, clinical pelvimetry, estimated fetal weight, and operator experience. There are **no circumstances where OVD is definitely indicated. Alternatives, including allowing the patient to labor longer, oxytocin augmentation, and CD, should always be considered.** OVD is usually considered for the following [3]:

- Maternal:
  - **Prolonged second stage:** At least 3 hours in nulliparous women and at least 2 hours in multiparous women (longer duration on individualized basis, e.g., with the use of epidural analgesia) [4].
  - **Shortening of the second stage of labor for maternal benefit (e.g., underlying medical condition precluding pushing).**
  - **Inefficient maternal effort** (e.g., exhaustion or underlying medical condition precluding pushing).
- Fetal:
  - **Suspicion of fetal compromise.**

"Elective" forceps delivery, that is, without an indication, is associated with increased maternal perineal trauma, and given the other potential maternal and neonatal complications, should not be preferred to spontaneous vaginal delivery [5].

CONTRAINDICATIONS TO OVD
Contraindications to OVD are listed in Table 12.1. Severe scalp trauma and unexplained active bleeding may be relative contraindications in individual cases. OVD should be used with extreme caution in women with maternal diabetes, prolonged labor, and fetal macrosomia, with appropriate preparations due to an increased risk of shoulder dystocia.

RISKS FOR FAILED OVD
Risks for failed vacuum or forceps vaginal delivery include increased maternal age, increased body mass index, diabetes, polyhydramnios, African-American race, induction of labor, occiput posterior (also increases rates of third- and fourth-degree perineal lacerations), dysfunctional labor, and prolonged labor [6].

Table 12.1 Contraindication to Operative Vaginal Delivery

- Nonvertex presentation
- Unengaged fetal head
- Unknown fetal head position
- Fetal prematurity such as <34 weeks (vacuum)
- Known fetal coagulation disorders (e.g., hemophilia and NAIT)
- Known fetal bone demineralization conditions (e.g., osteogenesis imperfecta)

Source: Modified from Committee on Practice Bulletins—Obstetrics, *Obstet Gynecol*, 126(5), e56–e65, 2015.
Abbreviation: NAIT, neonatal alloimmune thrombocytopenia.

CLASSIFICATION OF OVD

- **Outlet:** Scalp is visible at introitus without separating the labia, fetal skull has reached pelvic floor, sagittal suture is anteroposterior (AP) diameter or right or left occiput anterior or posterior position, fetal head is at or on perineum, and rotation ≤45° [3].
- **Low:** Leading point of the fetal skull is at station ≥+2 cm and not on the pelvis floor, rotation is ≤45° (left or right occiput anterior to occiput anterior or left or right occiput posterior to occiput posterior), or rotation is >45°.
- **Mid:** Station is above +2 cm but head is engaged.

Originally devised for forceps, this classification is valid for any OVD, including vacuum [7].

TYPES OF FORCEPS

There are many different designs for forceps, but all consist of two separate halves that each have the same four basic components: blade, shank, lock, and handle. **There is insufficient evidence to compare different types of forceps and it is recognized that the choice is often subjective.** In the only small trial performed, severe facial abrasion was decreased from 4.1% to 1.9% from the regular forceps compared with soft forceps, as were minimal markings (from 61% to 34%, respectively) [8]. Unfortunately successful delivery rates for the two different forceps were not reported, and the soft forceps were self-made. Given the paucity of data, **choice of forceps type is operator dependent**.

- **Classical forceps:** These have cephalic and pelvic curvatures. Usually indicated when no rotation of the fetal head is necessary before delivery. Common types include the following: Simpson forceps (fenestrated blades and nonoverlapping shanks), Tucker–McLane forceps (nonfenestrated blades and overlapping shanks), and Elliot forceps (fenestrated blades, overlapping shanks, and largest cephalic curvature). Many of these forceps have been modified with a Luikart pseudofenestration of the blade.
- **Rotational forceps:** These have cephalic curvature but lack a pelvic curvature. Also have a sliding lock to allow forceps to slide to correct asynclitism of the fetal head if present. After rotation of the fetal head is accomplished classical forceps should be used to complete the delivery. Types include Kielland, Luikart, Barton, and Salinas forceps.
- **Forceps for breech delivery:** These are indicated to help with the aftercoming head in a breech delivery. These forceps lack a pelvic curvature and have blades that are beneath the plane of the shank. Types include Piper and Laufe forceps.

TYPES OF VACUUM EXTRACTORS

Vacuum extractors were originally designed with a rigid metal cup. Subsequently, soft cups have been developed. **Several types of rigid (metal or plastic) and soft (silicone plastic or rubber) vacuums are in clinical use** [9–11]. Among different types of vacuums, **the metal cup is more likely to result in a successful vaginal birth** than the soft cup (9% vs. 17%), with **more cases of scalp injury** (41% vs. 30%) **and cephalohematoma** (14% vs. 8%). The handheld ventouse is associated with more failures than the metal ventouse, and a trend to fewer than the soft ventouse [9–12].

Rigid cups may be better for occiput posterior and other more difficult deliveries, while **soft cups are better suited for less complicated, routine deliveries** [9]. Maternal injury, low Apgar scores at 1 or 5 minutes, umbilical artery pH < 7.20, hyperbilirubinemia/phototherapy, retinal/intracranial hemorrhage, and perinatal death do not differ between soft and rigid vacuum cups [9,12]. Soft vacuum cups have largely replaced the rigid cup in routine clinical practice. For a comprehensive review of vacuum delivery see Vacca, 2009 [13].

Possible Complications of Operative Vaginal Deliveries

1. **Maternal**
   - Forceps use is associated with a **sixfold increase in third- and fourth-degree perineal tears** compared with a spontaneous vaginal delivery [14].
   - Vacuum use is associated with a **twofold increase in third- and fourth-degree lacerations compared with spontaneous vaginal deliveries** [14].
   - Forceps delivery has an increased risk of **anal sphincter injury compared with vacuum delivery** [9].
   - Urinary, flatus, liquid and solid incontinence is similar at 1 year in women who had OVD compared with women who had a second stage CD [15].
   - Pelvic floor and sexual function do not differ at 1 year postpartum compared with women who had CD [16].
   - In the absence of anal sphincter injury, anal incontinence rates at 5–10 years are similar to those in women who had a spontaneous vaginal delivery [17].

2. **Neonatal**
   - Intracranial hemorrhage rate is increased in OVD, but the absolute risk is low [18].
   - The rates of intracranial hemorrhage and neonatal encephalopathy compared with second stage CD are similar [18,19].
   - Cephalohematoma, fetal scalp lacerations, retinal hemorrhages, subgaleal hematoma, and intracranial hemorrhages have been reported in **vacuum deliveries**.
   - **Facial lacerations, facial nerve palsy, and corneal abrasion** are more common *with forceps delivery*.
   - Long-term cognitive outcomes are similar to spontaneous vaginal deliveries [20,21].

COMPARISON OF FORCEPS VERSUS VACUUM-ASSISTED DELIVERY
Safety/Complications

Maternal
- There is a trend for less regional (37% vs. 40%) and significantly less general anesthesia (1% vs. 10%) with vacuum compared with forceps-assisted deliveries. We do not use general anesthesia for operative delivery [9].

- **Third- and fourth-degree perineal** [14% vs. 7.5%; relative risk (RR) 1.89, 95% confidence interval (CI) 1.51–2.37] **and vaginal wall lacerations** (26% vs. 8%; RR 2.48, 95% CI 1.59–3.87) **(maternal trauma) are significantly increased with forceps** compared with vacuum.
- **Severe perineal pain at 24 hours is decreased (9% vs. 15%) with vacuum** compared with forceps-assisted deliveries.
- Flatus incontinence or altered continence is more common with forceps compared with vacuum in a small trial (59% vs. 33%; RR 1.77, 95% CI 1.19–2.62). **In one randomized controlled trial (RCT) comparing forceps and vacuum delivery there was no difference in either bowel or urinary dysfunction 5 years postpartum** [22].
- Rates of moderate/severe pain at delivery, endoanal ultrasound abnormalities [22], and other maternal outcomes are similar.
- Rotational forceps does not increase adverse maternal outcome compared with rotational vacuum delivery [23].

Fetal/Neonatal
- **Facial injury** is more likely with **forceps** (1.7% vs. 0.2%; RR 5.10, 95% CI 1.12–23.25).
- Using a random effects model because of heterogeneity between studies, there was a trend toward **fewer cases of cephalohematoma with forceps** (5% vs. 9%; RR 0.64, 95% CI 0.37–1.11). Rates of cephalohematomas occur in about 10% versus 4% in vacuum and forceps, respectively [9]. Cephalohematomas have an overall rate of 2.5% in the general population [24]. However, the diagnosis of cephalohematoma can be falsely positive in up to 75% of cases [25].
- **Retinal hemorrhages** trended to be **less common in forceps** than vacuum deliveries (5% vs. 8%; RR 0.68, 95% 0.43–1.06) [11]. One study found retinal hemorrhages occurred in 18% in spontaneous vaginal deliveries [26]. The clinical significance of retinal hemorrhages remains unclear [24].
- Rates of scalp/face injury other than cephalohematoma, use of phototherapy, perinatal death, readmission to hospital, and hearing or vision disability are similar between forceps and vacuum-assisted vaginal deliveries [9,27].
- Other possible uncommon fetal complications associated with OVD include facial nerve injury, corneal abrasions, facial bruising, and lacerations. Very rare findings include facial nerve palsy, skull fractures, cervical spine injury, and intracranial hemorrhage. **With vacuum-assisted delivery,** life-threatening neonatal injuries include **subgaleal (subaponeurotic) hematoma** (0%–4%). **Intracranial hemorrhage** is a rare complication of OVD (0%–2.5%).

Efficacy
Both vacuum- and forceps-assisted delivery have high delivery success rates (with vacuum from 83% to 94% and with forceps from 78% to 92%) [9,25]. **Forceps are less likely than the vacuum to fail to achieve a vaginal birth with the allocated instrument** (9% vs. 14%; RR 0.65, 95% CI 0.45–0.94) [9].

CD occurred in 4.5% of forceps, and 2.6% of vacuum deliveries, as in these studies unfortunately failed vacuum would at times be followed by forceps, which, in general, should not be done [9].

Alternatives to Operative Vaginal Delivery
Alternative management should always be discussed with the patient. This includes continued **expectant management for prolonged second stage in the presence of a reassuring fetal status, oxytocin augmentation or proceeding with a CD**. However, the appropriate use of OVD is encouraged by American Congress of Obstetricians and Gynecologists (ACOG) to safely prevent the primary CD [4].

Summary
There is a recognized place for forceps and all types of vacuum in clinical practice [9]. The role of operator training with any choice of instrument must be emphasized. The **increasing risks of failed delivery with the chosen instrument from forceps to metal cup to handheld to soft cup vacuum, and trade-offs between risks of maternal and neonatal trauma** (see Table 12.2) need to be considered when choosing an instrument. **Overall forceps or the metal cup appears to be most effective at achieving a vaginal birth, but with increased risk of maternal trauma with forceps and neonatal trauma with the metal cup** [9].

MANAGEMENT
Preoperative Assessment
Counseling
Review with the patient the indication, risks (possible complications) and benefits, and type of instrument to be used for OVD. The option of CD, including its risks and benefits, should also be reviewed. Obtain verbal or written informed consent prior to OVD.

Preparation/Documentation
  Maternal. Sufficient analgesia, clinical assessment of pelvis, lithotomy position, ± empty bladder (Table 12.3).
  Fetal. Vertex presentation, head engaged (lower part of bony vertex—not caput—at or lower than level of ischial spines), knowledge of the position of the head, asynclitism, and estimated fetal weight. Suboptimal instrument placement increases maternal and neonatal morbidity [28]. In a recent RCT, **the use of ultrasound significantly decreased the incidence of incorrect diagnosis of fetal head position** [29].

Table 12.2 Comparison of Forceps vs. Vacuum for Operative Vaginal Delivery

Fetal		Maternal	
Favors Forceps	Favors Vacuum	Favors Vacuum	Favors Forceps
		Less third- and fourth-degree perineal tears (7.5% vs. 14%) and vaginal wall (8% vs. 26%) lacerations	Less likely to fail to deliver the baby vaginally (9% vs. 14%)
	Less facial injury (0.2% vs. 1.7%)	Less severe perineal pain postpartum (9% vs. 15%)	

Source: Modified from O'Mahony F et al., *Cochrane Database Syst Rev*, (11), CD005455, 2010.

Table 12.3 Preoperative Checklist before Operative Delivery

Maternal Criteria	Fetal Criteria	Uteroplacental Criteria	Other Criteria
Sufficient analgesia	Vertex presentation	Cervix fully dilated	Obtain patient's informed consent. Alert nursing, anesthesia, and neonatology
Patient in the lithotomy position	The fetal head must be engaged in the pelvis	Membranes ruptured	An experienced operator who is fully acquainted with the use of the instrument
Bladder has been emptied	The position of the fetal head must be known with certainty	No placenta previa	Ability to monitor fetal well-being continuously
Clinical pelvimetry must be adequate in dimension and size to facilitate an atraumatic delivery	The station of the fetal head must be +2 or more		The capability to perform an emergency cesarean delivery if required

Uteroplacental: Cervix completely dilated, ruptured membranes, absence of placenta previa, or other contraindications.

Other: Alert nursing, anesthesia, and neonatology of plan for OVD. Be prepared for possible shoulder dystocia. Willingness to discontinue the procedure if it does not proceed as planned [2].

Episiotomy

There is insufficient evidence (no trials) to assess the benefits and risks of episiotomy in operative deliveries. Lateral episiotomy has been shown to be protective against anal sphincter injuries in vacuum deliveries, compared with mediolateral and median episiotomies, in a meta-analysis [30]. In a large observational study, mediolateral episiotomy protected significantly for anal sphincter damage in both vacuum extraction (odds ratio [OR] 0.11, 95% CI 0.09–0.13) and forceps delivery (OR 0.08, 95% CI 0.07–0.11), compared with no episiotomy. The number of mediolateral episiotomies needed to prevent one sphincter injury in vacuum extractions was 12, whereas five mediolateral episiotomies could prevent one sphincter injury in forceps deliveries [31,32]. Episiotomy should not be routinely performed, as it is associated with perineal lacerations in nonoperative vaginal deliveries. However, episiotomy should not be used as an obstetric quality measure in assisted vaginal deliveries, as this could decrease further the use of OVD and increase CD rate [33].

Antibiotic Prophylaxis

Antibiotic prophylaxis cannot be recommended solely for the indication "OVD." Two grams cefotetan IV at the time of vacuum or forceps delivery are associated with a nonsignificant decrease (0% vs. 3.5%) in endometritis [34].

Vacuum Application

Vacuum application, if performed, should begin with low suction and be slowly increased to vacuum of about 0.7–0.8 kg/cc^2 (500–600 mmHg). Compared with stepwise negative pressure for vacuum delivery, rapid negative pressure application is associated with reduced duration (by 6 minutes) of vacuum procedure, but no other maternal or perinatal effects, in a small trial [23]. No torque or rocking motions should be applied to the vacuum. Traction should only be in the direct line of the vaginal canal. The risk of cephalohematoma increases as the time of vacuum application increases. There is no evidence that reducing pressure between contractions decreases risk of fetal injuries [35]. Most deliveries are achieved with one to three pulls with increased neonatal trauma (45%) after three pulls [36]. The risk of cephalohematoma is increased after 5 minutes of vacuum application [37].

Failed Operative Delivery

Attempting to use a different extraction instrument after failing with one should be avoided, as cephalopelvic disproportion may be present, and the highest incidence of neonatal intracranial hemorrhage, as well as other neonatal injuries, is highest among infants delivered using forceps and vacuum sequentially [27,38–40]. At that point, cesarean is usually offered and performed.

Postpartum

It is essential to examine carefully both the fetus and the maternal perineum after OVD.

REFERENCES

1. Stephenson PA, Bakoula C, Hemminki E, et al. Patterns of use of obstetrical interventions in 12 countries. *Paediatr Perinat Epidemiol*, 1993;7:45–54. [II-3]
2. Center for Disease Control. Births: Final data for 2013. *Nat Vital Stat Rep.*, 2015;64(1):1–65. [Epidemiologic Data]
3. Committee on Practice Bulletins—Obstetrics. ACOG Practice Bulletin No. 154: Operative vaginal delivery. *Obstet Gynecol.* 2015;126(5):e56–65. [Guideline]
4. American College of Obstetricians and Gynecologists. Obstetric care consensus no. 1: Safe prevention of primary caesarean delivery. *Obstet Gynecol.* 2014;123:693–711. [Guideline]
5. Yancey MK, Herpolsheimer A, Jordan GD, et al. Maternal and neonatal effects of outlet forceps delivery compared with spontaneous vaginal delivery in term pregnancies. *Obstet Gynecol.* 1991;78:646–650. [II-2]
6. Gopalani S, Bennett K, Critchlow C. Factors predictive of failed operative vaginal delivery. *Am J Obstet Gynecol.* 2004;191:896–902. [II-3]
7. Weinstein L, Calvin S, Trofatter KR. Operative vaginal delivery: Risks and benefits. *ACOG.* Update 2001;27:5. [Review]
8. Roshan DF, Petrikovski B, Sichinava L, et al. Soft forceps. *Int J Obstet Gynecol.* 2005;88:249–252. [II-2]
9. O'Mahony F, Hofmeyr GJ, Menon V. Choice of instruments for assisted vaginal delivery. *Cochrane Database Syst Rev.* 2010;(11):CD005455. [I-Meta-Analysis]
10. Attilakos G, Sibanda T, Winter C, et al. A randomized controlled trial of a new handheld vacuum extraction device. *Br J Obstet Gynecol.* 2005;112:1510–1515. [RCT; I]

11. Groom KM, Jones BA, Miller N, et al. A prospective randomized controlled trial of the Kiwi OmniCup versus conventional ventouse cups for vacuum-assisted vaginal delivery. *Br J Obstet Gynecol*. 2006;113:183–189. [RCT; I]
12. Ismail NAM, Saharan WSL, Zaleha MA, et al. Kiwi OmniCup versus Malmstrom metal cup in vacuum assisted delivery: A randomized comparative trial. *J Obstet Gynaecol Res*. 2008;34:350–353. [RCT; I]
13. Vacca A. *Handbook of Vacuum Delivery in Obstetric Practice*. Brisbane, Australia: Vacca Research, 2009. [Review]
14. Gurol-Urganci I, Cromwell DA, Edozien LC, et al. Third- and fourth-degree perineal tears among primiparous women in England between 2000 and 2012: Time trends and risk factors. *BJOG*. 2013;120:1516–1525. [II-3]
15. Macleod M, Goyder K, Howarth L, et al. Morbidity experienced by women before and after operative vaginal delivery: Prospective cohort study nested within a two-centre randomised controlled trial of restrictive versus routine use of episiotomy. *BJOG*. 2013;120:1020–1026. [II-2]
16. Crane AK, Geller EJ, Bane H, et al. Evaluation of pelvic floor symptoms and sexual function in primiparous women who underwent operative vaginal delivery versus cesarean delivery for second-stage arrest. *Female Pelvic Med Reconstr Surg*. 2013;19:13–6. [II-2]
17. Evers EC, Blomquist JL, McDermott KC, Handa VL. Obstetrical anal sphincter laceration and anal incontinence 5–10 years after childbirth. *Am J Obstet Gynecol*. 2012;207:425.e1–6. [II-3]
18. Towner D, Castro MA, Eby-Wilkens E, Gilbert WM. Effect of mode of delivery in nulliparous women on neonatal intracranial injury. *N Engl J Med*. 1999;341:1709–1714. [II-2]
19. Walsh CA, Robson M, McAuliffe FM. Mode of delivery at term and adverse neonatal outcomes. *Obstet Gynecol*. 2013;121(1):122–128. [II-3]
20. Wesley BD, van den Berg BJ, Reece EA. The effect of forceps delivery on cognitive development. *Am J Obstet Gynecol*. 1993;169:1091–1095. [II-3]
21. Ngan HY, Miu P, Ko L, Ma HK. Long-term neurological sequelae following vacuum extractor delivery. *Aust N Z J Obstet Gynaecol*. 1990;30:111–114. [II-2]
22. Fitzpatrick M, Behan M, O'Connel PR, et al. Randomized clinical trial to assess anal sphincter function following forceps or vacuum assisted vaginal delivery. *Br J Obstet Gynecol*. 2003;110:424–429. [RCT, n = 130]
23. Al Wattar BH, Al Wattar B, Gallos I, Pirie AM. Rotational vaginal delivery with Kielland's forceps: A systematic review and meta-analysis of effectiveness and safety outcomes. *Curr Opin Obstet Gynecol*. 2015;27(6):438–444. [Meta-Analysis; I]
24. Uhing M. Management of birth injuries. *Clin Perinatol*. 2005;32(1):19–38. [II-3]
25. Williams M, Knuppel R, O'Brien W, et al. A randomized comparison of assisted vaginal delivery by obstetric forceps and polyethylene vacuum cup. *Obstet Gynecol*. 1991;78:789–794. [RCT; I]
26. Williams M, Knuppel R, O'Brien W, et al. Obstetric correlates of neonatal retinal hemorrhage. *Obstet Gynecol*. 1993;81:688–694. [II-2]
27. Bofill JA, Rust OA, Schorr SJ, et al. A randomized prospective trial of the obstetric forceps versus the M-cup vacuum extractor. *Am J Obstet Gynecol*. 1996;175:1325–1330. [RCT; I]
28. Ramphul M, Kennelly MM, Burke G, Murphy DJ. Risk factors and morbidity associated with suboptimal instrument placement at instrumental delivery: Observational study nested within the instrumental delivery & ultrasound randomised controlled trial. *BJOG*. 2015;122(4):558–563. [II-1]
29. Ramphul M, Ooi PV, Burke G, et al. Instrumental delivery and ultrasound: A multicentre randomised controlled trial of ultrasound assessment of the fetal head position versus standard care as an approach to prevent morbidity at instrumental delivery. *BJOG*. 2014;121(8):1029–1038. [RCT; I]
30. Sagi-Dain L, Sagi S. Morbidity associated with episiotomy in vacuum delivery: A systematic review and meta-analysis. *BJOG*. 2015;122(8):1073–1081. [Meta-Analysis]
31. De Leeuw J, De Wit C, Kuijken J, et al. Mediolateral episiotomy reduces the risk for anal sphincter injury during operative vaginal delivery. *Br J Obstet Gynecol*. 2008;115:104–108. [II-3]
32. de Vogel J, van der Leeuw-van Beek A, Gietelink D, et al. The effect of a mediolateral episiotomy during operative vaginal delivery on the risk of developing obstetrical anal sphincter injuries. *Am J Obstet Gynecol*. 2012;206(5):404. [II-3]
33. Committee on Obstetric Practice. Committee Opinion No. 647: Limitations of perineal lacerations as an obstetric quality measure. *Obstet Gynecol*. 2015;126(5):e108–e111. [Guideline]
34. Heitmann JA, Benrubi GI. Efficacy of prophylactic antibiotics for the prevention of endomyometritis after forceps delivery. *South Med J*. 1989;82:960–962. [I]
35. Bofill JA, Rust OA, Schorr SJ, et al. A randomized trial of two vacuum extraction techniques. *Obstet Gynecol*. 1997;89(5 Pt 1):758–762. [RCT; I]
36. Murphy DJ, Liebling RE, Patel R, et al. Cohort study of operative delivery in the second stage of labour and standard of obstetric care. *BJOG*. 2003;110:610–615. [II-2]
37. Bofill JA, Rust OA, Devidas M, et al. Neonatal cephalohematoma from vacuum extraction. *J Reprod Med*. 1997;42:565–569. [II-3]
38. Edozien LC, Williams JL, Chattopadhyay I, et al. Failed instrumental delivery: How safe is the use of a second instrument? *J Obstet Gynaecol*. 1999;19:460–462. [II-3]
39. Demissie K, Rhoads GG, Smulian JC, et al. Operative vaginal delivery and neonatal and infant adverse outcomes: Population based retrospective analysis. *BMJ*. 2004;329(7456):24–29. [II-2]
40. Murphy DJ, Macleod M, Bahl R, Strachan B. A cohort study of maternal and neonatal morbidity in relation to use of sequential instruments at operative vaginal delivery. *Eur J Obstet Gynecol Reprod Biol*. 2011;156(1):41–5. [II-3]

Cesarean delivery

A. Dhanya Mackeen

See also specific chapters on Anesthesia (Chapter 11), Trial of Labor after Cesarean Section (TOLAR) (Chapter 14), and Postpartum Care (Chapter 30).

KEY POINTS
- A **cesarean delivery on maternal request (CDMR)** or a planned repeat CD without other indication should not be performed before 39 weeks.
- Prophylactic antibiotics should be administered before every CD. The evidence suggests that a **single dose of cefazolin or ampicillin intravenous (IV)** be given 30–60 minutes prior to skin incision.
- All women undergoing CD should receive mechanical venous thromboembolism (VTE) prophylaxis with either pneumatic compression devices or compression stockings. These should be **applied preoperatively and continued until full ambulation**.
- **Left lateral tilt** is associated with a lower incidence of hypotension.
- Skin should be cleansed with chlorhexidine-alcohol immediately prior to skin incision.
- Compared with no scrub, **vaginal irrigation with povidone-iodine (p-i) immediately before CD** significantly reduces the incidence of postcesarean endometritis.
- **Adhesive drapes** for CD are associated with a **higher incidence of wound infection**.
- A **transverse skin incision** with either the Joel–Cohen or Pfannenstiel technique is the preferred one for CD.
- **Routine development of a bladder flap may not be necessary.**
- The **uterine incision should be performed with the scalpel in a transverse fashion and expanded cephalocaudad bluntly with fingers.**
- **Tranexamic acid (TA)** should be used for prevention of postpartum hemorrhage.
- **Carbetocin**, when available, is superior to oxytocin for prevention of postpartum hemorrhage.
- **Uterine massage**, associated with cord traction, is associated with less blood loss.
- **Spontaneous placental removal** should be preferred to manual removal given the significant decrease in blood loss and endometritis.
- The **uterus should be repaired with sutures with full-thickness bites, in a continuous fashion.**
- Compared with two (double) layer closure, one (single) layer of suture for uterine incision repair is associated with a statistically significant reduction in mean blood loss; duration of the operative procedure; and presence of postoperative pain; but also with poorer healing and thinner residual myometrium. It might be reasonable to omit the second layer if the woman is planning no more pregnancies (e.g., receives tubal ligation). For women planning future pregnancies, the uterus can be closed in two layers.
- There is no evidence to justify the time taken and the cost of peritoneal closure, so avoid it.
- The evidence supports routine subcutaneous suture closure in women with a subcutaneous tissue depth ≥2 cm.
- Suture closure of the skin incision is associated with a significant decrease in wound complications, especially separation, compared to staple closure; it is therefore the preferred closure method for the transverse skin incision.
- **Gum chewing three times/day for at least 30 minutes each time** after CD is associated with earlier return of bowel sounds (by 5 hours), earlier passage of flatus (by about 5 hours), and less (12% vs. 21%) symptoms of mild ileus.
- There is insufficient evidence for a strong recommendation, but early oral fluids and even food after CD seem to be safe and possibly beneficial.
- **Reclosure of the disrupted laparotomy wound of CD** is associated with success in >80% of women, faster healing times, and fewer office visits.

HISTORIC NOTES
The word cesarean is probably derived either from the "Lex Regia," later called "Cesarea," which allowed the postmortem abdominal delivery of the child in ancient Rome, or from the Latin "caesare," which means "to cut." Until the late 1800s, most CDs were done after maternal death, for attempt at fetal salvage. In 1882, the era of modern CD began when Saenger advocated closing all uterine incisions immediately after surgery. The lower uterine segment incision was introduced by Kronig in 1912 and popularized in the United States by DeLee in 1922. The transverse uterine incision was described by Munro-Kerr in 1926 [1]. CD has been associated with relatively low maternal mortality for about 100 years. Safety has improved in the last 50 years, as the above techniques have become more widely used, and antibiotics have been introduced.

DIAGNOSIS/DEFINITION
Birth via abdominal route by laparotomy.

EPIDEMIOLOGY/INCIDENCE
CD is now the most common surgical procedure in the United States with over 1 million performed each year. Its incidence has increased to 33% of deliveries in the United States in 2013 [2]. This increase has been fueled at least in part by the increased incidence of multiple gestations and decreased incidences of vaginal births after CD and vaginal breech deliveries. Women's demand for scheduled CD (CDMR) has increased as cesarean complications diminish, women have fewer children, and fear or concerns about vaginal delivery do not abate.

INDICATIONS

Common accepted indications for CD are **failure to progress** (aka failure to dilate, failure to descend, suspected cephalopelvic disproportion [CPD], dystocia, etc.), **nonreassuring fetal heart rate tracing** (NRFHT), **nonvertex presentation**, etc. (Figure 13.1). See Chapters 7, 8, 10, and 24.

There is insufficient evidence (lack of any trial) to assess the benefits and risks of a policy of CDMR (only indication: woman's desire; also called elective CD, a term which should be avoided) compared with trial of labor in women with term singleton gestations in cephalic presentation. The most common reason for a request for CDMR is fear of labor pain. CDMR should not be motivated by the unavailability of effective pain medication. There is also no randomized controlled trial (RCT) to evaluate the obstetrician's recommendation for CD without indication. As there are no such trials, **there is insufficient evidence to assess the long-term maternal and neonatal morbidity and mortality of planned CD versus trial of labor**. There is insufficient evidence on the impact of counseling during pregnancy with the aim of reducing the incidence of CDMR, but counseling reduces anxiety and concerns related to pregnancy and birth [5]. The incidence of women (without prior CD) preferring CDMR in a systematic review of studies is about 10%, and even less in low-income countries [6]. A practitioner is not obligated to perform a CDMR, but should appropriately refer the woman as necessary.

A CDMR or a planned repeat CD without other indication should not be performed before 39 weeks.

OPTIMAL CD RATE

The optimal CD rate is unknown. Per the World Health Organization (WHO), there were no reductions in maternal and neonatal mortality with CD rates higher than 10% [7]. However, it is important to note that this is based on an ecological analysis at the population level and does not provide information that can be used at an institutional or individual physician level [7]. **Maternal and neonatal morbidity and mortality are the important outcomes, not CD rate per se.** What is most important is that a woman/fetus who needs a cesarean is able to have one. A recent study on the relationship between CD rate and maternal and neonatal mortality in 194 WHO member states revealed that about **19% was the CD rate associated with lower maternal and neonatal mortality** [8]. CD rates of less that 15%–20% have been associated instead with higher neonatal mortality rates [9].

In centers which have excessive CD rates, strategies to decrease the CD rate should focus on the three main indications for CD: arrest (or dystocia, CPD); NRFHT; and malpresentation. These strategies include using 6 cm for active labor, not performing CD for arrest before 6 cm, not performing a CD for prolonged latent phase, reserving consideration for CD for arrest in the first stage of labor only for women ≥6 cm dilation with rupture of membranes who failed to progress despite ≥4 hours of adequate uterine activity, or ≥6 hours of inadequate uterine activity and no cervical change, calling a failed induction in the latent phase one which requires ≥18–24 hours of oxytocin after membrane rupture, using secondary means (e.g., scalp stimulation) to assure normal fetal status in cases of NRFHT, routine use of external cephalic version for nonvertex presentations, use of operative vaginal delivery as appropriate, offering trial of labor after CD, and others [4,10].

There are **limited data of nonclinical interventions aimed at decreasing the unnecessary CD rate** [11]. Implementation of guidelines with **mandatory second opinion** can lead to a small reduction in CD rates, predominately in **intrapartum CD** [12]. **Peer review** [13], **including precesarean consultation, mandatory secondary opinion, postcesarean surveillance, and audit** [13] can lead to a reduction in repeat cesarean delivery rates. **Guidelines** disseminated with endorsement and support from local opinion leaders may increase the proportion of women with previous CD being offered a trial of labor in certain settings (see also Chapter 14). **Nurse-led relaxation classes and birth preparation classes** may reduce CD rates in low-risk pregnancies [11]. **Primary midwifery antenatal** [14] **and labor** [15] **care** in low-risk patients may help decrease CD. There is insufficient evidence that prenatal education and support programs, computer-based patient decision aids, decision-aid booklets, and intensive group therapy are effective. There

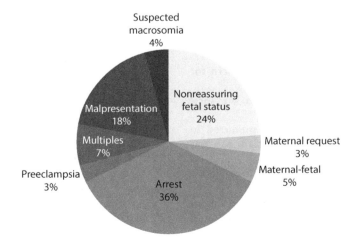

Figure 13.1 Primary cesarean delivery indications. (Adapted from American College of Obstetricians and Gynecologists, Society for Maternal-Fetal Medicine, *Obstet Gynecol*, 123(3), 693–711, 2014; Barber, E. L. et al., *Obstet Gynecol*, 118(1), 29–38, 2011.)

is insufficient evidence that training of public health nurses, insurance reform, and legislative changes are effective.

TIMING OF DELIVERY

In a study of 23,794 women, planned repeat CD at 37 or 38 weeks gestation has a significantly increased risk of adverse neonatal outcomes when compared with planned repeat CD at 39 or 40 weeks or expectant management [16]. A planned repeat CD should in general be performed at 39 0/7–39 6/7 weeks, unless there is a medical indication to perform it earlier (Table 56.9, Chapter 56, Antenatal Testing chapter in *Maternal-Fetal Evidence Based Guidelines*).

PREOPERATIVE CONSIDERATIONS

See Tables 13.1 and 13.2 for summary of recommendations on how to perform a CD [17].

Consent should always be obtained *after* counseling. Counseling should include a discussion of indication, benefits, risks including possible complications, and alternatives.

A checklist, including possibly pre-, intra-, and postoperative steps aimed at preventing complications, has been associated with benefits in general surgery [18] and should probably be implemented at CD [19] (Table 13.2).

Prophylactic Antibiotics

Who to Give Them to
Prophylactic antibiotics should be administered before every CD [20,21]. They are associated with decreased incidence of endometritis by 62%, wound infection by 60%, fever by 55%, and serious maternal infectious complications by 69%. Urinary tract infections (UTI) are also markedly decreased [21]. These results are similar for elective, scheduled CDs.

Which Antibiotics to Use and How
Comparing which antibiotic to give, the **efficacy of a first generation cephalosporin such as cefazolin (Ancef) appears equivalent to that of ampicillin** [22–25]; however, the former is preferred [26]. These are the recommended agents to use unless there are drug allergies to them. A seemingly equally efficacious alternative is penicillin [27], though sample size may have been too small to show a difference. Later-generation (e.g., second or third), or more expensive broad-spectrum agents, do not improve efficacy further [27]. A multiple-dose regimen for prophylaxis appears to offer no added benefit over a single-dose regimen [21,24,28]. Systemic administration after cord clamping versus lavage routes of antibiotic administration seems to have similar efficacy to each other [21,28]. If ampicillin or a first-generation cephalosporin has already been given in labor (e.g., for chorioamnionitis), there may be no need for additional prophylactic antibiotics at CD [26]. If preoperative antibiotics were not given, prophylaxis should include an extended-spectrum regimen, involving azithromycin or metronidazole in the setting of chorioamnionitis [29]. Obese women may benefit from higher doses, e.g., Ancef 2–4 g) [26,30–34] (see Chapter 3 in *Maternal-Fetal Evidence Based Guidelines*).

When to Give the Antibiotics
Compared with after cord clamp, **administration of antibiotics within 1 hour (optimally about 30 minutes) before skin incision is associated with a lower incidence of endometritis and wound infection** [20,35–39]. In a meta-analysis of 10 trials, antibiotics administered preoperatively as compared with after neonatal cord-clamp are associated with a 46% decreased incidence of endometritis and 41% decreased incidence of wound infection [20]. Pharmacokinetic studies demonstrate that adequate cefazolin tissue concentration is attained 30 minutes after administration [20,40,41].

Summary
This evidence suggests the use of a **single dose of IV cefazolin or ampicillin given within 1 hour (about 30 minutes) prior to skin incision.**

Table 13.1 Standard Recommendation Language and Quality of Evidence

Recommendation:
A. Strongly recommend that clinicians provide (the service) to eligible patients. There is good evidence that (the service) improves important health outcomes and concludes that benefits substantially outweigh harms.
B. Recommend that clinicians provide (this service) to eligible patients. There is at least fair evidence that (the service) improves important health outcomes and concludes that benefits outweigh harms.
C. No recommendation for or against routine provision of (the service). There is at least fair evidence that (the service) can improve health outcomes but concludes that the balance of benefits and harms is too close to justify a general recommendation.
D. Recommend against routinely providing (the service) to asymptomatic patients. There is at least fair evidence that (the service) is ineffective or that harms outweigh benefits.
I. Evidence is insufficient to recommend for or against routinely providing (the service). Evidence that the (service) is effective is lacking, of poor quality, or conflicting and the balance of benefits and harms cannot be determined.

Quality of evidence:
Good: Evidence includes consistent results from well-designed, well-conducted studies in representative populations that directly assess effects on health outcomes.
Fair: Evidence is sufficient to determine effects on health outcomes, but the strength of the evidence is limited by the number, quality, or consistency of the individual studies, generalizability to routine practice, or indirect nature of the evidence on health outcomes.
Poor: Evidence is insufficient to assess the effects on health outcomes because of limited number or power of studies, important flaws in their design or conduct, gaps in the chain of evidence, or lack of information on important health outcomes.

Source: Adapted from the Method Outlined by the U.S. Preventive Services Task Force (USPSTF) U.S. Preventive Services Task Force, Agency for Health Care Research and Quality, Available at www.ahcpr.gov, Updated 2015.

Table 13.2 Evidence-Based Recommendations for CD

CD Technical Aspect	Recommendation[a]	Quality[a]	Comment
Prophylactic antibiotics			
Yes or no	A	Good	Yes for all CD
Antibiotic type	A	Good	First generation cephalosporin or ampicillin preoperatively
Route of administration	A	Good	IV
Single dose	B	Good	[b]
Timing	A	Good	Administer 30–60 minutes before skin incision
Prophylaxis for VTE	C	Poor	Mechanical prophylaxis with graduated compression stockings or a pneumatic compression device during and after CD
Lateral tilt	B	Fair	15° to left
No indwelling bladder catheterization	C	Poor	No complications with its avoidance
Hair removal	B	Fair	Hair does not need to be removed. If the decision is made to remove hair, use hair clippers (not razors) on the morning of the surgery
Skin cleansing	B	Fair	Use chlorhexidine-alcohol[b]
Vaginal irrigation	C	Fair	Povidone-iodine[b]
Adhesive drapes	B	Fair	Avoid Use nonadhesive drapes
Skin incision			
Type	C	Fair	Transverse, Pfannenstiel or Joel–Cohen
Length	I	Poor	15 cm
Changing to a second knife	C	Fair	No need to change knife after skin incision[b]
Subcutaneous dissection	I	Poor	we prefer bluntly[b]
Fascial incision	I	Poor	[b]
No rectus muscle cutting	B	Fair	Avoid
Dissection of fascia off rectus	I	Poor	[b]
Opening of peritoneum	I	Poor	[b]
Bladder flap	C	Fair	Routine use not necessary for term deliveries
Uterine incision			
Type	B	Fair	Low transverse uterine incision preferred
Stapling device	B	Fair	Not recommended
Expansion of uterine incision	A	Good	Use blunt uterine incision expansion, with cephalad-caudad traction
Fetal delivery			
Delayed cord clamping	B	Good	Delay cord clamping for 30–120 seconds for all infants <37 weeks[b]
Prevention of uterine atony			
Oxytocin[c]	I	Poor	IV or IM[b]
Oxytocin infusion rate	C	Poor	Optimal rate unclear[b]
Carbetocin	B	Fair	Carbetocin superior to oxytocin, should be used if available[b]
Misoprostol	C	Fair	[b]
Tranexamic acid	A	Good	Use to prevent postpartum hemorrhage[b]
Uterine massage	B	Fair	Perform with cord traction
Placental removal			
Spontaneous	A	Good	Avoid manual removal
Glove change	B	Fair	Not recommended
Uterine exteriorization	C	Fair	Suggested to facilitate better visualization
Cleaning of uterus	I	Poor	[b]
Cervical dilation	I	Poor	Avoid[b]
Closure of uterine incision			
Two vs. one layers	B	Fair	Double layer generally though single layer can be considered if bilateral tubal ligation performed concurrently[b]; continuous stitches
Sharp vs. blunt needles	I	Poor	[b]
Intra-abdominal irrigation	B	Fair	Not recommended
Peritoneal closure	A	Good	Not recommended (for both parietal and visceral)
Reapproximation of rectus muscles	I	Poor	[b]
Fascial closure	I	Poor	[b]
Subcutaneous tissue closure			
≥2 cm thickness	A	Good	Close subcutaneous space if ≥2 cm
Subcutaneous tissue drain	A	Good	Routine use not recommended
Closure of skin			
Staples vs. subcuticular suture	A	Good	Close transverse skin incision with suture.[b]

[a]Level of evidence was based on the U.S. Preventive Services Task Force recommendations (Table 13.1).
[b]See text for more details.
[c]Based on trials of women with vaginal delivery, not CD.
Abbreviations: CD, cesarean delivery; IV, intravenous; IM, intramuscular; VTE, venous thromboembolism.

Prophylactic Agents to Prevent VTE

There is insufficient evidence to give strong recommendations for thromboprophylaxis during pregnancy and the early postnatal period [42]. The three most commonly used interventions are pneumatic compression devices, compression stockings, and anticoagulants such as unfractionated (UH) or low-molecular-weight heparin (LMWH).

Pneumatic compression devices have been recommended based on retrospective data [43–46]. They appear to be safe and effective.

While there are two RCTs on UH versus placebo, two RCTs of LMWH versus placebo, and four RCTs on LMWH versus UH given antenatally, the RCTs are, in general, small and the data are insufficient to make any recommendation [44,45]. It is not possible to assess the effects of any of these interventions on most outcomes, and especially on rare outcomes such as VTE, death, and osteoporosis, because of small sample sizes and the small number of RCTs making the same comparisons. There was some evidence of side effects associated with thromboprophylaxis. In summary, given the higher risk of VTE at CD compared with vaginal delivery, **all women undergoing CD should receive at least mechanical VTE prophylaxis with either pneumatic compression devices or compression stockings** [45]. These should be **applied preoperatively and continued until full ambulation**.

In women undergoing CD with body mass index (BMI) > 50 kg/m^2, previous VTE, or two or more additional risk factors for VTE (such as smoking, multiple gestation, BMI ≥ 30 kg/m^2, prolonged immobility, and infection), pharmacological VTE prophylaxis, with either enoxaparin 40 mg daily or UH 5000 every 12 hours in addition to mechanical prophylaxis, should be considered. This pharmacological prophylaxis can start at 6–12 hours postoperatively, after concerns for hemorrhage have decreased, and can continue until full ambulation [45].

Fetal Heart Monitoring

1. If *external monitoring* has been employed, it should be continued up until the abdominal prep has begun. This includes the time when regional anesthesia is administered. If continuous fetal monitoring is not possible, reapply the external monitor for 2–3 minutes if feasible after completion of the regional anesthesia to determine the postanesthesia fetal status.
2. If *internal monitoring* has been employed, the scalp electrode can be kept on until delivery of the fetal head, at which point the lead can be cut and the fetus delivered or the fetus delivered with the electrode attached. The operating room team will be responsible to document on the count sheet the location of the scalp electrode after delivery.
3. If the CD is done for **nonreassuring fetal status**, all attempts should be made to perform continuous fetal monitoring until the delivery occurs. This may not apply when the CD is done in an emergent manner.

There is no trial regarding optimal *time of* **"decision to incision"** for CD. Thirty minutes for CD for NRFHT and 60 minutes for CD for dystocia and most other indications have been proposed but are not based on trials [47,48]. Additionally, studies have shown that while many cesareans are not performed within this time frame, neonatal outcomes are not adversely affected by longer intervals from decision to delivery [49,50], unless significant neonatal compromise is suspected (such as with fetal bradycardia).

Steroids for Fetal Maturity

If delivery by cesarean is necessary before 37 weeks, **betamethasone** 12 mg intramuscular (IM) × 2 doses, 24 hours apart *(or dexamethasone 6 mg IM × 4 doses, 12 hours apart)* should be given for fetal maturity [51,52]. **There is new evidence that steroids are associated with neonatal benefits also ≥34 weeks,** as three RCTs have been done on steroids administered between 34 and 36 6/7weeks [51,53,54] in women at risk of preterm birth (PTB), and two RCTs in women at ≥37 weeks [55,56]. Women who received antenatal corticosteroids ≥34 weeks had a significantly lower incidence of respiratory distress syndrome (RDS) (relative risk [RR] 0.76, 95% confidence interval [CI] 0.62–0.93), mild RDS (RR 0.40, 95% CI 0.23–0.69), moderate RDS (RR 0.39, 95% CI 0.18–0.89), severe RDS (RR 0.66, 95% CI 0.53–0.82), transient tachypnea of the newborn (RR 0.62, 95% CI 0.50–0.77), use of surfactant (RR 0.61, 95% CI 0.38–0.99), mechanical ventilation (RR 0.62, 95% CI 0.41–0.94), significantly less time on oxygen (mean difference [MD] –2.06 hours, 95% CI –2.17 to –1.95), lower maximum inspired oxygen concentration (MD -0.66%, 95% CI –0.69 to –0.63), shorter length of stay (LOS) in neonatal intensive care unit (NICU) (MD –7.64 days, 95% CI –7.65 to –7.64), higher Apgar scores at 1 and at 5 minutes (MD 0.06, 95% CI 0.05–0.07) compared with those who did not [57]. Steroids should be considered to decrease respiratory and other neonatal morbidities in women at high risk of preterm birth between 34 0/7 to 36 6/7 weeks [51]. **Betamethasone** 12 mg × 2 doses 24 hours apart at 37 weeks or beyond before planned CD has been also shown to reduce the incidence of RDS, to 0.2% from 1.1% in one RCT [58]. However, as this trial was not blinded, or placebo controlled, these data are insufficient for a definite recommendation. Steroids for fetal maturity should in general not be given at ≥39 weeks since the incidence of RDS is small.

Music

Playing music preoperatively significantly increases positive emotions and decreases negative emotions [59]. Playing music during planned CD under regional anesthesia may improve pulse rate and birth satisfaction score. However, the magnitude of these benefits is small and the methodological quality of the one included trial is questionable. Therefore, the clinical significance of music is unclear [60,61].

PREPARATIONS ON THE OPERATIVE TABLE
Maternal Position

There is **insufficient evidence to support or clearly disprove the value of the use of tilting or flexing the table, the use of wedges and cushions, or the use of mechanical displacers at CD** [62]. Most of the results below are from small single RCTs. The incidence of air embolism is not affected by head up versus horizontal position. **Lateral tilt** involves tilting the woman toward her left side 10°–15° to avoid vena caval compression by the gravid uterus. There are no changes in hypotensive episodes when comparing left lateral tilt (RR 0.11, 95% CI 0.01–1.94), right lateral tilt (RR 1.25, 95% CI 0.39–3.99), and head down tilt (MD –3.00; 95% CI –8.38 to 2.38) with horizontal positions or when comparing full lateral tilt with 15° tilt (RR 1.20, 95% CI 0.80–1.79) [62]. **Hypotensive episodes are** decreased with manual displacers (RR 0.11, 95% CI 0.03–0.45), a right lumbar wedge compared with a right pelvic wedge (RR 1.64, 95% CI 1.07–2.53), and increased right lateral tilt (RR 3.30, 95% CI 1.20–9.08) versus **left lateral tilt** [62]. Position does not affect systolic blood pressure when comparing left lateral tilt or head down tilt to horizontal positions, or full lateral tilt to 15° tilt. Manual displacers resulted in a decreased fall in mean systolic blood pressure compared with left lateral tilt. Position does not affect diastolic blood pressures when comparing left lateral tilt versus horizontal positions. The mean diastolic pressure is a bit lower in head down tilt when compared with horizontal positions. There are no statistically significant changes in maternal pulse rate, 5-minute Apgars, maternal blood pH, or cord blood pH when comparing different positions [62].

Indwelling Bladder Catheterization
Compared with use of indwelling urinary catheters inserted pre-CD and removed ≥12 hours after CD, a systematic review of three trials showed that nonuse is associated with a lower incidence of urinary tract infection (UTI) (RR 0.08, 95% CI 0.01–0.64), lower rate of discomfort at first voiding (RR 0.06, 95% CI 0.03–0.12), less time to first voiding (by 16 minutes), and less time until ambulation (by about 6 minutes) [63]. No differences in intraoperative difficulties, complications (including urinary retention), or operative time were seen [63]. Given that these studies were not powered to assess differences in bladder or ureteral injury, were both performed in developing countries, that the quality of the RCTs were poor, and the use of prophylactic antibiotics and other important confounders were not reported, there is still insufficient evidence to justify the routine use of bladder catheterization, but **its avoidance does not seem to be associated with complications.**

Hair Removal
Based on a meta-analysis of 1343 patients, shaving was associated with twice the number of surgical site infections as compared with clipping. Therefore, **electric clipper** the morning of the surgery is preferred [64,65] (see Chapter 7).

Skin Cleansing
Skin is impossible to sterilize. In nonpregnant adults, there are no differences in wound infection with different types and times of scrubs. **Skin cleansing** techniques for CD have been insufficiently studied for an evidence-based recommendation. Compared with standard preparation of 7.5% p-i scrub and then p-i 10% solution, the addition of preceding parachlorometaxylenol scrub for 5 minutes, in the women who had received prophylactic antibiotics for CD, is not associated with differences in incidences of endometritis or wound infection in a small, likely underpowered trial [66]. Chlorhexidine-alcohol scrub results in less wound infections than p-i scrub (9.5% vs. 16.1%, RR 0.59; 95% CI 0.41–0.85) in patients undergoing clean-contaminated surgeries [67]. Additionally, one small study showed that chlorhexidine scrub is associated with less bacterial contamination of the cesarean skin incision 18 hours after application as compared with p-i scrub [68,69]. In a recent RCT, p-i with alcohol, chlorhexidine with alcohol, or both, were associated with similar and low (3.9%–4.6%) incidences of surgical site infections [70]. Overall, the use of **chlorhexidine** is currently **preferred** to iodine solution.

Vaginal Irrigation
Compared with no scrub, **vaginal irrigation with p-i immediately before CD** significantly reduces the incidence of postcesarean endometritis from 8.3% in control groups to 4.3% in vaginal cleansing groups (RR 0.45., 95% CI 0.25–0.81) [71]. The risk reduction was particularly strong for women with ruptured membranes (4.3% in the vaginal cleansing group vs. 17.9% in the control group; RR 0.24, 95% CI 0.10–0.55) and those already in labor at the time of cesarean (7.4% in the vaginal cleansing group vs. 13.0% in the control group; RR 0.56, 95% CI 0.34–0.95). No other outcomes were significantly different between the vaginal cleansing and control groups. No adverse effects were reported with the p-i vaginal cleansing [71]. Most, but not all, of these studies used p-i skin cleansing and prophylactic antibiotics so **it is difficult to determine if vaginal preparation is necessary in women who receive the current recommendations for preoperative antibiotics**; however, as a simple, generally inexpensive intervention, providers should consider implementing preoperative vaginal cleansing with p-i. Compared with matching placebo, metronidazole gel 5 g intravaginally before CD is associated with a decrease from 17% to 7% in the incidence of endometritis, but no other significant changes in important outcomes [72].

Adhesive Drapes
Adhesive drapes for CD are associated with a **higher incidence of wound infection** (13.8%) compared with the control group (10.4%) [73,74]. Therefore, adhesive drapes should be avoided.

Oxygen Administration
A Cochrane review of supplemental oxygen in adult surgical patients found no firm evidence that a high fraction of inspired oxygen (60%–90%) reduces all-cause mortality or surgical site infection as compared with 30%–40% inspired oxygen [75]. In pregnancy, several RCTs have been done. An RCT of 585 women showed no difference in the rate of infectious morbidity when comparing 2 L oxygen via nasal cannula versus 10 L oxygen by nonrebreather during CD [76]. An RCT of 831 women showed no difference in rate of surgical site infection or endometritis when comparing 30% versus 80% supplemental oxygen after cord clamp and for 1 hour post-CD [77]. In summary, so far there is **no evidence that supplemental oxygen affects outcomes** at CD.

Anesthesia
For anesthesia, see Chapter 11. Metoclopramide 10 mg IV before spinal and ondansetron 4 mg IV after neonatal cord clamping are associated with less intraoperative and early postoperative nausea and vomiting as compared with placebo [78].

SURGICAL TECHNIQUE
Skin Incision
Skin incision techniques for CD have been evaluated separately from other aspects of CD in limited studies [79,80]. In general, a **transverse skin incision** is recommended, since this is associated with less postoperative pain and improved cosmesis compared with a vertical incision. The **Pfannenstiel** (slightly curved, 2–3 cm or two fingerbreadths above the symphysis pubis, with the midportion of the incision lying within the shaved area of the pubic hair) and **Joel–Cohen** (straight, 3 cm below the line joining the anterior superior iliac spines, and therefore slightly more cephalad than the Pfannenstiel) are the preferred transverse incisions. Most RCTs not only evaluate type of skin incision, but also other technical aspects of CD,

making it often impossible to evaluate the effect of only the type of skin incision [81]. The better designed, larger trial revealed no differences in total operative time (32 vs. 33 minutes), intra- and postoperative complications, and neonatal outcomes, with the extraction time 50 seconds shorter for the Joel–Cohen group [79,82]. Considering the absence of clinical benefits to the mother and fetus, **there is no clear indication for preferring either a Pfannenstiel or a Joel–Cohen incision for CD.** In contrast, a smaller, less well-designed trial [80] shows significantly shorter operating times, reduced blood loss and postoperative discomfort associated with the Joel–Cohen compared with the Pfannenstiel incision [82].

There are probably **no absolute indications for performing a vertical skin incision.** Compared with transverse skin incision, vertical skin incision is associated with slightly shortened incision-to-delivery intervals of about 1 minute for primary and about 2 minutes for repeat CD [83].

Skin incision length has not been studied in a trial. Abdominal surgical incision size should probably provide about 15 cm (size of a standard Allis clamp) of exposure to assure optimal outcome of both mother and term fetus [1,84].

Changing to a second scalpel after the first scalpel has been used for skin incision versus no such change has never been evaluated in a trial, or in any obstetrical literature. From general surgery data, one scalpel is probably adequate to use throughout the whole surgical procedure.

Subcutaneous Tissue Opening

There is limited data on whether the subcutaneous tissue should be opened with blunt or sharp technique. We use the scalpel as little as possible, opening layers bluntly from medial to lateral to avoid injury to tissue and the inferior epigastric vessels. Blunt dissection has been associated with shorter operating times. In one RCT, use of diathermy (Bovie) for CD abdominal wall opening from subcutaneous tissue until the peritoneum was associated with lower blood loss, lower skin-to-peritoneum incision time, and lower post-CD pain compared with the use of No. 22 disposable scalpel blade [85].

Fascial Incision

Fascial incision has **not been studied separately in a trial.** A transverse incision is usually performed with the scalpel, and then extended with scissors. Digital extension can alternatively be accomplished by separating the forefingers in a cephalad-caudad direction after inserting the fingers into a small, midline transverse fascial incision. In an RCT evaluating entry into the abdomen, **blunt entry with rectus sheath incision extended manually** and parietal peritoneum entered and extended bluntly (manually) was associated with less blood loss, shorter operative time, and less post-CD fever and pain, compared with sharp entry [86].

Rectus Muscle Cutting

Rectus muscle cutting with Maylard technique is not associated with any difference in operative morbidity, difficult deliveries, or postoperative complications compared with Pfannenstiel (no muscle cutting) technique [84,87,88], but abdominal muscle strength at 3 months tends to be better in the Pfannenstiel group [88]. Pain scores also did not differ between the groups, but this may have been due to a sample size of only 97 women [88]. Therefore, **rectus muscle cutting is probably not necessary** [82].

Dissection of Fascia off the Rectus Muscles

Nondissection of the fascia off the recti muscles inferiorly may result in less pain and similar blood loss as compared with dissection of the rectus sheath inferiorly during cesarean [89]. There seems to be no necessity of this commonly used technical step of CD [1].

Extraperitoneal versus Transperitoneal CD

There is insufficient evidence to compare maternal and perinatal outcomes between extraperitoneal versus transperitoneal CD, as only one small RCT has been performed [90]. The current standard is to perform CD transperitoneally.

Opening of the Peritoneum

Opening of the peritoneum has not been studied separately in a trial. The peritoneum is usually carefully opened with blunt or sharp dissection, and blunt expansion, high above the bladder, avoiding injury to organs below. As compared with sharp entry, blunt entry and extension of the rectus sheath incision and parietal peritoneum was associated with less blood loss, shorter operative time, and less post-CD fever and pain [86].

Retractors

There is insufficient evidence for comparing different types of retractors in CD.

Bladder Flap

Four RCTs of 581 women have compared development of a bladder flap versus direct uterine incision above the bladder fold [91]. There were no differences in the rate of bladder injury, estimated blood loss or hospitalization. Though the skin incision to delivery was 1.27 minutes longer for bladder flap formation, overall operative time did not differ [91]. However, one study was unpublished, two were judged to be of poor methodological quality, populations were heterogeneous, emergency cesareans were excluded from analysis and the majority of fetuses were >32 weeks gestation [91]. Based on the trial that was of better quality, there is some evidence that omission of the bladder flap shortened incision to delivery time in primary CD by 1 minute, though there was no difference in total operating time [92]. These results may not be able to be extrapolated to preterm and emergency CD since they were typically not included in these RCTs. No long-term effects (e.g., adhesions, bladder function, and fertility) have been evaluated. As bladder injury at CD is an uncommon event (1–3/1000), a sample size over 40,000 women would be required to show a difference in this outcome [93]. **Developing a bladder flap at CD may not be necessary at term.**

The use of a bladder blade to protect the bladder has not been studied separately in a trial.

Uterine Incision

Uterine incision type has not been studied separately in a trial. The **transverse incision of the lower uterine segment** is usually recommended because there is less blood loss and it allows for TOLAC in subsequent pregnancies [1,94]. Some experts advocate the classical vertical or at least low vertical incision if the lower uterine segment is not large enough to allow a transverse incision, for example, for the very preterm (<28 weeks) uterus or fibroids, but this has been associated with increased blood loss compared with low transverse incision [95].

Uterine Stapling

Use of uterine stapling (autosuture) device for opening and closing of the uterus has been assessed in two trials of 300 women. There is no difference in febrile morbidity between the groups [96]. One trial showed a nonsignificant increase in the duration of the procedure (by about 3 minutes) [96,97]. **There is not enough evidence to justify the routine use of stapling devices** to extend the uterine incision of the lower segment, especially since there is a possibility that stapling **could cause harm** by prolonging the time to deliver the baby.

Expansion of Uterine Incision

Expansion of the uterine incision with fingers (blunt) is associated with significantly decreased blood loss (by about 55 mL) and need for transfusion (RR 0.24; 95% CI 0.09–0.62) [96]. As it is also quicker, and associated with less risk of inadvertently cutting the neonate or cord, **blunt should be preferred to sharp expansion of the uterine incision** [98].

Compared with transverse expansion, **cephalad-caudad expansion** of the low transverse uterine incision is associated with significantly lower incidence of blood loss >1500 mL (0.2% vs. 2%) [99], less unintended uterine extensions (3.7% vs. 7.4%) [99] and less blood loss overall [100]. A meta-analysis of these two RCTs showed that women who were randomized in the cephalad-caudad group had lower incidences of postpartum blood loss (MD −67.64 mL, 95% CI −102.85 to −32.43), hemoglobin drop (MD −0.26 g/dL, 95% CI −0.37 to −0.14) and hematocrit drop 24 hours after CD (MD −1.20 g/dL, 95% CI −1.87 to −0.53), unintended extension (4.8% vs. 8.9%; RR 0.51, 95% CI 0.30–0.88), injury of uterine vessels (1.5% vs. 2.8%; RR 0.52, 95% CI 0.20–1.37), blood loss >1500 mL (0.2% vs. 1.7%; RR 0.12, 95% CI 0.02–0.99) and need for additional stiches (20.3% vs. 29.2%; RR 0.60, 95% CI 0.44–0.82). Therefore, cephalad-caudad uterine incision expansion by fingers should be preferred to transverse expansion [101].

Instrumental Delivery

Instrumental delivery of the fetal head by either vacuum or forceps compared with manual means has been insufficiently evaluated for a firm recommendation in women with cephalic [102] or breech presentation undergoing CD. As instrumentation has been associated with maternal (especially for forceps) or fetal (especially for vacuum) harm in vaginal deliveries, the principle of "primum non nocere" (first do no harm) should be applied in this setting, therefore *favoring* **manual delivery of the fetal head whenever possible** until further data are available.

Tocolysis for assisting in delivery of the fetal head at CD has been insufficiently studied [103].

Delivery of the Impacted Fetal Head

Though a strong recommendation cannot be made based on the available evidence, in cases where the fetal vertex is wedged into the maternal pelvis, vaginal displacement of the presenting part upward has been associated with longer operating time, more extension of the uterine incision and postpartum endometritis as compared with **reverse breech extraction ("pull" method)** in a small RCT [104]. A meta-analysis of RCT and non-RCT data confirmed reductions in uterine incision extension, blood loss and operative time with reverse breech extraction [105].

Family-Oriented CD

One study showed that allowing the parents to directly visualize delivery of the baby's body (after head is delivered), to cut umbilical cord and to perform early skin to skin contact, improves birth satisfaction without increased blood loss [106].

Skin-to-Skin

Early skin to skin contact is beneficial for both mothers and babies and can be performed at time of CD [106–108]. Professional supervision is warranted to ensure neonatal well-being.

Collection and Drainage of Cord Blood

At CD, drainage of fetal blood from the umbilical cord is associated with less incidence of feto-maternal transfusion (measured by Kleihauer–Betke test) compared with no drainage [109]. The clinical significance of this finding is unknown.

Delayed cord clamping (DCC) for 30–120 seconds (or milking) increases neonatal blood volume by approximately 30% and decreases morbidity including intraventricular hemorrhage in preterm infants [110,111]. In term infants, it is associated with higher hematocrit, but also higher bilirubin levels. Therefore DCC is **indicated routinely in preterm infants** [112].

Prevention of Uterine Atony and Postpartum Hemorrhage

Prevention of uterine atony and postpartum hemorrhage has not been comprehensively studied for CD, but has been studied extensively for the third stage of labor after vaginal delivery (see Chapter 9).

Oxytocin

In the setting of vaginal delivery, **both IV and IM oxytocin effectively reduce postpartum hemorrhage** and the need for therapeutic uterotonics by at least 40% compared with placebo or no routine prophylactic agent. **Oxytocin is as effective and has fewer side effects than ergot alkaloids.**

Regarding oxytocin infusion rates at CD, patients required fewer additional uterotonics (19% vs. 36%) when treated with 80 international units (IU) oxytocin/500 mL infused over 30 minutes as compared with those who received 10 IU/500 mL infused over 30 minutes [113]. One study showed lower rates of excessive blood loss (EBL) >1000 cc, need for uterotonics and blood transfusion in those that received 5 IU oxytocin bolus and 30 IU infusion as compared with those who received 5 IU bolus and placebo [114]. Other lower oxytocin doses have been studied with nonsignificant differences between treatment groups [115]; **the optimal infusion rate for oxytocin at CD is still unclear.** For CD, oxytocin 20 IU IV is as effective as ergometrine plus oxytocin, with less vomiting, in a small RCT [116].

Carbetocin

For CD, **carbetocin as a single 100-g dose is associated with more effective prevention of uterine atony and lower need for additional uterotonics compared with oxytocin 8- or 16-hour infusion** [117,118]. Carbetocin (where available) may be recommended over oxytocin for prevention of uterine atony.

Misoprostol

There is **insufficient evidence** to compare misoprostol to oxytocin for prevention of uterine atony and postpartum hemorrhage at CD, as the seven RCTs compared different regimens of misoprostol and oxytocin. In single RCTs, **either sublingual misoprostol or rectal misoprostol were associated with lower post-CD blood loss compared with oxytocin** [119,120]. Given that misoprostol and oxytocin appear equally efficacious based on this limited evidence and that side effects such as shivering and pyrexia [119] are more common with misoprostol, oxytocin for now remains preferred [121].

Misoprostol combined with oxytocin (e.g., 400 μg sublingual after cord clamping, or rectal) was associated with **less post-CD blood loss, fall in hematocrit and need for additional uterotonics agents** when compared with oxytocin alone. In women at high-risk for post-CD hemorrhage, the combination of both misoprostol and oxytocin should be considered.

Tranexamic acid
TA inhibits fibrinolysis that potentiates the clotting system and can be used to prevent bleeding. Its half-life is 2–10 hours and it typically works immediately after IV administration. Side effects include gastrointestinal upset, but additional rare complications have been reported. TA was administered pre-cesarean though the time frame varied among trials (three out of nine studies administered it 10 minutes prior to incision). Dose also varied but was typically 1 g of TA in 20 mL of 5% glucose given IV over 5–10 minutes [122]. There was significantly less postpartum hemorrhage (PPH) (odds ratio [OR] 0.43) and mean blood loss (72 mL) in those treated with TA compared with those that were not [122]. Four trials reported no cases of maternal death or severe morbidity (including thromboembolism, seizure, ICU admission) among 1511 women. The most recent meta-analysis showed that all women in the nine RCTs received standard oxytocin prophylaxis; in addition the TA group received **TA 1 gram or 10 mg/kg IV 10–20 minutes before skin incision or spinal anesthesia**. Women who received TA experienced *less postpartum blood loss* (MD-167.50 mL, 95% CI −225.79, −109.20) compared with controls. Women who were randomized to the TA group had a significantly **lower incidence of postpartum hemorrhage**, i.e., blood loss more than 500 mL, (3.9% vs. 41.9%; RR 0.06, 95% CI 0.04–0.10) **and of severe postpartum hemorrhage**, i.e., blood loss more than 1000 mL (1.3% vs. 3.0%; RR 0.42, 95% CI 0.19–0.92), compared with controls. The **number of women who needed additional uterotonic agents was significantly lower in the TA group** compared with controls (3.9% vs. 6.6%; RR 0.59, 95% CI 0.38–0.92). Women who received TA had a **significantly lower hemoglobin drop as compared with controls** (1.1 g/dL vs. 1.8 g/dL; MD −0.61 g/dL, 95% CI −1.04, −0.18). The percentage of women who required **blood transfusions at or immediately after CD was significantly lower** in the TA group compared with controls (2.1% vs. 5.7%; RR 0.36, 95% CI 0.20–0.64). There was no difference in the incidence of thromboembolic events in the two groups [123]. Therefore, **TA should be recommended for preventing PPH in all women undergoing CD** [122].

Uterine Massage
Uterine massage, associated with cord traction, is associated with less blood loss compared with no such interventions [124]. Uterine massage has not been studied by itself in an RCT for CD.

Placental Removal
In a meta-analysis of 4694 women, manual removal of the placenta is associated with greater morbidity than spontaneous expulsion with gentle cord traction: increased endometritis (RR 1.64, 95% CI 1.42–1.90); greater blood loss (by 94 mL); increased postpartum hemorrhage (RR 1.81, 95% CI 1.44–2.28); and decreased hematocrit after delivery (by 1.6%) [124]. Blood loss may be increased in manual removal because dilated sinuses in the uterine wall are not closed yet. Bacterial contamination of the lower uterine segment and incision may contaminate the surgeon's dominant hand, and therefore the upper segment in manual removal, or the glove itself may be contaminated. Therefore, **uterine massage with gentle cord traction resulting in spontaneous expulsion should be utilized for delivery of the placenta** given the significant decrease in blood loss and endometritis as compared with manual placental removal.

Change of Gloves
Changing the operator's glove before manual removal of the placenta does not alter the incidence of endometritis [125].

Uterine Exteriorization
Meta-analyses have showed there are no significant differences in blood loss, intraoperative hypotension, nausea/vomiting or pain, blood transfusion, endometritis or wound infection, with uterine exteriorization (extra-abdominal uterine incision repair) versus repair in situ [126,127]. The Cochrane review showed that there was less febrile morbidity (RR 0.41; 95% CI 0.17–0.97) and 0.24 day longer hospital stay with extra-abdominal closure [126]. So **the balance of the benefits and harms is too close to justify a strong recommendation,** but many obstetricians subjectively prefer to exteriorize the uterus for easier uterine incision repair.

Uterine Cooling
Uterine cooling after uterine exteriorization and during uterine closure is associated with a decrease in blood loss and postpartum hemorrhage in one RCT [128].

Cleaning the Uterus
Cleaning any placental remnants or blood clots from the uterus with a sponge or other means is a technique frequently used after placental removal, but not studied in any trial.

Cervical Dilation
Routine cervical dilation at CD before uterine incision repair has been insufficiently studied, but it is not associated with an effect on infectious morbidity (UTI, wound infection, endometritis) or change in hemoglobin [42,129].

Closure of Uterine Incision
At least one-layer uterine closure is always done, as the uterus should not be left open. Closure of uterine incision involves several decisions. These include use of blunt versus sharp needles; type of suture; full- versus split-thickness repair; continuous versus interrupted sutures; locking versus nonlocking of sutures; and whether or not to imbricate the second layer if it is even closed.

Blunt needles for closure of the uterus, peritoneum, and rectus sheath are associated with similar outcomes compared with sharp needles in one RCT [130]. In another RCT, glove perforation was significantly less with use of blunt compared with sharp needles, especially for the assistant surgeon. However, physicians reported decreased satisfaction performing CD with blunt needles [131]. In summary, there is **still limited evidence to recommend blunt versus sharp needles at CD.**

In one RCT, placing the sutures with the left hand and pulling the suture in a caudal direction was associated with lower need for additional sutures, shorter operative times, and lower decrease in hemoglobin compared with placing and pulling the suture with the right hand [132].

There is insufficient evidence to compare different **sutures** at closure at CD (no RCTs). In the only RCT comparing different sutures for uterine incision repair, polyglactin-910 was associated with generally similar outcomes compared with chromic catgut [86]. Compared with split-thickness repair (avoiding the endometrium), **full-thickness uterine incision repair** is associated with a lower incidence of incomplete healing (documented by split in uterine muscle seen on transvaginal ultrasound about 40 days after the CD) of the uterine incision after CD [96,133].

Continuous single-layer closure may save operating time and reduce blood loss compared with interrupted single-layer closure [134]. **Locking of sutures** in the first layer has been insufficiently studied, but associated with **poorer healing and possibly thinner residual myometrium**, as is single layer closure [135].

Compared with two (double) layers, one (single) layer of suture for low transverse uterine incision repair is associated with no differences in febrile morbidity (13,980 women; RR 0.98). Although there was a **reduction in mean blood loss for single layer closure,** there were no differences in blood transfusion and heterogeneity was high for included studies [86,96]. Unfortunately, the women followed-up are too few to detect a significant difference in rare but extremely important long-term outcomes such as rates of rupture in the next pregnancy [42,96,134–137], with contradictory results of retrospective studies. Since there is, as of yet, no trial demonstrating benefit from two- versus one-layer uterine closure, **it might be reasonable to omit the second layer if the woman is planning no more pregnancies (e.g., receives tubal ligation). For women planning future pregnancies, the uterus can be closed in two layers** [138]. Vertical uterine incisions require a double or triple layer closure [139].

Intra-Abdominal Irrigation
Intra-abdominal irrigation with 500–1000 mL of normal saline before abdominal wall closure **should not be routinely performed** since it provides no significant differences in blood loss, intrapartum complications, hospital stay, return of gastrointestinal function, or incidence of infectious complications versus no irrigation [140]. In another RCT, 500–1000 mL of warm normal saline irrigation before the closure of the abdominal wall was associated with increased intraoperative nausea, but similar incidences of post-CD infectious morbidities [141].

Adhesion Formation Prevention
There is **insufficient evidence** to assess if any intervention is effective at adhesion prevention at CD. In one RCT, hyaluronate carboxymethylcellulose (Seprafilm®) adhesion barrier applied at CD did not reduce adhesion formation at the subsequent CD [142]. Evidence from non-CD abdominal surgery shows that oxidized regenerated cellulose (Interceed®) and hyaluronate carboxymethylcellulose (Seprafilm®) safely reduce clinically relevant consequences of adhesions [143].

Intraoperative Interventions to Reduce Postoperative Pain
One study of 370 patients who underwent primary CD showed that intraperitoneal instillation of 10 mL of 2% lidocaine significantly decreased persistent pain postoperatively from 21% to 11%; parietal peritoneum was closed [144].

Appendectomy
Performing a planned appendectomy without indication at CD is not associated with inpatient morbidity in a small RCT [145]. However, no clear benefits were shown. The evidence is insufficient to make a recommendation regarding this nonindicated procedure.

Intra-Abdominal Drain
There is insufficient evidence to evaluate the effect of placing a drain in the abdominal cavity at CD. In one RCT, liberal use of a subrectus sheath drain was not associated with any effect compared with the restricted use of such intervention [146].

Peritoneal Nonclosure
Observational studies have shown that the peritoneum regenerates in 5–6 days. Compared with closure, **peritoneal nonclosure** is associated with a reduction in operating time whether both or either visceral or parietal peritoneal layers were not sutured. For nonclosure of both layers, the operating time was reduced by about 6 minutes [147]. While nonclosure of visceral peritoneum versus closure of both peritoneal surfaces showed an increase risk of adhesion formation, one of the two included studies had a high risk of bias. Peritoneal nonclosure is also associated with significantly **less postoperative pain and shorter operative time** as compared with closure of both layers. Nonclosure of the visceral peritoneum when the parietal peritoneum is closed is associated with **decreased urinary symptoms of urgency, frequency and stress incontinence** [147].

Long-term follow-up in one trial showed no significant differences. Long-term follow-up [148] after 7 years showed no differences in pain, fertility, urinary symptoms, and adhesions. Long-term studies following CD are limited; there is therefore no definite evidence for nonclosure until long-term data become available [147]. A review of general surgery and gynecological data concluded that "we encourage clinicians not to close both parietal and visceral peritoneum." [149] The hypothetical benefits of closing these layers for anatomic barrier, reduction of wound dehiscence, and minimization of adhesion have not been proven, and in fact have been invalidated by trials. **There is no evidence to justify the time taken and the cost of peritoneal closure.**

Reapproximation of Rectus Muscles
Reapproximation of rectus muscles has not been studied in any trial. Most clinicians agree that they do go back to their original anatomic place, and suturing them together can cause unnecessary pain when the woman starts to move postoperatively.

Fascial Closure
Techniques of fascial closure have not been studied in any trial of CD. Most experts suggest continuous nonlocking closure with delayed absorbable suture at about 1cm intervals. Recent non-CD evidence instead has shown that small fascial tissue bites of 5 mm every 5 mm are associated with prevention of incisional hernia in midline incisions and is not associated with a higher rate of adverse events, compared with large fascial bites of 1 cm every 1 cm [150].

Subcutaneous Tissue
Irrigation
Irrigation of the subcutaneous tissue to minimize wound infections and other complications has not been studied versus no irrigation in a trial of CD. The type of irrigation, with saline or antibiotic solution, has also not been studied in a trial.

Suture Closure
Subcutaneous tissue closure versus nonclosure by suture should be analyzed by the thickness of the subcutaneous tissue, as results differ according to <2 cm versus ≥2 cm of subcutaneous tissue thickness [151,152]. Most studies used 3-0 Vicryl for suture closure.

Any subcutaneous thickness: *Suture closure* of subcutaneous fat in women with *any subcutaneous thickness* is overall associated with less wound disruption *versus nonclosure,* but inclusion of both women with <2 cm and ≥2 cm thickness (which can have differing outcomes), and inability to blind represent a possible source of confounding and bias [152].

Less than 2 cm subcutaneous thickness: Routine subcutaneous tissue closure in women with a depth <2 cm has been insufficiently studied. It is not associated with any effects on outcome, and therefore cannot be recommended [151].

Greater than or equal to 2 cm subcutaneous thickness: *Suture closure* of subcutaneous fat in women with ≥2 *cm thickness* is associated with a significant decrease in wound disruptions, defined as any wound complication that required intervention, and seromas, compared with nonclosure. **The evidence supports routine subcutaneous suture closure in women with a subcutaneous tissue depth ≥2 cm** [151]. We find that many obstetricians underestimate subcutaneous thickness, so consider measuring this space if close to 2 cm.

Drainage
Some RCTs have evaluated drainage of subcutaneous tissue, compared with no drainage, or compared with tissue closure.

In meta-analyses of all RCTs, there is no evidence of a difference in the risk of wound infection, other wound complications, febrile morbidity, or endometritis in women who had wound drains compared with those who did not [153,154]. Drainage of subcutaneous tissue (i.e., wound drainage) in women with any thickness and who did not receive prophylactic antibiotics with a 2-cm corrugated rubber drain, left to drain open, coming out of one end of incision, and removed the following day is associated with a trend toward increased wound infection [153]. Drainage is also not as effective as tissue closure for women with ≥2 cm of subcutaneous fat. Drainage was usually performed with a 7-mm Jackson–Pratt drain [153]. Therefore, **routine subcutaneous tissue drainage in women undergoing CD cannot be recommended** [149]. These trials do not answer the question of whether wound drainage is of benefit when hemostasis is not felt to be adequate.

Closure of Skin
Closure of skin at CD has been most commonly performed with either absorbable sutures or nonabsorbable metal staples. In a meta-analysis of 3112 women, compared with sutures, staple closure is associated with higher rates of wound complications (13.0% vs. 4.8%), separation (9.4% vs. 2.5%), and a shorter duration of surgery by 7 minutes [155–157]. This decrease in wound complications persists even when only examining obese patients as suture was still associated with less complications (6.7% vs. 12.8%) [156]. Though the incidences were small, there were no significant differences in hematoma, seroma and readmission between groups. Additionally, there were no significant differences between groups with regards to pain perception, patient satisfaction, and incision cosmesis. **Therefore, the low transverse cesarean skin incision should be closed with suture.**

There is insufficient evidence to compare different sutures for CD skin closure. The suture most commonly used in the RCTs showing superiority of suture compared with staples was poliglecaprone [156]; though the largest of these studies used poliglecaprone or polyglactin [157]. Neither of these sutures has been shown to be superior to the other. In one small RCT, polyglycolic acid suture was associated with a higher incidence of hypertrophic scarring compared with interrupted nylon suture [158]. In one RCT, barbed suture was associated with similar rates of wound dehiscence, infection and other adverse outcomes, compared with 3-0 polydioxanone suture [159].

If staples are used, they should probably be removed on or after day 7, as early (day 3) removal is associated with a non-significant trend for higher rate of wound dehiscence (15.2% vs. 11.5%) compared with delayed (days 7–10) removal [160]. In one RCT, absorbable staples were associated with similar outcomes compared with metallic staples, except for a longer closure time [161].

There is insufficient evidence to evaluate the effectiveness of a new wound closure device, Leukosan® Skinlink, for skin closure at CD. The one small RCT comparing it to Prolene suture closure showed similar cosmetic results [162].

POSTOPERATIVE CARE
Gum Chewing
Compared with no gum chewing, **gum chewing typically three times/day for at least 30 minutes each time after CD is associated with earlier return of bowel sounds (by 4.4 hours), earlier passage of flatus (by about 7.9 hours)** [163] **and stool (9.1 hours)** [163] **and less ileus (OR 0.36)** [164,165].

Early Oral Fluids and Feeding
A meta-analysis of 11 somewhat heterogeneous studies showed that compared with delayed (usually after 8 hours or upon passage of flatus) oral fluids or food, *early oral fluids or food* are associated with reduced time (by about 8.8 hours) to return of bowel sounds; reduced time to flatus (7.3 hours) and decreased time to bowel movement (6.3 hours) [166]. No significant differences were identified with respect to nausea, vomiting, abdominal distention, and mild ileus [166,167]. Typically feeding was initiated within 6–8 hours with water, clear liquids or solid foods (4 studies) [168]. In summary, **there is insufficient evidence for a strong recommendation, but early oral fluids and even food within 6–8 hours after CD seem to be safe and possibly beneficial.**

Pain Relief after CD
Nonsteroidal anti-inflammatory drugs (NSAIDs; e.g., ibuprofen) and/or **narcotics** (e.g., oxycodone) are commonly used in the United States for post-CD pain relief (see also Chapter 11). There is no RCT evaluating oral narcotic use or oral NSAIDs use. **Local analgesia wound infiltration** and **abdominal nerve blocks** as adjuncts to regional analgesia and general anesthesia seem to be of benefit in CD by reducing opioid consumption in small RCTs. NSAIDs (even as a wound infiltration) as an adjuvant may confer additional pain relief [169]. In women who had CD performed under regional analgesia, wound infiltration is associated with a decrease in morphine consumption at 24 hours compared with placebo. In women with regional analgesia and also a local anesthetic, NSAID cocktail wound infiltration is associated with less morphine use compared with local anesthetic control. Women who have regional analgesia with

abdominal nerves blocked have decreased opioid consumption. In women under general anesthesia, with CD wound infiltration and peritoneal spraying with local anesthetic, the need for opioid rescue is reduced [169].

DISCHARGE
A study of almost 3000 women who were randomized to be discharged at 24 hours versus 72 hours postcesarean with their newborn showed that **those discharged at 24 hours were more likely to report mood swings and less success with breastfeeding**. Additionally, although there was no difference in maternal readmission, there were **increased neonatal admissions (typically due to jaundice) in those discharged at 24 hours** [170]. After a planned CD, discharge on the first as compared with the second day is not associated with any difference in maternal or perinatal immediate or 6-week outcomes [171]. For women who are discharged early, a home health registered nurse (RN) visit is advised.

MANAGEMENT OF COMPLICATIONS
Disrupted (Open) Laparotomy Wound
Compared with healing by secondary intention, **reclosure of the disrupted laparotomy wound is associated with success in >80% of women, faster healing times** (16–23 vs. 61–72 days), **and fewer office visits** [172]. No serious morbidity or mortality is associated with either method. There is insufficient evidence to assess optimal timing (probably 4–6 days after disruption if noninfected) and technique (superficial vertical mattress or "en bloc" reclosure of entire wound thickness with absorbable sutures, or adhesive tape) of reclosure, as well as utility of antibiotics. **Compared with reclosure using sutures, reclosure using permeable, adhesive tape** (Cover-Roll; Biersdorf, Inc., Norwalk, CT) is associated with faster procedure, less pain scores, and similar healing times in a small RCT [173].

Postoperative Counseling
Interval until next pregnancy after a CD should be about 18–23 months, as shorter intervals have been associated with increased risk of uterine rupture [174,175] (see also Chapter 14).

SHORT- AND LONG-TERM OUTCOMES FOR THE BABY
Scheduled CD compared with vaginal delivery (but not compared with unscheduled CD) has been associated with a small absolute increased risk of childhood asthma requiring hospital admission, salbutamol inhaler prescription at age 5 years, and all-cause death by age 21 years (0.40% vs. 0.32%; difference, 0.08% [95% CI, 0.02%–1.00%]; adjusted HR, 1.41 [95% CI, 1.05–1.90]) [176].

SHORT- AND LONG-TERM OUTCOMES FOR THE MOTHER
The dominant maternal risk in subsequent pregnancies is placenta accreta and its associated complications (Chapter 28). Pregnancies following CD also have increased risk for other types of abnormal placentation, reduced fetal growth, preterm birth, and possibly stillbirth. Chronic maternal morbidities associated with CD include pelvic pain and adhesions. Adverse reproductive effects may include decreased fertility and increased risk of spontaneous abortion and ectopic pregnancy [177].

FOR FUTURE RESEARCH
In order to make comparisons of CD rates over time, it is important that everyone use a similar classification scheme. Robson proposed a scheme that is mutually exclusive and totally inclusive and takes into consideration category of pregnancy (singleton cephalic/breech/other lie, multiples), prior obstetric record (nulliparous, multiparous with or without uterine scar), course of labor (spontaneous, induced, CD before labor), and gestational age (based on completed weeks at time of delivery) [178].

REFERENCES
1. Berghella V, Baxter JK, Chauhan SP. Evidence-based surgery for cesarean delivery. *Am J Obstet Gynecol.* 2005;193:1607–1617. [Systematic review].
2. Martin JA, Hamilton BE, Osterman MJ, et al. Births: Data for 2013. *Nat Vital Stat Rep.* 2015;64(1):1–68. [Data review].
3. American College of Obstetricians and Gynecologists, Society for Maternal-Fetal Medicine. Obstetric care consensus no. 1: Safe prevention of the primary cesarean delivery. *Obstet Gynecol.* 2014;123(3):693–711.
4. Barber EL, Lundsberg LS, Belanger K, et al. Indications contributing to the increasing cesarean delivery rate. *Obstet Gynecol.* 2011;118(1):29–38.
5. Saisto T, Salmela-Aro K, Nurmi JE, et al. A randomized controlled trial of intervention in fear of childbirth. *Obstet Gynecol.* 2001;98(5):820–826. [RCT, $n = 176$].
6. Mazzoni A, Althabe F, Liu NH, et al. Women's preference for caesarean section: A systematic review and meta-analysis of observational studies. *Br J Obstet Gynecol.* 2011;118:391–399. [Meta-analysis of 23 observational studies, $n = 13,922$].
7. Betran AP, Torloni MR, Zhang JJ, et al. for the WHO Working Group on Caesarean Section. WHO statement on caesarean section rates. *BJOG.* 2015;123(5):667–70. Published online [Review, Guideline].
8. Molina G, Weiser TG, Lipsitz SR, et al. Relationship between cesarean delivery rate and maternal and neonatal mortality. *JAMA.* 2015;314(21):2263–2270. [I-2].
9. Matthews TG, Crowley P, Chong A, et al. Rising caesarean section rates: A cause for concern? *BJOG.* 2003;110(4):346–349. [II-2].
10. Boyle A, Reddy UM, Landy HJ, et al. Primary cesarean delivery in the United States. *Obstet Gynecol.* 2013;122(1):33–40. [II-2].
11. Khunpradit S, Tavender E, Lumbiganon P, et al. Non-clinical interventions for reducing unnecessary caesarean section. *Cochrane Database Syst Rev.* 2011;(6):CD005528. [Meta-analysis: 16 RCTs].
12. Althabe F, Belizan JM, Villar J, et al. Mandatory second opinion to reduce rates of unnecessary caesarean sections in Latin America: A cluster randomized controlled trial. *Lancet.* 2004;363:1934–1940. [RCT].
13. Chaillet N, Dumont A, Abrahamowicz M, et al. A cluster-randomized trial to reduce cesarean delivery rates in Quebec. *N Engl J Med.* 2015;372(18):1710–1721.
14. McLachlan HL, Forster DA, Davey MA, et al. Effects of continuity of care by a primary midwife (caseload midwifery) on caesarean section rates in women of low obstetric risk: The COSMOS randomised controlled trial. *BJOG.* 2012;119(12):1483–1492.
15. Kashanian M, Javadi F, Haghighi MM. Effect of continuous support during labor on duration of labor and rate of cesarean delivery. *Int J Gynaecol Obstet.* 2010;109(3):198–200.
16. Chiossi G, Lai Y, Landon MB, et al. Timing of delivery and adverse outcomes in term singleton repeat cesarean deliveries. *Obstet Gynecol.* 2013;121(3):561–569. [Review].
17. U.S. Preventive Services Task Force. Agency for Health Care Research and Quality. Available at: www.ahcpr.gov. Accessed on August 31, 2016. Updated 2015 [Guideline].
18. Haynes AB, Weiser TG, Berry WR, et al. A surgical safety checklist to reduce morbidity and mortality in a global population. *N Engl J Med.* 2009;360:491–499. [II-2].

19. American College of Obstetricians and Gynecologists. Patient safety checklist no. 4: Preoperative planned cesarean delivery. *Obstet Gynecol.* 2011;118(6):1471–1472. [Checklist; III].
20. Mackeen AD, Packard RE, Ota E, et al. Timing of intravenous prophylactic antibiotics for preventing postpartum infectious morbidity in women undergoing cesarean delivery. *Cochrane Database Syst Rev.* 2014;(12):CD009516. [Meta-analysis: 10 RCT, n = 5041].
21. Smaill FM, Grivell RM. Antibiotic prophylaxis versus no prophylaxis for preventing infection after cesarean section. *Cochrane Database Syst Rev.* 2014;(10):CD007482. [95 RCTs and quasi RCTs, n > 15,000].
22. Alekwe LO, Kuti O, Orji EO, et al. Comparison of ceftriaxone versus triple drug regimen in the prevention of cesarean section infectious morbidities. *J Matern Fetal Neonatal Med.* 2008;21(9):638–642. [RCT, n = 2000].
23. Rudge MV, Atallah AN, Peracoli JC, et al. Randomized controlled trial on prevention of postcesarean infection using penicillin and cephalothin in brazil. *Acta Obstet Gynecol Scand.* 2006;85(8):945–948. [RCT, n = 600].
24. Mackeen AD, Packard RE, Ota E, et al. Antibiotic regimens for postpartum endometritis. *Cochrane Database Syst Rev.* 2015;(2):CD001067. [Meta-analysis, 40 RCTs, n = 4240].
25. Mivumbi VN, Little SE, Rulisa S, et al. Prophylactic ampicillin versus cefazolin for the prevention of post-cesarean infectious morbidity in Rwanda. *Int J Gynaecol Obstet.* 2014;124(3):244–247. [RCT, n = 132].
26. American College of Obstetricians and Gynecologists. ACOG Practice Bulletin No. 120: Use of prophylactic antibiotics in labor and delivery *Obstet Gynecol.* 2011;117:1472–1483.
27. Gyte GM, Dou L, Vazquez JC. Different classes of antibiotics given to women routinely for preventing infection at caesarean section. *Cochrane Database Syst Rev.* 2014;(11):CD008726. [Meta-analysis: 31 RCTs, n = 7697].
28. Hopkins L, Smaill F. Antibiotic prophylaxis regimens and drugs for cesarean section. *Cochrane Database Syst Rev.* 2000;(2):CD001136. [51 RCTs, n = >10,000].
29. Tita AT, Rouse DJ, Blackwell S, et al. Emerging concepts in antibiotic prophylaxis for cesarean delivery: A systematic review. *Obstet Gynecol.* 2009;113(3):675–682. [Meta-analysis of RCTs].
30. Pevzner L, Swank M, Krepel C, et al. Effects of maternal obesity on tissue concentrations of prophylactic cefazolin during cesarean delivery. *Obstet Gynecol.* 2011;117(4):877–882.
31. Stitely M, Sweet M, Slain D, et al. Plasma and tissue cefazolin concentrations in obese patients undergoing cesarean delivery and receiving differing pre-operative doses of drug. *Surg Infect (Larchmt).* 2013;14(5):455–459.
32. Swank ML, Wing DA, Nicolau DP, et al. Increased 3-gram cefazolin dosing for cesarean delivery prophylaxis in obese women. *Am J Obstet Gynecol.* 2015;213(3):415.e1–415.e8.
33. Young OM, Shaik IH, Twedt R, et al. Pharmacokinetics of cefazolin prophylaxis in obese gravidae at time of cesarean delivery. *Am J Obstet Gynecol.* 2015;213(4):541.e1–541.e7.
34. Maggio L, Nicolau DP, DaCosta M, et al. Cefazolin prophylaxis in obese women undergoing cesarean delivery: A randomized controlled trial. *Obstet Gynecol.* 2015;125(5):1205–1210.
35. Gordon HR, Phelps D, Blanchard K. Prophylactic cesarean section antibiotics: Maternal and neonatal morbidity before or after cord clamping. *Obstet Gynecol.* 1979;53:151–154. [RCT, n = 114].
36. Cunningham FG, Leveno KJ, DePalma RT, et al. Perioperative antimicrobials for cesarean delivery: Before or after cord clamping? *Obstet Gynecol.* 1983;62:151–154. [RCT, n = 305].
37. Wax JR, Hersey K, Philput C, et al. Single dose cefazolin prophylaxis for postcesarean infections: Before vs. after cord clamping. *J Matern Fetal Med.* 1997;6(1):61–65. [RCT, n = 90].
38. Thigpen BD, Hood WA, Chauhan S, et al. Timing of prophylactic antibiotic administration in the uninfected laboring gravida: A randomized clinical trial. *Am J Obstet Gynecol.* 2005;192(6):1864–8; discussion 1868–1871 [RCT, n = 303].
39. Clark SL, Belfort MA, Dildy GA, et al. Maternal death in the 21st century: Causes, prevention, and relationship to cesarean delivery. *Am J Obstet Gynecol.* 2008;199(1):36.e1–5; discussion 91-2. e7-11 [II-1].
40. Fiore MT, Pearlman MD, Chapman RL, et al. Maternal and transplacental pharmacokinetics of cefazolin. *Obstet Gynecol.* 2001;98(6):1075–9. [Prospective, n = 26].
41. Elkomy MH, Sultan P, Drover DR, et al. Pharmacokinetics of prophylactic cefazolin in parturients undergoing cesarean delivery. *Antimicrob Agents Chemother.* 2014;58(6):3504–3513. [Prospective n = 20].
42. Dahlke JD, Mendez-Figueroa H, Rouse DJ, et al. Evidence-based surgery for cesarean delivery: An updated systematic review. *Am J Obstet Gynecol.* 2013;209(4):294–306. [Review].
43. Casele H, Grobman WA. Cost-effectiveness of thromboprophylaxis with intermittent pneumatic compression at cesarean delivery. *Obstet Gynecol.* 2006;108(3 Pt 1):535–540. [III].
44. Bain E, Wilson A, Tooher R, et al. Prophylaxis for venous thromboembolic disease in pregnancy and the early postnatal period. *Cochrane Database Syst Rev.* 2014;2:001689. [Meta-analysis, 16 RT, n = 2592].
45. SMFM Publications Committee, with Varner MW. Thromboprophylaxis for cesarean delivery. *Cont Obstet Gynecol.* 2011;6:30–33. [Review].
46. Clark SL, Christmas JT, Frye DR, et al. Maternal mortality in the united states: Predictability and the impact of protocols on fatal postcesarean pulmonary embolism and hypertension-related intracranial hemorrhage. *Am J Obstet Gynecol.* 2014;211(1):32. e1–32.e9. [II-2].
47. Chauhan SP MG. ACOG Practice Bulletin no. 62: Intrapartum fetal heart rate monitoring. *Obstet Gynecol.* 2005;105(5 Pt 1):1161–1169. [Review].
48. American Academy of Pediatrics, American College of Obstetricians and Gynecologists. *Guidelines for Perinatal Care.* 5th ed. Washington, DC: Elk Grove Village (IL), AAP, 2002:147. [Guideline].
49. Bloom SL, Leveno KJ, Spong CY, et al. Decision-to-incision times and maternal and infant outcomes. *Obstet Gynecol.* 2006;108(1):6–11. [Prospective, Observational].
50. Tolcher MC, Johnson RL, El-Nashar SA, et al. Decision-to-incision time and neonatal outcomes: A systematic review and meta-analysis. *Obstet Gynecol.* 2014;123(3):536–548. [Meta-analysis, 34 studies, n > 20,000].
51. Gyamfi-Bannerman C. Antenatal late preterm steroids (ALPS): A randomized trial to reduce neonatal respiratory morbidity. *AJOG.* 2016;214(1):S2.
52. Roberts D, Dalziel S. Antenatal corticosteroids for accelerating fetal lung maturation for women at risk of preterm birth. *Cochrane Database Syst Rev.* 2006;(3):CD004454.
53. Balci O, Ozdemir S, Mahmoud AS, et al. The effect of antenatal steroids on fetal lung maturation between the 34th and 36th week of pregnancy. *Gynecol Obstet Invest.* 2010;70(2):95–99.
54. Porto AM, Coutinho IC, Correia JB, et al. Effectiveness of antenatal corticosteroids in reducing respiratory disorders in late preterm infants: Randomised clinical trial. *BMJ.* 2011;342:d1696.
55. Ahmed MR, Sayed Ahmed WA, Mohammed TY. Antenatal steroids at 37 weeks, does it reduce neonatal respiratory morbidity? A randomized trial. *J Matern Fetal Neonatal Med.* 2015;28(12):1486–1490.
56. Stutchfield P, Whitaker R, Russell I for Antenatal Steroids for Term Elective Caesarean Section (ASTECS) Research Team. Antenatal betamethasone and incidence of neonatal respiratory distress after elective caesarean section: Pragmatic randomised trial. *BMJ.* 2005;331(7518):662.
57. Saccone G, Berghella V. Antenatal corticosteroids for term or near-term fetal maturity: A systematic review and meta-analysis of randomized controlled trials. *BMJ.* 2016;355:i5044. [Meta-analysis; 6 RCTs, n = 5698].
58. Stuchfield P, Whitaker R, Russell I, et al. Antenatal betamethasone and incidence of neonatal respiratory distress after

elective caesarean section: Pragmatic randomized trial. *Br Med J.* 2005;331:662–668. [RCT; n = 942].
59. Kushnir J, Friedman A, Ehrenfeld M, et al. Coping with preoperative anxiety in cesarean section: Physiological, cognitive, and emotional effects of listening to favorite music. *Birth.* 2012;39(2):121–127. [RCT, n = 60].
60. Laopaiboon M, Lumbiganon P, Martis R, et al. Music during caesarean section under regional anaesthesia for improving maternal and infant outcomes. *Cochrane Database Syst Rev.* 2009;(2):CD006914. doi(2):CD006914. [Meta-analysis: 1 RCT, n = 76].
61. Bradt J, Dileo C, Shim M. Music interventions for preoperative anxiety. *Cochrane Database Syst Rev.* 2013;(6):CD006908.
62. Cluver C, Novikova N, Hofmeyr GJ, et al. Maternal position during caesarean section for preventing maternal and neonatal complications. *Cochrane Database Syst Rev.* 2013;(3):CD007623. [Meta-analysis, 11 RCT, n = 857].
63. Li L, Wen J, Wang L, et al. Is routine indwelling catheterisation of the bladder for caesarean section necessary? A systematic review. *BJOG.* 2011;118(4):400–409. [Meta-analysis: 2 RCTs, n = 690].
64. Alexander JW, Fischer JE, Boyajian M, et al. The influence of hair-removal methods on wound infections. *Arch Surg.* 1983;118(3):347–352. [RCT, n = 1013].
65. Tanner J, Norrie P, Melen K. Preoperative hair removal to reduce surgical site infection. *Cochrane Database Syst Rev.* 2011;(11):CD004122. doi(11):CD004122. [Meta-analysis, 14 CTs, n = 3528].
66. Magann EF, Dodson MK, Ray MA, et al. Preoperative skin preparation and intraoperative pelvic irrigation: Impact on postcesarean endometritis and wound infection. *Obstet Gynecol.* 1993;81(6):922–925. [RCT, n = 50].
67. Darouiche RO, Wall MJ Jr, Itani KM, et al. Chlorhexidine-alcohol versus povidone-iodine for surgical-site antisepsis. *N Engl J Med.* 2010;362(1):18–26. [RCT, n = 849].
68. Kunkle CM, Marchan J, Safadi S, et al. Chlorhexidine gluconate versus povidone iodine at cesarean delivery: A randomized controlled trial. *J Matern Fetal Neonatal Med.* 2015;28(5):573–577. [RCT, n = 60].
69. Hadiati DR, Hakimi M, Nurdiati DS. Skin preparation for preventing infection following caesarean section. *Cochrane Database Syst Rev.* 2012;(9):CD007462. [Meta-analysis, 6 RCTs, n = 1522].
70. Ngai IM, Van Arsdale A, Govindappagari S, et al. Skin preparation for prevention of surgical site infection after cesarean delivery: A randomized controlled trial. *Obstet Gynecol.* 2015;126(6):1251–1257. [RCT, n = 1404].
71. Haas DM, Morgan S, Contreras K. Vaginal preparation with antiseptic solution before cesarean section for preventing postoperative infections. *Cochrane Database Syst Rev.* 2014;(12):CD007892. [Meta-analysis, 7 RCTs, n = 2635].
72. Pitt C, Sanchez-Ramos L, Kaunitz AM. Adjunctive intravaginal metronidazole for the prevention of postcesarean endometritis: A randomized controlled trial. *Obstet Gynecol.* 2001;98(5 Pt 1):745–750. [RCT, n = 224].
73. Cordtz T, Schouenborg L, Laursen K, et al. The effect of incisional plastic drapes and redisinfection of operation site on wound infection following caesarean section. *J Hosp Infect.* 1989;13(3):267–272. [RCT, n = 1340].
74. Ward HR, Jennings OG, Potgieter P, et al. Do plastic adhesive drapes prevent post caesarean wound infection? *J Hosp Infect.* 2001;47(3):230–234. [RCT, n = 605].
75. Wetterslev J, Meyhoff CS, Jorgensen LN, et al. The effects of high perioperative inspiratory oxygen fraction for adult surgical patients. *Cochrane Database Syst Rev.* 2015;(6):CD008884. [Meta-analysis, 28 RCTs, n = 9330].
76. Scifres CM, Leighton BL, Fogertey PJ, et al. Supplemental oxygen for the prevention of postcesarean infectious morbidity: A randomized controlled trial. *Am J Obstet Gynecol.* 2011;205(3):267.e1–267.e9. [RCT, n = 535].
77. Duggal N, Poddatoori V, Noroozkhani S, et al. Perioperative oxygen supplementation and surgical site infection after cesarean delivery: A randomized trial. *Obstet Gynecol.* 2013;122(1):79–84. [RCT, n = 831].
78. Habib AS, George RB, McKeen DM, et al. Antiemetics added to phenylephrine infusion during cesarean delivery: A randomized controlled trial. *Obstet Gynecol.* 2013;121(3):615–623. [RCT, n = 300].
79. Franchi M, Ghezzi F, Raio L, et al. Joel-Cohen or Pfannenstiel incision at cesarean delivery: Does it make a difference? *Acta Obstet Gynecol Scand.* 2002;81:1040–1046. [RCT, n = 366].
80. Mathai M, Ambersheth S, George A. Comparison of two transverse abdominal incisions for cesarean delivery. *Int J Gynaecol Obstet.* 2002;78(1):47–49. [RCT, n = 101 (411 total)].
81. Hofmeyr GJ, Mathai M, Shah A, et al. Techniques for caesarean section. *Cochrane Database Syst Rev.* 2008;(1):CD004662. doi(1):CD004662. [Meta-analysis: 8 RCTs, n = 412].
82. Mathai M, Hofmeyr GJ, Mathai NE. Abdominal surgical incisions for caesarean section. *Cochrane Database Syst Rev.* 2013;(5):CD004453. [Meta-analysis, 4 RCTs, n = 666].
83. Wylie BJ, Gilbert S, Landon MB, et al. Comparison of transverse and vertical skin incision for emergency cesarean delivery. *Obstet Gynecol.* 2010;115(6):1134–1140. [II-1].
84. Ayers JW, Morley GW. Surgical incision for cesarean section. *Obstet Gynecol.* 1987;70:706–708. [RCT, n = 97].
85. Elbohoty AE, Gomaa MF, Abdelaleim M, et al. Diathermy versus scalpel in transverse abdominal incision in women undergoing repeated cesarean section: A randomized controlled trial. *J Obstet Gynaecol Res.* 2015;41(10):1541–1546. [RCT, n = 130].
86. CORONIS Collaborative Group, Abalos E, Addo V, et al. Caesarean section surgical techniques (CORONIS): A fractional, factorial, unmasked, randomised controlled trial. *Lancet.* 2013;382(9888):234–248. [RCT, n = 15,935].
87. Berthet J, Peresse JF, Rosier P, et al. Comparative study of Pfannenstiel's incision and transverse abdominal incision in gynecologic and obstetric surgery. *Presse Med.* 1989;18(29):1431–1433. [RCT].
88. Giacalone PL, Daures JP, Vignal J, et al. Pfannesteil versus maylard incision for cesarean delivery: A randomized controlled trial. *Obstet Gynecol.* 2002;99:745–750. [RCT, n = 97].
89. Kadir RA, Khan A, Wilcock F, et al. Is inferior dissection of the rectus sheath necessary during pfannenstiel incision for lower segment caesarean section? A randomised controlled trial. *Eur J Obstet Gynecol Reprod Biol.* 2006;128(1–2):262–266. [RCT, n = 120].
90. Tappauf C, Schest E, Reif P, et al. Extraperitoneal versus transperitoneal cesarean section: A prospective randomized comparison of surgical morbidity. *Am J Obstet Gynecol.* 2013;209(4):338.e1–338.e8. [RCT, n = 54].
91. O'Neill HA, Egan G, Walsh CA, et al. Omission of the bladder flap at caesarean section reduces delivery time without increased morbidity: A meta-analysis of randomised controlled trials. *Eur J Obstet Gynecol Reprod Biol.* 2014;174:20–26. [Meta-analysis, 4 RCT, n = 581].
92. Tuuli MG, Odibo AO, Fogertey P, et al. Utility of the bladder flap at cesarean delivery: A randomized controlled trial. *Obstet Gynecol.* 2012;119(4):815–821.
93. Hohlagschwandtner M, Ruecklinger E, Husslein P, et al. Is the formation of a bladder flap at cesarean necessary? A randomized trial. *Obstet Gynecol.* 2001;98(6):1089–1092. [RCT, n = 102].
94. American College of Obstetricians and Gynecologists. ACOG practice bulletin 115: Vaginal birth after previous cesarean delivery. *Obstet Gynecol.* 2010;116(2 Pt 1):450–463. [Review].
95. Lao TT, Halpern SH, Crosby ET, et al. Uterine incision and maternal blood loss in preterm caesarean section. *Arch Gynecol Obstet.* 1993;252(3):113–117. [II-2].
96. Dodd JM, Anderson ER, Gates S, et al. Surgical techniques for uterine incision and uterine closure at the time of caesarean section. *Cochrane Database Syst Rev.* 2014;(7):CD004732. [Meta-analysis, 27 RCTs, n = 17,808].

97. Villeneuve MG, Khalife S, Marcoux S, et al. Surgical staples in cesarean section: A randomized controlled trial. *Am J Obstet Gynecol*. 1990;163(5 Pt 1):1641–1646. [RCT, n = 200].
98. Saad AF, Rahman M, Costantine MM, et al. Blunt versus sharp uterine incision expansion during low transverse cesarean delivery: A meta-analysis. *Am J Obstet Gynecol*. 2014;211(6):684. e1–684.11. [Meta-analysis, 6 RCTs, n = 2908].
99. Cromi A, Ghezzi F, Di Naro E, et al. Blunt expansion of the low transverse uterine incision at cesarean delivery: A randomized comparison of 2 techniques. *Am J Obstet Gynecol*. 2008;199(3):292. e1–292.e6. [RCT, n = 811].
100. Ozcan P, Ates S, Can MG, et al. Is cephalad-caudad blunt expansion of the low transverse uterine incision really associated with less uncontrolled extensions to decrease intra-operative blood loss? A prospective randomised-controlled trial. *J Matern Fetal Neonatal Med*. 2016;29(12):1952–1956. [RCT, n = 112].
101. Xodo S, Saccone G, Cromi A, et al. Cephalad-caudad versus transverse blunt expansion of the low transverse uterine incision during cesarean delivery: A systematic review and meta-analysis. *BJOG* 2016;202:75–80.
102. Bofill JA, Lencki SG, Barhan S, et al. Instrumental delivery of the fetal head at the time of elective repeat cesarean: A randomized pilot study. *Am J Perinatol*. 2000;17(5):265–269. [RCT, n = 44].
103. David M, Halle H, Lichtenegger W, et al. Nitroglycerin to facilitate fetal extraction during cesarean delivery. *Obstet Gynecol*. 1998;91(1):119–124. [RCT, n = 97].
104. Fasubaa OB, Ezechi OC, Orji EO, et al. Delivery of the impacted head of the fetus at caesarean section after prolonged obstructed labour: A randomised comparative study of two methods. *J Obstet Gynaecol*. 2002;22(4):375–378. [RCT, n = 108].
105. Berhan Y, Berhan A. A meta-analysis of reverse breech extraction to deliver a deeply impacted head during cesarean delivery. *Int J Gynaecol Obstet*. 2014;124(2):99–105. [Meta-analysis, 11 studies].
106. Armburst R, Hinkson L, von Weizsacker K, et al. The Charite cesarean birth: A family orientated approach of cesarean section. *J Matern Fetal Neonatal Med*. 2016;29(1):163–168. [RCT, n = 185].
107. Moore ER, Anderson GC, Bergman N, et al. Early skin-to-skin contact for mothers and their healthy newborn infants. *Cochrane Database Syst Rev*. 2012;(5):CD003519. [Meta-analysis, 34 RCTs, n = 2177].
108. Yuksel B, Ital I, Balaban O, et al. Immediate breastfeeding and skin-to-skin contact during cesarean section decreases maternal oxidative stress, a prospective randomized case-controlled study. *J Matern Fetal Neonatal Med*. 2015:1–6. [RCT, n = 90].
109. Leavitt BG, Huff DL, Bell LA, et al. Placental drainage of fetal blood at cesarean delivery and feto maternal transfusion: A randomized controlled trial. *Obstet Gynecol*. 2007;110(3):608–611. [RCT, n = 86].
110. Rabe H, Diaz-Rossello JL, Duley L, et al. Effect of timing of umbilical cord clamping and other strategies to influence placental transfusion at preterm birth on maternal and infant outcomes. *Cochrane Database Syst Rev*. 2012;(8):CD003248. [Meta-analysis, 15 RCTs, n = 738].
111. Backes CH, Rivera BK, Haque U, et al. Placental transfusion strategies in very preterm neonates: A systematic review and meta-analysis. *Obstet Gynecol*. 2014;124(1):47–56. [Meta-analysis, 12 RCTs, n = 531].
112. McDonald SJ, Middleton P, Dowswell T, et al. Effect of timing of umbilical cord clamping of term infants on maternal and neonatal outcomes. *Evid Based Child Health*. 2014;9(2):303–397. [Meta-analysis, RCT, n = 3911].
113. Munn MB, Owen J, Vincent R, et al. Comparison of two oxytocin regimens to prevent uterine atony at cesarean delivery: A randomized controlled trial. *Obstet Gynecol*. 2001;98(3):386–390.
114. Gungorduk K, Asicioglu O, Celikkol O, et al. Use of additional oxytocin to reduce blood loss at elective caesarean section: A randomised control trial. *Aust N Z J Obstet Gynaecol*. 2010;50(1):36–39. [RCT, n = 720].
115. Roach MK, Abramovici A, Tita AT. Dose and duration of oxytocin to prevent postpartum hemorrhage: A review. *Am J Perinatol*. 2013;30(7):523–528. [Review].
116. Balki M, Dhumme S, Kasodekar S, et al. Oxytocin-ergometrine co-administration does not reduce blood loss at caesarean delivery for labour arrest. *Br J Obstet Gynecol*. 2008;115:579–584. [RCT, n = 48].
117. Boucher M, Horbay GL, Griffin P, et al. Double-blind, randomized comparison of the effect of carbetocin and oxytocin on intraoperative blood loss and uterine tone of patients undergoing cesarean section. *J Perinatol*. 1998;18(3):202–207. [RCT, n = 57].
118. Dansereau J, Joshi AK, Helewa ME, et al. Double-blind comparison of carbetocin versus oxytocin in prevention of uterine atony after cesarean section. *Am J Obstet Gynecol*. 1999;180(3 Pt 1):670–676. [RCT, n = 694].
119. Conde-Agudelo A, Nieto A, Rosas-Bermudez A, et al. Misoprostol to reduce intraoperative and postoperative hemorrhage during cesarean delivery: A systematic review and meta-analysis. *Am J Obstet Gynecol*. 2013;209(1):40.e1–40.e17. [Meta-analysis, 17 RCTs, n = 3174].
120. Hua J, Chen G, Xing F, et al. Effect of misoprostol versus oxytocin during caesarean section: A systematic review and meta-analysis. *BJOG*. 2013;120(5):531–540.
121. Elsedeek MS. Impact of preoperative rectal misoprostol on blood loss during and after elective cesarean delivery. *Int J Gynaecol Obstet*. 2012;118(2):149–152. [RCT, n = 200].
122. Novikova N, Hofmeyr GJ, Cluver C. Tranexamic acid for preventing postpartum haemorrhage. *Cochrane Database Syst Rev*. 2015;(6):CD007872. [Meta-analysis, 12 RCTs, n = 3285].
123. Simonazzi G, Bisulli M, Saccone G, et al. Tranexamic acid for preventing postpartum blood loss after cesarean delivery: A systematic review and meta-analysis of randomized controlled trials. *Acta Obstet Gynecol Scand*. 2016;95(1):28–37.
124. Anorlu RI, Maholwana B, Hofmeyr GJ. Methods of delivering the placenta at caesarean section. *Cochrane Database Syst Rev*. 2008;(3):CD004737. doi: 10.1002/14651858.CD004737.pub2. [Meta-analysis: 15 RCTs, n = 4694].
125. Atkinson MW, Owen J, Wren A, et al. The effect of manual removal of the placenta on post-cesarean endometritis. *Obstet Gynecol*. 1996;87(1):99–102. [RCT, n = 643].
126. Jacobs-Jokhan D, Hofmeyr G. Extra-abdominal versus intra-abdominal repair of the uterine incision at caesarean section. *Cochrane Database Syst Rev*. 2004;(4):CD000085. [Meta-analysis: 6 RCTs, n = 1221].
127. Walsh CA, Walsh SR. Extraabdominal vs intraabdominal uterine repair at cesarean delivery: A meta-analysis. *Am J Obstet Gynecol*. 2009;200(6):625.e1–625.e8. [Meta-analysis: 11 RCTs, n = 3183].
128. Mitchell J, Stecher J, Crowson J. Uterine cooling during cesarean delivery to reduce blood loss and incidence of postpartum hemorrhage: A randomized controlled trial. *Obstet Gynecol*. 2015;125:9.–10s. [RCT, n = 200].
129. Liabsuetrakul T, Peeyananjarassri K. Mechanical dilatation of the cervix at non-labour caesarean section for reducing postoperative morbidity. *Cochrane Database Syst Rev*. 2011;(11):CD008019. doi(11): CD008019. [Meta-analysis, 3 RCTs, n = 735].
130. Stafford MK, Pitman MC, Nanthakumaran N, et al. Blunt-tipped versus sharp-tipped needles: Wound morbidity. *J Obstet Gynaecol*. 1998;18(1):18–19. [RCT, n = 203].
131. Sullivan S, Williamson B, Wilson LK, et al. Blunt needles for the reduction of needlestick injuries during cesarean delivery: A randomized controlled trial. *Obstet Gynecol*. 2009;114(2 Pt 1):211–216. [RCT, n = 194].
132. Kostu B, Ercan O, Ozer A, et al. A comparison of two techniques of uterine closure in caesarean section. *J Matern Fetal Neonatal Med*. 2016;29(10):1573–1576.
133. Yazicioglu F, Gokdogan A, Kelekci S, et al. Incomplete healing of the uterine incision after caesarean section: Is it preventable? *Eur J Obstet Gynecol Reprod Biol*. 2006;124(1):32–36. [RCT, n = 78].

134. Hohlagschwandtner M, Chalubinski K, Nather A, et al. Continuous vs interrupted sutures for single-layer closure of uterine incision at cesarean section. *Arch Gynecol Obstet.* 2003;268(1):26–28. [II-2, $n = 81$].
135. Roberge S, Demers S, Berghella V, et al. Impact of single- vs double-layer closure on adverse outcomes and uterine scar defect: A systematic review and metaanalysis. *Am J Obstet Gynecol.* 2014;211(5):453–460. [Meta-analysis, 20 RCTs, $n > 13,000$].
136. Enkin MW, Wilkinson C. Single versus two layer suturing for closing the uterine incision at caesarean section. *Cochrane Database Syst Rev.* 2000;(2). [Meta-analysis: 2 RCTs, $n = 1006$].
137. Chapman SJ, Owen J, Hauth JC. One- versus two-layer closure of a low transverse cesarean: The next pregnancy. *Obstet Gynecol.* 1997;89(1):16–18. [Follow-up of RCT].
138. Bujold E, Goyet M, Marcoux S, et al. The role of uterine closure in the risk of uterine rupture. *Obstet Gynecol.* 2010;116(1):43–50. [II-2, $n = 98$ cases of uterine rupture].
139. Gabbe S, ed. *Obstetrics: Normal and Problem Pregnancies.* 5th ed. Philadelphia, PA: Churchill Livingstone, 2007.
140. Harrigill KM, Miller HS, Haynes DE. The effect of intraabdominal irrigation at cesarean delivery on maternal morbidity: A randomized trial. *Obstet Gynecol.* 2003;101(1):80–85. [RCT, $n = 196$].
141. Viney R, Isaacs C, Chelmow D. Intra-abdominal irrigation at cesarean delivery: A randomized controlled trial. *Obstet Gynecol.* 2012;119(6):1106–1111. [RCT, $n = 236$].
142. Kiefer DG, Muscat JC, Santorelli J, et al. Effectiveness and short-term safety of modified sodium hyaluronic acid-carboxymethylcellulose at cesarean delivery: A randomized trial. *Am J Obstet Gynecol.* 2015;214(3):373.e1–373.e12. doi: S0002-9378(15)01275-2 [pii].
143. ten Broek RP, Stommel MW, Strik C, et al. Benefits and harms of adhesion barriers for abdominal surgery: A systematic review and meta-analysis. *Lancet.* 2014;383(9911):48–59. [Meta-analysis; 28 RCTs, $n = 5191$].
144. Shahin AY, Osman AM. Intraperitoneal lidocaine instillation and postcesarean pain after parietal peritoneal closure: A randomized double blind placebo-controlled trial. *Clin J Pain.* 2010;26(2):121–127. [RCT, $n = 370$].
145. Pearce C, Torres C, Stallings S, et al. Elective appendectomy at the time of cesarean delivery: A randomized controlled trial. *Am J Obstet Gynecol.* 2008;199(5):491.e1–491.e5 [RCT, $n = 93$].
146. The CAESAR Study Collaborative Group. Caesarean section surgical techniques: A randomized factorial trial. *Br J Obstet Gynecol.* 2010;117:1366–1376. [RCT, $n = 3033$].
147. Bamigboye AA, Hofmeyr GJ. Closure versus non-closure of the peritoneum at caesarean section: Short- and long-term outcomes. *Cochrane Database Syst Rev.* 2014;(8):CD000163. [Meta-analysis, 21 RCTs, $n > 17,000$].
148. Roset E, Boulvain M, Irion O. Nonclosure of the peritoneum during caesarean section: Long-term follow-up of a randomised controlled trial. *Eur J Obstet Gynecol Reprod Biol.* 2003;108(1):40–44. [Follow-up of RCT].
149. Tulandi T, Al-Jaroudi D. Nonclosure of peritoneum: A reappraisal. *Am J Obstet Gynecol.* 2003;189(2):609–612. [Review].
150. Deerenberg EB, Harlaar JJ, Steyerberg EW, et al. Small bites versus large bites for closure of abdominal midline incisions (STITCH): A double-blind, multicentre, randomised controlled trial. *Lancet.* 2015;386(10000):1254–1260. [RCT, $n = 560$].
151. Chelmow D, Rodriguez EJ, Sabatini MM. Suture closure of subcutaneous fat and wound disruption after cesarean delivery: A meta-analysis. *Obstet Gynecol.* 2004;103(5):974–980. [Meta-analysis, 3 RCTs, $n = 875$].
152. Anderson ER, Gates S. Techniques and materials for closure of the abdominal wall in caesarean section. *Cochrane Database Syst Rev.* 2004;(4):CD004663. [Meta-analysis, 7 RCTs, $n = 2056$].
153. Gates S, Anderson ER. Wound drainage for caesarean section. *Cochrane Database Syst Rev.* 2013;(12):CD004549. [Meta-analysis, 10 RCT, $n = 5248$].
154. Hellums EK, Lin MG, Ramsey PS. Prophylactic subcutaneous drainage for prevention of wound complications after cesarean delivery—A metaanalysis. *Am J Obstet Gynecol.* 2007;197(3):229–235. [Meta-analysis: 6 RCTs].
155. Mackeen AD, Berghella V, Larsen ML. Techniques and materials for skin closure in caesarean section. *Cochrane Database Syst Rev.* 2012;(11):CD003577. [Meta-analysis, 11 RCTs].
156. Mackeen AD, Schuster M, Berghella V. Suture versus staples for skin closure after cesarean: A meta-analysis. *Am J Obstet Gynecol.* 2015;212(5):621.e1–621.10. [Meta-analysis, 12 RCTs, $n = 3112$].
157. Mackeen AD, Khalifeh K, Fleisher J, et al. Suture compared with staple skin closure after cesarean delivery: A randomized controlled trial. *Obstet Gynecol.* 2014;123(6):1169–1175. [RCT, $n = 746$].
158. Roungsipragarn R, Somboonsub O. Hypertrophic cesarean section scarring: Polyglycolic acid and nylon sutures in a randomized trial. *J Obstet Gynecol.* 2001;13:19–21. [RCT, $n = 62$].
159. Murtha AP, Kaplan AL, Paglia MJ, et al. Evaluation of a novel technique for wound closure using a barbed suture. *Plast Reconstr Surg.* 2006;117(6):1769–1780. [RCT, $n = 188$].
160. Nuthalapaty FS, Lee CM, Lee JH, et al. A randomized controlled trial of early versus delayed skin staple removal following caesarean section in the obese patient. *J Obstet Gynaecol Can.* 2013;35(5):426–433. [RCT, $n = 295$].
161. Feese CA, Johnson S, Jones E, et al. A randomized trial comparing metallic and absorbable staples for closure of a pfannenstiel incision for cesarean delivery. *Am J Obstet Gynecol.* 2013;209(6):556.e1–556.e5. [RCT, $n = 100$].
162. Juergens S, Maune C, Kezze F, et al. A randomized, controlled study comparing the cosmetic outcome of a new wound closure device with prolene suture closing caesarean wounds. *Int Wound J.* 2011;8(4):329–335. [RCT, $n = 61$].
163. Short V, Herbert G, Perry R, et al. Chewing gum for postoperative recovery of gastrointestinal function. *Cochrane Database Syst Rev.* 2015;(2):CD006506. [Meta-analysis, 81 RCTs, $n = 9072$].
164. Craciunas L, Sajid MS, Ahmed AS. Chewing gum in preventing postoperative ileus in women undergoing caesarean section: A systematic review and meta-analysis of randomised controlled trials. *BJOG.* 2014;121(7):793–799; discussion 799. [Meta-analysis, 7 RCTs, $n = 1462$].
165. Zhu YP, Wang WJ, Zhang SL, et al. Effects of gum chewing on postoperative bowel motility after caesarean section: A meta-analysis of randomised controlled trials. *BJOG.* 2014;121(7):787–792. [Meta-analysis, 6 RCTs, $n = 939$].
166. Huang H, Wang H, He M. Early oral feeding compared with delayed oral feeding after caesarean section: A meta-analysis. *J Matern Fetal Neonatal Med.* 2016;29(3):423–429. [Meta-analysis, 11 RCTs, $n = 1800$].
167. Mangesi L, Hofmeyr GJ. Early compared with delayed oral fluids and food after caesarean section. *Cochrane Database Syst Rev.* 2002;(3):CD003516. [Meta-analysis, 6 RCTs, $n =$ about 500].
168. Hsu YY, Hung HY, Chang SC, et al. Early oral intake and gastrointestinal function after caesarean delivery: A systematic review and meta-analysis. *Obstet Gynecol.* 2013;121(6):1327–1334. [Meta-analysis, 17 RCTs, $n = 2966$].
169. Bamigboye AA, Hofmeyr GJ. Local anaesthetic wound infiltration and abdominal nerves block during caesarean section for postoperative pain relief. *Cochrane Database Syst Rev.* 2009;(3):CD006954. [Meta-analysis: 20 RCTs, $n = 1150$].
170. Bayoumi YA, Bassiouny YA, Hassa AA, et al. Is there a difference in the maternal and neonatal outcomes between patients discharged after 24h versus 72h following cesarean section? A prospective randomized observational study on 2998 patients. *J Matern Fetal Neonatal Med.* 2016;29(8):1339–1343. [Randomized, Observational, $n = 2998$].
171. Tan PC, Norazilah MJ, Omar SZ. Hospital discharge on the first compared with the second day after a planned cesarean delivery: A randomized controlled trial. *Obstet Gynecol.* 2012;120(6):1273–1282. [RCT, $n = 360$].
172. Wechter ME, Pearlman MD, Hartmann KE. Reclosure of the disrupted laparotomy wound: A systematic review. *Obstet Gynecol.* 2005;106(2):376–383. [Meta-analysis, 8 RCTs, $n = 324$. Includes both CDs, gyn and GI laparotomies].

173. Harris RL, Magann EF, Sullivan DL, et al. Extrafascial wound dehiscence: Secondary closure with suture versus noninvasive adhesive bandage. *J Pelvic Surg.* 1995;1:88–91. [RCT, $n = 27$].
174. Zhu BP, Rolfs RT, Nangle BE, et al. Effect of interval between pregnancies on perinatal outcomes. *N Engl J Med.* 1999;340:589–594. [Review].
175. Bujold E, Gauthier RJ. Risk of uterine rupture associated with an interdelivery interval between 18 and 24 months. *Obstet Gynecol.* 2010;115(5):1003–1006. [Retrospective, $n = 1768$].
176. Black M, Bhattacharya S, Philip S, et al. Planned cesarean delivery at term and adverse outcomes in childhood health. *JAMA.* 2015;314(21):2271–2279. [II-1].
177. Clark EA, Silver RM. Long-term maternal morbidity associated with repeat cesarean delivery. *Am J Obstet Gynecol.* 2011;205(6 Suppl):S2–S10.
178. Robson MS. Classification of caesarean sections. *Fetal Matern Med Rev.* 2001;12(1):23–39. [Review].

14

Trial of labor after cesarean delivery

Amen Ness and Amanda Yeaton-Massey

KEY POINTS

- A woman with a prior cesarean delivery (CD) has two options for mode of delivery in the subsequent pregnancy: a planned repeat cesarean delivery (PRCD) or a trial of labor after cesarean (TOLAC) to try to achieve a vaginal birth after cesarean (VBAC).
- There is insufficient evidence (no large randomized controlled trial) to compare the safety, complications, maternal, and fetal/neonatal morbidity and mortality between these two options.
- TOLAC is a "reasonable option" for most women with a single prior low transverse CD with no other contraindications to a vaginal birth.
- Absolute contraindications to TOLAC are as follows:
  - Medical or obstetrical complications that preclude vaginal delivery
  - Inability to perform emergency CD
  - Vertical (classical) uterine scar or fundal or perifundal complete (from endometrium to serosa) uterine scar from other surgery (e.g., myomectomy)
  - Prior uterine rupture
- Successful VBAC rates in the general population of women with previous low transverse uterine incisions vary from 40% to 80%.
- No screening tool is sensitive enough to be clinically useful in predicting an unsuccessful trial of labor. One available for clinical use is at www.bsc.gwu.edu/mfmu/vagbirth.html.
- Rates of **maternal and perinatal complications** are in general similar and low with both TOLAC and PRCD, except for the **risk of uterine rupture, which confers both maternal and perinatal risks.**
- Uterine rupture is the main complication associated *with TOLAC*. Most maternal and perinatal morbidity results from repeat CD after TOLAC.
- **The overall risk of uterine rupture during a TOLAC at term is 0.7% after one prior low transverse CD, versus 0.26% after PRCD.** The lowest risk (0.4%) of rupture is with spontaneous labor TOLAC. With prior VBAC, TOLAC has also a very low (about 0.5%) risk of rupture. **The risk is increased with >1 prior CD, prior vertical scar, prior rupture, induction of labor with no prior vaginal deliveries** (especially when using prostaglandin ripening agents), augmentation with higher doses of oxytocin, interval between deliveries <18 months, maternal age >30-year-old, fetal macrosomia, single-layer closure, fever at time of prior CD, etc. (Table 14.2).
- **With term uterine rupture, the risks of fetal/neonatal morbidity/mortality are** about 33% risk of **pH < 7.00**, 40% admission to neonatal intensive care unit (NICU), 6% risk of **hypoxic–ischemic encephalopathy (HIE)**, and 1.8% risk of **neonatal death** (rupture-related risk of neonatal death: **1/10,000 TOLAC**) in equipped academic centers. In other centers, these risks are higher, including risk of neonatal death from rupture up to 10%–25%.
- **Compared with PRCD, TOLAC is associated with slightly higher rates of adverse perinatal outcome:** cord pH <7.00 (1.5/1000 TOLAC), HIE (5–8/10,000 TOLAC), and perinatal death (13/10,000 with TOLAC vs. 1/10,000 for PRCD) (Table 14.3). The overall risk of adverse perinatal outcome is 1/2000 with TOLAC, slightly higher than with PRCD.
- When compared with women without a previous CD (instead of with those having a planned primary CD), the perinatal mortality for TOLAC is higher than PRCD (10/10,000 vs. 0.4/10,000 births), but this rate is twice as high as that of a non-VBAC multipara in labor and the same as that of a nullipara in labor.
- **Appropriate counseling including risks as described** should be provided to the woman with a prior CD deciding on subsequent mode of delivery. **The ultimate decision regarding TOLAC or PRCD is up to the patient.**
- **To minimize risks, an experienced obstetrician in addition to anesthesia, nursing, and operating room (OR) personnel in a facility equipped to perform emergency CD must be immediately available throughout the TOLAC.**

HISTORICAL PERSPECTIVE

Each year almost 1.5 million childbearing U.S. women have CDs. Most of these are primary CDs but, the largest single indication for CD is prior CD, accounting for over half a million CDs each year [1]. In order to reduce this trend, there is a need to both prevent the first CD and increase the rate of TOLAC in appropriate candidates.

Until the late 1970s, "Once a cesarean always a cesarean" was the general rule among most obstetricians. This phrase did not derive from formal studies and was clearly not evidence based. A classical uterine incision was used until the 1920s when the low transverse incision was first introduced. The low transverse incision was associated with a tenfold decreased rate of uterine rupture in labor than the classical incision. On the basis of studies in the 1970s, when the VBAC rate was very low, the National Institutes of Health (NIH) in 1980 and then the American College of Obstetricians and Gynecologists (ACOG) in 1988 and again in 1994 suggested that a trial of labor (TOL) after a previous low transverse CD is a reasonable option [2]. ACOG encouraged all women with a single prior low transverse cesarean section to consider a TOLAC. In response to these recommendations, the VBAC rate in the United States increased from 3.5% in 1980 to 28.3% in 1996 (Figure 14.1).

As more VBACs were attempted, more ruptures were seen and litigation for complications of a TOL also increased. In 1999, ACOG addressed these risks and added the requirements of a "readily available" physician "throughout labor" and "availability of anesthesia and personnel for emergency

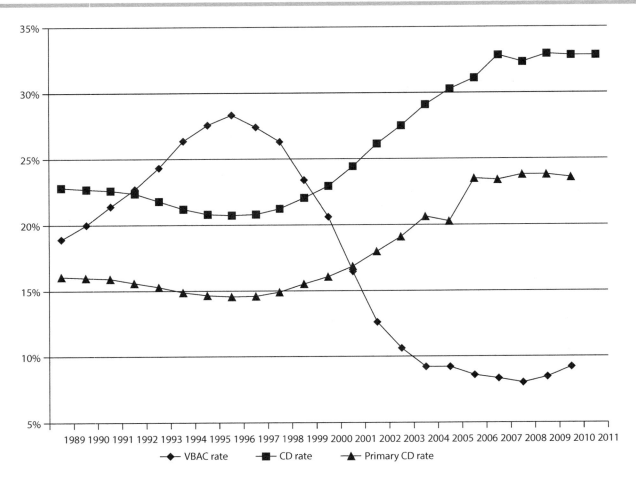

Figure 14.1 Rates of vaginal birth after cesarean (VBAC), total cesarean deliveries (CD), primary cesarean deliveries (primary CD), and repeat cesarean delivery (RCD). (From Caughey, AB et al., *Am J Obstet Gynecol*, 210(3), 179–193, 2014.)

CD." Since that time, after declining until about 1997, CDs have increased globally, 33% in the United States in 2013 and 26% in England in 2013–2014 [4,5].

At the same time, **VBAC rates have decreased rapidly to just 9% in the United States in 2011** (Figure 14.1), although they have remained relatively high in the United Kingdom at 33% (range 6%–64%) [6]. The ACOG requirement for "immediately available" personnel for women undergoing a TOLAC, but not for other laboring women, eliminated the option of TOLAC/VBAC in many community hospitals. Since 1996, about one-third of hospitals and one-half of physicians have stopped offering TOLAC/VBAC in the United States [6].

DEFINITIONS

TOLAC: Trial of labor after cesarean.
VBAC: Vaginal birth after cesarean.
PRCD: Planned repeat CD (before labor).
VBAC rate: Number of vaginal births after previous CD per 100 live births to all women with a previous CD (Same denominator as the CD rate).
TOLAC rate: If the average success rate of a TOLAC is about 70%, then the TOLAC rate is the VBAC rate/0.7.
Adjusted VBAC rate: Number of women with prior CD and no contraindications to TOL who had a VBAC per 100 live births to all women with a previous CD.
Successful VBAC rate: Percentage of women with prior CD who attempted a TOLAC achieving VBAC.
Successful adjusted VBAC rate: Percentage of women with prior CD **and no contraindications to TOLAC** achieving a VBAC.
Failed TOLAC (failed VBAC): TOLAC that results in a repeat CD.
Uterine dehiscence: Disruption of the uterine muscle **with intact serosa** [6]. It can include asymptomatic opening if the uterine scar is from prior surgery, without protrusion of fetus/fetal organs outside the uterus.
Uterine rupture: Disruption or tear of the uterine muscle and visceral peritoneum, or separation of the uterine muscle with extension to the bladder or broad ligament [6]. It includes symptomatic gross rupture of the uterine scar from prior surgery, with or without protrusion of fetus/fetal parts outside the uterus.

GENERAL CONSIDERATIONS

A woman with a prior CD has two options for mode of delivery in a subsequent pregnancy: a **PRCD or a TOLAC** to try to achieve a VBAC. There are two randomized controlled trials examining outcomes for women who underwent PRCD versus TOLAC [7,8]. Only one of these studies reported clinical outcomes and was quite small with a sample size of 22 [8]. The other, while larger, looked at maternal psychometric outcomes [7]. There is also a small prospective cohort study to compare these two options which also focuses on psychological outcomes, not maternal and fetal safety and complications [9]. Virtually all studies on VBAC, with a few exceptions [10], are retrospective and often use differing criteria for patient selection and differ in their ability to correctly ascertain (make sure all cases are included) and define uterine rupture. Most studies also include women at various gestational ages and may therefore not specifically apply to women at term considering their options of delivery after a prior CD. Studies with <1000 TOLAC cannot adequately assess maternal and fetal/neonatal morbidity and mortality, as these complications are rare, and meta-analyses [11–13] might compound errors from different retrospective studies. Many studies do not differentiate between asymptomatic uterine dehiscence and true acute symptomatic uterine rupture.

The **main issues** regarding TOLAC are the following: (1) Which women are **candidates** for TOLAC, and which should instead be recommended a PRCD? (2) Among women who attempt a TOLAC, what is the **VBAC rate** (successful TOLAC), and which factors that influence it? (3) What are the short- and long-term **maternal and perinatal benefits and harms** of attempting TOLAC versus PRCD, and what factors influence benefits and harms? Complications and safety are especially related to the risk of **uterine rupture.**

These issues are important in order to **properly counsel** women who are considering a TOLAC [6]. This information should be shared with the woman in a way best suited to her understanding. When a TOLAC and a PRCD are medically equivalent options, the woman's preference should be honored if possible [1].

CANDIDATES FOR TOLAC

The choice of candidates for TOLAC should be based on an acceptable balance between the chance of achieving a VBAC and maternal and fetal risks. The ACOG and the 2010 NIH consensus statement acknowledged that **TOLAC is a reasonable option for most women with a single prior low transverse CD with no other contraindications to a vaginal birth** [2,6]. Criteria to be a candidate, and absolute and relative contraindications for TOLAC are shown in Table 14.1.

FACTORS FOR SUCCESSFUL TOLAC

Vaginal delivery rates for TOLAC in the general population of women with previous low transverse uterine incisions vary from 60% to 80% [10,13–15]. In tertiary care centers the rates may be higher, about 73%–76% [10,16]. The rate is highly dependent on demographic and obstetric factors (Table 14.2). Based on these factors, **women with a probability for VBAC of at least 60%–70% have similar or less maternal and perinatal morbidity with a TOLAC than a PRCD** [20,33]. Conversely, women with less than a 60% probability of VBAC have a greater likelihood of morbidity with TOLAC than if they had a PRCD. One study demonstrated that composite neonatal morbidity is similar between TOLAC and PRCD for the women with the greatest probability of achieving VBAC [2,20]. Factors that influence the likelihood of VBAC after TOLAC, and their effect of success rates, are shown in Table 14.2, and described below.

Table 14.1 Candidates, and Absolute and Relative Contraindications for TOLAC

- Singleton gestation
- Clinically adequate pelvis
- One (or two) prior low transverse CD(s)
- No other uterine scars or previous rupture

Limited evidence
- A twin pregnancy who is a candidate for VBAC
- Unknown uterine scar (low clinical suspicion of prior classical uterine incision)

Absolute contraindications
- Medical or obstetrical complications that preclude vaginal delivery
- Inability to perform emergency CD
- Vertical (classical) uterine scar
- Fundal or perifundal complete (from endometrium to serosa) uterine scar from other surgery (e.g., myomectomy)
- Prior uterine rupture

Relative contraindications
- Multiple uterine scars (e.g., ≥ three prior CDs)
- Any other factor associated with a risk of rupture of >1% (see text)

Abbreviations: CDs, cesarean deliveries; TOLAC, trial of labor after CD; VBAC, vaginal birth after cesarean.

Maternal Demographics
Age
There is inconsistent evidence regarding the effect of age on successful VBAC after a TOLAC. Recent prospective studies did not show any relationship although overall there appears to be a small inverse association between maternal age and the likelihood of vaginal delivery [1].

Race/Ethnicity
Race and ethnicity are the strongest demographic predictors of VBAC. **Hispanic and African-American women have lower rates of VBAC** than non-Hispanic white women.

Obesity
Obese women attempting a VBAC have **lower vaginal delivery rates.** This appears to be true whether measured at first prenatal visit (per body mass index [BMI] unit) or at delivery (BMI > 30) (adjusted ORs [aORs] 0.94, 95% confidence interval [CI] 0.93–0.95 and 0.55, 95% CI 0.51–0.60, respectively) [17,34]. **Obese women, weighing ≥300 lb, had rates of VBAC of only 15%, while women weighing 200–300 lb had rates of 56%** [35]. **Greater maternal height and BMI < 30 kg/m2 are associated with an increased likelihood of VBAC.**

Others
Single marital status and less than 12 years of education also have been associated with lower rates of VBAC.

Obstetric History
Prior Vaginal Delivery
A prior vaginal delivery, either before or after a prior CD, is the strongest predictor of a VBAC after a TOLAC. A previous successful VBAC is the most predictive [28]. **The VBAC rate is >85% for women with a prior VBAC**, compared with 65% for women without a prior vaginal delivery [36,37]. The rate of VBAC increases with each prior VBAC [38]. Women with zero, one, two, three, and four or more prior VBACs have likelihoods of VBAC of 63%, 88%, 91%, 91%, and 91% ($p < .001$), respectively [38].

Table 14.2 Factors Associated with Success and Risk of Uterine Rupture Associated with TOLAC

Factor	Effect on Success Rates[a]	Effect on Risk of Uterine Rupture with TOLAC (% risk)	Comment (References)
Maternal Demographics			
Older age	↓	↑	
Obesity	↓↓	NA	
Obstetric History			
Prior vaginal delivery	↑↑	↓↓ (0.2%)	Especially prior VBAC. Recommend TOLAC [5,17,18]
No prior uterine scars	NA	NA (<0.01%)	
Prior nonrecurring indication for CD	↑		For example, prior CD for malpresentation [19]
Labor before primary CD		↓	
More than one prior CDs	↓	↑ (see below)	10%–15% lower success rate per CD
1 Prior LT CD (no prior VBAC)		(0.7%, range 0.5–1.0)[b]	[5,6]
1 Prior LT CD (prior VBAC)		↓ (<0.5%)	[20,21,22]
2 Prior LT CD (no prior VBAC)		↑ (1.8%, 1%–3.7%)	[13,46,47]
2 Prior LT CD (prior VBAC)		↓ (0.5%)	[46]
Prior vertical (classical) CD		↑↑ (4%–10%)	Avoid TOLAC [6]
Prior low-vertical CD		↑ (1%–2%)	[5,9]
Prior "unknown uterine scar" CD		(0.5%–2%)	[5]
1-Layer uterine closure		↑ (1%–2%)	[9,48,49][c]
Fever at prior CD		↑	If both intra- and postpartum fever
Prior preterm CD		↑ (1%)	
Prior uterine rupture		↑↑ (6% if lower segment rupture; 32% if upper segment rupture)	Avoid TOLAC [6]
Short interpregnancy interval		↑↑ (2%–5%)	<18 months; avoid TOLAC [61,62]
Current Labor Factors			
PRCD	NA	(0%–0.15% in labor) (0.5 risk of dehiscence)	[5,72]
Favorable cervical status	↑↑	↓↓	Bishop score >8, or CL <15 mm
Postdates	↓	–	Uterine rupture rate increased if induced/ augmented
Fetal macrosomia (e.g., BW >4000–4500 g)	↓	↑	Uterine rupture rate increased by relative risk 2.3 [22]
Induction/augmentation of labor	↓	↑ (mostly 1%–2%)	Avoid misoprostol; avoid PGE2 followed by oxytocin; avoid oxytocin >20 mU/minute. See below [5,51–55]
Misoprostol induction		↑↑ (>5%)	Avoid
PGE2 only induction		↑ (1%)	Cannot predict if PGE2 will be sufficient
PGE2 then oxytocin induction		↑ (1%–3%)	Probably avoid
Foley induction		–	Probably safe
Oxytocin only induction		↑ (1.1%)	
Oxytocin augmentation		↑ (0.9%)	

Abbreviations: BW, birth weight; CL, cervical length; LT, low transverse; NA, not applicable; PGE2, prostaglandin E2; PRCD, planned repeat CD.
[a]*Chance of achieving vaginal birth after CD.*
[b]*Used as reference.*
[c]*See Chapter 13.*

Prior Indication for Cesarean
Breech presentation or other **nonrecurring indication** (e.g., nonreassuring fetal monitoring) for the prior CD significantly increase the chances for a vaginal delivery (85%) compared with CD done for a recurring indication such as dystocia or failure to progress. These rates are similar to vaginal delivery rates in nulliparous women. Nevertheless, about 60%–70% of women undergoing a TOLAC for *dystocia* (failure to progress) deliver vaginally [1]. In addition, most studies show no reduction in the rates for a successful TOLAC after a **prior CD done for failure to progress in the second stage of labor** (75%–80%), with no increased risk of operative vaginal delivery [1,39–41].

Uterine Scar Type
Vaginal delivery rates appear to be *similar* for low transverse, low vertical, and for unknown incision types [12,34]. Most women with unknown scar types have had low transverse incisions.

Number of Prior CDs
Previous studies had reported that 75%–80% of women attempting a VBAC with a single prior cesarean will deliver vaginally versus about **60%–70% with more than one prior cesarean**. Recent studies have shown that **the greater the number of prior CDs, the lower the chances for a vaginal delivery (about 10%–15% lower per CD)** [12]. But a large retrospective multicenter study found similar rates of vaginal delivery after TOL in women with two versus one prior CD (75%) [42], while a recent meta-analysis of six studies that compared outcomes between women having a TOL after one or two CD found similar vaginal delivery rates of 77% and 72%, respectively [43].

Interdelivery Interval
Interdelivery interval of <18 months may be associated with similar success rates of TOL after CD compared with longer intervals [12], but in one study, rates were lower with induction [44].

Current Labor Factors
Cervical Status
Labor factors associated with a higher VBAC rate include greater cervical dilation at admission or at rupture of membranes. The more **favorable** the **cervix**, the greater the odds for a vaginal delivery. Fetal head engagement and a lower station also increase the likelihood of VBAC [1].

Gestational Age
Preterm patients with prior CD have a slightly higher VBAC success rate than term patients (82% vs. 74%) [45].

Gestational age greater than 40 weeks is associated with a decreased rate of VBAC. There is conflicting data regarding the chance of VBAC after TOLAC in *postterm* pregnancy. Successful VBAC rates of 65%–82% have been reported for women past 40 weeks, with the higher rates in women with prior vaginal deliveries [1]. In the MFMU cohort, women >41 weeks had a lower chance for vaginal delivery than women less than 41 weeks (aOR 0.61, 95% CI 0.55–0.68) [34]. **If VBAC is still desired after 40 weeks, awaiting the onset of spontaneous labor may be a better option than induction before 40 weeks for women planning a VBAC given the lower success rates with induction in this population, particularly for women with an unfavorable cervix** [34,46].

Induction/Augmentation of Labor
The overall estimated rate of vaginal birth with a TOLAC after any method of labor induction is 63% [1]. **Women with a prior CD who are induced have lower rates of successful TOLAC (about 10%) than those who labor spontaneously** [11,12,47]. Studies demonstrate that the rate of VBAC ranges from 54% for induction of labor with mechanical (transcervical balloon catheter) to 69% for induction with pharmacologic methods. There are no high-quality studies comparing VBAC rates with different induction methods [1].

Fetal Macrosomia
The most consistent infant factor associated with an increased likelihood of VBAC is birth weight less than 4000 g. As expected, large for gestational age/macrosomia, especially birth weight >4000 g, decreases the odds of a VBAC after TOLAC [48]. The success rates for VBAC in women with a previous CD and no other births is about **60% in the >4000 g group and 71% in the ≤4000 g group** [49]. There is a progressive reduction in VBAC success rates as birth weight increases. **With a prior VBAC or a vaginal delivery, there is no success rate below 63% for any of the birth weight strata. But with no previous vaginal delivery, VBAC success rates can drop below 50% as neonatal weight exceeds 4000 g** [36,48]. This success rate can decrease further if the indication for the previous CD is cephalopelvic disproportion or failure to progress. **There is limited data regarding prenatal estimated fetal birth weight and VBAC success.** Even so, VBAC rates after TOL were noted to be 60%–70% in fetuses suspected to be macrosomic [36]. This is likely due to the limitations of estimating birth weight by ultrasound. Thus, suspected macrosomia alone should not rule out a TOLAC [2].

Multiple Gestations
Vaginal delivery rates of both twins after prior CD generally range from 65% to 84% [12,50,51]. In most series, rates do not seem to differ from success rates in singletons, without increased risk for maternal morbidity or uterine rupture [50,51].

Prediction Tools for Vaginal Delivery
Given the associations above, several different scoring systems have been proposed to predict the likelihood of vaginal delivery or cesarean in women undergoing a TOLAC [17,36,45,52,53]. The best studies used scoring systems that were validated in separate data sets and in external studies [1]. These scoring systems performed as well in the validation testing as they did in the original data set. Unfortunately, although these models are accurate at predicting which women will have a VBAC, they are limited in their ability to predict who will have a repeat cesarean following a TOLAC [54,18]. Half of women with unfavorable risk factors had a vaginal delivery.

One available tool can be found at http://www.bsc.gwu.edu/mfmu/vagbirth.html but this tool only includes factors known at the beginning of pregnancy [33]. This model has been validated [55].

The authors of the NIH-sponsored review of prediction tools recommend clinicians use a sequential approach to screening [18] (Table 14.2). Initially, prenatal predictors such as previous vaginal delivery and previous indication for CD and possibly patient demographics and estimated fetal weight should be considered. This can then be modified by intrapartum predictors such as onset of spontaneous labor or the need for induction, and cervical status can be used to reevaluate the likelihood of vaginal delivery [17,54]. A variable that can be added to prediction of successful TOLAC is transvaginal ultrasound cervical length (CL) done at 19–23 weeks. Women with a CL <45mm have a 81% VBAC rate, while those with a CL ≥45mm have a 43% success rate [56].

Nevertheless, **none of these screening tools is sensitive enough to be clinically helpful in predicting an unsuccessful trial of labor, and none have been validated prospectively to improve outcomes.**

UTERINE RUPTURE
Complications and safety of TOLAC are especially related to the risk of *uterine rupture*. Uterine rupture is the most serious complication associated with TOLAC. It is defined as a complete separation through the entire thickness of the uterine wall (including serosa). At all gestational ages, pooled data from one review indicate that uterine rupture occurs in approximately 470/100,000 (0.47%, 95% CI 0.28–0.47) of women undergoing TOLAC and in 26/100,000 (0.026%, 95%

CI 0.009–0.082) of women undergoing a PRCD (RR 20.74, 95% CI 9.77–44.02; $p < 0.001$) [1]. At term, the overall risk for rupture is 778/100,000 (0.78%, 95% CI 0.62–0.96). This means that overall there are about 5 to 6 additional ruptures per 1000 in women undergoing a TOLAC [1]. No maternal deaths due to uterine rupture have been reported [1,57]. **Perinatal death occurs in about 6% of women with uterine rupture, which translates to an overall rate of intrapartum fetal death of about 20/100,000,** and a risk of perinatal death at term of about 0%–2.8% in women undergoing a TOLAC [1].

Risk Factors for Uterine Rupture

The risk for rupture is modified by a number of important factors [21] listed in Table 14.2 and described below. Prior vaginal delivery and prior VBAC reduce the risk of uterine rupture, while number of prior CDs, vertical scars, single-layer closure, induction or augmentation, greater maternal age, fever, prior preterm CD, and TOLAC at ≥40 weeks are associated with higher rupture rates.

Maternal Age

Maternal age (>30 years old) is associated with an increased risk (1.4%) of uterine rupture [22].

Prior Vaginal Delivery

Prior vaginal delivery significantly **reduces the risk for rupture during TOLAC from 1.1%, in women with no prior vaginal deliveries, to 0.2%.** After controlling for maternal demographics and labor characteristics, prior vaginal delivery reduced the risk for rupture fivefold (OR 0.2, 95% CI 0.04–0.08) [23]. This protective effect was also confirmed by recent large retrospective (OR 0.30, 95% CI 0.23–0.62) [24] and prospective (OR 0.66, 95% CI 0.45–0.95) studies [10].

Number of Prior Cesareans

Women with ≥2 prior low transverse CD may be at increased risk of uterine rupture compared with women with one prior CD, but the absolute risk is small (1.36%), while the success rate is high (71%) [43]. **Current ACOG recommendations allow this option regardless of whether there is a prior vaginal delivery** [2]. **Most ruptures occur in women undergoing induction or augmentation and in those without a prior vaginal delivery** [42]. Earlier data had indicated an overall relative increased risk of rupture (about two- to threefold) in women having a TOL after two low transverse CD compared with one [29,57,58]. A meta-analysis confirmed these findings **(0.9% one prior CD vs. 1.8% two prior CD)** [42]. A follow-up case-control analysis of the study by Macones et al. [58] showed no increased risk (OR 1.46, 95% CI 0.87–2.44), and in the MFMU cohort [21] there was no difference in the incidence of rupture after two CDs compared with one (0.9% vs. 0.7%). Furthermore, the rupture rate in women with a prior vaginal delivery and two prior CD is only 0.5%, no greater than a VBAC with only one prior CD [58].

Prior CD Characteristics

Labor Before Primary CD
Labor before the primary CD has been associated with a lower risk of uterine rupture in a future TOLAC compared with no labor before the primary CD [19].

Direction of Scar
Classical and low vertical uterine scars have higher rates of rupture compared with low transverse uterine incisions (4%–10%, and 1%–2%, respectively) [2]. **Records regarding the prior CD(s) should be obtained, with special care in documentation of direction of scar. If a woman has had a prior vertical (classical) CD, PRCD at 36 to 37 weeks is recommended** [2,30].

Layers of Closure
There is insufficient evidence to assess whether the numbers of layers performed at prior uterine closure affects the outcomes, specifically the rate of uterine rupture, for future pregnancies. Randomized trials have insufficient follow-up numbers (see Chapter 13). Compared with women who had double-layer closure, women with a single-layer closure have been reported to have anywhere from similar to a fourfold increased risk of uterine rupture compared with those with a double-layer closure [31,32,59]. One large multi-center case-controlled study that examined operative reports found a four-fold increase in uterine rupture for women with a single layer uterine closure compared with those with a double layer uterine closure (OR 3.95; 95% CI, 1.35–11.49) [31]. However, a more recent study showed no difference in uterine rupture by layers of closure (OR 1.17; 95% CI 0.78–1.76) [32].

Fever
The presence of both intrapartum and postpartum fever at CD, but not either alone, may increase the risk of uterine rupture in a subsequent pregnancy [60].

Previous Preterm CD
The Maternal-Fetal Medicine Units Network (MFMU Network) data showed a **higher risk of rupture** in women with a prior preterm CD compared with in those with a prior term CD (1% vs. 0.68%; aOR 1.6, 95% CI 1.01–2.50) [61]. No difference in rupture rates were found in a secondary analysis of the recent retrospective, multicenter cohort study comparing prior CD before and after 34 weeks (aOR 1.5, 95% CI 0.7–3.5) [62].

Prior CD for Twins
Compared with women with prior CD for singletons, women with prior CD for twins have similar risk of uterine rupture and TOLAC success [63].

Prior Uterine Rupture
As prior uterine rupture is associated with **high rates (6%–32%) of recurrent rupture** with TOLAC, these pregnancies should have a **PRCD before labor,** possibly around 36 to 37 weeks [30].

Interval between Deliveries
Interval between deliveries *of* **<18 months** is associated with an **increased risk of uterine rupture** (2.3%–4.8%) compared with longer intervals (1.1%–1.3%) in a number of studies [25,26].

Post Dates
The risk of uterine rupture does not increase substantially after 40 weeks, but is increased with induction of labor regardless of gestational age [64,65].

Preterm
In one study there was a trend toward a lower uterine rupture rate in preterm patients who attempted a VBAC [45].

In the large MFMU cohort the rates of uterine rupture and dehiscence were lower in preterm TOL versus term; 0.34% versus 0.74%, $p = .03$ and 0.26% versus 0.67%, $p = .02$ respectively [66]. On the other hand women with a very preterm delivery (<26 weeks) with a prior low transverse CD may have an increased rate of rupture with subsequent TOL compared with women with a prior term low transverse CD, 1.8% versus 0.4%, respectively [67].

Macrosomia >4000 g
Macrosomia >4000 is associated with a slightly increased risk of rupture [48]. A recent multicenter case-control study showed that birth weight >3500 g had twice the risk for rupture (OR 2.03, 95% CI 1.21–3.38) [48].

Twins
The risk of rupture or maternal mortality is not increased with prior CD and subsequent TOL with twins, with uncommon perinatal morbidity at ≥34 weeks [50,68].

Induction/Augmentation
The rate of uterine rupture in women with one prior low transverse CD undergoing TOLAC with spontaneous labor is about 0.4%. Almost all studies compare women undergoing induction with those in spontaneous labor instead of expectant management. These studies (including the large prospective MFMU observational trial) reported **higher rates of uterine rupture (up to 1%–2%) with induction** at any gestational age and of any kind [10,67,69]. There are no randomized controlled trials (RCTs) comparing these two groups but a recent meta-analysis of 8 studies comparing women with prior CD undergoing induction to those in spontaneous labor showed lower rates of vaginal delivery and higher rates of rupture among women undergoing induction but no differences in overall maternal or neonatal morbidity [70].

At term, the risk of rupture is not statistically significantly greater than women with spontaneous labor (OR 1.42, 95% CI 0.57–3.52). But women induced at >40 weeks have higher risk of rupture than those induced between 37 and 40 weeks (3.2% vs. 1.5%) [1]. In the MFMU cohort, induction increased the risk of rupture **only in women without a prior vaginal delivery** (induced 1.5%, vs. spontaneous 0.8%). In women with a prior vaginal delivery, the incidence of rupture was similar (0.6% vs. 0.4%) [46]. A recent case control study including 111 cases of uterine rupture did not find an increase in rupture compared with spontaneous labor even after controlling for labor duration. But the risk was slightly higher with an unfavorable cervix (<4cm) [71].

Recently two studies compared induction to expectant management instead of spontaneous labor, a more clinically appropriate comparison. One was a secondary analysis of the MFMU data and showed that induction had higher rates of vaginal delivery (73.8% vs. 61.3%) but also had higher rates of rupture (1.4% vs. 0.5%) [72]. The other was a secondary analysis of the Consortium on Safe Labor and found lower rates of vaginal delivery at 37–39 weeks but not at 40 weeks and no difference in uterine rupture [47].

Type of Induction
The risks of uterine rupture with induction in women who had one prior CD may also depend on the **type of induction**. Risk of rupture may be as high as **1.4%–2.5% with induction with prostaglandin** (with or without oxytocin) [10,27], and about **1.1% with oxytocin alone** [73]. The MFMU data, which included all prostaglandins, and Grobman et al. [46], which excluded misoprostol, did not find an increased risk for rupture when prostaglandins were used alone, but they did note a **threefold increased risk with sequential use of prostaglandins and oxytocin versus spontaneous labor.** The recent Cochrane review concluded that there is insufficient evidence from RCTs regarding method of induction (only two small RCTs comparing two different types of prostaglandins to oxytocin). One study was stopped due to two ruptures in the misoprostol group (2/17) [74].

ACOG therefore advises that induction with **sequential use of prostaglandins and oxytocin be avoided** [2].

ACOG considers the use of a Foley bulb for cervical ripening an acceptable method of labor induction as limited data appears to show no increased rates for rupture [2]. There are no randomized trials comparing induction to elective repeat cesarean delivery (ERCD). Women with prior CD should be made aware of these higher risks of rupture associated with induction.

Second Trimester Induction of Labor
Induction of labor in the second trimester with misoprostol is associated with **0.4% risk of uterine rupture** (with 0% risk of hysterectomy and 0.2% risk of transfusion) **after one prior low transverse CD,** and about 50% risk with a prior classical CD [75]. There is insufficient evidence to assess the safety of mifepristone induction in women with a prior CD.

Augmentation of Labor
Augmentation may be associated with an increased risk of rupture, up to about 1%, but the risk is mainly related to higher doses of oxytocin [10,74,76]. A secondary analysis of a large retrospective cohort and a follow-up nested case-control study reported a dose-response relationship between the maximum oxytocin dose and increased risk for uterine rupture (fourfold increased risk with 21–30 mU/minute vs. no oxytocin; attributable risk of 2.9%–3.6%) [76,77]. **Oxytocin should be used judiciously in women undergoing TOLAC, with a possible maximum dose of 20 mU/minute.**

BENEFITS AND HARMS ASSOCIATED WITH TOLAC

The majority of benefits and the least morbidity of a TOLAC are dependent on having a VBAC, while the potential harms of a TOLAC are associated with an unsuccessful TOLAC resulting in CD. Studies comparing TOLAC to PRCD usually include both VBAC and TOLAC ending in CD. Thus, the outcomes for women who have a TOLAC reflect both of these possibilities. These data are therefore appropriate for women with a previous CD who are deciding on the mode of delivery for the current pregnancy. Most studies show rates of all maternal and perinatal complications except rupture are infrequent and similar with both TOL and PRCD but these are small studies with few events [15,16,78,79].

One study of 2345 women with one prior CD compared outcomes among those with a planned ERCD and planned TOL and noted lower rates of serious perinatal complications (0.9% vs. 2.4%) and major maternal hemorrhage (0.8% vs. 2.3%) in the ERCD group. The vaginal delivery rate was 56.8% in the TOL group with similar rates of uterine rupture in both groups (0.1% vs. 0.2%) [8].

Maternal

Surgical Complications
Overall rates of surgical injury are low, but may be **slightly higher with TOLAC** compared with PRCD. This is primarily due to those women who have a TOLAC but deliver with a repeat CD in labor [8–10,20,80,81]. There are no studies that specifically evaluated the risks of complications due to subsequent surgery after a TOLAC or PRCD. Nevertheless, increasing number of abdominal surgeries is commonly associated with increased risks of adhesions, injury to bowel and bladder, and other complications at the time of subsequent CD or nonpregnancy-related hysterectomy (Table 14.3).

Hysterectomy
The risk of hysterectomy is about 1–2/1000 TOLAC, and similar to PRCD [9,10,13,16,27,79,82].

Transfusion
The risk of transfusion is very low, and in most studies not significantly different for TOLAC or PRCD (0.9% vs. 1.2%) [1,10]. It has been estimated at about 2 units packed red blood cells (pRBC)/1000 TOLAC [13]. The risk is higher when labor is induced with no prior vaginal deliveries, and it is related to the need for CD following a TOLAC [10].

Venous Thromboembolism
The risk is about 4/10,000 with TOLAC, similar to PRCD (1/1000) [10].

Endometritis
The risk is very similar for TOLAC or PRCD with a 6% versus 7%–8% rate of fever [11]; or 3% versus 2% in academic centers [10]. The overall absolute risk for any fever with TOLAC is 6.5% [1]. Morbid obesity, cesarean after TOLAC, and increased number of CDs increase infection rates.

Hospitalization
Overall, because most women deliver vaginally, a TOLAC results in a shorter **hospitalization** compared with PRCD. This benefit does not apply to morbidly obese women.

Maternal Mortality
The risk of **maternal mortality is lower overall for women having a TOLAC** (3–4/100,000) compared with PRCD (13.4/100,000). This compares to the overall U.S. maternal mortality rate of 11–15/100,000. At term, maternal mortality is lower: 1.9 for TOLAC versus 9.6 PRCD per 100,000 live births [1]. Based on limited evidence, mortality is lower for TOLAC in high-volume hospitals (more than 500 deliveries per year) [7].

Short-Term Satisfaction
Anxiety, depression, psychological well-being, and satisfaction scores are similar between women who choose TOLAC and those who elect for PRCD [9].

Long-Term Maternal Risks
There is a clear association between the number of CDs and abnormal placentation as well as other surgical complications [80]. This complication is an important consideration for the 28% of women who have more than two births. For each CD, the risk for placenta previa significantly increases, occurring in 900, 1,700, and 3,000 per 100,000 women who have one, two, and three or more prior CDs. The overall risk for placenta accreta also increases (0.2% in the first CD to 0.3%, 0.6%, 2.1%, 2.3%, and 6.7% for second, third, fourth, fifth, and more than or equal to sixth CD). In the presence of placenta previa, the risk for abnormal placentation is markedly increased for each additional CD (3.3%,

Table 14.3 Maternal and Perinatal Risks of TOLAC versus PRCD

	Favors	PRCD	TOLAC 1 prior CD	TOLAC ≥2 prior CDs
Maternal complications				
Uterine rupture	PRCD	1/200–250	1/111–140	1/55–140
Operative injury	PRCD	1/166–200	1/250	1/250
Hysterectomy	–	0–1/250	1/200–500	1/166
Transfusion	–	1/71–100	1/58–140	1/31
VTE	–	1/1,000	4/10,000	NA
Endometritis	–	1/47–66	1/34	1/32
Hospitalization	TOLAC			
Death	–	1/2,500–5,000	1/5,000	NA
Satisfaction	–			
Long-term risks	a			
Perinatal complications				
Stillbirth	PRCD	1/1,000	2–4/1,000	NA
Low cord pH	NA	NA	1.5/1,000	NA
Neonatal death	–	5/10,000	8/10,000	NA
Perinatal death	PRCD	1/10,000	13/10,000	NA
Respiratory morbidity	TOLAC	1–5/100	0.1–1.8/100	NA
Hyperbilirubinemia	TOLAC	5.8/100	2.2/100	NA
HIE	PRCD	1/10,000	5–8/10,000	NA

Sources: Data from American College of Obstetricians and Gynecologists, *Obstet Gynecol*, 104(1), 203–212, 2004; Landon MB et al., *N Engl J Med*, 351(25), 2581–2589, 2004; Macones GA et al., *Am J Obstet. Gynecol*, 193(5), 1656–1662, 2005; Eden KB et al., *Obstet Gynecol* 116(4), 967–981, 2010.

Abbreviations: HIE, hypoxic–ischemic encephalopathy; VTE, venous thromboembolism; NA, not available; PRCD, planned repeat cesarean delivery; CD, cesarean delivery.

Note: Some numbers may contradict each other as they are from different sources.

aSee text.

11%, 40%, and >60% for the first, second, third, and more than or equal to fourth CDs, respectively) [83]. Even without a placenta previa, the incidence of abnormal placentation, although much lower, increases with the number of CDs (see Chapter 25). **The major benefit of TOLAC is the about >70% chance of a VBAC and avoidance of multiple CDs.**

In addition, as noted above, women who undergo multiple CDs are at increased risk for many complications unrelated to placentation, including hysterectomy, adhesions, injury to bowel and bladder, transfusion of >4 units of pRBCs, need for postoperative ventilation, ICU admission, and increased operative time and hospital stay [83]. There is insufficient evidence regarding long-term pelvic floor function comparing TOLAC with PRCD. PRCD should not be used as a way to prevent pelvic floor disorders [1].

A decision analysis evaluating both the immediate and subsequent risks of the delivery decision for women with a prior CD suggested that **for women planning only one additional pregnancy, PRCD results in fewer hysterectomies than TOLAC,** while for women planning two or more additional pregnancies, a TOL provides the lowest risk [84].

Therefore, when counseling women about risks and benefits of a TOLAC compared with PRCD, the discussion should address her plans for future pregnancies.

Perinatal

The overall risk of serious **perinatal complications** is about 1 in 2000 *TOLAC*, which is **slightly greater** than that of PRCD [10]. Combining all poor perinatal outcomes, **more than 600 PRCD would need to be performed to prevent one poor perinatal outcome.** Although a woman with a TOLAC is at higher risk of uterine rupture than any other group, the risk of perinatal death is similar to that of any nulliparous woman in labor [16]. **The most serious fetal risk in women with prior CD is from uterine rupture during TOLAC.** Risks of fetal/neonatal morbidity/mortality with term uterine rupture are **33% risk of pH < 7.00, 40% admission to NICU, 6% risk of HIE, and 1.8% risk of neonatal death. The rupture-related risk of neonatal death is 1/10,000 in equipped academic centers** [10]. **In other centers, these risks are higher, including risk of neonatal death from rupture up to 10%–25%.**

Stillbirth
The rates of stillbirths are **2 to 6/1000 for TOLAC versus 1 to 2/1000 for PRCD.** At 39 weeks or more, the rate of antepartum stillbirth in the MFMU cohort was 1/1000 with TOLAC and 3/10,000 with PRCD [10,79]. This difference might be due to stillbirths occurring at ≥39 weeks with TOLAC, and/or to encouragement for TOLAC with diagnosis of stillbirth [10].

Low Cord pH
The risk of cord pH < 7.00 is about 1.5/1000 TOLAC [13].

Neonatal Death
Neonatal death rates are similar between the TOLAC and PRCD (0.08% vs. 0.05%, respectively) in academic centers, with the neonatal death rate associated with a rupture at term of about 1.8% [10].

Perinatal Death
Perinatal death rates at term (excluding malformations) are **1.3/1000 with TOLAC versus 0.5/1000 for PRCD** [11]. **Overall risk of adverse perinatal outcome is 1/2000 with TOLAC, slightly higher than with PRCD** [10]. In one study of women at term with vertex presentations, the risk of delivery-related perinatal mortality with a TOLAC was 11 times that of PRCD (OR 11.6, 95% CI 1.6–86.7). When compared with women **without a previous CD** (instead of to those having a PRCD), the **perinatal mortality for TOLAC was the same as that of a nullipara in labor,** but about twice as high as that of a non-TOLAC multipara in labor [16].

Respiratory Complications
Rates of **respiratory complications,** transient tachypnea of the newborn, and need for oxygen and ventilator support may be **slightly higher in infants delivered by PRCD versus those delivered by VBAC** [1,85]. It is unclear if there is a difference in respiratory outcomes in infants born by PRCD versus those born by repeat CD after a TOLAC.

Hypoxic–Ischemic Encephalopathy
Aside from perinatal death, HIE is the most serious adverse outcome of uterine rupture and is one of the primary concerns regarding the decision to have a TOLAC. The incidence is **46/100,000 live births for TOLAC,** versus none in the PRCD [10]. The overall risk of rupture-related HIE is 1 in 2,500 TOLAC. In term infants, the overall incidence for HIE is less than 10/100,000 live births.

MANAGEMENT

Patients with contraindications (Table 14.1) **to TOLAC should receive a PRCD at 39 weeks, or earlier if labor starts or in certain cases (e.g., prior early uterine rupture). TOLAC can be offered if the risk of uterine rupture is estimated to be <2%, possibly <1%** (Table 14.2), **and if spontaneous labor starts by 40 weeks. If the patient reaches her EDC with no labor and an unfavorable cervix, a PRCD should be recommended.**

Counseling

TOLAC can be offered to most women with a single or even two prior low transverse CDs, but several safety and success factors should be considered and discussed with the woman (Tables 14.1 through 14.3).

The composite of **maternal complications is slightly higher with TOLAC compared with PRCD group primarily due to the risk of rupture, and the increased risks of a CD in labor.** These estimates do not take into account the long-term increased risks of repeat CD and the associated risks of placenta previa and accreta. This is why **counseling should take into account how many future pregnancies are planned.**

The overall risk of serious **perinatal complications** is about 1 in 2000 *TOLAC*, which is **slightly greater** than that of PRCD [10]. Combining all poor perinatal outcomes, **more than 600 PRCD would need to be performed to prevent one poor perinatal outcome.** Although a woman with a TOLAC is at higher risk of uterine rupture than any other group, the risk of perinatal death is similar to that of any nulliparous woman in labor [16].

For the approximately 60%–80% of women having TOLAC **who will deliver vaginally,** the maternal and perinatal morbidity and mortality are lower than PRCD.

All women with a single prior low transverse CD without other indications for a CD are candidates for a TOLAC.

Women with two prior CD can also be considered for TOLAC, but induction should be avoided.

For women in whom the chance of having a vaginal delivery with a TOLAC is over 60%, the maternal and perinatal morbidity and mortality are lower than PRCD. **About 50% of women with prior CD have a 70% or higher chance of** successful VBAC (http://www.bsc.gwu.edu/mfmu/vagbirth.html), and they have no higher risk of maternal or perinatal morbidity and mortality compared with those who have PRCD. PRCD is safer than a TOLAC that results in a CD [15].

Although the overall risks of TOLAC for all women are higher than PRCD, the absolute risks are small and comparable to other potential complications of labor. Efforts to reduce the frequency of the first CD reduce the need for a TOLAC or repeat CD. Women at **lowest risk for adverse outcomes and highest chance for a vaginal delivery** include those with a prior vaginal delivery (especially a prior VBAC), in spontaneous labor, with a favorable cervix (Table 14.2). Other factors include younger age, normal BMI, prior CD for reason other than dystocia, and smaller fetus.

TOLAC should be approached with caution in those with the lowest chance of vaginal delivery and highest risk of rupture: for example, induction of labor in obese women over age 40 with an unfavorable cervix and no prior vaginal deliveries.

The ultimate decision regarding whether to have a TOLAC or PRCD should be based on the patient choice, after appropriate counseling and the availability of adequate resources and personnel to respond to obstetric emergencies. Most women should begin the decision process before term, and their decision should be documented in the medical record. The decision can then be modified at term in women to assess if spontaneous labor and/or favorable cervix make their chances of complications lower and of success higher. There is no evidence that examining the adequacy of the pelvis benefits outcomes.

Prenatal Education
Women who have had a prior CD need information and guidance to help them decide whether to have a TOL or an ERCD. Individualized prenatal education directed toward avoidance of a PRCD does not increase the rate of VBAC [86]. The Cochrane review evaluated three RCTs of decision support tools to help assist women in choosing ERCD or TOLAC and found no differences in the planned mode of birth or the percentage of women who remained unsure about their final decision [87]. A subsequent RCT showed that interactive or written evidenced based decision tools helped reduce conflict around the birth decision compared with baseline [88]. A recent study surveying a **woman's level of knowledge** prior to TOLAC or ERCD showed most women had a poor understanding of the risks, benefits and likelihood of success of either option; they also were most likely to choose the mode of delivery favored by their provider [89].

Consent
Specific consent for TOL after CD or PRCD should be signed by the woman after appropriate counseling.

Checklist
A patient safety checklist is publicly available through ACOG at http://www.acog.org/-/media/Patient-Safety-Checklists/psc009.pdf?la=en.

Nonvertex Presentation
External cephalic version (ECV) can safely be performed in women with a prior CD. The success rate for ECV is similar or higher in women with a prior CD compared with controls without a prior CD (82% vs. 61%) [90]. Women with a successful version have successful VBAC rates of 65%–76% [90,91].

Ultrasound of Lower Uterine Segment
Due to the uncommon nature of rupture, several thousand women need to be studied to assess whether measuring the thickness of the lower uterine segment predicts complications in women with a prior CD who elect TOLAC, and therefore there is insufficient evidence to assess the clinical utility of this screening test. No women with a lower uterine segment thickness of ≥4.5 mm in the late third trimester seem to have dehiscence or rupture, while the proportion of these complications rises as this thickness decreases, with **women with large defects, or lower uterine thickness <3.5 mm (especially <2.0 mm), or myometrial layer <2.0 mm (especially <1.4 mm) in the third trimester, possibly benefiting from PRCD** [29,73]. A recent meta-analysis of 21 studies looking at data for 2776 women provided support for using ultrasound measurement of the lower uterine segment in assessing for the presence of a uterine defect [92].

Requirements to Minimize Risks [1]
To minimize risks, the following must be immediately available throughout TOLAC:

- Experienced obstetrician
- Anesthesia
- Nursing and OR personnel
- Ability to perform emergency CD

Labor and delivery units with >500 to 1000 births per year have lower risks of uterine rupture and complications compared with units with less volume [9,88]. If centers cannot provide the above resources, this does not mean TOLAC should not be offered. Referral should be made to adequate facilities early during prenatal care so that TOLAC is safely available.

Detecting and Managing Rupture Intrapartum
Fetal heart rate (FHR) disturbances are the most common (but not universal) sign of uterine rupture (55%–85%) [93]. The most commonly reported FHR disturbance is repetitive progressively severe variable decelerations and prolonged bradycardia, although in most cases they are not caused by rupture. Nevertheless, **in women with a prior CD, in the presence of such FHR disturbances, uterine rupture must be considered.**

Abdominal pain over the area of the prior uterine scar is a poor predictor of uterine rupture. Epidural usually does not mask rupture. Epidural should not be withheld in women attempting TOL after prior CD. Intrauterine pressure catheter (IUPC) monitoring has not been shown to be helpful [94]. Significant loss of fetal station especially in the second stage may occur with rupture, but is of limited predictive value. There is insufficient data to assess the utility of uterine exploration after a successful VBAC.

Neonates delivered within 18 minutes after a suspected uterine rupture have the best outcome, with all normal umbilical pH levels and 5-minute Apgar scores in a recent series, while those with a decision-to-delivery time >30 minutes have poor outcomes [95].

Cost-Effectiveness
Multiple cost-effectiveness analyses have been performed to examine the relative cost of TOLAC versus PRCD. For women with at least a 47% likelihood of successful vaginal delivery TOLAC appears to be more cost-effective than ERCD [96,97]. In a recent analysis, TOLAC has similar cost-effectiveness for the first TOL but becomes less costly and more effective with subsequent deliveries [98].

REFERENCES

1. Guise JM, Eden K, Emeis C, et al. Vaginal birth after cesarean: New insights. *Evid Rep Technol Assess (Full Rep)*. 2010;(191): 1–397. [Review]
2. American College of Obstetricians and Gynecologists. ACOG Practice Bulletin No. 54: Vaginal birth after previous cesarean. *Obstet Gynecol*. 2004;104(1):203–212. [Review]
3. Caughey AB, Cahill AG, Guise JM, et al. for American College of Obstetricians and Gynecologists, Society for Maternal-Fetal Medicine. Safe prevention of the primary cesarean delivery. *Am J Obstet Gynecol*. 2014;210(3):179–193. [III]
4. Martin JA, Hamilton BE, Osterman MJ, et al. Births: Final data for 2013. *Natl Vital Stat Rep*. 2015;64(1):1–65. [Epidemiologic data]
5. Hospital Episode Statistics. NHS Maternity StatisticsEngland, 2013–14. Available at: http://digital.nhs.uk/catalogue/PUB16725. Accessed on August 31, 2016. [Epidemiologic data]
6. National Institutes of Health. National Institutes of Health Consensus Development Conference Statement: Vaginal birth after cesarean: New insights March 8–10, 2010. *Semin Perinatol*. 2010;34(5):351–365. [Review]
7. Law LW, Pang MW, Chung TK, et al., Randomised trial of assigned mode of delivery after a previous cesarean section—Impact on maternal psychological dynamics. *J Matern Fetal Neonatal Med*. 2010;23(10):1106–1113. [RCT, n = 298]
8. Crowther CA, Dodd JM, Hiller JE, et al. Planned vaginal birth or elective repeat caesarean: Patient preference restricted cohort with nested randomised trial. *PLoS Med*. 2012;9(3):e1001192. [RCT, n = 22]
9. McMahon MJ, Luther ER, Bowes WA Jr, et al. Comparison of a trial of labor with an elective second cesarean section. *N Engl J Med*. 1996;335(10):689–695. [II-2, n = 6138]
10. Landon MB, Hauth JC, Leveno KJ, et al. Maternal and perinatal outcomes associated with a trial of labor after prior cesarean delivery. *N Engl J Med*. 2004;351(25):2581–2589. [II-2, n = 33,699]
11. Guise JM, Berlin M, McDonagh M, et al. Safety of vaginal birth after cesarean: A systematic review. *Obstet Gynecol*. 2004;103(3):420–429. [Review]
12. Guise JM, Hashima J, Osterweil P. Evidence-based vaginal birth after caesarean section. *Best Pract Res Clin Obstet Gynaecol*. 2005;19(1):117–130. [Review]
13. Chauhan SP, Martin JN Jr, Henrichs CE, et al. Maternal and perinatal complications with uterine rupture in 142,075 patients who attempted vaginal birth after cesarean delivery: A review of the literature. *Am J Obstet Gynecol*. 2003;189(2):408–417. [Review]
14. Knight HE, Gurol-Urganci I, van der Meulen JH, et al. Vaginal birth after caesarean section: A cohort study investigating factors associated with its uptake and success. *BJOG*. 2014;121(2): 183–192. [II-2]
15. Miller DA, Diaz FG, and Paul RH. Vaginal birth after cesarean: A 10-year experience. *Obstet Gynecol*. 1994;84(2):255–258. [II-2, n = 17,322]
16. Smith GC, Pell JP, Cameron AD, Dobbie R, et al. Risk of perinatal death associated with labor after previous cesarean delivery in uncomplicated term pregnancies. *JAMA*. 2002;287(20):2684–2690. [II-2, n = 15,515]
17. Grobman WA, Lai Y, Landon MB, et al., Development of a nomogram for prediction of vaginal birth after cesarean delivery. *Obstet Gynecol*. 2007;109(4):806–812. [II-2; prospective, n = 7660]
18. Eden KB, McDonagh M, Denman MA, et al. New insights on vaginal birth after cesarean: Can it be predicted? *Obstet Gynecol*. 2010;116(4):967–981. [Meta-analysis, 203 total, 16 using scored models]
19. Algert CS, Morris JM, Simpson JM, et al. Labor before a primary cesarean delivery: Reduced risk of uterine rupture in a subsequent trial of labor for vaginal birth after cesarean. *Obstet Gynecol*. 2008;112(5):1061–1066. [II-1]
20. Cahill AG, Stamilio DM, Odibo AO, et al. Is vaginal birth after cesarean (VBAC) or elective repeat cesarean safer in women with a prior vaginal delivery? *Am J Obstet Gynecol*. 2006;195(4):1143–1147. [II-2, n = 6619]
21. Landon MB, Spong CY, Thom E, et al. Risk of uterine rupture with a trial of labor in women with multiple and single prior cesarean delivery. *Obstet Gynecol*. 2006;108(1):12–20. [II-2; prospective, n = 17,898]
22. Shipp TD, Zelop C, Repke JT, et al. The association of maternal age and symptomatic uterine rupture during a trial of labor after prior cesarean delivery. *Obstet Gynecol*. 2002;99(4):585–588. [II-2]
23. Zelop CM, Shipp TD, Repke JT, et al. Effect of previous vaginal delivery on the risk of uterine rupture during a subsequent trial of labor. *Am J Obstet Gynecol*. 2000;183(5):1184–1186. [II-2]
24. Macones GA, Cahill AG, Stamilio DM, et al. Can uterine rupture in patients attempting vaginal birth after cesarean delivery be predicted? *Am J Obstet Gynecol*. 2006;195(4):1148–1152. [II-2]
25. Shipp TD, Zelop CM, Repke JT, et al. Interdelivery interval and risk of symptomatic uterine rupture. *Obstet Gynecol*. 2001;97(2): 175–177. [II-2, n = 2409]
26. Bujold E, Gauthier RJ. Risk of uterine rupture associated with an interdelivery interval between 18 and 24 months. *Obstet Gynecol*. 2010;115(5):1003–1006. [II-2, n = 1768]
27. Lydon-Rochelle MT, Cahill AG, Spong C.Y. Birth after previous cesarean delivery: Short-term maternal outcomes. *Semin Perinatol*. 2010;34(4):249–257. [Review]
28. Hendler I, Bujold E. Effect of prior vaginal delivery or prior vaginal birth after cesarean delivery on obstetric outcomes in women undergoing trial of labor. *Obstet Gynecol*. 2004;104(2):273–277. [II-2, n = 2204]
29. Caughey AB, Shipp TD, Repke JT, et al. Rate of uterine rupture during a trial of labor in women with one or two prior cesarean deliveries. *Am J Obstet Gynecol*. 1999;181(4):872–876. [II-2, n = 3981]
30. Spong CY, Mercer BM, D'alton M, et al. Timing of indicated late-preterm and early-term birth. *Obstet Gynecol*. 2011;118(2 Pt 1):323–333. [Review]
31. Bujold E, Goyet M, Marcoux S, et al. The role of uterine closure in the risk of uterine rupture. *Obstet Gynecol*. 2010;116(1):43–50. [II-2]
32. Hesselman S, Högberg U, Ekholm-Selling K, et al. The risk of uterine rupture is not increased with single-compared with double-layer closure: A Swedish cohort study. *BJOG*. 2015;122 (11):1535–1541. [II-2]
33. Grobman WA, Lai Y, Landon MB, et al. Can a prediction model for vaginal birth after cesarean also predict the probability of morbidity related to a trial of labor? *Am J Obstet Gynecol*. 2009; 200(1):56.e1–e6. [Review: Prediction]
34. Landon MB, Leindecker S, Spong CY, et al. The MFMU Cesarean Registry: Factors affecting the success of trial of labor after previous cesarean delivery. *Am J Obstet Gynecol*. 2005;193(3 Pt 2): 1016–1023. [II-2; prospective, n = 14,529]
35. Durnwald CP, Ehrenberg HM, Mercer BM. The impact of maternal obesity and weight gain on vaginal birth after cesarean section success. *Am J Obstet Gynecol*. 2004;191(3):954–957. [II-2, n = 510]
36. Flamm BL, Geiger AM. Vaginal birth after cesarean delivery: An admission scoring system. *Obstet Gynecol*. 1997;90(6): 907–910. [II-2]
37. Caughey AB, Shipp TD, Repke JT, et al. Trial of labor after cesarean delivery: The effect of previous vaginal delivery. *Am J Obstet Gynecol*. 1998;179(4):938–941. [II-2, n = 800]
38. Mercer BM, Gilbert S, Landon MB, et al. Labor outcomes with increasing number of prior vaginal births after cesarean delivery. *Obstet Gynecol*. 2008;111(2 Pt 1):285–291. [II-2; prospective, n = 13,532]
39. Jongen VH, Halfwerk MG, Brouwer WK. Vaginal delivery after previous caesarean section for failure of second stage of labour. *Br J Obstet Gynaecol*. 1998;105(10):1079–1081. [II-2]
40. Kwon JY, Jo YS, Lee GS, et al. Cervical dilatation at the time of cesarean section may affect the success of a subsequent vaginal delivery. *J Matern Fetal Neonatal Med*. 2009;22(11):1057–1062. [II-2]

41. Lewkowitz AK, Nakagawa S, Thiet MP, Rosenstein MG. Effect of stage of initial labor dystocia on vaginal birth after cesarean success. *Am J Obstet Gynecol.* 2015;213(6):861.e1–e5. [II-2, n = 238]
42. Macones GA, Peipert J, Nelson DB, et al. Maternal complications with vaginal birth after cesarean delivery: A multicenter study. *Am J Obstet Gynecol.* 2005;193(5):1656–1662. [II-2; multicenter, n = 25,005]
43. Tahseen S, Griffiths M. Vaginal birth after two caesarean sections (VBAC-2)—A systematic review with meta-analysis of success rate and adverse outcomes of VBAC-2 versus VBAC-1 and repeat (third) caesarean sections. *BJOG.* 2010;117(1):5–19. [Meta-analysis, 20 studies]
44. Huang WH, Nakashima DK, Rumney PJ, et al. Interdelivery interval and the success of vaginal birth after cesarean delivery. *Obstet Gynecol.* 2002;99(1):41–44. [II-2]
45. Quinones JN, Stamilio DM, Paré E, et al. The effect of prematurity on vaginal birth after cesarean delivery: Success and maternal morbidity. *Obstet Gynecol.* 2005;105(3):519–524. [II-2]
46. Grobman WA, Gilbert S, Landon MB, et al. Outcomes of induction of labor after one prior cesarean. *Obstet Gynecol.* 2007;109(2 Pt 1):262–269. [II-2; prospective, n = 11,778]
47. Lappen JR, Hackney DN, Bailit JL. Outcomes of term induction in trial of labor after cesarean delivery: Analysis of a modern obstetric cohort. *Obstet Gynecol.* 2015;126(1):115–123. [II-2]
48. Elkousy MA, Sammel M, Stevens E, et al. The effect of birth weight on vaginal birth after cesarean delivery success rates. *Am J Obstet Gynecol.* 2003;188(3):824–830. [II-2, n = 9,960]
49. Zelop CM, Shipp TD, Repke JT, et al. Outcomes of trial of labor following previous cesarean delivery among women with fetuses weighing >4000 g. *Am J Obstet Gynecol.* 2001;185(4):903–905. [II-2]
50. Varner MW, Leindecker S, Spong CY, et al. The Maternal-Fetal Medicine Units Cesarean Registry: Trial of labor with a twin gestation. *Am J Obstet Gynecol.* 2005;193(1):135–140. [II-2, n = 186]
51. Cahill A. Stamilio DM, Paré E, et al. Vaginal birth after cesarean (VBAC) attempt in twin pregnancies: Is it safe? *Am J Obstet Gynecol.* 2005;193(3 Pt 2):1050–1055. [II-2, n = 535]
52. Hashima JN, Eden KB, Osterweil P, et al. Predicting vaginal birth after cesarean delivery: A review of prognostic factors and screening tools. *Am J Obstet Gynecol.* 2004;190(2):547–555. [Review: Prediction]
53. Dinsmoor MJ, Brock EL. Predicting failed trial of labor after primary cesarean delivery. *Obstet Gynecol.* 2004;103(2):282–286. [Review: Prediction]
54. Metz TD, Stoddard GJ, Henry E, et al. Simple, validated vaginal birth after cesarean delivery prediction model for use at the time of admission. *Obstet Gynecol.* 2013;122(3):571–578. [II-2]
55. Constatine M, Fox K, Byers B et.al. Validation of the prediction model for success of vaginal birth after cesarean. *Obstet Gynecol.* 2009;114:1029–33. [II-3]
56. Nicholas SS, Orzechowski KM, Berghella, et al. Second trimester cervical length and its association with vaginal birth after cesarean delivery. *Am J Perinatol.* 2016;33(1):20–3. [II-2]
57. Guise JM, McDonagh MS, Osterweil P, et al. Systematic review of the incidence and consequences of uterine rupture in women with previous caesarean section. *BMJ.* 2004;329(7456):19–25. [Review]
58. Macones GA, Cahill A, Pare E, et al. Obstetric outcomes in women with two prior cesarean deliveries: Is vaginal birth after cesarean delivery a viable option? *Am J Obstet Gynecol.* 2005;192 (4):1223–1228; discussion 1228–1229. [II-2, n = 20,175 with 1 prior CD and 3970 with 2 prior CD]
59. Bujold E, Bujold C, Hamilton EF, et al. The impact of a single-layer or double-layer closure on uterine rupture. *Am J Obstet Gynecol.* 2002;186(6):1326–1330. [II-2, n = 1980 with 1 or 2 layers]
60. Shipp TD, Zelop C, Cohen A, et al. Post-cesarean delivery fever and uterine rupture in a subsequent trial of labor. *Obstet Gynecol.* 2003;101(1):136–139. [II-2, n = 2409]
61. Sciscione AC, Landon MB, Leveno KJ, et al. Previous preterm cesarean delivery and risk of subsequent uterine rupture. *Obstet Gynecol.* 2008;111(3):648–653. [II-2; prospective, n = 41,367]
62. Harper LM, Cahill AG, Stamilio DM, et al. Effect of gestational age at the prior cesarean delivery on maternal morbidity in subsequent VBAC attempt. *Am J Obstet Gynecol.* 2009;200(3):276. e1–e6. [II-2]
63. Varner MW, Thom E, Spong CY, et al. Trial of labor after one previous cesarean delivery for multifetal gestation. *Obstet Gynecol.* 2007;110(4):814–819. [II-1]
64. Zelop CM, Shipp TD, Cohen A, et al. Trial of labor after 40 weeks' gestation in women with prior cesarean. *Obstet Gynecol.* 2001;97(3):391–393. [II-2]
65. Coassolo KM, Stamilio DM, Paré E, et al. Safety and efficacy of vaginal birth after cesarean attempts at or beyond 40 weeks of gestation. *Obstet Gynecol.* 2005;106(4):700–706. [II-2]
66. Durnwald CP, Rouse DJ, Leveno DJ, Gabbe SG. The Maternal-Fetal Medicine Units Cesarean Registry: Safety and efficacy of a trial of tabor in preterm pregnancy after a prior cesarean delivery. *Am J Obstet Gynecol.* 2006;195(4):1119–1126. [II-2, n= 510]
67. Lannon SM, Guthrie KA, Vanderhoeven JP, et al. Uterine rupture risk after periviable cesarean delivery. *Obstet Gynecol.* 2015;125(5):1095–1100. [II-2]
68. Aaronson D, Harlev A, Sheiner Eet al. Trial of labor after cesarean section in twin pregnancies: Maternal and neonatal safety. *J Matern Fetal Neonat Med.* 2010;23(6):550–554. [II-2]
69. McDonagh MS, Osterweil P, Guise JM. The benefits and risks of inducing labour in patients with prior caesarean delivery: A systematic review. *BJOG*, 2005;112(8):1007–1015. [Review]
70. Rossi AC, Prefumo F. Pregnancy outcomes of induced labor in women with previous cesarean section: A systematic review and meta-analysis. *Arch Gynecol Obstet.* 2015;291(2):273–380. [Meta-analysis]
71. Harper LM, Cahill AG, Boslaugh S, et al. Association of induction of labor and uterine rupture in women attempting vaginal birth after cesarean: A survival analysis. *Am J Obstet Gynecol.* 2012;206(1):51.e1–e5. [II-2]
72. Palatnik A, Grobman WA. Induction of labor versus expectant management for women with a prior cesarean delivery. *Am J Obstet Gynecol.* 2015;212(3):358.e1–e6. [II-2]
73. Bujold E, Jastrow N, Simoneau J, et al. Prediction of complete uterine rupture by sonographic evaluation of the lower uterine segment. *Am J Obstet Gynecol.* 2009;201(3):320.e1–e6. [II-2]
74. Jozwiak M, Dodd JM. Methods of term labour induction for women with a previous caesarean section. *Cochrane Database Syst Rev.*2013;(3):CD009792. [Cochrane review]
75. Berghella V, Airoldi J, O'Neill AM, et al. Misoprostol for second trimester pregnancy termination in women with prior caesarean: A systematic review. *BJOG.* 2009;116(9):1151–1157. [Review]
76. Cahill AG, Waterman BM, Stamilio DM, et al. Higher maximum doses of oxytocin are associated with an unacceptably high risk for uterine rupture in patients attempting vaginal birth after cesarean delivery. *Am J Obstet Gynecol.* 2008;199(1): 32.e1–e5. [II-2]
77. Cahill AG, Stamilio DM, Odibo AO, et al. Does a maximum dose of oxytocin affect risk for uterine rupture in candidates for vaginal birth after cesarean delivery? *Am J Obstet Gynecol.* 2007;197(5):495.e1–e5. [II-2, n = 13,523]
78. Nair M, Soffer K, Noor N, et al. Selected maternal morbidities in women with a prior caesarean delivery planning vaginal birth or elective repeat caesarean section: A retrospective cohort analysis using data from the UK Obstetric Surveillance System. *BMJ Open.* 2015;5(6):e007434. [II-2]
79. Dodd JM, Crowther CA, Huertas E, et al. Planned elective repeat caesarean section versus planned vaginal birth for women with a previous caesarean birth. *Cochrane Database Syst Rev.* 2013;(12):CD004224. [Cochrane review]

80. Silver RM, Landon MB, Rouse DJ, et al. Maternal morbidity associated with multiple repeat cesarean deliveries. *Obstet Gynecol.* 2006;107(6):1226–1232. [II-2, n = 30,132]
81. Spong CY, Landon MB, Gilbert S, et al. Risk of uterine rupture and adverse perinatal outcome at term after cesarean delivery. *Obstet Gynecol.* 2007;110(4):801–807. [II-2; prospective, n = 39,117]
82. Wen SW, Rusen ID, Walker M, et al. Comparison of maternal mortality and morbidity between trial of labor and elective cesarean section among women with previous cesarean delivery. *Am J Obstet Gynecol.* 2004;191(4):1263–1269. [II-2, n = 308,755 with 5839 prior preterm CD]
83. Silver RM. Delivery after previous cesarean: Long-term maternal outcomes. *Semin Perinatol.* 2010;34(4):258–266. [Review]
84. Pare E, Quiòones JN, Macones GA. Vaginal birth after caesarean section versus elective repeat caesarean section: Assessment of maternal downstream health outcomes. *BJOG.* 2006;113(1):75–85. [II-2]
85. Kamath BD, Todd JK, Glazner JE, et al. Neonatal outcomes after elective cesarean delivery. *Obstet Gynecol.* 2009;113(6):1231–1238. [II-1]
86. Fraser W, Maunsell E, Hodnett E, et al. Randomized controlled trial of a prenatal vaginal birth after cesarean section education and support program. Childbirth Alternatives Post-Cesarean Study Group. *Am J Obstet Gynecol.* 1997;176(2):419–425. [RCT, n = 1275]
87. Horey D, Kealy M, Davey MA, et al. Interventions for supporting pregnant women's decision-making about mode of birth after a caesarean. *Cochrane Database Syst Rev.* 2013;(7):CD010041. [Cochrane review]
88. Eden KB, Perrin NA, Vesco KK, et al. A randomized comparative trial of two decision tools for pregnant women with prior cesareans. *J Obstet Gynecol Neonatal Nurs.* 2014;43(5):568–579. [RCT, n = 131]
89. Bernstein SN, Matalon-Grazi S, Rosenn BM. Trial of labor versus repeat cesarean: Are patients making an informed decision? *Am J Obstet Gynecol.* 2012;207(3):204.e1–e6. [II-2, n = 155 with 87 TOL and 68 PRCD]
90. Flamm BL, Fried MW, Lonky NM, et al. External cephalic version after previous cesarean section. *Am J Obstet Gynecol.* 1991;165(2):370–372. [II-2]
91. de Meeus JB, Ellia F, Magnin G. External cephalic version after previous cesarean section: A series of 38 cases. *Eur J Obstet Gynecol Reprod Biol.* 1998;81(1):65–68. [II-2]
92. Kok N, Wiersma IC, Opmeer BC, et al. Sonographic measurement of lower uterine segment thickness to predict uterine rupture during a trial of labor in women with previous cesarean section: A meta-analysis. *Ultrasound Obstet Gynecol.* 2013;42(2):132–139. [Meta-analysis]
93. Ridgeway JJ, Weyrich DL, Benedetti TJ. Fetal heart rate changes associated with uterine rupture. *Obstet Gynecol.* 2004;103(3):506–512. [II-2]
94. Devoe LD, Croom CS, Youssef AA, Murray C. The prediction of "controlled" uterine rupture by the use of intrauterine pressure catheters. *Obstet Gynecol.* 1992;80(4):626–629. [II-2]
95. Holmgren C, Scott JR, Porter TF, et al. Uterine rupture with attempted vaginal birth after cesarean delivery: Decision-to-delivery time and neonatal outcome. *Obstet Gynecol.* 2012;119(4):725–731. [Meta-analysis]
96. Gilbert SA, Grobman WA, Landon MB, et al. Cost-effectiveness of trial of labor after previous cesarean in a minimally biased cohort. *Am J Perinatol.* 2013;30(1):11–20. [Cost-effectiveness analysis]
97. Gilbert SA, Grobman WA, Landon MB, et al. Lifetime cost-effectiveness of trial of labor after cesarean in the United States. *Value Health.* 2013;16(6):953–964. [Cost-effectiveness analysis]
98. Wymer KM, Shih YCT, Plunkett BA. The cost-effectiveness of a trial of labor accrues with multiple subsequent vaginal deliveries. *Am J Obstet Gynecol.* 2014;211(1):56.e1–56.e12. [Cost-effectiveness analysis]

Early pregnancy loss

Lisa K. Perriera, Beatrice A. Chen, and Aileen M. Gariepy

KEY POINTS

- The diagnosis of early (e.g., first trimester) pregnancy loss may be suspected based on symptoms, but is usually made by **transvaginal ultrasound,** and/or serial beta human chorionic gonadotrophin (BHCG) levels.
- **Early pregnancy loss (EPL)** is an inclusive term that comprises the following: incomplete, inevitable, or complete spontaneous abortion (SAB); anembryonic gestation (blighted ovum); and embryonic/fetal demise (missed abortion). Early pregnancy failure (EPF) is a term that should be avoided as it contributes to internalization of blame for patients.
- There are **three options** for management of EPL: **expectant, medical, and surgical management.** Choice of management for EPL **does not affect future fertility.**
- **Patient preference should guide treatment choice.**
- **Successful management** of EPL consists of complete evacuation of the uterus. The success of each management option depends on several factors, for example, the type of loss (e.g., with or without symptoms).
- Threatened pregnancy loss can be defined as vaginal bleeding in pregnancy before 20 weeks of gestation. Several **interventions** have been studied, but **none has been confirmed to be beneficial.**

Medical management

- **Medical management** is a **safe and effective** alternative to expectant management or surgical curettage for EPL.
- Medical management of EPL is more effective than expectant management.
- **Misoprostol 800 µg vaginally, with a repeat dose on day 3 if complete evacuation is not confirmed,** has a success rate of 93% **with incomplete or inevitable abortion, 88% with embryonic or fetal death, and 81% with anembryonic gestation** in women at **<13 weeks** of gestation.
- Misoprostol 800 µg vaginally is the most studied regimen for medical management of EPL. Success of medical management of EPL increases with **multiple dose** regimens. Whether there is added benefit from adding **mifepristone** to misoprostol is still uncertain.
- Women choosing medical management of EPL report an **average of 12 days of bleeding.** Hemorrhage after medical management of EPL is rare.
- **Follow-up:** Transvaginal ultrasound after medical management of EPL can be used to **confirm successful expulsion of the gestational sac. Measurement of endometrial thickness is not predictive of success.**
- **Advantages of medical management** of EPL: Avoidance of surgery and anesthesia, perception of more natural treatment, increased privacy, and increased control.

Surgical management

- Surgical management has a high (>97%) success rate.
- Endometritis or hemorrhage rates are <1%.
- Maternal safety is highest with vacuum aspiration, when regional or general anesthesia can be avoided.

DEFINITIONS

- **Pregnancy loss (PL):** Spontaneous loss of pregnancy from conception to <20 weeks.
- **Miscarriage:** Lay term signifying PL.
- **Early pregnancy loss:** Inclusive medical term describing inevitable abortion, incomplete abortion, anembryonic pregnancy, and embryonic/fetal demise at **<14 weeks** [1]. It can also be called "first-trimester" PL. Early first-trimester PL is a loss of pregnancy between conception and 9 6/7 weeks. Late first-trimester PL is a loss of pregnancy between 10 and 13 6/7 weeks. The terms EPL, miscarriage, and SAB are often used interchangeably in the first trimester [2].
  - **Spontaneous abortion** (aka loss): The term **spontaneous abortion** is often used as an equivalent term for EPL but should be avoided since women may associate negative feelings with this term. This guideline does not discuss voluntary (elective) termination (induced abortion).
  - **Complete abortion:** Clinical definition describing an EPL that is characterized by a history of a positive pregnancy test, vaginal bleeding with passage of tissue, and a closed cervical os at the time of diagnosis. Transvaginal ultrasound examination shows absence of a gestational sac.
  - **Incomplete abortion:** Clinical definition describing a history of positive pregnancy test, vaginal bleeding, and a cervical os that is open. Transvaginal ultrasound examination shows heterogeneous tissue distorting the endometrial canal with or without a gestation sac. There is no agreement on a measurement of endometrial thickness that can distinguish incomplete from complete abortion [3].
  - **Inevitable abortion:** Clinical definition describing an EPL that is characterized by a history of a positive pregnancy test, vaginal bleeding without passage of tissue, gestational sac in the uterus, and an open cervical os.
  - **Anembryonic pregnancy:** Previously described as "blighted ovum." This is a gestational sac without a visible yolk sac and/or embryo (with no heart motion) in relationship to the mean sac diameter (MSD) size (Table 15.1). It occurs when the embryonic disk has failed to develop or has already been resorbed [5].

- **Embryonic/fetal demise:** Previously described as "missed abortion." It is defined by the failure of a previously identified embryo to grow and/or retain cardiac activity over time (Table 15.1).
- **Expectant management:** No intervention. Awaiting natural passage of tissue.
- **Medical management:** The use of medications to expel the products of conception.
- **Surgical management:** The mechanical removal of the products of conception.

DIAGNOSIS
Transvaginal Ultrasound
To ensure 100% specificity to confirm EPL, the diagnostic criteria shown in Table 15.1 were adopted by the Society of Radiologists in Ultrasound Multispecialty Panel on Early First Trimester Diagnosis of Miscarriage and Exclusion of a Viable Intrauterine Pregnancy [4].

It is important to recognize that not all patients may desire 100% certainty of PL [2]. The wishes of the patient must be considered when determining the level of diagnostic certainty that will be used. Table 15.2 lists the sensitivity and specificity of different diagnostic cutoffs that can be used to counsel patients [4,6].

Beta Human Chorionic Gonadotropin
In a clinically stable patient with a highly desired pregnancy, a single BHCG level ≥ 3000 mIU/mL cannot differentiate between an ectopic pregnancy or EPL if a gestational sac is not visualized in the uterus [4]. If the pregnancy is desired, ectopic precautions should be given and intervention should be avoided until additional testing is performed.

SYMPTOMS
Symptoms of EPL include vaginal bleeding, lower abdominal cramping, and dilation of cervix. Women with EPL may also be asymptomatic.

EPIDEMIOLOGY/INCIDENCE
Fifteen to twenty percent of clinically recognized pregnancies end in EPL [7]. It is estimated that up to 60% of conceptions become an EPL, and most are not clinically recognized (e.g., "late cycle"). Human reproduction is relatively inefficient. Only 30% of fertilized eggs result in a viable pregnancy. Sporadic early PL is very common in humans. At least 15%–20% of clinically identified pregnancies (implanted) physiologically end with early PL, and only 50%–60% of all conceptions advance to >20 weeks [8]. Most PLs represent failure of implantation and are difficult to recognize clinically. Oocyte quality and normal karyotype are most important for normal implantation, a lot more than uterine factors. The prognosis after one uncomplicated early PL in a healthy young woman is for >70%–80% chance of a viable pregnancy in the successive pregnancy. Therefore, no workup or therapy is usually indicated after one PL. For women with 2 or more EPLs, see Chapter 16, "Recurrent Pregnancy Loss."

ETIOLOGY
Chromosomal abnormalities are responsible for >50% of all spontaneous EPL, most commonly aneuploidy. When tissue from EPLs <13 weeks (81% < 9 weeks) obtained by chorionic villus sampling (CVS) and manual vacuum aspiration (MVA) is analyzed, about 72% of cases revealed aneuploidy, with trisomy being the most common [9]. Many spontaneous losses may be secondary to other genetic defects that are impossible to discern by simple karyotype. Many other factors are also associated with spontaneous losses (see Chapter 16).

Table 15.1 Diagnostic Criteria for EPL

Diagnosis	Ultrasound Findings
Anembryonic pregnancy (any of the three)	• A gestational sac ≥25 mm MSD without an embryo • Absence of an embryo with cardiac activity ≥11 days after an ultrasound showed a gestational sac with a yolk sac • Absence of an embryo with cardiac activity ≥2 weeks after an ultrasound showing a gestational sac without a yolk sac
Embryonic/fetal demise	• Absence of cardiac motion in an embryo measuring ≥7 mm

Source: Adapted from Doubilet P et al., *N Engl J Med*, 369(15), 1443–1451.
Abbreviations: EPL, early pregnancy loss; MSD, mean sac diameter.

Table 15.2 Sensitivity, Specificity, and False Positive Rates When Diagnosing EPL

	Sensitivity (95% CI)	Specificity (95% CI)	FPR (%)
CRL >5 mm without cardiac activity	0.50 (0.12–0.88)	1.00 (0.90–1.00)	0
CRL >6 mm without cardiac activity	0.50 (0.07–0.93)	1.00 (0.87–1.00)	0
CRL >7 mm without cardiac activity	NA	1.00 (NA)	NA
MSD ≥13 mm without yolk sac	0.96 (0.92–0.99)	1.00 (0.69–1.00)	0
MSD ≥16 mm without yolk sac	0.50 (NA)	1.00 (0.88–1.00)	NA
MSD ≥20 mm without yolk sac	0.41 (0.30–0.52)	1.00 (0.96–1.00)	0
MSD ≥25 mm without yolk sac	NA	1.00 (NA)	NA

Sources: Modified from Doubilet P et al., *N Engl J Med*. 369(15), 1443–1451, 2013; Jeve Y et al., *Ultrasound Obstet Gynecol*, 38(5), 489–496, 2011.
Abbreviations: CI, confidence interval; CRL, crown rump length; FPR, false positive rate; NA, not available.

RISK FACTORS

The risk of EPL increases with maternal age, ranging from 9% at 22 years old, to 84% at 48 years old [10]. Other risk factors include smoking, alcohol, excessive caffeine intake, African racial origin, previous EPL, previous stillbirth, medical complications such as diabetes, ART, and vaginal bleeding [11]. A recent meta-analysis showed that caffeine and coffee consumption, especially more than three servings per day, during pregnancy are significantly associated with PL [12].

THREATENED PL

Threatened PL can be defined as vaginal bleeding in pregnancy before 20 weeks of gestation. Several **interventions** have been studied, but **none has been confirmed to be beneficial**.

Complications

- **Vaginal bleeding in the first trimester** has been associated with several complications in pregnancy, including antepartum hemorrhage (odds ratio [OR] 2.47), preterm premature rupture of membranes (PPROM) (OR 1.78), preterm birth (PTB) (OR 2.05), intrauterine growth restriction (IUGR) (OR 1.54), low birth weight (LBW) (OR 1.83), and perinatal mortality (OR 2.15) [13].
- The presence of a **subchorionic hematoma** detected on ultrasound (usually between 5 and 20 weeks) is associated with increased risks of SAB (OR 2.18), abruptio (OR 5.71), intrauterine fetal demise (IUFD) (OR 2.09), PPROM (OR 1.64), and PTB (OR 1.40) [14].

Prevention

- *Lifestyle modifications*
  - Epidemiologic studies suggest that lifestyle modifications can increase fertility potential, although these have not been definitively testing in randomized controlled trials (RCTs). These modifications include eliminating use of tobacco products, alcohol, and caffeine and reduction in body mass index (BMI) [15].
- *Multivitamins*
  - In non-high-risk women, multivitamin supplementation before 20 weeks is associated with similar total fetal loss (early/late miscarriage and stillbirth), early or late miscarriage or stillbirth, and most other outcomes compared with controls [16]. Multivitamin supplementation is associated with a 38% higher incidence to have a multiple pregnancy, probably associated with vitamin A as well as folic acid supplementation. Therefore, **vitamin supplementation cannot be recommended for prevention of miscarriage**.
- *Progesterone*
  - There is **no evidence to support the routine use of progesterone (synthetic or natural) to prevent miscarriage in early to midpregnancy**. The meta-analysis of all women, regardless of gravidity and number of previous miscarriages, showed no statistically significant difference in the risk of miscarriage between progesterone and placebo or no treatment groups (OR 0.99; 95% confidence interval [CI] 0.78–1.24) and no significant difference in the incidence of adverse effects in either mother or baby [17].
  - However, in a subgroup analysis of four trials involving women who had recurrent miscarriages (3+ consecutive miscarriages; four trials, 225 women), progesterone treatment showed a statistically significant decrease in the miscarriage rate compared with placebo or no treatment (OR 0.39; 95% CI 0.21–0.72) though these studies were of poorer quality.
  - **While progesterone supplementation cannot be recommended for prevention of miscarriage, there may be benefit in women with a history of recurrent miscarriage. Treatment for these women may be warranted** (see Chapter 16).

Therapy

- *Bed rest*
  - There is insufficient evidence of high quality that supports a policy of bed rest to prevent miscarriage in women with confirmed fetal viability and vaginal bleeding in the first half of pregnancy. There is no statistically significant difference in the risk of miscarriage in the bed rest group versus the no bed rest group (placebo or other treatment) (relative risk [RR] 1.54, 95% CI 0.92–2.58). Neither bed rest in a hospital nor bed rest at home shows a significant difference in the prevention of miscarriage. There is a higher risk of miscarriage in those women in the bed rest group than in those in the hCG therapy group with no bed rest (RR 2.50, 95% CI 1.22–5.11). The small number of participants included in these studies makes these analyses inconclusive [18].
  - **Bed rest cannot be recommended for prevention of miscarriage.** In fact, it might be harmful, given the higher rates of venous thromboembolism (VTE), muscle atrophy, and other detriments associated with bed rest.
- *Progesterone*
  - **There is insufficient evidence to assess the effect of progesterone supplementation in women with threatened miscarriage.** There was no evidence of effectiveness with the use of vaginal progesterone compared with placebo in reducing the risk of miscarriage (RR 0.47, 95% CI 0.17–1.30) [19].
- *Human chorionic gonadotropin*
  - **The current evidence does not support the routine use of hCG in the treatment of threatened miscarriage.** There is no statistically significant difference in the incidence of miscarriage between hCG and "no hCG" (placebo or no treatment) groups (RR 0.66, 95% CI 0.42–1.05). There were no reported adverse effects of hCG on the patient or fetus [20].
- *Muscle relaxant*
  - There is **insufficient evidence** to support the use of uterine muscle relaxant drugs for women with threatened miscarriage, and **therefore they should not be used**. In one poor-quality RCT, compared with placebo, buphenine (a β-agonist) was associated with a lower risk of intrauterine death (RR 0.25, 95% CI 0.12–0.51). PTB was the only other outcome reported (RR 1.67, 95% CI 0.63–4.38) (9) [21].

MANAGEMENT OF EPL
General Principles

- There are **three main options** for the woman with EPL (unless the spontaneous loss is complete): **expectant, medical,** and **surgical management**.
- Successful management of EPL entails complete evacuation of the uterus. The success of each management option depends on several factors, for example, the type of loss (e.g., with or without symptoms).

- Failure of expectant or medical management results in the need for surgical evacuation.
- There are **several types of medical management approaches and several surgical approaches.**

Principles of Surgical Management
- **Procedure:** Surgical management of EPL can be accomplished via **vacuum aspiration or sharp curettage.**
- When comparing vacuum aspiration versus sharp curettage, **vacuum aspiration is preferred,** as it is associated with [22]
  - Less blood loss (mean difference [MD] −17.10 mL, 95% CI −24.05 to −10.15 mL).
  - Less pain during the procedure (RR 0.74, 95% CI 0.61.0.90)
  - Shorter duration of the procedure (MD −1.20 minutes, 95% CI −1.53 to −0.87 minutes).
  - The small sample sizes of the trials were too small to evaluate rare complications such as uterine perforation and other morbidity.
- Vacuum aspiration can be accomplished with **electric vacuum aspiration (EVA) or MVA.** Both EVA and MVA are types of dilation and curettage (D&C).
- **Location:** Vacuum aspiration can be accomplished in the operating room or in the office.
- **MVA is a safe alternative** for gestations 6–12 weeks with EPL, and can be performed in the **office under local anesthesia** [23]. This should be strongly preferred at these gestational ages instead of an operating room procedure necessitating general anesthesia [24].
- **There is no significant difference in the success or complication rates for MVA versus EVA** [25].

Principles of Medical Management
Medications used
- **Misoprostol** is a prostaglandin E1 analog. It is a uterotonic that results in cervical softening and contractions that expel the products of conception. Routes of administration include vaginal, oral, buccal, or sublingual. Side effects vary, based on route of administration [26].
- **Mifepristone** is an antiprogestin that results in weakening of the uterine attachment of a pregnancy. This results in capillary breakdown and synthesis of prostaglandins [27].
- **Methotrexate** (intramuscularly or oral) antagonizes folic acid, a cofactor needed for synthesis of nucleic acids. It is toxic to the rapidly dividing cells of the trophoblast. There is no role for methotrexate in the treatment of EPL [28].
- **Success** of medical management is determined by the absence of significant symptoms and absence of the gestational sac on transvaginal ultrasound. Studies that use an endometrial thickness of >15 mm to define failure of medical management may underestimate success rates of expectant and medical management [4].
- **Success** of medical management is **higher in patients with symptoms,** such as cramping and bleeding [29].

Contraindications
The contraindications listed in Table 15.3 apply to medical management but can also apply to expectant management [25,30,31].

Complications
- Complications are rare. The incidence of gynecologic infection after surgical, expectant, or medical management of EPL is low (2%–3%). There is no evidence to show a differential risk of infection by management choice [32].

Table 15.3 Contraindications to Medical (or Expectant) Management

- Hemodynamically or medically unstable patients
- Signs of pelvic infection and/or sepsis
- Suspected molar or ectopic pregnancy
- Caution should be used in women with hemoglobin <9.5 g/dL
- History of coagulopathy or current use of anticoagulants
- Allergy to prostaglandins[a]

Sources: Modified from Zhang J et al., *N Engl J Med*, 353(8), 761–769, 2005; Royal College of Obstetricians and Gynaecologists (RCOG). *Green-Top Guideline No. 25: The Management of Early Pregnancy Loss,* RCOG, London, United Kingdom, 2006.
[a] Specific to medical management.

- In the largest RCT (*n* = 652) comparing medical with surgical management, there was no difference in the following complications [25]:
  - Hemorrhage requiring hospitalization with or without blood transfusion (1%)
  - Hospitalization for endometritis (<1%)
  - Fever (3%–4%)
  - Emergency visit to hospital within 24 hours of treatment (2%–3%)
  - Unscheduled hospital visits (17%–23%)
  - Decrease in hemoglobin ≥2 g/dL (4%–9%)
  - Decrease in hemoglobin ≥3 g/dL (1%–5%)

Principles of Expectant Management
Expectant management of EPL is an option for women who would like to avoid surgical or medical treatment of EPL; however, time until resolution of EPL is unpredictable and may take as long as 6 weeks. Success of expectant management can range from 25% to 83%, depending on length of time of follow-up, definition of "failed" expectant management, and inclusion criteria [33–35].

Medical versus Surgical Management
- **Cochrane review** [36]
  - Twelve RCTs were included in this Cochrane review of **incomplete abortion before 13 weeks** with *N* = 2894.
  - Misoprostol routes varied, including six studies via oral, four studies via vaginal, one study via sub-lingual, and one study via both vaginal and oral.
  - There was a slightly lower incidence of complete miscarriage in the misoprostol group (RR 0.97, 95% CI 0.95–0.99), but high success in both groups.
  - Women using misoprostol had fewer surgical procedures (RR 0.06, 95% CI 0.02–0.13).
  - Risk of unplanned procedure was higher with misoprostol (RR 5.82, 95% CI 2.93–11.56).
  - Deaths and "serious complications" with either management are too rare to compare.
- **Largest multicenter RCT** [25]
  - *N* = 652; 491 treated with **800 mg vaginal misoprostol** versus 161 by vacuum aspiration
  - Participant characteristics:
    - 58% embryonic/fetal demise
    - 36% anembryonic gestation
    - 6% incomplete/inevitable abortion
  - **Medical regimen: 800 mg vaginal misoprostol, repeated on day 3 if incomplete expulsion (diagnosed by persistence of gestational sac or endometrial lining greater than 30 mm on transvaginal ultrasound), vacuum aspiration on day 8 if still incomplete**

- **Success**
  - 97% success with vacuum aspiration
  - **84% success with misoprostol overall**
  - **71% success with one dose misoprostol**
  - Success increases to 84% with second dose of 800 mg vaginal misoprostol if gestational sac still present on ultrasound on day 3
- **Success by type of EPL**
  - 93% for incomplete/inevitable abortion
  - 88% embryonic/fetal demise
  - 81% anembryonic pregnancy
- Success did not vary by gestational age
- Increased rates of nausea, vomiting, and diarrhea and abdominal pain in misoprostol group
- No difference in hemorrhage or endometritis between groups (<1%)
- Success of medical management associated with cramping, vaginal bleeding, and nulliparity [29]

Conclusion: Medical management with misoprostol is an acceptable alternative to surgical evacuation. Patient preference should guide decision making [36].

Medical versus Expectant Management

Medical management commonly uses vaginal misoprostol [28]. There are several additional studies looking at mifepristone followed by vaginal or oral misoprostol [37–39].

- **Cochrane review** [28]
  - Twenty-four RCTs, $n = 1888$, of embryonic/fetal demise or anembryonic pregnancy.
  - **Vaginal misoprostol** compared with expectant management:
    - Shortens the time to achieve complete uterine evacuation:
      - At less than 24 hours after treatment (RR 4.73, 95% CI 2.70–8.28)
      - At less than 48 hours after treatment (RR 5.74, 95% CI 2.70–12.19)
    - Results in less need for uterine curettage
    - Does not show a significant difference in need for blood transfusion (RR 0.2, 95% CI 0.01–4.0)
    - Does not have a significant increase in nausea (RR 1.38, 95% CI 0.43–4.40) or diarrhea (RR 2.21, 95% CI 0.35–14.06)
  - **Dosage** of vaginal misoprostol: When compared with lower dosages, **800 mg** vaginal misoprostol is more effective at completing uterine emptying (RR 0.85, 95% CI 0.72–1.00) with similar incidence of nausea.
  - No advantage of "wet" versus "dry" preparation of vaginal misoprostol or of adding methotrexate.
  - Oral misoprostol is less effective than vaginal misoprostol in emptying the uterus (RR 0.90, 95% CI 0.82–0.99).
  - Sublingual misoprostol is equivalent to vaginal misoprostol in inducing complete uterine emptying but was associated with more frequent diarrhea.
- **Mifepristone**
  - Efficacy of mifepristone followed by misoprostol for treatment of miscarriage ranges from 65.5% to 80% [37–39].
  - In a Cochrane review published in 2006, two trials of mifepristone added to misoprostol show conflicting results [28].
  - One small RCT ($n = 115$) found that mifepristone in addition to misoprostol did not improve efficacy [39], though one retrospective study did find increased expulsion rates with mifepristone plus misoprostol versus misoprostol alone [40].

Conclusion: Medical management with 800 mg of vaginal misoprostol is significantly more effective than expectant management. Mifepristone and misoprostol appear to have similar success rates to misoprostol alone though data are conflicting, thus based on available evidence, it is uncertain whether there is any advantage to adding mifepristone to misoprostol for medical management.

Expectant versus Surgical Management

In a Cochrane review of seven RCTs, $n = 1521$: [41]

- Expectant management has a higher incidence of the following:
  - Incomplete miscarriage by 2 weeks (RR 3.98, 95% CI 2.94–5.38) or by 6–8 weeks (RR 2.56, 95% CI 1.15–5.69).
  - Need for unplanned or additional surgical emptying of the uterus (RR 7.35, 95% CI 5.04–10.72).
  - Surgical management is required in 28% in expectant group, while only 4% in surgical group require additional surgery.
  - More days of bleeding (weighted mean difference [WMD] 1.59, 95% CI 0.74–2.45).
  - Need for blood transfusion (RR 6.45, 95% CI 1.21–34.42).
- There was no difference in infection risk.
- Cost was lower in the expectant management group.

Conclusion: After counseling regarding the data above, patient preference should guide decision making.

Misoprostol: Route, Dose, and Safety

There is published literature on a wide range of therapeutic regimens [4,30,42]. Optimal doses and routes of administration of misoprostol have not been determined by randomized trials.

- **Misoprostol 800 µg per vagina** is the most studied regimen for medical management of EPL. Success of medical management of EPL increases with **multiple-dose regimens** [25].
- A single RCT showed that there is equivalent efficacy between a multidose regimen of vaginal misoprostol 400 and 800 µg with a lower incidence of fever/rigors and higher satisfaction in the lower dose group [43].
- An international panel of experts recommends a single oral dose of 600 µg misoprostol for medical management of incomplete abortion [30] and a single vaginal dose of 800 µg misoprostol for medical management of anembryonic pregnancy and embryonic/fetal demise [44]. Misoprostol 600 µg sublingual is an alternative regimen [44].
- Overall, misoprostol is safe and well tolerated. Side effects of prostaglandins include diarrhea, nausea, and vomiting. These side effects are increased when misoprostol is given orally. Patients receiving misoprostol vaginally have decreased gastrointestinal side effects and prolonged duration of action when compared with oral administration [26].

Antibiotics

There is insufficient evidence to recommend or to abandon prophylactic antibiotics for surgical evacuation in women with an incomplete abortion. Clinical judgment is recommended [30,45].

There is insufficient evidence to recommend prophylactic antibiotics for women undergoing surgical evacuation of the uterus for embryonic/fetal demise or anembryonic gestation but the risk of infection is thought to be similar to risk of infection for induced termination of pregnancy. American Congress of Obstetricians and Gynecologists (ACOG) recommends the use of a single preoperative dose of doxycycline in cases of EPL, but acknowledges the lack of data [2]. If provided, **doxycycline 100 mg 1 hour before the procedure** and 200 mg after the procedure is a low cost regimen [46].

Rh Negative
Women who are Rh(D) negative and unsensitized should receive Rh(D)-immune globulin within 72 hours of the EPL [2].

PATIENT COUNSELING
Patients choosing medical management of EPL should have appropriate counseling regarding expected symptoms.

- Bleeding with medical management is heavier and longer in duration than with surgical management, and rarely requires intervention [47].
- Women experienced approximately 12 days of bleeding after medical management of EPL [47]. Bleeding will most likely be heavy for about 3–4 days, followed by light bleeding or spotting for several weeks [31].
- Patients should be counseled to contact their physician if they experience heavy vaginal bleeding (soaking through more than two extra large sanitary pads per hour for 2 consecutive hours) or signs of infection [31].
- Some women experience fever and/or chills during the first 24 hours after misoprostol use. Patients should call their doctor and be evaluated for infection if fever and/or chills persist beyond 24 hours after using misoprostol [31].
- **Nausea and vomiting** may occur with use of misoprostol and will usually resolve 2–6 hours after taking misoprostol [31].
- **Pain should be expected with medical or expectant management and patients should be given a narcotic pain medication and non-steroidal anti-inflammatory drugs to treat pain** [2].

PATIENT ACCEPTABILITY
- In one study, the majority of women would prefer medical management of EPL with misoprostol to surgical management if its efficacy is >65% [48].
- In a large RCT comparing medical versus surgical management of EPL, women receiving medical management had significantly higher reports of treatment-related symptoms (cramping and bleeding), but overall quality of life and treatment acceptability were similar [49].
- In a large RCT comparing medical versus surgical management of EPL, 83% of women with EPL randomized to medical management with misoprostol would recommend medical management to others and 78% would probably/absolutely use medical management again [25].

PATIENT PREFERENCE
Most women have strong preferences regarding management of EPL [50]. Preferences are diverse and different women place different values on the advantages and disadvantages of avoiding the OR or of miscarrying at home, for example. Patient preference will depend on individual circumstances, expectations, and awareness of the advantages and disadvantages of each management option. Women have greater satisfaction when treated according to their preferences.

Due to the comparable safety and efficacy of all current treatment options for EPL, patient preference should be the guiding force deciding management of EPL.

COST
Expectant management has a lower cost when compared with surgical management [41]. In a decision analysis comparing surgical and expectant management to an expanded care option (expectant management, surgical management in the office or OR, and medical management), there was a cost savings of $241.39 per case in the expanded care option [51].

Follow-Up
There are no RCTs to assess optimal management of follow-up after EPL. **Transvaginal ultrasound** is the most common follow-up after medical or expectant management of EPL, typically done within 7–14 days [2]. Absence of the gestational sac indicates success [2]. Endometrial thickness after medical or expectant management is not predictive of retained products of conception and/or need for surgical evacuation [52].

If chorionic villi or a gestational sac is obtained at D&C, there is usually no need for BHCG follow-up. After expectant or medical management of a known intrauterine pregnancy, BHCG levels, in general, do not need to be followed. Ultrasound can be used to confirm expulsion of the gestational sac. BHCG can be used in patients with limited access to ultrasound [2].

FUTURE FERTILITY
There is no need for a work-up after one EPL. If >1 EPL has occurred, see Chapter 16, *Recurrent PL*. There is insufficient data to suggest an optimal interpregnancy interval between an EPL and the next conception [2]. There seems to be no improvement in outcome associated with waiting 3 months of more, as previously recommended [53]. There are no contraindications to the placement of an intrauterine device immediately after surgical (or other) management of EPL, as long as septic abortion is ruled out [54]. Choice of management for EPL does not affect future fertility. In long-term follow-up of women participating in an RCT of expectant, medical, or surgical management of EPL, there was no significant difference in the live birth rate 5 years after the index miscarriage [55].

- Expectant management: 177/224 (79%, 95% CI 73%–84%)
- Medical management: 181/230 (79%, 95% CI 73%–84%)
- Surgical management: 192/235 (82%, 95% CI 76%–86%)

REFERENCES
1. National Collaborating Centre for Women's and Children's Health (UK). *Ectopic Pregnancy and Miscarriage: Diagnosis and Initial Management in Early Pregnancy of Ectopic Pregnancy and Miscarriage*. London, United Kingdom: RCOG, 2012. [Guideline; 240 references]
2. American College of Obstetricians and Gynecologists. Committee on Practice Bulletins-Gynecology. Practice Bulletin No. 150: Early pregnancy loss. *Obstet Gynecol*. 2015;125(5):1258–1267. [Guideline; 60 references]
3. Perriera L, Reeves MF. Ultrasound criteria for diagnosis of early pregnancy failure and ectopic pregnancy. *Semin Reprod Med*. 2008;26(5):373–382. [Review]
4. Doubilet P, Benson C, Bourne T, et al. Diagnostic criteria for nonviable pregnancy early in the first trimester. *N Engl J Med*. 2013;369(15):1443–1451. [Review]

5. Chen BA, Creinin MD. Medical management of early pregnancy failure: Efficacy. *Semin Reprod Med.* 2008;26(5):411–422. [Review]
6. Jeve Y, Rana R, Bhide A, Thangaratinam S. Accuracy of first-trimester ultrasound in the diagnosis of early embryonic demise: A systematic review. *Ultrasound Obstet Gynecol.* 2011;38(5):489–496. [Review]
7. Hemminki E. Treatment of miscarriage: Current practice and rationale. *Obstet Gynecol.* 1998;91(2):247–253. [Review]
8. American College of Obstetricians and Gynecologists. ACOG Practice Bulletin No. 24: Management of recurrent pregnancy loss. *Int J Gynaecol Obstet.* 2002;78(2):179–190. [Review]
9. Nicholas S, Orzechowski K, Potti S, et al. Early pregnancy failure as a training tool for chorionic villus sampling. *Prenat Diagn.* 2013;33(11):1110–1112. [II-2]
10. Nybo Andersen AM, Wohlfahrt J, Christens P, et al. Maternal age and fetal loss: Population based register linkage study. *BMJ.* 2000;320(7251):1708–1712. [II-1]
11. Borrell A, Stergiotou I. Miscarriage in contemporary maternal-fetal medicine: Targeting clinical dilemmas. *Ultrasound Obstet Gynecol.* 2013;42(5):491–497. [Review]
12. Li J, Zhao H, Song J, et al. A meta-analysis of risk of pregnancy loss and caffeine and coffee consumption during pregnancy. *Int J Gynecol Obstet.* 2015;130(2):116–122. [II-2]
13. Saraswat L, Bhattacharya S, Maheshwari A. Maternal and perinatal outcome in women with threatened miscarriage in the first trimester: A systematic review. *BJOG.* 2010;117(3):245–257. [Systematic review]
14. Tuuli MG, Norman SM, Odibo AO, et al. Perinatal outcomes in women with subchorionic hematoma: A systematic review and meta-analysis. *Obstet Gynecol.* 2011;117(5):1205–1212. [Meta-analysis, $n = 1735$]
15. Sharma R, Biedenharn KR, Fedor JM, Agarwal A. Lifestyle factors and reproductive health: Taking control of your fertility. *Reprod Biol Endocrinol.* 2013;11(66):1–15. [Review]
16. Rumbold A, Middleton P, Pan N, Crowther CA. Vitamin supplementation for preventing miscarriage. *Cochrane Database Syst Rev.* 2011;(19):CD004073. [Meta-analysis: 28 RCTs, $n = 96{,}674$]
17. Haas DM, Ramsey PS. Progestogen for preventing miscarriage. *Cochrane Database Syst Rev.* 2013;(10):CD003511. [Meta-analysis: 14 RCTs, $n = 2158$]
18. Aleman A, Althabe F, Belizán JM, et al. Bed rest during pregnancy for preventing miscarriage. *Cochrane Database Syst Rev.* 2005;(2):CD003576. [Meta-analysis: 2 RCTs, $n = 84$]
19. Wahabi HA, Fayed AA, Esmaeil SA et al. Progestogen for treating threatened miscarriage. *Cochrane Database Syst Rev.* 2011;(12):CD005943. [Meta-analysis: 2 RCTs, $n = 84$]
20. Devaseelan P, Fogarty PP, Regan L. Human chorionic gonadotrophin for threatened miscarriage. *Cochrane Database Syst Rev.* 2010;(5):CD007422. [Meta-analysis: 3 RCTs, $n = 312$]
21. Soltan M. Buphenine and threatened abortion. *Eu J Obstet Gynecol Reprod Biol.* 1986;22(5):319–324. [RCT, $n = 170$]
22. Tunçalp O, Gulmezoglu A, Souza J. Surgical procedures to evacuating incomplete abortion. *Cochrane Database Syst Rev.* 2010;(9):CD001993. [Meta-analysis: 2 trials, $n = 550$]
23. Dalton VK, Harris L, Weisman CS, et al. Patient preferences, satisfaction, and resource use in office evacuation of early pregnancy failure. *Obstet Gynecol.* 2006;108(1):103–110. [II-2]
24. Farooq F, Javed L, Mumtaz A, Naveed N. Comparison of manual vacuum aspiration, and dilatation and curettage in the treatment of early pregnancy failure. *J Ayub Med Coll Abbottabad.* 2011;23(3):28–31. [II-1]
25. Zhang J, Gilles JM, Barnhart K, et al. A comparison of medical management with misoprostol and surgical management for early pregnancy failure. *N Engl J Med.* 2005;353(8):761–769. [RCT, $n = 652$]
26. Tang O, Gemzell-Danielsson K, Ho P. Misoprostol: Pharmacokinetic profiles, effects on the uterus and side-effects. *Int J Gynecol Obstet.* 2007;99:S160–S167. [Review]
27. Paul M, Lichtenberg S, Borgatta L, et al. *Management of Unintended and Abnormal Pregnancy: Comprehensive Abortion Care.* Oxford, United Kingdom: John Wiley & Sons, 2011. [Book]
28. Neilson JP, Hickey M, Vazquez J. Medical treatment for early fetal death (less than 24 weeks). *Cochrane Database Syst Rev.* 2006;(3):CD002253. [Meta-analysis: 24 trials, $n = 1888$]
29. Creinin MD, Huang X, Westhoff C, et al. Factors related to successful misoprostol treatment for early pregnancy failure. *Obstet Gynecol.* 2006;107(4):901–907. [II-2]
30. Royal College of Obstetricians and Gynaecologists (RCOG). *Green-Top Guideline No. 25: The Management of Early Pregnancy Loss.* London, United Kingdom: RCOG, 2006. [Guideline; 75 references]
31. Blum J, Winikoff B, Gemzell-Danielsson K, et al. Treatment of incomplete abortion and miscarriage with misoprostol. *Int J Gynecol Obstet.* 2007;99:S186–S189. [Review]
32. Trinder J, Brocklehurst P, Porter R, et al. Management of miscarriage: Expectant, medical, or surgical? Results of randomised controlled trial (miscarriage treatment (MIST) trial). *BMJ.* 2006;332(7552):1235–1240. [RCT]
33. Blohm F, Fridén B, Platz-Christensen J, et al. Expectant management of first-trimester miscarriage in clinical practice. *Acta Obstet Gynecol Scand.* 2003;82(7):654–658. [II-2]
34. Jurkovic D, Ross J, Nicolaides K. Expectant management of missed miscarriage. *BJOG.* 1998;105(6):670–671. [II-2]
35. Luise C, Jermy K, May C, et al. Outcome of expectant management of spontaneous first trimester miscarriage: Observational study. *BMJ.* 2002;324(7342):873–875. [II-2]
36. Neilson JP, Gyte GM, Hickey M, et al. Medical treatments for incomplete miscarriage. *Cochrane Database Syst Rev.* 2013;(3):CD007223. [Meta-analysis: 20 trials, $n = 4208$]
37. Kollitz KM, Meyn LA, Lohr PA, Creinin MD. Mifepristone and misoprostol for early pregnancy failure: A cohort analysis. *Obstet Gynecol.* 2011;204(5):386. [II-2]
38. Torre A, Huchon C, Bussieres L, et al. Immediate versus delayed medical treatment for first-trimester miscarriage: A randomized trial. *Obstet Gynecol.* 2012;206(3):215. [RCT]
39. Stockheim D, Machtinger R, Wiser A, et al. A randomized prospective study of misoprostol or mifepristone followed by misoprostol when needed for the treatment of women with early pregnancy failure. *Fertil Steril.* 2006;86(4):956–960. [RCT]
40. van den Berg J, van den Bent, Johan M, et al. Sequential use of mifepristone and misoprostol in treatment of early pregnancy failure appears more effective than misoprostol alone: A retrospective study. *Eur J Obstet Gynecol Reprod Biol.* 2014;183:16–19. [II-2]
41. Nanda K, Lopez LM, Grimes DA, et al. Expectant care versus surgical treatment for miscarriage. *Cochrane Database Syst Rev.* 2012;(3): CD003518. [Meta-analysis: 5 trials, $n = 689$]
42. Dempsey A, Davis A. Medical management of early pregnancy failure: How to treat and what to expect. *Semin Reprod Med.* 2008;26(5):401–410. [Review]
43. Petersen SG, Perkins A, Gibbons K, et al. Can we use a lower intravaginal dose of misoprostol in the medical management of miscarriage? A randomised controlled study. *Aust N Z J Obstet Gynaecol.* 2013;53(1):64–73. [RCT]
44. Gemzell-Danielsson K, Ho P, de León, et al. Misoprostol to treat missed abortion in the first trimester. *Int J Gynecol Obstet.* 2007;99:S182–S185. [Review]
45. May W, Gulmezoglu A, Ba-Thike K. Antibiotics for incomplete abortion. *Cochrane Database Syst Rev.* 2007;(4):CD001779. [Meta-analysis: 1 trial, $n = 140$]
46. American College of Obstetricians and Gynecologists. ACOG Committee on Practice Bulletins-Gynecology. ACOG Practice Bulletin No. 104: Antibiotic prophylaxis for gynecologic procedures. *Obstet Gynecol.* 2009;113(5):1180–1189. [Guideline; 55 references]
47. Davis AR, Hendlish SK, Westhoff C, et al. Bleeding patterns after misoprostol vs surgical treatment of early pregnancy failure: Results from a randomized trial. *Obstet Gynecol.* 2007;196(1):31. [RCT]

48. Graziosi GC, Bruinse HW, Reuwer PJ, et al. Women's preferences for misoprostol in case of early pregnancy failure. *Eur J Obstet Gynecol Reprod Biol.* 2006;124(2):184–186. [II-3]
49. Harwood B, Nansel T. Quality of life and acceptability of medical versus surgical management of early pregnancy failure.* *BJOG.* 2008;115(4):501–508. [II-2]
50. Wallace RR, Goodman S, Freedman LR, et al. Counseling women with early pregnancy failure: Utilizing evidence, preserving preference. *Patient Educ Couns.* 2010;81(3):454–461. [II-3]
51. Dalton VK, Liang A, Hutton DW, et al. Beyond usual care: The economic consequences of expanding treatment options in early pregnancy loss. *Obstet Gynecol.* 2015;212(2):177. [II-3]
52. Reeves MF, Lohr PA, Harwood BJ, et al. Ultrasonographic endometrial thickness after medical and surgical management of early pregnancy failure. *Obstet Gynecol.* 2008;111(1):106–112. [II-3]
53. Wong LF, Schliep KC, Silver RM, et al. The effect of a very short interpregnancy interval and pregnancy outcomes following a previous pregnancy loss. *Obstet Gynecol.* 2015;212(3):375. [II-1]
54. World Health Organization. Reproductive Health. *Medical Eligibility Criteria for Contraceptive Use.* Geneva, Switzerland: World Health Organization, 2010. [III]
55. Smith LF, Ewings PD, Quinlan C. Incidence of pregnancy after expectant, medical, or surgical management of spontaneous first trimester miscarriage: Long term follow-up of miscarriage treatment (MIST) randomised controlled trial. *BMJ.* 2009;339:b3827. [II-1]

Recurrent pregnancy loss

Reshama Navathe and Michela Villani

KEY POINTS

- Diagnosis of recurrent pregnancy loss (RPL) is more than or equal to two consecutive losses or three nonconsecutive losses of pregnancy <20 weeks.
- *Workup* includes *uterine study, antiphospholipid antibodies* **(APAs)**, and **parental karyotypes**, as well as **karyotype of products of conception (POC)** (if available).
- Prognosis with negative workup is for a 60%–70% subsequent successful pregnancy in women <35 years old and 40%–50% in women ≥35 years old.
- Women with **RPL and APA** should be **treated** with **low-dose aspirin and heparin** in subsequent pregnancy (see Chapter 26 in *Maternal-Fetal Evidence Based Guidelines*). Women with unexplained RPL should not receive anticoagulant therapy.
- Women with **RPL and uterine septum, synechiae, or submucous myomata** can consider *hysteroscopic resection* of these abnormalities.
- Couples with abnormal parental karyotype can be offered genetic counseling, prenatal diagnosis, and/or gamete donation.
- There is insufficient evidence for universal screening for diabetes mellitus (DM), thyroid disease, progesterone deficiency (luteal phase defect [LPD]), infections, thrombophilia, etc.
- Women should **not be tested for alloimmunization or receive any of the immune therapies**, since they are ineffective and at times detrimental.
- Women should **not receive estrogen supplementation**, as this is unsafe, as it is detrimental to the future offspring, and ineffective.
- There is very limited evidence that supportive care and progesterone are beneficial interventions.
- Women with RPL, **especially more than or equal to three losses, should be offered progesterone until 10 weeks gestation** in subsequent pregnancies.
- There is insufficient evidence to support human chorionic gonadotropin (hCG), aspirin, and vitamins as interventions.

DIAGNOSIS/DEFINITIONS

For diagnoses of pregnancy loss, miscarriage, spontaneous and other kind of abortions, anembryonic pregnancy, embryonic demise, etc., please see Chapter 15.

RPL: either two consecutive pregnancy losses, or three nonconsecutive pregnancy losses before the twentieth week of gestation [1], excluding ectopic and molar pregnancies.

The definition of RPL varies in different publications, which makes diagnosing and treating this entity more challenging for physicians and couples. Early pregnancy loss is usually defined as a pregnancy loss <14 weeks, and these make up the majority of RPL.

There are several guiding committees with slightly different variations on this definition (Table 16.1) [2–4].

CLASSIFICATION

Primary RPL: no intervening live births; secondary RPL: intervening live births. The prognosis is better with secondary RPL [5].

INCIDENCE

As seen in Chapter 15, most fertilized eggs do miscarry, often without a recognized clinical pregnancy. Approximately 15% of pregnant women experience loss of a clinically recognized pregnancy. It is estimated that **fewer than 5% of women experience two consecutive pregnancy losses, and only 1% experience 3 or more** [6].

ETIOLOGY

Etiology of RPL is not established in at least 50% of cases after workup (see below). General categories include: genetic, anatomic, endocrine, immunologic, thrombophilic, and environmental (Table 16.2) [7,8].

RISK FACTORS/ASSOCIATIONS

Advancing maternal age is associated with a higher rate of RPL. Rate of clinically recognized miscarriage is 20% at age 35 years, 40% at age 40 years, and up to 80% at age 45 years [9]. Other risk factors include maternal medical diseases, especially poorly controlled, such as hypertension and diabetes (see Chapter 15).

A previous PL is a risk factor for a subsequent PL (Table 16.3) [6,10]. Women with only unsuccessful pregnancy history have a greater risk of future miscarriage than primigravidas and women with a history of previous successful pregnancy [11].

RECURRENT PREGNANCY LOSS
Counseling
The frequency of PL should be reviewed with the patient and partner (see Chapter 15), as well as the prognosis after one or more PLs (Table 16.3) [6,10].

Workup (Screening)
Appropriate diagnostic workup of RPL is essential for choosing the proper intervention (Table 16.4) [12]. Screening tests should not only discover diagnosis (etiology) but also lead to interventions effective in increasing the incidence of

Table 16.1 Definitions of RPL

Committee	Number of Pregnancies	Consecutive?	Specifics
RCOG 2011 [2]	3	Yes	Not required to be intrauterine
ASRM 2013 [3]	2	No	Clinical pregnancies confirmed by histology or ultrasonography
ESHRE 2014 [4]	Not specified	No	Intrauterine, confirmed by histology or ultrasonography

Abbreviations: ASRM American Society of Reproductive Medicine; ESHRE: European Society of Human Reproduction and Embryology; RCOG, Royal College of Obstetricians and Gynecologists; RPL, recurrent pregnancy loss.

Table 16.2 Etiology, Diagnostic Considerations, and Treatment in RPL

Etiology	Percentage	Diagnostic Evaluation	Therapy
Genetic	2–5	Karyotype—parental Karyotype—POC	Genetic counseling Genetic counseling, PGD
Anatomic	12–22	3D ultrasound Hysterosalpingogram SIS	Correction of anatomic defect
Endocrinology	20	TSH Prolactin HgbA1c	Levothyroxine Bromocriptine Diabetic optimization
Immunologic/thrombophilic	15–25	APLAS	Aspirin + heparin
Environmental		Tobacco, EtOH Exposure	Eliminate exposures
Unknown	40–50		

Sources: Adapted from Kutteh WH, *Cur Opin Obstet Gynecol*, 11(5), 435–439, 1999; Carp HJ, *Recurrent Pregnancy Loss: Causes, Controversies and Treatment*, London, United Kingdom, Informa UK Ltd., 290 p., 2007.
Abbreviations: 3D, three-dimensional; APLAS, antiphospholipid antibody syndrome; EtOH, ethyl alcohol; HgbA1c, hemoglobin A1c; PGD, preimplantation genetic diagnosis; POC, products of conception; SIS, saline infusion sonogram; TSH, thyroid stimulating hormone.

Table 16.3 Miscarriage Risk after Prior PL

Prior PL (n)	Risk of Miscarriage in Subsequent Pregnancy (%)
0	10–15
1	13–25
2	17–35
3	25–45
4	60–65

Sources: Adapted from Stirrat GM, *Lancet*, 336(8716), 673–675, 1990; Nybo Andersen, A. M. et al. *BMJ*, 320(7251), 1708–1712, 2000.
Abbreviation: PL, pregnancy loss.

subsequent live birth. **The following women should be offered evaluation:**

1. Women with more than or equal to two consecutive miscarriages
2. Women with more than or equal to three nonconsecutive miscarriages

Initial part of workup consists of **history** (smoking, alcohol and caffeine, illicit drug use, environmental exposures, working conditions, as well as detailed obstetrical and gynecological history) and **physical examination** (pelvic). Eliciting the gestational age of miscarriage is important, as often RPL occurs at a similar gestational age in subsequent pregnancies, and the most common cause of RPL varies by gestational age. Sometimes, though, obstetrical history is mixed, with early PL, second-trimester PL, preterm birth (PTB), and/or fetal death, so that workup may include other tests (see specific chapters, including Chapter 55 in *Maternal-Fetal Evidence Based Guidelines*).

RECOMMENDED SCREENING TESTS
Genetic Evaluation
Parental Karyotype
Three to four percent of couples with RPL have one parent with balanced translocation, or less commonly a chromosome inversion. Although these couples experience increased reproductive loss rates, most will have successful pregnancies without intervention [13]. Available intervention includes preimplantation genetic screening (PGS), and donor gametes.

POC Karyotype
Management of women with more than or equal to two RPLs should also be based on genetic evaluation of POCs (Figure 16.1) [14]. Most sporadic pregnancy losses in the first trimester result from random numeric chromosomal errors. When tissue of anembryonic pregnancies <9 weeks obtained by chorionic villus sampling (CVS) and manual vacuum aspiration (MVA) is analyzed, about **72% of cases revealed aneuploidy**, with trisomy being most common [15]. This novel approach in the management of RPL includes CVS before evacuation. When compared with POCs, CVS is more successful in achieving a cytogenetic result, as omitting culturing of cells eliminates the potential for maternal contamination [16]. Additionally, miscarriage associated with aneuploidy increases with increasing maternal age; up to 80% in those over 35 years of age [17]. Aneuploidy is present in >50% of embryos tested preimplantation in women

Table 16.4 Evaluation of a Woman with Recurrent Miscarriages

Assessment	Comment
Medical History	
Determine pattern and gestational age of preembryonic, embryonic, or fetal death, if such information is available.	Preembryonic and embryonic losses before 10 weeks of gestation are the most common type of miscarriage, although the onset of symptoms may be later.
Evaluate for features suggestive of the antiphospholipid syndrome.	Features include thrombosis, fetal death, autoimmune disease, and thrombocytopenia.
Assess whether patient has history of uterine malformations (e.g., seen on previous ultrasonographic examination or during intra-abdominal surgery).	Previous obstetrical complication such as preterm labor or breech presentation suggests possibility of uterine malformation.
Assess whether patient has had another fetus or infant with congenital anomaly.	A congenital anomaly suggests the possibility of a parental karyotype abnormality, although these abnormalities may be present in the absence of such a history.
Determine whether patient has history of symptoms suggestive of thyroid disease or diabetes.	
Physical Examination	
Perform pelvic examination with particular focus on findings compatible with uterine or cervical abnormalities.	
Examine patient for other physical findings suggestive of thyroid disease or diabetes.	
Recommended Tests[a]	
Lupus anticoagulant, anticardiolipin antibodies, and anti-β_2-glycoprotein 1 antibodies	Tests for lupus anticoagulant are reported as either positive or negative; levels of anticardiolipin and anti-β_2-glycoprotein 1 antibodies are clinically significant only in medium-to-high titers as defined by the laboratory; antiphospholipid syndrome is diagnosed when tests are repeatedly positive at least 12 weeks apart.[b]
Sonohysterography	Sonohysterography and hysterosalpingography are noninvasive screening tests used to evaluate uterine cavity and shape; MRI, hysteroscopy, or both may be more informative but are more expensive and invasive, respectively; all are useful in detecting a uterine abnormality.
Chromosome analyses of father and mother	Parental karyotyping is expensive and not always covered by third-party payers; because treatment options are limited and do not surpass results of spontaneous conception, some couples may choose to forgo this testing.
Chromosome analysis of products of conception	Karyotype testing of the conceptus is somewhat controversial, but an aneuploid conceptus indicates a more favorable outcome of a subsequent pregnancy and may avert further unnecessary evaluation and treatment.
Other laboratory tests (e.g., thyrotropin measurement or screening for diabetes), if suggested by history or physical examination	

Source: Adapted from Stirrat GM, *Lancet*, 336(8716), 673–675, 1990.
Abbreviation: MRI, magnetic resonance imaging.
[a]Routine testing for thyroid disease, diabetes, the polycystic ovary syndrome, heritable thrombophilias, bacteria and viruses, and alloimmune abnormalities is not recommended.
[b]See also Chapter 26 in *Maternal-Fetal Evidence Based Guidelines*.

with RPL. More than 50% of aneuploidies are trisomies; most common single aneuploidy is 45XO. 46XX karyotype is often associated with maternal cell contamination, so that caution is necessary; microsatellite analysis decreases this confusion. This test can identify probable etiology and decrease further workup; this provides the couple with explanation and has been shown to **decrease self-blame** [18].

Anatomic Evaluation

A maternal **uterine study** (e.g., three-dimensional [3D] or two-dimensional [2D] sonohysterogram [days 8–10 of follicular phase], hysterosalpingogram [HSG], hysteroscopy, or magnetic resonance imaging [MRI]) is recommended. **Ten to fifteen percent** of women with RPL have uterine anomalies. **The most common congenital anomaly associated with RPL is septate uterus** (spontaneous abortion [SAB] rate is high, about 65%) [19], followed by didelphys and bicornuate. Arcuate uterus has not been consistently associated with RPL. Uterine synechiae (Asherman's syndrome) and diethylstilbestrol (DES) exposure are associated with RPL. Myomata have been associated with decreased implantation rates in the in vitro fertilization (IVF) literature [20], but have not been consistently associated with RPL. Available intervention is hysteroscopic resection of septum, synechiae, or submucous myomata. **Surgical correction of these and other uterine anomalies has not been studied in trials.**

Endocrine Evaluation

Endocrine factors may contribute to **8%–12% of RPL**. Basic evaluation should consistent of **diabetes screening** (hemoglobin A1c [HgbA1c], fasting glucose, glucose tolerance testing), screening for **thyroid** dysfunction (thyroid-stimulating

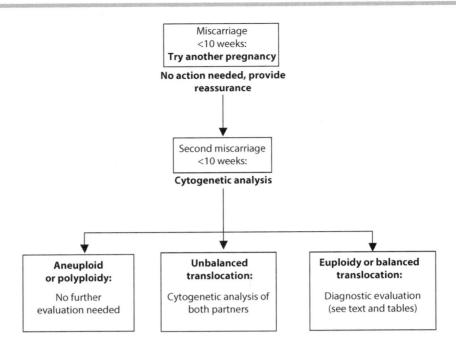

Figure 16.1 Evaluation of patients with early pregnancy loss based on cytogenetic analysis of POC. (From Carp HJ, *Recurrent Pregnancy Loss: Causes, Controversies and Treatment*, London, United Kingdom, Informa UK, p. 290, 2007.)

hormone [TSH] and free thyroxine [T4]); prolactin levels only if clinically suspicious.

Immunologic Evaluation

Three to fifteen percent of women with RPL have APAs. Tests should be positive twice, ≥12 weeks apart. See Chapter 26 in *Maternal-Fetal Evidence Based Guidelines* for tests (lupus anticoagulant, anticardiolipin antibodies [ACAs], and β-2 glycoprotein 1) and effective intervention (e.g., low-dose aspirin and prophylactic heparin).

TESTS THAT CANNOT BE ROUTINELY RECOMMENDED
Products of Conception

- POC molecular genetic abnormalities (e.g., X-chromosome inactivation)
  Commercially available tests are not widely available for this testing.

Mother
Endocrine

- Endometrial biopsy or progesterone levels
  - *Hypothesis:* The corpus luteum fails to make enough progesterone to sustain early decidua for placentation (LPD). It is normal to have at least two consecutive out-of-phase (≥2 days discrepancy) biopsies (diagnosis of LPD) on endometrial histology (late luteal phase—day 25 or 26—after presumed ovulation) in 50% of menstrual cycles; there is also high interobserver variation on interpretation of endometrial biopsies. There is insufficient evidence that intervention (such as progesterone supplementation—17P, micronized progesterone tablets 100 mg by mouth twice a day [po bid] or Crinone cream [8%] one application per vagina daily [beginning 2 days after ovulation until 10 weeks' gestation or menses]) improves outcomes specifically in women with RPL and LPD [21,22]. 17P is efficacious in improving pregnancy outcomes in women with IVF, and in decreasing PTB in women with prior PTB (see Chapter 17).

- Thyroid antibodies
  No consistent association and no intervention studies.

Immunologic

- Alloimmune tests (includes fecal occult blood [FOB])
  No consistent association and no efficacious intervention—see below.

- Antinuclear antibody (ANA)
  No consistent association and no intervention studies.

Both
Thrombophilic

Inherited thrombophilias (factor V Leiden [FVL], prothrombin G20210A gene mutation [PTM], antithrombin III deficiency, protein S, and protein C deficiencies) have not been consistently associated with RPL in the best designed prospective studies. However, a higher frequency of FVL carrier state has recently been shown in women with early RPL [23]. Second-trimester PL has been associated with thrombophilic mutations. There is **insufficient evidence regarding any interventions in women with PL and thrombophilias** (see Chapter 27 in *Maternal-Fetal Evidence Based Guidelines*).

Infectious

No infectious agent has been proven to cause RPL. *Listeria, Toxoplasma gondii,* and many viruses have been associated with sporadic early PL. Chlamydia, mycoplasma/ureoplasma (proposed diagnosis with endometrial biopsy, with treatment of woman and partner with either doxycycline 100 mg po bid or ciprofloxacin 250 mg po bid), and bacterial vaginosis are associated with sporadic PL, not RPL.

MANAGEMENT
Prevention
Optimize preconception medical care of all maternal diseases.

Preconception Care
Informative and sympathetic counseling should be provided. **Workup is best done preconception** (Table 16.4). When workup is positive, counsel regarding specific association. If workup is negative (>50% of couples), counseling should include the fact that 60%–70% of couples with unexplained RPL have successful pregnancies in the next gestation (Table 16.3). This percentage decreases to 40%–50% in women ≥40 years old. Offer all women with RPL a support group. UNITE provides the opportunity for emotional support, through parent-to-parent sharing on issues related to grieving. The groups are guided by trained facilitators, but the meetings are not group therapy sessions. UNITE can assist in referral if additional professional support is needed [24].

Prenatal Care
See subsection "Preconception Care."

Therapy (Specific for Workup)
Abnormal Parental Chromosomes
Offer genetic counseling, prenatal diagnosis, and gamete donation. PGS with IVF is not supported by randomized controlled trials (RCTs) and should therefore not be recommended [12].

Abnormal Uterine Cavity
Septum, synechiae, and/or submucous myomata can be resected hysteroscopically, but **there are no trials regarding this intervention**. There is a high likelihood of successful pregnancy in women with unrepaired septa, so that some suggest against surgical repair in nulligravid women with uterine septa [12]. **Repair of the bicornuate or unicornuate uterus is also usually not suggested in these women, as outcomes are usually good without repair, whereas surgical correction is associated with higher risk of complications**. Consider referral to reproductive endocrinology specialist if necessary. **There is unfortunately insufficient evidence to give a recommendation for women with fibroids and RPL**.

Medical Condition
If a medical condition is identified (e.g., DM, thyroid disease), treat as indicated (see specific chapters in *Maternal-Fetal Evidence Based Guidelines*). Metformin has not been shown to reduce the risk of miscarriage in women with RPL and polycystic ovary syndrome [12].

Antiphospholipid Syndrome
Heparin and aspirin (see Chapter 26 in *Maternal-Fetal Evidence Based Guidelines*)
 Therapy is usually begun once fetal viability is established. **Low-dose aspirin** is usually about **75–100 mg** daily. For prophylactic **unfractionated heparin (UFH):** **5,000–7,500 U first trimester, 7,500–10,000 U second trimester, and 10,000 U third-trimester SQ q12h**. Heparin used in positive trials against placebo was UFH, and even if low-molecular-weight heparin (LMWH) is associated with fewer side effects in nonpregnant adults, RCTs of LMWH in pregnancy for RPL in antiphospholipid syndrome (APS) women have not shown benefit compared with low-dose aspirin [25,26]. Nonetheless, two small RCTs have directly compared LMWH to UFH, and despite the small number of patients recruited, effectiveness of LMWH appears comparable with that of UFH [27,28], and therefore either UGH or LMWH can probably be used (see Chapter 26 and Table 26.3).
 UFH combined with aspirin is associated with a significant reduction in PL compared with aspirin alone (risk ratio [RR] 0.46, 95% confidence interval [CI] 0.29–0.71; three trials, $n = 140$). There is no advantage in high-dose, over low-dose, UFH (one trial, $n = 50$).
 LMWH combined with aspirin compared with aspirin does not significantly reduce PL (odds ratio [OR] 0.70, 95% CI 0.34–1.45; 5 trials, $n = 398$) [29]. For prophylactic LMWH either enoxaparin (Lovenox) 30–40 mg subcutaneously every 12 hours (SQ q12h) or dalteparin (Fragmin) 5000 U SQ q12h were used in RCTs, and clinicians may adjust prophylaxis in high-risk cases to heparin (anti-Xa) level range of 0.2–0.3.
 Three trials of **aspirin alone** ($n = 135$) show no significant reduction in PL (RR 1.05, 95% CI 0.66–1.68).
 Prednisone and aspirin (three trials, $n = 286$) result in a significant increase in prematurity when compared with placebo, aspirin, and heparin combined with aspirin, and an increase in gestational diabetes, but no significant benefit.
 Intravenous immunoglobulin (IVIG) ± UFH and aspirin (two trials, $n = 58$) is associated with an increased risk of PL or premature birth when compared with UFH or LMWH combined with aspirin (RR 2.51, 95% CI 1.27–4.95). When compared with prednisone and aspirin, IVIG (one trial, $n = 82$) is not significantly different in outcomes [30].
 In summary, **therapy with UFH and aspirin can be recommended to the woman with RPL and APS**, as it reduces the chance of PL by 54% compared with aspirin alone.
 In women with RPL and APA, available guidelines recommend a combined therapy with low-dose aspirin and prophylactic doses of heparin, although the available RCTs include heterogeneous groups of patients [31].

Inherited Thrombophilia
As stated above, a workup for inherited thrombophilia is not indicated. If positive inherited **thrombophilia** is incidentally or previously identified, no intervention has been consistently shown to improve outcomes. Please also refer to Chapter 15, and to Chapter 27 in *Maternal-Fetal Evidence Based Guidelines*.

Negative Workup
Progesterone. In women who had more than or equal to three consecutive miscarriages, progesterone treatment is associated with a **statistically significant reduction in miscarriage rate** (OR 0.39, 95% CI 0.21–0.72) compared with placebo or no treatment in four small trials [32–35]. No statistically significant differences, probably because of small numbers, were found between the route of administration of progesterone (oral, intramuscular, and vaginal) and placebo or no treatment [32–35], so the best route and dose of progesterone for prevention of RPL are still unknown. In summary, **progesterone treatment for women**

with RPL may be warranted given the reduced rates of miscarriage in the treatment group and the finding of no statistically significant difference between treatment and control groups in rates of adverse effects suffered by either mother or baby [32].

Supportive care. **Consider** intensive supportive early prenatal care, focusing on antenatal counseling and psychological support. There are **no properly controlled trials to assess the effect of this intervention**. Three studies (not RCTs) showed improved outcome versus standard or no prenatal care [10,36,37].

Human chorionic gonadotropin. There is **not enough evidence** to evaluate the use of hCG during pregnancy in order to prevent miscarriage in women with a history of unexplained recurrent spontaneous miscarriage because the trials are small, and have significant (especially two studies) limitations [38–42]. hCG is associated with a 74% reduced risk of miscarriage for women with a history of recurrent miscarriage [38–42]. All studies showed at least a trend favoring benefit of hCG. This result should be interpreted cautiously because the apparent effect is greatly influenced by the two methodologically weaker studies.

Low-dose aspirin. Compared with placebo, aspirin did not increase the chance of live birth (risk ratio [RR] 0.94, 95% CI 0.80–1.11) in a pooled analysis of 256 women with unexplained recurrent miscarriage with or without thrombophilia [43,44]. In one of these RCTs, aspirin 80 mg had effects similar to placebo in women with unexplained recurrent miscarriages [45]. Therefore, low-dose aspirin should not be recommended for women with recurrent unexplained early PLs.

UFH. There is **insufficient evidence** to assess the effect of UFH in women with unexplained RPL.

LMHW. There are several RCTs that show **no effect of LMWH on prevention of PL in women with unexplained RPL**. Compared with low-dose aspirin, enoxaparin (a LMWH) was associated with similar live birth rates, respectively 82% and 84% (RR 0.97, 95% CI 0.81–1.16), in 107 women with consecutive recurrent miscarriage (more than or equal to three consecutive first-trimester miscarriages or more than or equal to two consecutive second-trimester miscarriages) without any apparent cause and no hereditary thrombophilia [46]. In 340 women with more than or equal to three unexplained first-trimester RPLs, enoxaparin 20 mg daily from fetal viability until 34 weeks was associated with a slight nonsignificant reduction in both early (4.1% vs. 8.8%) and late (1.1% vs. 2.3%) miscarriages, but no other effects on other perinatal outcomes [47]. Additionally, a more recent multicenter trial with a minimization randomization scheme confirmed similar live birth rates (86% vs. 86.7%) in the intervention (LMWH) and control groups, respectively [48].

No reduction in PL was observed when LMWH and low-dose aspirin were used in combination to treat 297 women with idiopathic recurrent miscarriage (22% in pharmacologic intervention group vs. 20% in surveillance group) [49]. In women with 364 unexplained RPLs, nadroparin, and low-dose aspirin were associated with similar outcomes compared with either low-dose aspirin alone or to placebo [45].

Vitamins
There is no specific adequate trial on multivitamin supplementation of any kind for women with prior RPL.

Diethylstilbestrol
DES should not be used in pregnancy for any indication. Data are mostly from studies of women without risk factors, women with "threatened abortion" in the current pregnancy, or diabetics (most women with RPL). **DES use in pregnancy is significantly associated with several harmful consequences for both mother and baby.** DES given in the first trimester [50] leads to a 37% increased rate of miscarriage and 61% increased rate of PTB [51–58]. There is also a 48% increase in the numbers of babies weighing less than 2500 g. Stillbirth and neonatal death are not influenced by the intervention (DES) as compared with the control group. Preeclampsia is similar in the two groups. Exposed female offsprings have a nonsignificant trend toward more cancer of the genital tract and cancer other than of the genital tract. Primary infertility, adenosis of the vagina/cervix in female offsprings, and testicular abnormality in male offsprings are significantly higher in those exposed to DES before birth.

The vast use in the 1950s to 1970s of a medication with no benefit proven by evidence-based medicine is the best example of the importance of using data from trials and meta-analyses to guide effective practice.

Immunotherapy
The various forms of immunotherapy did not show significant differences between treatment and control groups in terms of subsequent live births [59]:

- Paternal cell immunization (12 trials, 641 women), OR 1.23, 95% CI 0.89–1.70 [60–70].
- Third-party donor cell immunization (3 trials, 156 women), OR 1.39, 95% CI 0.68–2.82 [50,61,63].
- Trophoblast membrane infusion (one trial, 37 women), OR 0.40, 95% CI 0.11–1.45 [71].
- IVIG (eight trials, 303 women), OR 0.98, 95% CI 0.61–1.58 [72–79]. More recently, another trial confirmed these results [80].

Immunization using viable mononuclear cells carries the **risk of any blood transfusion** such as hepatitis B virus or human immunodeficiency virus (HIV). Reactions have been uncommon but include soreness and redness at the injection site, fever, maternal platelet alloimmunization, blood group sensitization, and one cutaneous graft-versus-host-like reaction. Women who have received lymphocyte immune therapy may have a higher incidence of subsequent miscarriage than women who did not receive such cellular products [54]. The Director of the Office of Therapeutics Research and Review, U.S. Food and Drug Administration (FDA), sent a letter on January 30, 2002, to physicians believed to be using lymphocyte immune therapy to prevent miscarriages. He informed them that the injectable products used in lymphocyte immune therapy do not have the required FDA approval and are considered investigational new drugs that pose several significant safety concerns. Administration of such cells or cellular products in humans can only be performed in the United States as part of clinical investigations, and then only if there is an investigational new drug (IND) application in effect. IVIG therapy is expensive and in relatively short supply.

Immunotherapies should not be offered as treatment for unexplained RPL. Women should be spared the pain and grief associated with false expectations that an ineffective treatment might work.

ANTEPARTUM TESTING
No specific testing indicated.

DELIVERY
No specific precaution.

ANESTHESIA
No specific precaution.

POSTPARTUM/BREAST-FEEDING
No specific precaution.

FUTURE
Effective treatment of an alleged alloimmune cause of recurrent miscarriage awaits more complete knowledge of the underlying pathophysiology. A specific assay to diagnose immune-mediated early PL and a reliable method to determine which patients might benefit from manipulation of the maternal immune system are urgently needed. It is not presently known exactly how many REPLs are the results of anembryonic or chromosomally abnormal conceptuses, anatomic or structural abnormalities, and how many are embryonic or fetal deaths. It is likely that some unexplained early losses are due to as yet undefined subchromosomal genetic abnormalities impairing early development of the conceptus. New molecular techniques should be directed at understanding the factors responsible for successful pregnancy as well as PL.

REFERENCES
1. World Health Organization. WHO: Recommended definitions, terminology and format for statistical tables related to the perinatal period and use of a new certificate for cause of perinatal deaths. modifications recommended by FIGO as amended October 14, 1976. *Acta Obstet Gynecol Scand.* 1977;56(3):247–253. [III]
2. Royal College of Obstetricians and Gynaecologists. *Green-Top Guideline No. 17: Recurrent Miscarriage, Investigation and Treatment of Couples.* London, United Kingdom: RCOG, 2011. [III]
3. Practice Committee of the American Society for Reproductive Medicine. Definitions of infertility and recurrent pregnancy loss: A committee opinion. *Fertil Steril.* 2013;99(1):63. [III]
4. Kolte AM, Bernardi LA, Christiansen OB, et al. Terminology for pregnancy loss prior to viability: A consensus statement from the ESHRE early pregnancy special interest group. *Hum Reprod.* 2015;30(3):495–498. [III]
5. Ansari AH, Kirkpatrick B. Recurrent pregnancy loss. An update. *J Reprod Med.* 1998;43(9):806–814. [Review]
6. Stirrat GM. Recurrent miscarriage I: Definition and epidemiology. *Lancet.* 1990;336(8716):673–675. [III]
7. Kutteh WH. Recurrent pregnancy loss: An update. *Curr Opin Obstet Gynecol.* 1999;11(5):435–439. [III]
8. Carp HJ. *Recurrent Pregnancy Loss: Causes, Controversies and Treatment.* London, United Kingdom: Informa UK, 2007, p. 290 [III]
9. Nybo Andersen AM, Wohlfahrt J, Christens P, et al. Maternal age and fetal loss: Population based register linkage study. *BMJ.* 2000;320(7251):1708–1712. [II-2]
10. Clifford K, Rai R, Regan L. Future pregnancy outcome in unexplained recurrent first trimester miscarriage. *Hum Reprod.* 1997;12(2):387–389. [II-2]
11. Regan L, Braude PR, Trembath PL. Influence of past reproductive performance on risk of spontaneous abortion. *BMJ.* 1989;299(6698):541–545. [II-1]
12. Branch DW, Gibson M, Silver RM. Recurrent miscarriage. *N Engl J Med.* 2010;363(18):1740–1747. [Review]
13. Stephenson MD, Sierra S. Reproductive outcomes in recurrent pregnancy loss associated with a parental carrier of a structural chromosome rearrangement. *Hum Reprod.* 2006;21(4):1076–1082. [II-2]
14. Stephenson MD. Recurrent early pregnancy loss: Is miscarriage evaluation the missing link? *Contemp OB/GYN.* 2008:53(10):m50–m55. [Review]
15. Nicholas S, Orzechowski K, Potti S, et al. Early pregnancy failure as a training tool for chorionic villus sampling. *Prenat Diagn.* 2013;33(11):1110–1112. [II-2]
16. Borrell A, Stergiotou I. Miscarriage in contemporary maternal-fetal medicine: Targeting clinical dilemmas. *Ultrasound Obstet Gynecol.* 2013;42(5):491–497. [Review]
17. Marquard K, Westphal LM, Milki AA, et al. Etiology of recurrent pregnancy loss in women over the age of 35 years. *Fertil Steril.* 2010;94(4):1473–1477. [II-2]
18. Nikcevic AV, Tinkel SA, Kuczmierczyk AR, et al. Investigation of the cause of miscarriage and its influence on women's psychological distress. *BJOG.* 1999;106(8):808–813. [II-2]
19. Sugiura-Ogasawara M, Ozaki Y, Katano K, et al. Uterine anomaly and recurrent pregnancy loss. *Semin Reprod Med.* 2011;29(6):514–521. [Review]
20. Stovall DW, Parrish SB, Van Voorhis BJ, et al. Uterine leiomyomas reduce the efficacy of assisted reproduction cycles: Results of a matched follow-up study. *Hum Reprod.* 1998;13(1):192–197. [II-2]
21. Karamardian LM, Grimes DA. Luteal phase deficiency: Effect of treatment on pregnancy rates. *Obstet Gynecol.* 1992;167(5):1391–1398. [Meta-analysis: 1 RCT, $n = 44$ and 3 controlled studies]
22. Balasch J, Vanrell JA, Marquez M, et al. Dehydrogesterone versus vaginal progesterone in the treatment of the endometrial luteal phase deficiency. *Fertil Steril.* 1982;37(6):751–754. [RCT, $n = 44$]
23. Sergi C, Al Jishi T, Walker M. Factor V leiden mutation in women with early recurrent pregnancy loss: A meta-analysis and systematic review of the causal association. *Arch Gynecol Obstet.* 2015;291(3):671–679. [I, variable quality studies]
24. UNITE, Inc. Grief Support After Miscarriage, Stillbirth, and Infant Death. Available at: http://Unitegriefsupport.org/. Accessed on August 31, 2016.
25. Farquharson RG, Quenby S, Greaves M. Antiphospholipid syndrome in pregnancy: A randomized, controlled trial of treatment. *Obstet Gynecol.* 2002;100(3):408–413. [RCT $n = 98$]
26. Laskin CA, Spitzer KA, Clark CA, et al. Low molecular weight heparin and aspirin for recurrent pregnancy loss: Results from the randomized, controlled HepASA trial. *J Rheumatol.* 2009;36(2):279–287. [RCT $n = 88$]
27. Noble LS, Kutteh WH, Lashey N, et al. Antiphospholipid antibodies associated with recurrent pregnancy loss: Prospective, multicenter, controlled pilot study comparing treatment with low-molecular-weight heparin versus unfractionated heparin. *Fertil Steril.* 2005;83(3):684–690. [RCT $n = 50$]
28. Stephenson MD, Ballem PJ, Tsang P, et al. Treatment of antiphospholipid antibody syndrome (APS) in pregnancy: A randomized pilot trial comparing low molecular weight heparin to unfractionated heparin. *J Obstet Gynaecol Can.* 2004;26:729–734. [RCT $n = 26$]
29. Ziakas PD, Pavlou M, Voulgarelis M. Heparin treatment in antiphospholipid syndrome with recurrent pregnancy loss: A systematic review and meta-analysis. *Obstet Gynecol.* 2010;115(6):1256–1262. [Meta-analysis: 5 RCTs, $n = 398$]
30. Empson M, Lassere M, Craig J, et al. Prevention of recurrent miscarriage for women with antiphospholipid antibody or lupus anticoagulant. *Cochrane Database Syst Rev.* 2007:CD002859. [Meta-analysis: 13 RCTs, $n = 840$]
31. Grandone E, Villani M, Tiscia GL. Aspirin and heparin in pregnancy. *Expert Opin Pharmacother.* 2015;16(12):1793–1803. [III]
32. Haas DM, Ramsey PS. Progestogen for preventing miscarriage. *Cochrane Database Syst Rev.* 2013;(10):CD003511. [Meta-analysis: 14 RCTs, $n = 2158$]
33. Goldzieher JW. Double-blind trial of a progestin in habitual abortion. *JAMA.* 1964;188(7):651–654. [RCT, $n = 16$. Women who had either: never had a term pregnancy and who had had two or more miscarriages or who had had one or more term pregnancy followed by a minimum number of two consecutive miscarriages. All women had to have a urinary pregnanediol of <5 mg/day before 8 weeks' gestation and/or <7 mg/day by 14 weeks' gestation. 10 mg/day of oral medroxyprogesterone. Placebo: yes. Duration: not stated.]

34. Swyer GIM, Daley D. Progesterone implantation in habitual abortion. *Br Med J.* 1953;1(4819):1073–1077. [RCT, $n = 47$ (out of 113 total). Women having had two or more consecutive miscarriages before 12 weeks' gestation. 6 × 25 mg progesterone pellets inserted within the gluteal muscle either: *(i)* as soon as pregnancy was confirmed or (ii) not later than 10th week of gestation, or (iii) not later than the earliest previous miscarriage. Placebo: no but had a no-treatment control group.]
35. El-Zibdeh M. Dydrogesterone in the reduction of recurrent spontaneous abortion. *J Steroid Biochem Mol Biol.* 2005;97(5):431–434. [RCT $n = 180$]
36. Stray-Pedersen B, Stray-Pedersen S. Recurrent abortion: The role of psychotherapy. In: Beard RW, Sharp F (eds.). *Early Pregnancy Loss.* London, United Kingdom: Springer, 1988:433–440. [II-2]
37. Liddell H, Pattison N, Zanderigo A. Recurrent miscarriage-outcome after supportive care in early pregnancy. *Aust NZ J Obstet Gynaecol.* 1991;31(4):320–322. [II-1]
38. Scott JR, Pattison N. Human chorionic gonadotrophin for recurrent miscarriage. *Cochrane Database Syst Rev.* 2007:CD000101. [Meta-analysis: 4 RCTs, $n = 180$. Variable quality trials]
39. Harrison RF. Treatment of habitual abortion with human chorionic gonadotropin: Results of open and placebo-controlled studies. *Eur J Obstet Gynecol Reprod Biol.* 1985;20(3):159–168. [RCT, $n = $ spontaneous miscarriage of *three previous consecutive pregnancies without evidence of a cause*, normal investigative profile included: Chromosomal analysis of both partners; no systemic disease; normal bacteriological investigations of semen and cervical secretions; normal HSG, normal serum FSH, LH, estradiol, and prolactin; normal or low progesterone. Initially 10,000 IU hCG by IM injection followed by 5000 IU twice weekly up to 12 weeks, followed by 5000 IU weekly until 20 weeks.]
40. Harrison RF. Human chorionic gonadotrophin (hCG) in the management of recurrent abortion; results of a multi-centre placebo-controlled study. *Eur J Obstet Gynecol Reprod Biol.* 1992;47(3):175–179. [RCT. "Modus operandi" described as identical to Harrison 1985 study. hCG 10,000 IU IM starting before 8 weeks. hCG 5000 IU IM twice weekly until 12 weeks. hCG 5000 IU IM once weekly from 12 to 16 weeks. Identically packaged vs. placebo vials given as same regime]
41. Quenby S, Farquharson RG. Human chorionic gonadotropin supplementation in recurring pregnancy loss: A controlled trial. *Fertil Steril.* 1994;62(4):708–710. [RCT, $n = 104$. Two or more consecutive first-trimester miscarriages. Profasi (Serono) 10,000 U IM initially and 5000 U twice weekly until 14 weeks' gestation. Control group: placebo of normal saline IM "in an identical fashion."]
42. Svigos J. Preliminary experience with the use of human chorionic gonadotrophin therapy in women with repeated abortion. *Clin Reprod Fertil.* 1982;1(2):131–135. [RCT. Two unexplained (normal genital tract and chromosomes) miscarriages. Treatment group managed in one of two ways according to serum progesterone. A low progesterone precipitated compliance with the intended treatment. A normal progesterone precipitated no treatment (i.e., managed as a control). Groups analyzed on an intention-to-treat basis. 9000 IU, IM × 3 per week from 6 to 7 weeks until 12 weeks vs. no treatment.]
43. Tulppala M, Marttunen M, Soderstrom-Anttila V, et al. Low-dose aspirin in prevention of miscarriage in women with unexplained or autoimmune related recurrent miscarriage: Effect on prostacyclin and thromboxane A2 production. *Hum Reprod.* 1997;12(7):1567–1572.
44. de Jong PG, Kaandorp S, Di Nisio M, et al. Aspirin and/or heparin for women with unexplained recurrent miscarriage with or without inherited thrombophilia. *Cochrane Database Syst Rev.* 2014;(7):CD004734. [Meta-analysis: 9 RCTs, $n = 1228$, variable quality studies]
45. Kaandorp SP, Goddijn M, van der Post, et al. Aspirin plus heparin or aspirin alone in women with recurrent miscarriage. *N Engl J Med.* 2010;362(17):1586–1596. [RCT, $n = 364$]
46. Fawzy M, Shokeir T, El-Tatongy M, et al. Treatment options and pregnancy outcome in women with idiopathic recurrent miscarriage: A randomized placebo-controlled study. *Arch Gynecol Obstet.* 2008;278(1):33–38. [RCT $n = 160$, Women with ≥ 3 fetal losses randomized to enoxaparin $n = 57$, combination prednisone, aspirin, and progesterone $n = 53$, or placebo $n = 50$]
47. Badawy A, Khiary M, Sherif L, et al. Low-molecular weight heparin in patients with recurrent early miscarriages of unknown aetiology. *J Obstet Gynecol.* 2008;28(3):280–284. [RCT $n = 340$]
48. Schleussner E, Kamin G, Seliger G, et al. Low-molecular-weight heparin for women with unexplained recurrent pregnancy loss. *Ann Intern Med.* 2015;162(9):601–609. [RCT $n = 449$]
49. Clark P, Walker ID, Langhorne P, et al. SPIN (Scottish Pregnancy Intervention) study: A multicenter, randomized controlled trial of low-molecular-weight heparin and low-dose aspirin in women with recurrent miscarriage. *Blood.* 2010;115(21):4162–4167. [RCT, $n = 294$, multicenter, >2 recurrent pregnancy losses at 24 or fewer weeks, randomized to enoxaparin 40 mg SQ QD and aspirin 75 mg PO QD until 36 weeks, or to pregnancy surveillance only.]
50. Scott JR, Branch WD, Dudley D, et al. Immunotherapy for recurrent pregnancy loss: The University of Utah perspective. In: Dondero F, Johnson P (eds.). *Reproductive Immunology..* New York, NY: Serono Symposium Publications, Raven Press, 1997: 255–257. [RCT]
51. Bamigboye AA, Morris J. Oestrogen supplementation, mainly diethylstilbestrol, for preventing miscarriages and other adverse pregnancy outcomes. *Cochrane Database Syst Rev.* 2003;(3):CD004353. [Meta-analysis: 7 RCTs, $n = 2897$]
52. Bender S. The effect of diethylstilboestrol on recurrent miscarriage. Personal communication, February 1988. [RCT, $n = 58$ women with prior SAB. DES in one clinic vs. control in another clinic].
53. Crowder RE, Bills ES, Broadbent JS. The management of threatened abortion: A study of 100 cases. *Am J Obstet Gynecol.* 1950;60(4):896–899. [RCT, $n = 100$. Women admitted for threatened abortion and diabetic. DES 25 mg every 30 minutes for 6 hours then 100 mg daily until asymptomatic for 24 hours, then 50 mg daily until 28 weeks of pregnancy. Both DES and control group had phenobarbitone and demerol.]
54. Dieckmann WJ, Davis ME, Rynkiewcz LM, et al. Does the administration of diethylstilbestrol during pregnancy have therapeutic value? *Am J Obstet Gynecol.* 1953;66(5):1062–1081. [RCT, $n = 1646$ (all women). 5 mg of DES administered from 7 to 8 weeks in graduated fashion up to 150 mg at 34–35 weeks vs. placebo. Many long-term follow-up manuscripts]
55. Ferguson JH. Effect of stilbestrol on pregnancy compared to the effect of a placebo. *Am J Obstet Gynecol.* 1953;65(3):592–601. [RCT, $n = 393$ (all women). DES 6.3–137.5 mg depending on gestational age vs. placebo]
56. Reid D. The use of hormones in the management of pregnancy in diabetics. *Lancet.* 1955;2:833–836. [RCT, $n = 147$ (High-risk diabetic women). Incremental doses of 50–200 mg DES daily from about 16 weeks to term. Ethisterone, 25 mg/day from 16 weeks, incrementally to 250 mg/day at 32 weeks to term. Ethisterone was given incrementally. Graduated dosing with stilbestrol from 50 mg at 19 weeks or less to 200 mg at 32 weeks or more. Ethisterone from 25 mg/day at 19 weeks or less to 250 mg at 32 weeks or more vs. placebo]
57. Robinson D, Shettles LB. The use of diethylstilbestrol in threatened abortion. *Am J Obstet Gynecol.* 1952;63(6):1330–1333. [RCT, $n = 93$. Women admitted for threatened abortion. DES 5–125 mg depending on gestational age vs. placebo]
58. Swyer G, Law R. An evaluation of the prophylactic antenatal use of stilboestrol. Preliminary report. *J Endocrinol.* 1954;10(4):R6–R7. [RCT, $n = 460$ (all primigravidas). 5 mg of DES administered from 7 to 8 weeks in graduated fashion up to 150 mg at 34–35 weeks vs. placebo (as Dieckman).]
59. Wong LF, Porter TF, Scott JR. Immunotherapy for recurrent miscarriage. *CochraneDatabase Syst Rev.* 2014;(10):CD000112. [Meta-analysis: 20 RCTs]

60. Cauchi M, Lim D, Young D, et al. Treatment of recurrent aborters by immunization with paternal cells—Controlled trial. *Am J Reprod Immunol*. 1991;25(1):16–17. [RCT n = 46]
61. Christiansen OB, Mathiesen O, Husth M, et al. Placebo-controlled trial of active immunization with third party leukocytes in recurrent miscarriage. *Acta Obstet Gynecol Scand*. 1994;73(3):261–268. [RCT n = 66]
62. Gatenby PA, Cameron K, Simes RJ, et al. Treatment of recurrent spontaneous abortion by immunization with paternal lymphocytes: Results of a controlled trial. *Am J Reprod Immunol*. 1993;29(2):88–94. [RCT]
63. Ho H, Gill TJ, Hsieh H, et al. Immunotherapy for recurrent spontaneous abortions in a chinese population. *Am J Reprod Immunol*. 1991;25(1):10–15. [RCT]
64. Illeni MT, Marelli G, Parazzini F, et al. Immunotherapy and recurrent abortion: A randomized clinical trial. *Hum Reprod*. 1994;9(7):1247–1249. [RCT n = 44]
65. Mowbray J, Liddell H, Underwood J, et al. Controlled trial of treatment of recurrent spontaneous abortion by immunisation with paternal cells. *Lancet*. 1985;325(8435):941–943. [RCT n = 49]
66. Kilpatrick DC LW. Abstracts of contributors' individual data submitted to the worldwide prospective observation study on immunotherapy for treatment of recurrent spontaneous abortion. *Am J Reprod Immunol*. 1994;32:264. [I; RCT + Review]
67. Ober C, Karrison T, Odem RR, et al. Mononuclear-cell immunisation in prevention of recurrent miscarriages: A randomised trial. *Lancet*. 1999;354(9176):365–369. [RCT, n = 183]
68. Pandey MK, Thakur S, Agrawal S. Lymphocyte immunotherapy and its probable mechanism in the maintenance of pregnancy in women with recurrent spontaneous abortion. *Arch Gynecol Obstet*. 2004;269(3):161–172. [III]
69. Reznikoff-Etievant MF. Abstract of contributors' individual data submitted to the worldwide prospective observation study on immunotherapy for treatment of recurrent spontaneous abortion. *Am J Reprod Immunol*. 1994;32(4):266–267. [RCT]
70. Stray-Pederson S. Department of Obstetrics and Gynecology, University of Oslo, Oslo, Norway. Personal communication, 1994 (in Cochrane, Ref. 44 above). [RCT]
71. Johnson P, Ramsden G, Chia K, et al. A combined randomised double-blind and open study of trophoblast membrane infusion (TMI) in unexplained recurrent miscarriage. In: Chaouat, G, Mowbray, J F (eds.). *Cellular Molecular Biology of the Materno-Fetal Relationship*, Vol. 212. Paris, France: Colloque INSERM/John Libbey Eurotext Ltd, 1991:277–284. [RCT]
72. Christiansen OB, Mathiesen O, Husth M, et al. Placebo-controlled trial of treatment of unexplained secondary recurrent spontaneous abortions and recurrent late spontaneous abortions with i.v. immunoglobulin. *Hum Reprod*. 1995;10(10):2690–2695. [RCT, n = 34]
73. Christiansen OB, Pedersen B, Rosgaard A, et al. A randomized, double-blind, placebo-controlled trial of intravenous immunoglobulin in the prevention of recurrent miscarriage: Evidence for a therapeutic effect in women with secondary recurrent miscarriage. *Hum Reprod*. 2002;17(3):809–816. [RCT, n = 58]
74. Coulam CB, Krysa L, Stern JJ, et al. Intravenous immunoglobulin for treatment of recurrent pregnancy loss. *Am J Reprod Immunol*. 1995;34(6):333–337. [RCT, n = 95]
75. German RSA/IVIG Group. Intravenous immunoglobulin for treatment of recurrent miscarriage. *Br J Obstet Gynecol*. 1994;101:1072–1077. [RCT, n = 64]
76. Jablonowska B, Selbing A, Palfi M, et al. Prevention of recurrent spontaneous abortion by intravenous immunoglobulin: A double-blind placebo-controlled study. *Hum Reprod*. 1999;14(3):838–841. [RCT, n = 41]
77. Perino A, Vassiliadis A, Vucetich A, et al. Short-term therapy for recurrent abortion using intravenous immunoglobulins: Results of a double-blind placebo-controlled Italian study. *Hum Reprod*. 1997;12(11):2388–2392. [RCT, n = 46]
78. Stephenson MD, Dreher K, Houlihan E, Wu V. Prevention of unexplained recurrent spontaneous abortion using intravenous immunoglobulin: A prospective, randomized, Double-Blinded, Placebo-Controlled trial. *Am J Reprod Immunol*. 1998;39(2):82–88. [RCT, n = 62]
79. Stephenson MD, Kutteh WH, Purkiss S, et al. Intravenous immunoglobulin and idiopathic secondary recurrent miscarriage: A multicentered randomized placebo-controlled trial. *Hum Reprod*. 2010;25(9):2203–2209. [RCT]
80. Christiansen OB, Larsen E, Egerup P, et al. Intravenous immunoglobulin treatment for secondary recurrent miscarriage: A randomised, double-blind, placebo-controlled trial. *BJOG*. 2015;122(4):500–508. [RCT, n = 82]

Preterm birth prevention in asymptomatic women

Anju Suhag

KEY POINTS
- Gestational age (GA) determination is of utmost importance in prevention of preterm birth (PTB) and management of presumed threatened PTB.
- PTB is defined as birth between 20 0/7 and 36 6/7 weeks. It is the **number one cause of perinatal morbidity and mortality**, and these complications are inversely proportional to GA at birth. **Over 1 million babies die of the consequences of PTB every year in the world,** 1 every 30 seconds.
- An accurate history should be taken regarding risk factors for PTB, especially obstetric–gynecological (ob-gyn) history, maternal lifestyle, and prepregnancy weight (Table 17.1).
- **Primary prevention strategies** for PTB aimed at the general population include family planning, avoidance of lifestyle risks, and proper nutrition. A reproductive-age woman should **avoid** (as feasible) **extremes of age, of interpregnancy interval (18–23 months is optimal interval between last delivery and next conception), uterine evacuation of pregnancy without ripening, multiple gestations, illegal drugs (e.g., cocaine), physical abuse, sexually transmitted infections (STIs),** poverty, poor education, and **a prepregnancy weight of <50 kg (<120 lb).** A normal body mass index (BMI) at the start of pregnancy, not dieting but instead a balanced diet during pregnancy achieving weight gain of >5 kg by 30 weeks for underweight and normal-weight women, can certainly help avoid PTB.
- Screening with transvaginal ultrasound (TVU) cervical length (CL) at 18–23 6/7 weeks should be offered to all singleton gestations. In singleton gestations without a prior spontaneous PTB (SPTB), if CL ≤25 mm develops, vaginal progesterone (e.g., 200 mg suppositories daily until 36 weeks) should be recommended.
- Secondary prevention of PTB is based on identification and treatment (or avoidance) of risk factors. **A screening test aimed at prediction of PTB is only beneficial if an intervention reduces the outcome once the screening test is positive.** Secondary prevention of PTB has been shown in the following groups for the following interventions:
  - In women who **smoke, smoking cessation counseling/** support programs.
  - In women with ≥1 prior SPTBs, now carrying **a singleton gestation,** all the following intervention are associated with a significant decrease in recurrent PTB:
    - **17 α-hydroxyprogesterone caproate** (17P) 250 mg intramuscular (IM) each week starting at 16–20 weeks until 36 weeks.
    - Moderate **fish intake,** up to three meals per week, before 22 weeks.
    - **Cerclage if the CL is <25 mm between 16 and 23 6/7 weeks. Therefore, all singleton gestations should have TVU CL screening in the second trimester.**
  - In women with ≥3 prior SPTBs or second-trimester losses (STLs), history-indicated cerclage.
- In women with cervical dilatation ≥1 cm before 24 weeks, physical examination–indicated cerclage (PEIC) is associated with a significant decrease in PTB.
- In women with **asymptomatic bacteriuria of >100,000 bacteria/mL, appropriate antibiotics** are associated with a significant decrease in PTB.
- In women with **asymptomatic group B streptococcus (GBS) bacteriuria of any colony count,** appropriate antibiotics (usually **penicillin**) are associated with a significant decrease in PTB.
- All other screening and treatment interventions for prevention of PTB are not supported by evidence for recommending their clinical use.

BACKGROUND
Prevention of PTB is the number one issue in pregnancy, as being born preterm is the number one cause of neonatal mortality and the second leading cause of all under-five childhood mortality in many developed countries, including the United States [1,2]. This chapter reviews evidence-based guidelines for women without symptoms related to PTB. The following two chapters deal with women with symptoms of PTB: first preterm labor (PTL) (Chapter 18), then preterm premature rupture of membranes (PPROM) (Chapter 19).

DIAGNOSES/DEFINITIONS
Gestational age (GA) determination is of utmost importance in prevention of PTB and management of presumed threatened PTB (see Chapter 4 for best GA determination criteria).

Definitions regarding prematurity vary in different publications, but the ones most commonly accepted and used in trials are the following:

- **Preterm birth (PTB):** birth between 20 0/7 and 36 6/7 weeks [3]
- Very early PTB: birth between 20 0/7 and 23 6/7 weeks
- Early PTB: birth between 24 0/7 and 33 6/7 weeks
- Late PTB: birth between 34 0/7 and 36 6/7 weeks

Pregnancy loss (PL): spontaneous loss of pregnancy from conception to <20 weeks. The term spontaneous abortion is equivalent but should be avoided since women associate negative feeling with this term. Miscarriage is a lay term for PL (see also Chapters 15 and 16).

Second-trimester PL (aka STL): birth between 14 0/7 and 19 6/7 weeks.

Cervical insufficiency (CI) (formerly called incompetence): recurrent painless dilatation leading to STLs [4]. A better definition is a **CL <25 mm before 24 weeks in women with singleton gestations and prior SPTB <37 weeks.**

Preterm labor (PTL): uterine contractions (≥4/20 minutes or ≥8/hours) and documented cervical change with

Table 17.1 Selected Risk Factors for SPTB

History:
- Obstetrical–gynecological history: prior SPTB; prior STL; prior D&Es; prior LEEP; prior cone biopsy; uterine anomalies; DES exposure; myomatas; short interpregnancy interval (<6 months); ART; prior stillbirth <24 weeks; prior early twin SPTB; prior full-term cesarean delivery for second stage arrest
- Maternal lifestyle (smoking, drug abuse)
- Maternal prepregnancy weight <120 lb (<50 kg) or low BMI (<19.8 kg/m^2), short height (<53 inches or 3 SD below any race/ethnicity); poor nutritional status
- Maternal age (<19; >35)
- Race (especially African-American)
- Education (<12 grades)
- Certain medical conditions (e.g., DM, HTN, renal disease, and intrahepatic cholestasis of pregnancy)
- Low socioeconomic status
- Limited prenatal care
- Family history of SPTB (poorly studied)
- Vaginal bleeding (especially during second trimester, subchorionic hematoma)
- Social or psychological stress (mostly related to above risks)
- Infections (bacterial vaginosis, chlamydia, gonorrhea, asymptomatic bacteriuria, urinary tract infection, periodontal disease)
- Higher number of lifetime sexual partner

Identifiable by screening:
- Anemia
- Infections (STIs, periodontal disease)
- TVU CL <25 mm (especially <24 weeks)
- fFN positive ($\geq$50 ng/mL) (between 22 and 34 weeks)

Usually symptomatic:
- Uterine contractions

Not spontaneous (indicated/iatrogenic):
- Fetal demise/major fetal anomaly
- Multiple gestation/polyhydramnios
- Nonreassuring fetal heart tracing
- IUGR
- Placenta previa
- Placental abruption
- Major maternal disease (HTN complications, DM, etc.)

Abbreviations: ART, assisted reproductive technology; BMI, body mass index; CL, cervical length; D&Es, dilation and evacuations; DES, diethylstilbestrol; DM, diabetes mellitus; fFN, fetal fibronectin; HTN, hypertension; IUGR, intrauterine growth restriction; LEEP, loop electrosurgical excision procedure; SD, standard deviation; SPTB, spontaneous preterm birth; STI, sexually transmitted infection; STL, second-trimester loss; TVU, transvaginal ultrasound.

intact membranes at 20–36 6/7 weeks. A better definition is **uterine contractions ($\geq$4/20 minutes or $\geq$8/hour) with TVU CL <20 mm, or 20–29 mm with positive fetal fibronectin (fFN)** at 20–36 6/7 weeks (see Chapter 18).

Premature preterm rupture of membranes (PPROM): vaginal pooling, nitrazine, and/or ferning at 16–36 6/7 weeks (see Chapter 19).

- Early PPROM: PPROM between 24 and 33 6/7 weeks
- Very early PPROM: PPROM between 16 and 23 6/7 weeks

EPIDEMIOLOGY/INCIDENCE

Incidence of PTB <37 weeks varies between about 5% and 18% in different countries [5]. The rate of PTB in the United States steadily increased from 9.4% in 1981 and peaked in 2006 at 12.8%. Since then, the rate of PTB in the United States dropped to 9.6% in 2014 (25% decline) [6,7]. The incidence of PTB <32 weeks remains at about 2% in United States; and $\leq$1% in most other high-income countries. **Over 1 million babies die of the consequences of PTB every year in the world, 1 every 30 seconds** [1]. The high incidence of PTB in many high-income countries may be due to assisted reproductive technology (ART)-related multiple gestations, older and sicker mothers, earlier GA of registered births and neonatal improvements, better and earlier timing of births (related to ultrasound), worsening socioeconomic factors, and other factors. In addition to the use of progesterone and cerclage in women at high risk for PTB, there are several other demographic factors which lead to reducing national PTB rate. This decline in PTB in the United States appears to be related also to reduced teen birth rate, lower rate of higher order multiple births, smoking cessation counseling and bans, and improved institution/national policies of preventing non-medically indicated PTB <39 weeks [8].

GENETICS

While a genetic predisposition in certain ethnic groups and families has been reported, no clinical genetic studies are yet recommended for prediction/prevention of PTB due to insufficient evidence [9].

ETIOLOGY/BASIC PATHOPHYSIOLOGY

Just like cardiac disease, PTB is a final common manifestation of multifactorial, complex etiology. Several processes leading to PTB are shown in Figure 17.1.

CLASSIFICATION

PTB can be spontaneous, and follow PTL (50%; Chapter 18), PPROM (30%; Chapter 19), or, rarely, cervical insufficiency; or be iatrogenic (20%). Cervical insufficiency may comprise about 1% of spontaneous PTB (SPTB) and/or STLs (see below in the section "Prediction and Prevention of PTB"). Cervical insufficiency represents one extreme of SPTB, as PTB is continuous.

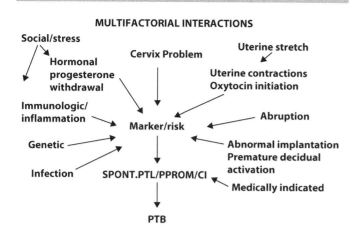

Figure 17.1 PTB is the final common pathway of many associated possible etiologies. CI, cervical insufficiency; SPONT.PTL, spontaneous preterm labor; PPROM, preterm premature rupture of membranes; PTB, preterm birth.

RISK FACTORS/ASSOCIATIONS

Most women who have a PTB have identifiable risk factors. Risk factors for SPTB (presenting as PTL, PPROM, or cervical insufficiency) are similar (Table 17.1). **All these risk factors should be reviewed in details with every pregnant woman at the first prenatal visit.** The vast majority of U.S. pregnant women (96% on in one study) has at least one risk factor for PTB [10]. For many of these risks, there are interventions associated with prevention of PTB.

COMPLICATIONS

PTB is the **number one cause of perinatal mortality.** Seventy-five percent of perinatal mortality occurs in preterm babies; more than two-third of perinatal mortality (60% of total) occurs in infants aged <32 weeks. **Mortality and morbidities are inversely associated with GA at birth** (Table 17.2) [11]. Morbidities include compared with (RDS), bronchopulmonary dysplasia (BPD), intraventricular hemorrhage (IVH), necrotizing enterocolitis (NEC), sepsis, apnea and retinopathy of prematurity [12]. The long-term neonatal morbidities from PTB include chronic lung disease, grade III/IV IVH, NEC, vision and hearing impairment, cerebral palsy, reduced cognition, academic difficulties, and attention deficit disorders [13,14].

PREDICTION AND PREVENTION OF PTB

A screening test aimed at prediction of PTB is only beneficial if an intervention (prevention) reduces the outcome once the screening test is positive. Several predictive strategies have poor sensitivity and specificity.

Prevention is preferable, rather than treatment once symptoms have been identified. Prevention can be divided into three categories (Table 17.3). Primary and secondary prevention are preferable, rather than tertiary prevention of symptomatic women with PTL or PPROM. This chapter refers to prevention of SPTB mostly in **singleton gestations,** unless otherwise specified. Prevention of PTB in multiple gestations is also discussed in Chapter 44 in *Maternal-Fetal Evidence Based Guidelines.*

For women at risk for **iatrogenic (indicated) PTB,** one should aim to keep the pregnant woman as healthy as nonpregnant adult. Appropriate prevention and therapy of any maternal medical or fetal/congenital anomaly disorder is paramount, as is appropriate prevention and therapy for preeclampsia and fetal growth restriction (FGR) (please refer specific chapters in *Maternal-Fetal Evidence Based Guidelines*) [1].

All **prepregnancy evaluations** of the cervix (e.g., hysterosalpingogram, no. 8 Hegar dilator passage, and catheter traction test) aimed at screening for cervical insufficiency have either been inadequately studied or been shown not to be sufficiently predictive and therefore useful in a prevention program (no trial ever reported).

An accurate history should be taken regarding risk factors for PTB, especially ob-gyn history, maternal lifestyle, and prepregnancy weight (Table 17.1). A detailed history should include whether the prior PTB was spontaneous or indicated (iatrogenic). Spontaneous PTB is defined as PTB prior to 37 weeks due to PTL, PPROM, advanced cervical dilation (ACD) or cervical insufficiency. It is also important to document the sequence of events (antepartum) leading to a PTB, as this could help **counsel these women about their risk of recurrent PTB and appropriate PTB prevention strategies** could be utilized. For example, women with a history of ACD are at an increased risk of having cervical shortening (50% vs. 14.6% vs. 15.6%, $p<.01$), recurrent PTB (55.2% vs. 27.2% vs. 32.2%, $p<.01$) and a lower GA at delivery (34.0 vs. 37.2 vs. 37.0 weeks, $p<.01$) in a subsequent pregnancy compared with women with prior PTB associated PPROM or PTL, respectively [15].

A Creasy's score or other similar history-based systems to predict PTB have been associated with a low (10%–30%) positive predictive value (PPV) for PTB, and not clinically useful given negative intervention trials (see below, in the last paragraph in this section and "Intervention: Weekly manual examinations, education"). There are **no trials on risk-scoring systems for predicting PTB** [16]. There is a need for prospective studies that evaluate the use of a risk-screening tool designed to predict PTB (in combination with appropriate consequent interventions) to prevent PTB, including qualitative and/or quantitative evaluation of their impact on women's well-being.

There are four main risk factors for which there are effective interventions for prevention of PTB: smoking; short TVU CL; prior SPTB; and asymptomatic bacteriuria (Table 17.4). **A TVU CL screening at 18–24 weeks is indicated in all women with a singleton gestation** (see "Risk: Short Cervix on Ultrasound" in the section "Secondary Prevention").

Current evidence does not support the use of home uterine activity monitoring (HUAM) [17] or bacterial vaginosis (BV) screening [18] in asymptomatic low-risk women. There are insufficient data to support the use of salivary estriol or fFN in asymptomatic women (even if fFN is one of the best predictive screening tests). Cytokines, matrix metalloproteinases, corticotropin-releasing hormone (CRH), salivary estriol, relaxin, human chorionic gonadotropin (HCG), prothrombin, fetal DNA, and many other tests remain research tools for prediction of PTB and are not yet clinically beneficial, given lack of intervention trials based on these screening tests.

Primary Prevention

Primary prevention includes prevention strategies aimed at **all asymptomatic pregnant women** at risk for PTB (i.e., aimed at all pregnant women). Unfortunately, many primary prevention interventions have been so far either insufficiently studied or found not to be effective.

Table 17.2 Preterm Neonatal Morbidity and Mortality

Outcome	All	Delivery Gestational Age (Weeks)														p-Value
		23	24	25	26	27	28	29	30	31	32	33	34	35	36	
Death	1.4	44.2	31.6	12.1	11.2	8.2	2.0	1.9	1.5	1.0	0.2	0.2	0.0	0.0	0.0	<.001
Major morbidity[a]	7.9	44.2	52.6	54.8	52.1	40.3	21.9	22.5	13.7	7.1	8.7	4.2	4.4	2.8	1.8	<.001
Minor morbidity[b]	37.6	9.3	15.8	31.5	34.9	48.4	73.5	69.0	78.6	81.7	76.3	63.5	51.0	27.2	15.9	<.001
Survival without any of above morbidities	53.1	2.3	0.0	1.6	1.8	3.1	2.6	6.6	6.1	10.3	14.9	32.1	44.6	69.9	82.4	

Source: Modified from Manuck TA et al., Am J Obstet Gynecol, 215(1), 103.e1–103.e14, 2016.
Note: Data presented as %; N = 8334.
[a]Includes persistent pulmonary hypertension, intraventricular hemorrhage grade 3/4, seizures, hypoxic–ischemic encephalopathy, necrotizing enterocolitis stage II/III, and bronchopulmonary dysplasia.
[b]Includes intraventricular hemorrhage grade 1/2, necrotizing enterocolitis stage 1, respiratory distress syndrome, hyperbilirubinemia requiring treatment, and hypotension requiring treatment.

Table 17.3 Definition of the Different Categories of Prevention of PTB

	Definition	Examples
Primary prevention	Prevention strategies aimed at *all asymptomatic* pregnant women at risk for PTB (i.e., aimed at all pregnant women).	Encourage optimal (18–23 months) interpregnancy interval. Limit higher order multiple births (ART).
Secondary prevention	Prevention strategies aimed at *identifying asymptomatic women at high risk for PTB through screening*. Screen for predictive risk factor (prediction) in asymptomatic women and avoid/treat (preventive intervention).	Obtain comprehensive OB history and offer preventive interventions (progesterone, cerclage, CL screening) to appropriate candidates. Smoking cessation. Screen for infection, and treat if indicated.
Tertiary prevention	Prevention strategies aimed at women with active *symptoms* of PTB.	Interventions for women with PTL (Chapter 18) or PPROM (Chapter 19).

Abbreviations: OB, obstetrical; PTB, preterm birth; PTL, preterm labor; PPROM, preterm premature rupture of membranes; ART, assisted reproduction technologies; CL, cervical length.

Table 17.4 Selected Effective Interventions for Prevention of PTB

Avoid (as feasible)	
	• Extremes of age
	• Interpregnancy interval <6 months
	• Induced termination of pregnancy without ripening
	• Multiple gestation
	• Illegal drugs (e.g., cocaine)
	• Physical abuse
	• STIs
	• Poverty
	• Poor education
	• Prepregnancy weight of <50 kg (<120 lb).
Risk	Intervention
Smoking	Smoking cessation programs
Short CL ≤ 20 mm (screen every singleton with TVU CL at 18–23-6/7 weeks)[a]	Vaginal progesterone (e.g., 200 mg daily)
Prior spontaneous PTB (SPTB)[b]	17-OH progesterone caproate, moderate (≥3 meals/week) fish intake
Prior SPTB and CL <25 mm between 16 and 23 6/7 weeks[b]	Ultrasound-indicated cerclage
Prior ≥3 PTB/STL[b]	History-indicated cerclage
Asymptomatic bacteriuria	Appropriate antibiotics

Abbreviations: STI, sexually transmitted infections; CL, cervical length; TVU, transvaginal ultrasound; SPTB, spontaneous preterm birth; STL, second trimester loss.
[a]For singleton gestations without prior PTB.
[b]For singleton gestations.

Preconception/Early Pregnancy

Family planning. There are no trials to assess interventions. **Avoiding extremes of age, avoiding short interpregnancy interval <6 months** (18–23 months is optimal interval between last delivery and next conception) [19], **and reducing the rate of multiple gestations** (through ART improvements) seem self-evident for efficacy in preventing PTB when feasible. Evidence suggests that risks of PTB, low birth weight (LBW), and small-for-gestational-age (SGA) infants are minimized when interpregnancy intervals are between 18–23 months [19,20]. For appropriate interpregnancy interval, physicians should pay close attention to plans for postpartum contraception. Improvements in postpartum contraceptive use have been associated with decreased incidence in PTB. For every month of contraception coverage, the odds of PTB <37 weeks decrease by 1.1% (odds ratio [OR] 0.98, 95% confidence interval [CI] 0.98–0.99) [21].

Induced termination of pregnancy (TOP) is associated with a higher risk of PTB, even if just one early TOP is performed [22]. Recent meta-analyses showed that dilation and curettage (D&C) compared with no D&C increase the risk of PTB <37 weeks (OR 1.29, 95% CI 1.17–1.42) [23,24]. Women who had even just one uterine evacuation for either spontaneous or induced abortion have a higher risk of PTB (OR 1.44, 95% CI 1.09–1.90) [24]. The risk of PTB <37 weeks is noted to be even higher in women with history of multiple D&Cs (OR 1.74, 95% CI 1.10–2.76) [23]. **Avoiding TOPs as feasible with effective contraception seems to be an effective preventive strategy to avoid PTB.** If TOP is unavoidable, the D&C should be performed with preoperative cervical ripening (e.g., misoprostol, mifepristone, or laminaria), as this is associated with no or very low risk for PTB [22].

Avoidance of lifestyle risks. There are no trials to assess interventions. **Avoiding illegal drugs** (e.g., cocaine and amphetamines), **physical abuse, and STIs** (chlamydia, gonorrhea, syphilis, human immunodeficiency virus [HIV], etc.) seem self-evident for efficacy in preventing PTB [25]. **Poverty, poor education,** lack of women's empowerment, and several other social stressors (Table 17.1) are all linked profoundly to an increased risk of PTB and should be avoided as possible, especially through political and social changes. Workplace conditions are only weakly related or are not related to adverse pregnancy outcomes. In the third trimester, >42 hours of work/week, >6 hours of standing/day, and pesticide use are associated with PTB [26]. There are no trials on modifying other potential risks, such as physically demanding job, prolonged standing, night work, or others.

Proper nutrition, weight gain. **A prepregnancy weight of <50 kg (<120 lb) should be avoided.** Recent meta-analysis of 17 randomized controlled trials (RCTs) showed benefit of **nutrition education to increase energy and protein intake in decreasing risk of PTB** (two trials, 449 women) (relative risk [RR] 0.46, 95% CI 0.21–0.98, *low-quality evidence*), **and LBW** (one trial, 300 women) (RR 0.04, 95% CI 0.01–0.14) **among undernourished women** [27]. **A normal BMI at the start of pregnancy, not dieting but instead a balanced diet during pregnancy achieving weight gain of >5 kg by 30 weeks for underweight and normal-weight women, can certainly help to avoid PTB.**

The available evidence shows no benefit of balanced protein/energy supplementation on prevention of PTB [28]. High-protein diet (>25% of total energy content) has no association with PTB prevention, and is not recommended in pregnancy because of increased risk of SGA [29] (see also Chapter 2).

Early Pregnancy

Fish intake. Shark, swordfish, king mackerel, or tilefish contain high levels of mercury and should be avoided or eaten infrequently (≤1/week) in pregnancy. **Canned light tuna, salmon, pollock, grouper, mussels, scallops, shrimp, and catfish are common fishes low in mercury, and two portions (6 oz = 1 portion) of these per week can** (and probably should) **be safely eaten in pregnancy.** Albacore (white) tuna has more mercury and should be consumed up to 6 oz/week. In general, for other fishes, smaller fishes have less mercury than larger ones. More information on fish and mercury intake in pregnancy is available at www.cfsan.fda.gov and www.epa. gov/ost/fish. There is **limited evidence suggesting potential benefit of maternal fish intake on reduction of PTB**. A recent prospective cohort study reported a significant reduction in risk of PTB, in women choosing a "prudent" or a "traditional" dietary pattern, characterized by, for example, vegetables, cooking oil, fruit, berries, olive oil, rice, water as beverage, whole grain cereals, yogurt, poultry, lean fish, and boiled potatoes, as well as low intake of processed meat products, white bread, and pizza/tacos [30].

Omega-3 fatty acids. Low-risk women without a prior PTB have a similar incidence of PTB <37 weeks when given 12 eggs with either 133 mg docosahexaenoic acid (DHA) or with 33 mg DHA per week starting at 24–28 weeks [31]. Supplementation has been shown to prolong pregnancy by 3–8 days in different populations. When all RCTs are examined, women allocated a marine oil supplement had a mean gestation that was 2.6 days longer than women allocated to placebo or no treatment. This was not reflected in a clear difference between the two groups in PTB <37 weeks, although women allocated marine oil did have a **lower risk of PTB <34** *weeks* (RR 0.69, 95% CI 0.49–0.99). Birth weight was slightly greater (47 g) in infants born to women in the marine oil group compared with controls. However, there were no overall differences between the groups in the proportion of LBW or small-for-GA babies. There was no clear difference in the relative risk of preeclampsia between the two groups [32]. A large RCT found that DHA 800 mg supplementation before 21 weeks was associated with a decrease in PTB <34 weeks (RR 0.49, 95% CI 0.25–0.94) [33]. In contrast, in a recent meta-analysis of nine randomized trials including over 3800 asymptomatic women with singleton pregnancies and no prior PTB, **women who received omega-3 had a similar rate of PTB <37 weeks as women who received either a placebo or no supplementation** (7.7% vs. 9.1%; RR 0.90, 95% CI 0.72–1.11) [34]. The evidence suggests **minimal or no benefit of omega-3 supplementation in reduction in PTB <37 weeks in asymptomatic low-risk singleton pregnancies.**

PrimaCare vitamin supplement contains 150 mg of omega-3 fatty acids and has not been evaluated in a trial. The possible beneficial effects of omega-3 fatty acids to later fetal/neonatal/infant cognition remain not fully proven. For omega-3 supplementation in high-risk women, see section "Risk: Prior PTB."

Probiotics. Women who report habitual intake of probiotic diary foods (e.g., yogurt) have been associated with lower incidence of PTB in non-RCT [35]. Currently, there are **insufficient data** from RCTs to demonstrate any impact of probiotic foods supplementation in low-risk women on PTB and its complications [36].

Other nutritional changes. There are no trials with specific aim of prevention of PTB to evaluate other nutritional changes, such as vitamin supplementation (see Chapter 2), HCG, and anticytokine supplements. **Prepregnancy weight <120 lb (<50 kg) is a very significant risk factor for PTB and should be avoided if possible.** Suggested pregnancy weight gain in pregnancy is 25–35 lb for women with normal BMI, but there are no trials on proper prepregnancy weight or pregnancy weight gain.

Vitamin C. Vitamin C supplementation alone is not associated with a reduced risk of PTB [37].

Vitamin E. Vitamin E supplementation alone or in combination with other supplements is not associated with prevention of PTB [38].

Vitamins C and E. Maternal supplementation with vitamin C 1000 mg and vitamin E 400 mg daily from 9 to 16 weeks until delivery in nulliparous low-risk women is **not associated with a reduction in PTB** [39].

Vitamin D. Level II evidence suggests protective effect of vitamin D supplementation in women with low 25-hydroxyvitamin D concentration (at or prior to 20 weeks) on rate of PTB in low-risk women [40]. Routine vitamin D level assessment and/or vitamin D replacement or supplementation is **not indicated** in women at risk for PTB, until a well-designed RCT confirms above findings.

Calcium supplementation. Maternal supplementation of calcium versus placebo is *not associated* with a reduction in PTB [41].

Magnesium supplementation. There is **insufficient high quality evidence** to show that dietary magnesium supplementation during pregnancy is not beneficial. In the analysis of all trials, oral magnesium treatment before 25 weeks showed no significant effect of magnesium on perinatal mortality, SGA, preeclampsia and PTB, compared with placebo [42]. Of the ten trials included in the review, only two were judged to be of high quality, and showed no association of magnesium and pregnancy outcomes.

Progesterone. The mechanism of action of progesterone for prevention of PTB is poorly understood but probably involves an anti-inflammatory action. Safety for the fetus/neonate has not been yet proven with 100% certainty, but progesterone is known not to be a teratogen, and long-term detrimental effects up to 18 years of age have not been shown. The effect of progesterone supplementation should be **evaluated according to different patient populations, and according to type of progesterone.** Here we review progesterone for low-risk women (see below for other risk groups).

In a small RCT including women in active military duty with only a 3% rate of prior PTB and unknown CL, 17P 1000 mg IM weekly starting at 16–20 weeks was **not associated with any effect** on incidence of PTB or perinatal outcomes compared with placebo [43]. No RCT has evaluated the effect of vaginal progesterone in this population.

In summary, there is **insufficient evidence to determine the impact on PTB of progesterone in singleton gestations with no prior PTB, with unknown or normal CL.**

Secondary Prevention

Secondary prevention strategies involve screening for a predictive risk factor (prediction) in asymptomatic women, and avoiding it or treating it (preventive intervention) (Table 17.3).

Risk: Smoking

Intervention: Smoking cessation programs. It is estimated that 10%–15% of PTBs may be due to smoking. In the United States, about 23% of women start pregnancy as a smoker, and 11% continue to smoke throughout pregnancy [44]. **Psychosocial interventions (e.g., counseling, health education, feedback, incentives, social support) to support women to stop smoking in pregnancy has been associated with an increase the proportion of women who stop smoking in late pregnancy, and reduce LBW** (RR 0.82, 95% CI 0.71–0.94) **and PTB** (18% reduction, RR 0.82, 95% CI 0.70–0.96) [45]. The American College of Obstetricians and Gynecologists (ACOG) has recommended use of the five As—ask, advice, assess, assist, arrange—approach [46]. The most effective intervention for smoking cessation in pregnancy is **social support and a reward component** (23% decrease) [47,48]. If above approach is not successful, consider nicotine replacement therapy (NRT) (see Chapter 22 in *Maternal-Fetal Evidence Based Guidelines*).

Intervention: Nicotine replacement therapy. NRT is associated with a trend for benefit in reduction in the incidence of smoking [49–51] (see Chapter 22 in *Maternal-Fetal Evidence Based Guidelines*). A recent RCT showed that NRT was associated with a higher validated smoking cessation rate 1-month postrandomization; however, there was no difference between group's smoking cessation rate at the time of delivery [52]. One concern about NRT use in pregnancy is the possibility of adverse effects of nicotine on the fetus, through alterations in uterine, placental, or blood flow, or directly on the brain. As there are still too few trials to assure it's safe use in pregnancy, and animal studies suggest nicotine may be toxic to the developing central nervous system, registries of women using NRT should be established to gather more outcome data. A 2-year follow up study showed that infants born to women who used NRT for smoking cessation in pregnancy were more likely to have unimpaired development [53]. **There is insufficient evidence to assess the safety of NRT, or nicotine gum, and also the effect on incidence of PTB.** No trial has been done using bupropion (see Chapter 22 in *Maternal-Fetal Evidence Based Guidelines*).

Other interventions. Interventions to increase smoking cessation among the partners of pregnant women, with the additional aim of facilitating cessation by the women themselves, have been insufficiently studied (only one trial) [45]. Stages of change, or feedback, do not show benefit [45]. A recent RCT showed no benefit of combining supervised exercise and physical activity counseling, to improve the effectiveness of behavioral support for smoking cessation in pregnancy [54]. There has been increased awareness and use of e-cigarette or electronic nicotine delivery system (ENDS) in adolescents (especially in middle and high school students), health impact of which is not clear [55,56]. E-cigarettes are marketed as smoking cessation devices and as better alternatives to regular cigarettes. This perception of harm reduction in comparison to regular cigarettes may be prevalent due to the lack of Food and Drug Administration (FDA) regulation on e-cigarette advertising and this potentially can further increase use of e-cigarette in adolescents/reproductive age women and in pregnant women as well [55,57]. ENDS device do not burn tobacco leaves, instead delivers liquid nicotine (with other ingredients and by-products from metals, plastics, rubbers, ceramics, fibers and foams) as an aerosol by heating and vaporizing the liquid components through a battery charged atomizer [58] (see Chapter 22 in *Maternal-Fetal Evidence Based Guidelines*).

Risk: Short Cervix on Ultrasound

Intervention: Activity restriction. Activity restriction is **not associated with prevention of PTB** in asymptomatic singleton gestations with a TVU CL <30 mm, and in fact is associated with a **237% increase in PTB** incidence [59].

Intervention: Progesterone. **Regarding 17P**, a multicenter RCT evaluating the effect of 17P in women with singleton gestations, no prior PTB, and short CL <30 mm compared with placebo showed no difference in rate of PTB <37 weeks (25.1% vs. 24.2%, RR 1.03, 95% CI 0.79–1.35) [60]. In another smaller RCT including women with singleton pregnancies (66% of which had no prior PTB) with CL <25 mm between 16 and 24 weeks, 17P was associated with similar incidences of PTB and neonatal morbidity and mortality compared with cerclage [61]. Cerclage was significantly more effective than 17P at reducing the incidences of PTB <35 and <37 weeks in the subgroup with CL ≤15 mm [61]. In summary, **17P cannot be recommended for prevention of PTB in singletons gestations (no prior PTB) with a short TVU CL.**

Regarding **vaginal progesterone**, there are several RCTs available. In 250 women with mostly (90%) singleton gestations and CL ≤15 mm at 20–25 weeks, of whom about 85% had no prior PTB, vaginal progesterone 200 mg nightly started at 24 weeks until 34 weeks was associated with a 44% significant decrease in SPTB <34 weeks (19% vs. 34%, RR 0.56, 95% CI 0.36–0.86), but no significant effects on neonatal morbidities (composite neonatal adverse outcomes: RR 0.57, 95% CI 0.23–1.31) [62]. A subgroup analysis of only women without prior PTB confirmed significant benefit of progesterone in preventing PTB <34 weeks (RR 0.54, 95% CI 0.34–0.88) [62]. The incidence of CL ≤15 mm was 1.7%. Based on the frequency of short CL and effectiveness for prevention of SPTB <34 weeks from the work of Fonseca et al., the number of women needed to be screened with CL in order to prevent one SPTB <34 weeks is approximately 387, if all women with a CL ≤15 mm receive vaginal progesterone. Once the short CL ≤15 mm is identified, the number needed to treat to prevent one PTB <34 weeks is 7.

In 458 women with singleton gestations and CL 10–20 mm at 19–23 6/7 weeks, of whom about 84% had no prior PTB, vaginal progesterone 90 mg daily started at 20–23 6/7 weeks until 36 6/7 weeks was associated with a 45% significant decrease in PTB <33 weeks (9% vs. 16%, RR 0.55, 95% CI 0.33–0.92) and 43% significant decrease in composite neonatal morbidity and mortality (8% vs. 14%, RR 0.57, 95% CI 0.33–0.99) [63]. The incidences of PTB <28 and <35 weeks, and RDS, were also significantly decreased. Analysis of only women without prior PTB confirmed significant benefit of progesterone in preventing PTB <33 weeks (8% vs. 15%, RR 0.50, 95% CI 0.27–0.90) [63]. The incidence of CL 10–20 mm was 2.3%. Based on the frequency of short CL and effectiveness for prevention of PTB <33 weeks from this study [63], the number of women needed to be screened with CL in order to prevent one PTB <33 weeks is approximately 604, if all women with a CL 10–20 mm receive vaginal progesterone. Once the short CL 10–20 mm is identified, the number needed to treat to prevent one PTB <33 weeks is 14.

A individual patient data meta-analysis of five high quality RCTs, also showed **benefit of vaginal progesterone in asymptomatic women with sonographic short cervix (≤25 mm) in reduction of PTB <33 weeks** (RR 0.58, 95% CI 0.42–0.80) and **composite neonatal morbidity and mortality** (RR 0.57, 95% CI 0.40–0.81) [64].

In summary, in women with singleton gestations, no prior SPTB, and short CL, vaginal progesterone is associated with reduction in PTB and composite perinatal morbidity and mortality. Based on these results, **if a TVU CL ≤ 25 mm is identified at ≤ 24 weeks, vaginal progesterone should be offered for prevention of PTB** [62–64]. There is insufficient evidence that any of the vaginal preparations or doses are superior, as they have not been compared. Vaginal progesterone 200 mg suppository has been used in the trial for CL ≤15 mm [62], and 90 mg gel for the trial for CL 10–20 mm [63]. Therefore, CL, but also cost, availability, and other factors may influence preferred dosing [65,66].

These results also support **universal screening with a single TVU assessment of CL at around 18–24 weeks in singleton gestations without prior SPTB** (Figure 17.2). TVU CL screening of singleton gestations fulfills all criteria for an effective screening program. [67]. For example, multiple cost-effectiveness analyses evaluating universal CL screening in singleton gestations, to identify those with short CL eligible for vaginal progesterone, have been published so far [65,66,68]. All reported that such a strategy would be cost-effective, and in fact cost-saving.

In one study, compared with other managements, including no screening, "universal" sonographic screening of CL in singletons was associated with a reduction of 95,920 PTBs <37 weeks annually in the United States, and was actually cost-saving (almost $13 billion saved) [65]. Even varying the variables (e.g., the cost of vaginal progesterone or of TVU screening), universal screening was the preferred strategy 99% of the time [65].

The other cost-effectiveness analysis, when analyzing universal screening of singleton gestations without prior PTB with TVU CL at 18–24 weeks, calculated over $12 million saved, 424 quality-adjusted life-years (QALY) gained, and 22 neonatal deaths or long-term neurologic deficits prevented for every 100,000 women screened, compared with no screening. Even varying the variables (e.g., the cost of vaginal progesterone or of TVU screening), universal screening was cost-effective over 99% of the time [66].

It should be noted that only 1.7%–2.3% of women were identified to have short CL in the two large trials published [62,63], and that the incidence of CL ≤20 mm at 18–24 weeks is even lower (about 0.8%) in singletons without prior SPTB [67]. There are more limited data to evaluate the effectiveness of vaginal progesterone for CL 21–25 mm [64].

Guidelines from Society for Maternal-Fetal Medicine (SMFM) and ACOG state that implementation of universal TVU CL screening should be viewed as reasonable, and can

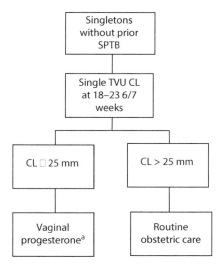

Figure 17.2 Transvaginal ultrasound (TVU) cervical length (CL) screening for the woman with a singleton gestation and no prior spontaneous preterm birth (SPTB) at 16–36 6/7 weeks. ᵃFor example, daily 200 mg suppository or 90 mg gel from time of diagnosis of short CL to 36 weeks. (Adapted from Romero R et al., *Am J Obstet Gynecol*, 206, 124.e1–e19, 2012; Society for Maternal-Fetal Medicine and Berghella V, *Am J Obstet Gynecol*, 206, 376–386, 2012.)

be considered by individual practitioners; third-party payers should not deny reimbursements for this screening [69,70]. International Federation of Gynecology and Obstetrics (FIGO) recommends TVU CL screening [71]. TVU CL examinations should be done following strict quality criteria, in the US via Cervical Length Education and Review (CLEAR) and the Perinatal Quality Foundation (https://clear.perinatalquality.org) [72], and in Europe through the Fetal Medicine Foundation [73]. **Only TVU, and not transabdominal (TA) ultrasound, should be used for CL screening** [69,70].

Screening with TVU CL at 18–24 weeks should be offered to all singleton gestations without prior SPTB. If CL ≤25 mm, vaginal progesterone (e.g., 200 mg suppositories daily until 36 weeks) should be recommended [62–64].

Intervention: Cerclage (ultrasound-indicated cerclage [UIC]). A UIC involves first screening of pregnancies with TVU of the cervix to determine during pregnancy the risk of PTB, since the majority of even women at high risk by obstetrical risk factors for PTB do not develop a short CL and deliver at term even without intervention. A short CL (<25 mm) on TVU in the second trimester (between 14 and 23 6/7 weeks) significantly increases the risk of PTB in all populations studied [74]. UIC is defined as a cerclage performed because a short CL has been detected on TVU during pregnancy, usually in the second trimester. This cerclage has also been called in the past therapeutic, salvage, or rescue cerclage, but these terms are confusing and should be avoided. UIC has differing effects in different populations.

In women with **singleton gestations, no prior PTB or other risk factors for PTB, and CL <25 mm** before 24 weeks, cerclage is associated with no significant effect of PTB <35 weeks RR (0.76, 95% CI 0.52–1.15) [75]. This is probably due to the relatively small numbers of women ($n = 235$) included in RCTs done so far. Therefore, cerclage cannot be recommended in this population, but more research is needed.

For singleton gestations with prior PTB and a short TVU CL, see under the section "Prior PTB and Short Cervix."

Intervention: Pessary. There is contradictory evidence regarding the efficacy of pessary to prevent PTB in women with singleton gestations and a short TVU CL ≤25 mm in the second trimester. All studies so far used the Arabin pessary. While the first RCT revealed a 82% decrease in PTB <34 weeks associated with pessary [76], subsequent, other (some larger) RCTs have not shown any benefit in PTB or neonatal outcomes [77,78]. All these RCTs included mostly (about 85%–90%) singletons without a prior SPTB. In summary, **pessary cannot be recommended for prevention of PTB in singleton gestations (without prior PTB) with a short TVU CL.**

Intervention: Indomethacin. There is **insufficient evidence** to eval-uate the effect of indomethacin on incidence of PTB in women with a short CL on TVU [79], as no RCTs have been performed.

Intervention: Antibiotics. There is **insufficient evidence** to eval-uate the effect of antibiotics on incidence of PTB in women with a short CL on TVU, as no RCTs have been performed.

Risk: "Pregnancy High-Risk for PTB"

Intervention: Activity restriction/bed rest. Activity restriction and/or bed rest are probably the most commonly prescribed intervention for PTB prevention despite no proven benefit and potential for increased maternal morbidity. There is no evidence supporting bed rest or activity restriction to prevent PTB [80,81]. Per ACOG, bed rest should not be routinely recommended for prevention of PTB [82]. **Bed rest (rest 1 hour tid) in (asymptomatic and symptomatic) "high-risk" singleton pregnancies is not associated with prevention of PTB over no bed rest** [83]. Bed rest can be associated with an increased incidence of complications; in-hospital extended strict bed rest for PTL or PPROM is associated with an up to 1%–2% incidence of thromboembolic disease. Moreover, muscle wasting, cardiovascular deconditioning, bone demineralization, impaired glucose tolerance, heartburn, constipation, failure of volume expansion, headaches, dizziness, fatigue, depression, anxiety, stress, as well as lost wages, lost domestic productivity, and other costs may be other detrimental consequences of bed rest.

It is true that rest decreases uterine activity, and exercise increases it, but these are small effects that do not change rates of PTB. In nonrandomized studies, **exercise in pregnancy has been associated with a decrease in PTB** [84], while physically demanding work, prolonged standing, shift and night work, and high cumulative work fatigue score have been associated with PTB. Despite its use in about 20% of pregnancies, **bed rest or any activity restriction for prevention of PTB cannot be recommended.** These interventions should be studied in trials before clinical use. If prescribed bed rest, women should be allowed to ambulate to the bathroom a few times a day to limit complications of strict bed rest. It is possible that women at real risk of PTB from the above or other risk factors have not been studied adequately with this intervention of bed rest.

Intervention: Support. Programs of additional support during at-risk pregnancy (varying definitions) usually by a professional (social worker, midwife, or nurse) **do not reduce PTB** or LBW [85]. "Additional support" was defined as some form of emotional support (e.g., counseling, reassurance, and sympathetic listening) with or without additional information/advice, occurring during home visits, clinic appointments, and/or by telephone; most of the times these were intensive programs started in the first or second trimesters to the end of pregnancy. Other significant outcomes are as follows: antenatal hospital admission and cesarean delivery are decreased [85].

Intervention: Weekly manual examinations, education. A program of weekly manual cervical examinations in addition to education for women at high-risk for PTB (≥10 on Creasy's score) **does not reduce PTB** [86–88].

Intervention: Antibiotics. See "Intervention: Antibiotics" in the section "Risk: Prior PTB."

Intervention: Cerclage. Different specific clinical scenarios have been studied for possible benefit of cerclage. For efficacy of history-indicated cerclage, TA cerclage, UIC, PEIC, as well as cerclage in twins (see below).

Risk: Prior PTB [89]

Intervention: Low-dose aspirin. A recent secondary analysis of an RCT (underpowered) showed no association of preconception low-dose aspirin in women with one or more prior pregnancy loss or PTB on overall PTB rates (Figures 17.3 and 17.4) [90].

Intervention: Fish intake. **Moderate fish intake, up to three meals per week, before 22 weeks is associated with a reduction in repeat PTB,** compared with women eating fish less than once per month (odds ratio [OR] 0.60, CI 0.38–0.95) [91]. **Moderate fish intake should be encouraged in women with prior PTB for prevention of recurrent PTB** (see the section "Primary Prevention").

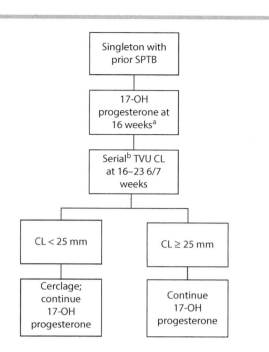

Figure 17.3 TVU CL screening for the woman with a singleton gestation and prior SPTB at 16–36 6/7 weeks. [a]250 mg intramuscularly (IM) every week from 16 to 20 weeks to 36 weeks; vaginal progesterone can be used as well as an alternative. [b]Every 2 weeks; if 26–29 mm, repeat in 1 week. (Adapted from Society for Maternal-Fetal Medicine and Berghella V, *Am J Obstet Gynecol*, 206, 376–386, 2012.)

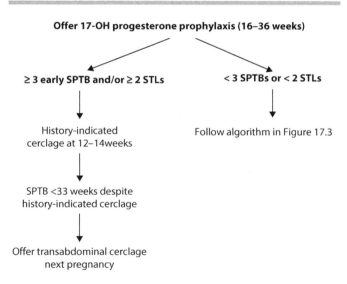

Figure 17.4 Clinical algorithm for care of asymptomatic women with multiple prior PTB or second-trimester losses (STLs) (see text). (Adapted from Iams JD and Berghella V, *Am J Obstet Gynecol*, 203(2), 89–100, 2010.)

Intervention: Omega-3 fatty acids. In one RCT, omega-3 fatty acids (fish oil, Pikasol: 32% eicosapentaenoic acid [EPA], 23% DHA, and 2 mg tocopherol/mL; 4 capsules/day: 1.3 g EPA and 0.9 g DHA, total 2.7 g/day; started ≥16 weeks at an average of 29–30 weeks) were associated with reduction in PTB <37 weeks by 46% and PTB <34 weeks by 68% in women with a prior PTB <37 weeks and a singleton gestation. The same omega-3 fatty acid regimen does not reduce PTB in women with twins [92]. In another larger RCT, in singleton gestations with prior SPTB and on 17P 250 mg IM, omega-3 supplementation (1200 mg EPA and 800 mg DHA) from 16 to 22 weeks until 36 weeks was associated with similar incidences of PTB <37 weeks (38% vs. 41%; RR 0.91, 95% 0.77–1.07) and PTB <35 weeks (RR 0.95, 95% CI 0.72–1.25) [93]. Meta-analysis of these two RCTs revealed that women who received omega-3 had similar rates of PTB at <37 weeks (34.5% vs. 39.8%; RR, 0.81; 95% CI, 0.59–1.12) and PTB at <34 weeks (12.0% vs. 15.4%; RR, 0.62; 95% CI, 0.26–1.46) compared with control. The omega-3 groups had a statistically significantly longer latency (mean difference, 2.10 days; 95% CI, 1.98–2.22) and higher birthweight (mean difference, 102 g; 95% CI, 20–185) compared with control subjects [94]. In summary, **in singleton gestations with prior SPTB on 17P, omega-3 supplementation does not seem to be beneficial in preventing recurrent PTB**. The benefits in longer latency and higher birth weight may deserve further study (see the section "Primary Prevention").

Intervention: Antibiotics. Antibiotics to prevent PTB in women with prior PTB have been evaluated either as preconception (one RCT) or as prenatal intervention.

In women with prior PTB <34 weeks, **preconception** oral azythromycin 1 g twice (4 days apart) and metronidazole 750 mg daily for 7 days are not associated with an effect of subsequent PTB or miscarriage rates [95].

Clindamycin cream 2% for 7 days at 26–32 weeks does not reduce PTB <37 weeks in women with a prior PTB 24–36 weeks but may increase PTB <34 weeks, especially in women without BV, so that antibiotics in this setting may actually be detrimental [96].

Cefetamet Pivoxil (not available in United States) 2 g × 1 at 28–32 weeks in women in Nairobi with prior PTB, fetal death, or LBW did not affect GA at delivery (PTB was not reported) [97].

Metronidazole 250 mg tid × 7 days and erythromycin base 333 mg tid × 14 days in women with a prior PTB or prepregnancy weight <50 kg do not prevent PTB <37 weeks but may increase PTB <34 weeks [98]. Antibiotic prophylaxis did not reduce the risk of PPROM or PTB (except in a subgroup of women with a prior PTB who had bacterial vaginosis in current pregnancy) [99].

In summary, **antibiotics given just because of a prior PTB do not prevent recurrent PTB**.

Intervention: Progesterone. The effect of progesterone supple-mentation should be evaluated according to different patient populations, and according to type of progesterone. Here we review progesterone for prior PTB.

For 17P, there are at least two RCTs available in women with prior PTB. In 43 women with mostly (>90%) singleton gestation and either prior PTB or prior >1 spontaneous abortion, 17P 250 mg IM weekly started as soon as prenatal care began was associated with significant reduction in PTB <37 weeks and perinatal mortality compared with placebo [100]. In 463 women with singleton gestation and prior SPTB at 20–36 6/7 weeks of a singleton gestation, compounded 17P 250 mg IM weekly started at 16–20 6/7 weeks was associated with reduction in the incidences of PTB <37 weeks (RR 0.66, 95% CI 0.54–0.81), PTB <35 weeks, and <32 weeks, as well as of supplemental oxygen, NEC and IVH, compared with placebo [101]. The number needed to treat to prevent one recurrent PTB was 5.4. Based mostly on this clinical trial, **17P 250 mg IM weekly**

started at 16–20 weeks is recommended for all women with prior SPTB 20–36 6/7 weeks [102–104] (Figure 17.3). The estimated number of prevented PTBs <37 weeks in the United States by this policy is about 9870.

For **vaginal progesterone**, there are at least two RCTs available in women with prior PTB. In 142 women with singleton gestations and mostly (>90%) prior PTB, vaginal progesterone 100 mg nightly from 24 to 34 weeks was associated with significant reduction in the incidences of PTB <37 weeks (RR 0.48, 95% CI 0.25–0.96) and <34 weeks, as well as contraction frequency, compared with placebo [105]. In 659 women with singleton gestation and prior SPTB 20–35 0/7 weeks, vaginal progesterone 90 mg every morning starting at 18–22 6/7 weeks until 37 0/7 weeks was not associated with significantly different rates of PTB <37, 36, 33, 29 weeks and neonatal morbidity and mortality [106]. Several women screened **for this trial were excluded from inclusion because of short** CL [106], therefore, **vaginal progesterone cannot be recommended for prevention of recurrent PTB** when data against placebo is considered.

For **comparison of 17P versus vaginal progesterone**, there are two RCTs. In 518 women with singleton gestation and prior PTB between 20 and 34 weeks, 17P 250 mg IM weekly was associated with similar incidences of PTB and neonatal morbidities and mortality compared with vaginal progesterone 90 mg (Crinone) daily, except for significant lower incidences of PTB 28–31 6/7 weeks, neonatal intensive care unit (NICU) admission, and maternal side effects in the vaginal progesterone group [107]. Another RCT reported similar outcomes, including incidence of PTB, with either vaginal progesterone or 17P in women with singleton gestations and prior PTB [108] Another recent nonblinded randomized trial of 78 singleton pregnancies from Iran, compared effectiveness of vaginal progesterone with 17P in women with either prior PTB or short cervix TVU CL <25 mm. The authors concluded that vaginal progesterone and IM progesterone have same level of effectiveness and reported similar rate of PTB in two groups [109]. Overall this RCT does not appear to be high quality and the study results should be used cautiously. **More data are necessary to evaluate how 17P and vaginal progesterone compare in efficacy in singletons with a prior PTB**, as other populations, but vaginal progesterone seems to be at least equivalent, if not possibly more efficacious, than 17P in women with prior SPTB.

For **oral progesterone**, there are two small RCTs. In 150 women with singleton gestation and prior SPTB 20–36 6/7 weeks, oral micronized progesterone 100 mg twice a day was associated with significantly reduced incidences of PTB <37 weeks (39.2% in the oral progesterone vs. 59.5% in the placebo group, $p = .002$) and NICU admission compared with placebo [110]. In 33 women with singleton gestation and prior PTB 20–36 6/7 weeks, oral progesterone 400 mg daily was associated with nonsignificant reductions in the incidence of PTB <37 weeks (26% vs. 57%) and ventilator use (0% vs. 21%) compared with placebo [111]. In summary, there is **insufficient evidence** to assess the efficacy of oral progesterone for prevention of PTB in women with prior PTB.

In summary, in women with prior SPTB and singleton gestation, progesterone administration is beneficial in preventing PTB. Although we have limited data comparing the different preparations of progesterone, there is at present **stronger evidence of effectiveness for 17P than for vaginal progesterone**, based on the two largest trials [101,106], but comparison RCTs seems to show vaginal guogesterone is an effective alternative [107,109]. **17P 250 mg IM weekly starting at 16–20 weeks until 36 weeks should be recommended to women with singleton gestations and prior SPTB 20–36 6/7 weeks** [101]. In cases in which 17P is unavailable, other progesterone preparations may be considered [105].

Intervention: Cerclage. A history-indicated cerclage is placed based solely on prior ob-gyn history (previously called a prophylactic or elective cerclage). Trials on women with only one or two prior PTBs have not shown benefit from history-indicated cerclage [112,113]. **A history-indicated cerclage has been associated with prevention of PTB in women with three or more STLs or PTBs** [114]. Cerclage decreases the incidence of PTB <37 weeks from 53% (with no cerclage) to 32%, and the incidence of PTB <32 weeks from 32% (with no cerclage) to 15% in women with three or more prior PTBs or STLs [114] (Figure 17.4).

The other clinical indication for history-indicated cerclage might include cervical insufficiency, defined by some as prior painless cervical dilatation leading to recurrent STLs. Unfortunately, **no trial has been done to confirm the efficacy of history-indicated cerclage in reducing PTB in women with a diagnosis of cervical insufficiency.** Other indications such as prior cone biopsy, Mullerian anomaly, diethylstilbestrol (DES) exposure, prior PTB are not associated with cervical insufficiency, and Ehler-Danlos have occasionally been used clinically but have not been confirmed by any trial as indications that benefit from history-indicated cerclage. History-indicated cerclage is usually performed at 12–15 weeks' gestation, and its techniques have been well described [74].

TA cerclage has been associated with less recurrent PTB compared with controls receiving transvaginal cerclage in women with a **history of a failed (SPTB <33 weeks despite cerclage) transvaginal history-indicated cerclage** in a case-control study [115]. It should be noted that in this study antibiotics and progesterone were uniformly given to the TA cerclage women. There is no RCT on TA cerclage. The efficacy of TA cerclage for other clinical scenarios such as a cervix with no intravaginal portion has not been adequately studied. TA cerclage can be performed prophylactically at around 10–12 weeks, and its technique has been well described [74,115]. TA cerclage has been successfully performed also laparoscopically and robotically, in particular prepregnancy, but also in the early first trimester [116].

In summary, **the vast majority of women with prior PTB (e.g., those with only 1 or 2 prior PTBs) do not benefit from universal history-indicated cerclage, and can instead be followed with TVU CL screening starting usually at 16 weeks.** A policy of TVU CL screening with cerclage for short CL is associated with similar incidences of PTB <37 weeks (31% vs. 32%; RR 0.97, 95% CI 0.73–1.29), PTB <34 weeks (17% vs. 23%; RR 0.76, 95% CI 0.48–1.20), and perinatal mortality (5% vs. 3%; RR 1.77, 95% CI 0.58–5.35) compared with universal history-indicated cerclage, and omits an obviously unnecessary cerclage in about 58% of these women [117]. **Therefore, all singleton gestations with a prior spontaneous PTB should be screened with TVU CL starting at 16 weeks, every 2 weeks, until 23 6/7 weeks. If the CL is 26–29 mm, repeat TVU CL can be done in 1 week instead of 2 weeks. If the CL <25 mm is detected before 24 weeks, singleton gestations with prior PTB should undergo UIC** [118] (Figure 17.3) (see also the section "Risk: Short Cervix on Ultrasound").

If cerclage is performed, it should be performed according to best technique. McDonald cerclage, with suture (usually mersilene tape) placed as close to the internal os as possible (as high as possible), under spinal anesthesia, is recommended. There is usually no need for preoperative antibiotics or tocolytics [119]. A double suture might improve outcomes compared with one suture, but the evidence is still insufficient for a recommendation [120]. Cervical occlusion has no significant additional effect on cerclage [121].

Intervention: Oral tocolytics. There is insufficient evidence (only 1 small old RCT) to support the use of prophylactic oral betamimetics for preventing PTB in women with prior PTB with a singleton pregnancy [122].

For a summary of care of pregnant women with prior PTB, see also Ref. [89].

Risk: Prior PTB and Short Cervix on Ultrasound

Intervention: Progesterone. In a secondary analysis of an RCT evaluating just 46 singleton gestations with prior SPTB <35 weeks and short CL <28 mm at 18–22 6/7 weeks, **vaginal progesterone 90 mg daily started at 18–23 6/7 weeks until 37 weeks was associated with significant decreases in incidences of both PTB <32 weeks and NICU admission compared with placebo** [123].

In a small RCT which did not recruit the planned sample size, **17P** in singleton gestation are at high risk for PTB (56% with prior PTB) with TVU CL <25 mm 20–31 6/7 weeks was noted to have no benefit in prolonging pregnancy compared with no 17P. The sample size was too small, and the intervention probably too late, to show significance [124].

In a randomized trial that did not recruit the planned sample size, **17P** and **cerclage** had similar effect in women for CL <25 mm for prevention of PTB, but cerclage was more effective in women with CL <15 mm [61]. So while cerclage seems to be more efficacious (lower RRs) as the CL is shorter [125,126], progesterone seems to be most efficacious in cases of "moderate" short CL [62,63].

Until further evidence is available, we suggest continuation of 17P in women with prior PTB and short cervix in the index pregnancy. Some instead have suggested switching from 17P to vaginal progesterone, but not based on RCT data [127]. There is no good evidence suggesting benefit of addition of vaginal progesterone in women with prior PTB on 17P who are noted to have short cervix [127]. In summary, **women with prior PTB should be screened with TVU CL from 16 to 24 weeks. 17P should be recommended to women with prior SPTB starting at 16 weeks**, as described above. If the cervix shortens, there is insufficient evidence to assess efficacy of a different progesterone therapy, and therefore it is reasonable to continue 17P until 36 weeks.

Intervention: Cerclage. In women with a **singleton gestation, prior SPTB, and CL <25 mm** before 24 weeks, **cerclage is associated with a significant 30% reduction in PTB <35 weeks** (28.4% vs. 41.3%; RR 0.70, 95% CI 0.55–0.89), **significant reductions also in PTB <37, <32, <28, and <24 weeks**, as well as a **significant 36% decrease in composite perinatal mortality and morbidity** (15.6% vs. 24.8%; RR 0.64, 95% CI 0.45–0.91), compared with no cerclage [118]. Therefore, **cerclage is recommended in women with a singleton gestation, prior SPTB, and CL <25 mm before 24 weeks** [69,70].

There are no randomized trials on **management of subsequent pregnancy in women who required UIC in their prior pregnancy**. Level II evidence suggests similar outcomes with TVU CL screening with UIC for short cervix of 25 mm or less, or planned HIC in the subsequent pregnancy, in singleton gestations with prior UIC. Authors reported less than 50% of the TVU CL screening group require a repeat UIC in the subsequent pregnancy [128]. Another retrospective study of women with prior UIC also reported that majority of women who underwent CL surveillance in the next pregnancy did not require intervention for short cervix. The authors reported higher rate of PTB in women who received HIC in the subsequent pregnancy, which was not justified based on their risk status [129]. Based on the available level II evidence, **TVU CL screening with UIC for short cervix is acceptable and possibly more effective than routine history-indicated cerclage in women with UIC in prior pregnancy.** A consideration can be given to **HIC in the small subset of women who delivered prior to 32 weeks in their prior pregnancy with UIC** [128].

If the TVU CL shortens again later after the UIC has been placed, a second "reinforcing" cerclage has not been associated with prevention of PTB [130,131].

For singleton gestations without a prior PTB and with a short TVU CL, see the sections "Risk: Short Cervix on Ultrasound" and "Intervention: Cerclage" (Ultrasound Indicated Cerclage).

Intervention: Vaginal progesterone versus cerclage. There is no RCT comparing directly vaginal progesterone to cerclage in this population, and therefore there is insufficient evidence for a recommendation. While an indirect meta-analysis reported that either vaginal progesterone or cerclage are equally efficacious in the prevention of PTB in women with a sonographic short cervix in the mid trimester, singleton gestation, and previous PTB, the populations compared were not similar, introducing significant bias [132]. We offer 17P based on the prior PTB, and cerclage for the short CL, based on data reviewed above.

Intervention: 17P versus cerclage

Intervention: progesterone in addition to cerclage. There is **insufficient evidence** *to assess the size of any cumulative effect of 17P for prior PTB in singletons already with cerclage for short CL. 17P was associated with reduction in PTB <35 weeks in women with UIC in the current pregnancy for TVU CL <25 mm, but sample size was too small to show significance* [133,134].

Intervention: cerclage in addition to progesterone. There is **insufficient evidence** to assess the size of any cumulative effect of cerclage for short CL in singletons already on 17P for prior PTB. UIC was associated with reduction in PTB <35 weeks in women already on 17P for prior PTB in the current pregnancy, but sample size was too small to show significance [135].

Risk: Cervical Insufficiency

Intervention: Cerclage. **No intervention has been specifically studied in this population** (see the section "Risk: Prior PTB"). There are no randomized trials evaluating the role of history-indicated cerclage in women with prior PTB or pregnancy loss due to cervical insufficiency. There is insufficient evidence to recommend a history-indicated cerclage in women with less than three prior PTBs or STLs. **A policy of TVU CL screening with UIC if CL shortens to <25 mm at <24 weeks has shown to be equivalent to a policy of universal history-indicated cerclage in women with a prior loss or PTB** [74,117,136].

Intervention: 17P in addition to cerclage. There is insufficient evidence to assess the possible cumulative effect of 17P on PTB <35 weeks in women with a history-indicated cerclage [137].

Risk: IVF ART

Intervention: Progesterone or HCG. 17P or HCG supplementation in the first trimester **is associated with an increase in the incidence of fetal heart activity on ultrasound by 238%, and of pregnancy ≥24 weeks' rate by 380%** compared with placebo [138].

Risk: Amniocentesis
   Intervention: Progesterone. Natural progesterone 200 mg IM q day for 3 days postamniocentesis followed by 17P 340 mg IM 2×/week until the second week after the amniocentesis **did not reduce PTB** <25 weeks in women undergoing amniocentesis [139].

Risk: Uterine Contractions Detected by Home Uterine Activity Monitoring (HUAM)
   Intervention: Varied, per obstetrician. Uterine contractions have been associated with PTB, but their predictive value is poor. HUAM usually consists of 1 hour of tocomonitoring twice daily at 24–36 weeks. **HUAM with or without nursing contact and education is not associated with prevention of PTB.** Some studies show earlier (at lower cervical dilatation) detection of PTL. The lack of benefit in prevention of PTB might have been secondary to lack of effective intervention (usually tocolysis) once PTL was diagnosed. Three different populations of women at high risk for PTB have been studied: singleton gestations with risk factors for PTB (e.g., prior PTB), twin gestations, and women status-post an episode of PTL. Unfortunately, there is no published meta-analysis of all trials, and most trials do not report results for each population specifically, and also report differing outcomes. A meta-analysis of published data shows no decrease in PTB <37 weeks in any of these three subgroups: mostly singletons at high risk (nine trials; $n = 3613$) [140–149]: RR 1.01, 95% CI 0.91–1.11; twins (five trials; $n = 998$) [64,67,69–71]: RR 0.91, 95% CI 0.80–1.04; or women s/p PTL episode (four trials; $n = 218$) [67,72–74]: RR 1.21, 95% CI 0.92–1.60. The largest study [149] and a recent meta-analysis [17] showed more unscheduled antenatal visits and prophylactic tocolytic use in the HUAM group compared with controls. Therefore, **HUAM should not be routinely provided for prevention of PTB.**

Risk: Cervical Dilatation
   Intervention: Physical Exam-Indicated Cerclage (PEIC). PEIC (aka emergency, or urgent) is the cerclage placed because of changes in the cervix (dilatation, effacement, etc.) detected by physical (manual) examination. Since about 50% of women with asymptomatic cervical dilatation ≥2 cm in the second trimester have microbial invasion of the amniotic cavity, **an amniocentesis should be considered before offering this cerclage.**

There are insufficient data to assess efficacy of PEIC in women with cervical dilatation in the second trimester, as only one small trial has been reported. In women with membranes at or beyond the external os at around 20–24 weeks, **PEIC (and indomethacin) is associated with a delay in delivery of about 4 weeks** compared with controls (30 vs. 26 weeks) [150]. The major limitations of this study are the small sample size and the inclusion of twins. Over 25 retrospective observational series, mostly with no controls, have claimed benefit of PEIC. The largest cohort study reported a significant decrease of 92% in prevention of PTB <28 weeks with PEIC, compared with no cerclage, in singletons with ≥1 cm of cervical dilatation before 26 weeks [151]. A recent meta-analysis reported that PEIC is associated with a significant increase in neonatal survival and prolongation of pregnancy of approximately 1 month when compared with no cerclage. The strength of this conclusion is limited by the potential for bias in the included studies [152]. For PEIC, perioperative indomethacin and antibiotics have been associated with a significant 28 days prolongation of pregnancy [153]. In summary, **PEIC in singleton gestations with a cervix dilated to ≥1 cm in the second trimester is associated with prevention in PTB and neonatal benefits.** Clearly a large, well-designed prospective randomized trial is needed to confirm these benefits.
   Intervention: Indomethacin. There is **insufficient evidence** to eval-uate the effect of indomethacin on incidence of PTB in women with a short CL on TVU [154], as no RCT has been performed. An RCT of perioperative indomethacin and antibiotics in women receiving a PEIC between 16–23 weeks, showed significant prolongation of gestation by 28 days compared with control [153].

Risk: Positive fFN
   Intervention: Antibiotics. fFN is a basement membrane protein present between the decidua/uterus and fetal membranes/placenta and produced by the trophoblast. Its presence (>50 ng/mL) at ≥22 weeks in the cervicovaginal canal has been associated with an increased risk for PTB. In fact fFN is one of the best predictors of PTB in all populations, including asymptomatic low-and high-risk women, twins, and women in PTL. Even at 13–22 weeks, higher (using 90th percentile) fFN levels are associated with two-to-threefold increase risk in subsequent SPTB. In women found to be fFN positive at 21–25 weeks, treatment with metronidazole 250 mg tid and erythromycin 250 mg qid × 10 days is associated with similar incidences of PTB <37 weeks to placebo. Among women with a prior SPTB, this antibiotic regimen is associated with a significantly higher incidence of PTB <37 weeks than the placebo group [155]. In women with at least one other risk factor for PTB (e.g., prior PTB), and positive fFN at 24–27 weeks, metronidazole 400 mg orally tid for 7 days was associated with no effect on reduction of PTB and maternal and perinatal outcomes compared with placebo, rather authors reported that metronidazole use can be detrimental due to a trend of higher PTB rate, antenatal admission and LBW in metronidazole group compared with placebo [156]. In summary, **screening low-risk or high-risk asymptomatic pregnant women for fFN is not effective,** as there is no intervention (the one tried has been antibiotics) shown to alter outcomes.

Risk: Prior Intrauterine Growth Restriction (IUGR) or Pre-eclampsia
   Intervention: Low-dose aspirin. Compared with no aspirin or placebo, **low-dose aspirin (usually 50–150 mg) is associated with decreased incidence of PTB** (RR 0.22, 95% CI 0.10–0.49) *in women at high risk for pregnancy complications, such as those with prior preeclampsia or prior IUGR* [157]. A large systematic review showed 8% reduction in rate of PTB <37 weeks in women (many with prior preeclampsia or IUGR) treated with antiplatelet agents (RR 0.92, 95% CI 0.88–0.97) [158]. **Low dose aspirin started between 12 and 28 weeks is recommended in women at high risk of recurrent preeclampsia** [159]. (See Chapters 1 and 45 in *Maternal-Fetal Evidence Based Guidelines*).

Risk: Periodontal Disease
   Intervention: Periodontal therapy. Periodontal disease has been associated with increased risk of PTB in several observational studies. Periodontal treatment such as scaling, root planning, plaque control, and daily rinsing have been evaluated as an intervention to decrease PTB in women with periodontal disease [160,161].

Periodontal treatment has not been associated with decrease in PTB in women with periodontal disease (RR 0.63, 95% CI 0.32–1.22), even when controlling for probing depth and attachment loss for periodontitis criteria, multiparity, prior PTB, or genitourinary infections [162].

Infections

Risk: Asymptomatic Bacteriuria

Intervention: Antibiotics. Asymptomatic bacteriuria occurs in 2%–10% of pregnancies, can lead to pyelonephritis, and is associated with an increased risk of PTB. **Screening for asymptomatic bacteriuria and treating for urine colony count of >100,000 bacteria/mL reduce the incidence of PTB** by 73% (RR 0.27, 95% CI 0.11–0.62, 2 studies, $n = 242$) [163]. The optimal time to perform the urine culture is unknown; it seems reasonable to perform the urine culture and treat, as done in most studies, at the first prenatal visit. Quantitative urine culture of a midstream or clean catch urine is the gold standard for detecting asymptomatic bacteriuria in pregnancy. The choices of a sulfonamide or sulfonamide-containing combination, a penicillin, or nitrofurantoin, based on the results of susceptibility testing, are appropriate regimens for the management of asymptomatic bacteriuria. A short (3–7 days) course therapy of asymptomatic bacteriuria has become accepted practice, as is as effective as longer therapy. A single-dose regimen of antibiotics may be less effective than a short course (4–7 day) regimen [164]. Women with asymptomatic bacteriuria in pregnancy should be treated by the standard regimen of antibiotics until more data becomes available on the cure rate of shorter course 3–5 days regimen compared with standard regimen. Although it is recommended that a urine culture be done following treatment, with retreatment as necessary, the evidence is insufficient to specifically evaluate the effectiveness of this strategy. Treatment of asymptomatic pregnant women with lower colony counts is not currently recommended, but further study of appropriate strategies to manage these women is warranted. **Asymptomatic women with even low (100+) colony-forming units (CFU) of GBS in the urine culture at 27–31 weeks have decreased PTB <37 weeks (5.4% in the penicillin group vs. 38% in the placebo group, p < .002) when treated with penicillin 1 million IU three times per day for 6 days** compared with placebo [165].

Antibiotic treatment compared with placebo or no treatment is effective in clearing asymptomatic bacteriuria. Antibiotic treatment of asymptomatic bacteriuria is then clinically indicated to reduce the risk of pyelonephritis in pregnancy. If untreated, the overall incidence of pyelonephritis is about 21%. Overall, the number of women needed to treat to prevent one episode of pyelonephritis is seven, and treatment of asymptomatic bacteriuria will lead to approximately a 75% reduction in the incidence of pyelonephritis (RR 0.23, 95% CI 0.13–0.41; 11 studies, $n = 1932$) [163]. The apparent reduction in PTB is consistent with current theories about the role of infection as a cause of PTB. Prevention of pyelonephritis, which in early studies prior to the availability of effective antimicrobial therapy was associated with PTB, may be a factor, but treatment of bacteriuria with antibiotics may also eradicate organisms colonizing the cervix and vagina that are associated with adverse pregnancy outcomes. The use of tetracycline is contraindicated in pregnancy. Insufficient data are available to determine the effectiveness of treatment to prevent recurrent bacteriuria during pregnancy. There is a need to define the appropriate frequency of follow-up cultures and retreatment strategies [163]. See Chapter 17 in *Maternal-Fetal Evidence Based Guidelines*.

Risk: BV

Intervention: Antibiotics. BV is a massive overgrowth of orga-nisms such as anaerobics, *Gardnerella*, *Mycoplasma*, and others in the vagina. Most of these organisms are normally present in the vagina, but are at higher concentrations in BV, while predominant normal flora such as lactobacilli is decreased.

The diagnosis of BV is usually made clinically with at least three out of four of these (Amsel's) criteria: pH >4.5 (most important), clue cells, thin homogenous discharge, and "amine" test, while in many studies Nugent's criteria (≥7 on Gram stain) are used for diagnosis. All these screening tests are not very accurate in predicting PTB (PPV 6%–49% depending on PTB prevalence and patient population) in both asymptomatic and symptomatic women.

Antibiotic therapy is effective at decreasing the presence of BV during pregnancy. In nonselected women, antibiotic treatment is not effective in reducing the incidence of PTB <37 weeks, PTB <34 weeks, PTB <32 weeks, or PPROM [166]. However, **treatment before 20 weeks** may reduce the risk of PTB <37 weeks (OR 0.72, 95% CI 0.55–0.95).

In women with a previous PTB, treatment did not affect the risk of subsequent PTB <37 weeks, with a 17%–25% nonsignificant trend for benefit [166,167]. It may decrease the risk of PPROM and LBW. Subgroup analysis of treatment with metronidazole or clindamycin does not alter incidence of PTB <37 weeks [167].

Risk: Trichomonas vaginalis

Intervention: Antibiotics. Antibiotics (**metronidazole** only one tested) **do not prevent PTB** in women with asymptomatic *T. vaginalis* (TV) infection [167–171]. In fact, metronidazole as studied (two 2-g doses 48 hours apart; possibly excessive dose) is associated with 78% higher incidence of PTB <37 weeks [170], and similar incidences of PTB <32 weeks and perinatal mortality [100]. Even in women with a prior PTB, metronidazole is associated with an 84% higher risk of PTB [167]. Metronidazole does eradicate TV in >90% of pregnant women with TV. Therefore, at least for the purpose of decreasing PTB, asymptomatic women should not be screened for TV and treated with metronidazole at doses studied so far if positive for TV. **Symptomatic** women with TV should still be adequately treated with metronidazole as a **single 2-g oral dose, or 500 mg twice a day for seven days** (see Chapter 36 in *Maternal-Fetal Evidence Based Guidelines*).

Risk: BV, Candida, and Trichomonas

Intervention: Antibiotics. In one large RCT, **screening for BV** (treatment clindamycin 2% vaginal cream for 6 days), **Candida** (treatment local clotrimazole 100 mg for 6 days), and **Trichomonas** (treatment local metronidazole 500 mg for 7 days) was **associated with lower risks of PTB <37 weeks** (3% vs. 5%; RR 0.55, 95% CI 0.41–0.75). The incidence of PTB for BW <2500 g and <1500 g were significantly lower in the intervention group (RR 0.48, 95% CI 0.34–0.66 and RR 0.34; 95% CI 0.15–0.75, respectively) compared with screening with results unavailable to the managing physician [172]. Very few women were positive for *Trichomonas*, while about 21% of women had either BV or candida, or both.

Risk: GBS Vaginal–Cervical Colonization

Intervention: Antibiotics. GBS colonization of the cervicovaginal tract is common in pregnancy (10%–20%), and has been associated with a slight (OR 1.5–3, usually) increased risk of PTB. Antibiotic therapy (with erythromycin) does not prevent PTB in women with GBS colonization, or affect stillbirths. Subanalysis by heavy colonization did not change results [173].

Risk: Ureoplasma Vaginal–Cervical Colonization

Intervention: Antibiotics. Ureoplasma urealyticum and/or mycoplasma hominis colonization of the cervicovaginal tract is common in pregnancy and has been associated with a possible increased risk of PTB. **There is insufficient evidence to show whether giving antibiotics to women with ureaplasma in the vagina prevents PTB.** The only trial did not report data on PTB [174]. Compared with placebo, erythromycin is associated with a nonsignificant 30% decrease in incidence of LBW <2500 g (RR 0.70, 95% CI 0.46–1.07). Although some studies appeared to meet the inclusion criteria for this review, in most studies ureaplasma was not an essential entry criterion or studies reported just a post hoc subgroup analysis of ureaplasma.

Multiple Gestations (See Chapter 44 in *Maternal-Fetal Evidence Based Guidelines*)

Intervention: Bed Rest
In uncomplicated twin pregnancies, **prophylactic bed rest in the hospital does not reduce PTB, perinatal mortality, LBW,** and other complications of pregnancy [175]. **In fact, the incidence of PTB <34 weeks is significantly increased by 84%** [176–180].

In **twin pregnancies with cervical dilatation, bed rest in the hospital does not decrease PTB** in women in Zimbabwe [181]. In the trial in which it was recorded, only 6% of women appreciated in-hospital bed rest. For complications, see the section "Intervention: Bed Rest" (singleton pregnancies).

Intervention: Mutifetal Reduction
There is no trial to assess the effect of multifetal reduction to prevent PTB. Compared with triplets/higher order multiples, triplets/higher order multiples reduced to twins have a higher incidence of loss <24 weeks, but lower incidences of PTB <32 weeks and better neonatal outcome of the remaining twins after reduction in case-control studies. See Chapter 44 in *Maternal-Fetal Evidence Based Guidelines*.

Intervention: CL Screening. Routine second-trimester TVU assessment of CL in twin gestation is not associated with improved outcomes when incorporated into the standard management of otherwise low-risk twin pregnancies in an RCT [182]. See below for progesterone, cerclage, and pessary as interventions for short CL in twins.

Intervention: Progesterone
17P. **17P is not associated with prevention of PTB or neonatal adverse outcomes** in the over 6 RCTs including twins [183–188]. A meta-analysis revealed no benefit of 17P in unselected twin pregnancies [189].

In **twins with short CL**, there was **no effect** of 17P on PTB rates, but numbers are limited [186,190]. A meta-analysis showed that 17-alpha-hydroxy progesterone caproate is not beneficial in reducing PTB or adverse perinatal outcome in 175 twin pregnancies (with >90% of mothers with no prior spontaneous PTB) with a TVU CL ≤25 mm before 24 weeks.

In women with **twins and prior PTB**, 17P did not affect incidence of PTB [187].

In **triplet gestations**, 17P is not associated with an effect on the incidence of PTB [191,192].

Intervention: Vaginal progesterone. **Vaginal progesterone** 90 mg daily starting at 24 weeks for 10 weeks, in 500 women with **unselected twin** gestation, was **not associated with significant effects in incidences of PTB** or perinatal morbidity and mortality [193]. Other RCTs showed also no effect of vaginal progesterone in unselected twins [194,195]. A recent double-blinded placebo controlled RCT on nonselected twin pregnancies with no prior PTB investigated use of daily vaginal progesterone or placebo from 18 to 21 weeks to 34 weeks for prevention of PTB <34 weeks [196]. There was no difference in mean GA at delivery, the rate of SPTB <34 weeks (18.5% in the progesterone group and 14.6% in the placebo group, OR 1.32, 95% CI 0.24–2.37), and no reduction of neonatal morbidity and mortality. Another RCT evaluated two different dose of vaginal progesterone (200 mg vs. 400 mg daily) to placebo in dichorionic multiple gestations, and showed no difference in rate of PTB <37 weeks in the three groups [197]. A meta-analysis revealed no benefit from vaginal progesterone in unselected twins [189]. **In summary, vaginal progesterone should not be given to unselected twin pregnancies for prevention of PTB.**

In women with **twin pregnancies and a short TVU CL**, a subgroup analysis of an individual patient data meta-analysis of **multiple gestations with TVU CL ≤25 mm** showed that vaginal progesterone is associated with a **non-significant reduction in PTB <33 weeks** (30.4% vs. 44.8%, RR 0.70, 95% CI 0.34–1.44), and **significant reduction in composite neonatal morbidity and mortality** (23.9% vs. 39.7%, RR 0.52, 95% CI 0.29–0.93) [64] Another meta-analysis found that vaginal progesterone was not beneficial in preventing PTB at <34 weeks in 58 twin pregnancies (with >95% of mothers with no prior spontaneous PTB) with a TVU CL ≤25 mm before 24 weeks, but was associated with a significant 43% decrease in adverse perinatal outcome [189]. **In summary, further trials are needed to evaluate the efficacy of vaginal progesterone in multiple gestations with short cervix.**

There is insufficient evidence to assess the effect of vaginal progesterone on unselected triplet gestations [194].

In summary, **the evidence is insufficient to recommend the use of any type of progesterone for prevention of PTB in unselected multiple gestations. The effect of vaginal progesterone in women with both multiple gestations and short CL deserves further study.** Therefore, TVU CL cannot be yet recommended as routine in multiple gestations. *In women with prior SPTB, and a current multiple gestation, some experts have suggested the use of 17P starting at 16 weeks based on the historic risk factor [89], but there is insufficient level 1 evidence to make this a strong recommendation.*

Intervention: Cerclage
History-indicated cerclage **does not prevent PTB** in unselected twin gestations in one small RCT [198].

There is insufficient evidence to assess the efficacy of **UIC** in twin pregnancies with a short TVU CL. UIC **does not prevent PTB** in a meta-analysis of the 49 twin gestations and TVU CL <25 mm included in the three RCTs published so far [75]. An individual patient level data meta-analysis of three RCTs showed no benefit of cerclage compared with no cerclage in preventing PTB <34 weeks [199]. For multiple gestations, there is no evidence that cerclage is an effective intervention for preventing PTBs and reducing perinatal deaths or neonatal morbidity [200]. A recent retrospective cohort study of asymptomatic twin gestation with short cervix (TVU CL ≤25 mm) between 16–24 weeks showed UIC was not associated with perinatal outcomes compared with controls. However, in the planned subgroup analysis of asymptomatic twin pregnancies with TVU CL ≤15 mm before 24 weeks, UIC was associated with a significant prolongation of pregnancy by almost 4 more weeks, significantly decreased SPTB <34 weeks by 49%, and admission to neonatal intensive care unit by 58% compared with controls [201]. Given these contradictory data, while UIC should not be recommended for twin gestations currently, further research is warranted.

There is **insufficient evidence** to assess the effectiveness of **PEIC** in twins, as no RCT has been done.

Intervention: Pessary

In unselected twin gestations, the largest RCT found no benefit of pessary use [202]. **In summary, there sufficient evidence to recommend against pessary for prevention of PTB in unselected twins.**

There is contradictory evidence regarding the efficacy of pessary to prevent PTB in women with **twin gestations and a short TVU CL** in the second trimester. All studies so far used the Arabin pessary. One RCT on twins with TVU CL ≤25 mm revealed that SPTB <34 weeks was significantly less frequent in the pessary than in the expectant management group (11/68 [16.2%] vs. 26/66 [39.4%]; RR: 0.41; 95% CI 0.22–0.76) [203]. A secondary analysis of an RCT suggests pessary use is associated with decreased rate of PTB <28 weeks and <32 weeks (but not <37 weeks) in twin pregnancies with TVU CL less than 38 mm before 23 weeks GA [204]. In the largest RCT so far, pessary on twins with TVU CL ≤25 mm was not associated with prevention of PTB ≤34 weeks (33/106 [31%], vs. 28/108 [26%]; RR 1.20; 95% CI 0.78–1.83) or other PTB or neonatal outcomes [202]. **In summary, there insufficient evidence to recommend pessary use for prevention of PTB in twins with short CL. In summary, pessary cannot be recommended for prevention of PTB in singleton gestations with a short TVU CL.**

For **preconception counseling, prenatal care, antepartum testing, mode of delivery, anesthesia, and postpartum/breastfeeding in multiple gestations**, see Chapter 44 in *Maternal-Fetal Evidence Based Guidelines*.

For PTL, see Chapter 18. For preterm premature rupture of membranes, see Chapter 19.

For consequences of PTB for the infant and child, see *The Neonate*, Chapter 31.

REFERENCES

1. Berghella V (ed.). *Preterm Birth: Prevention and Management*. Oxford, United Kingdom: Wiley-Blackwell, 2010. [Review book]
2. Lackritz EM, Wilson CB, Guttmacher AE, et al., A solution pathway for preterm birth: Accelerating a priority research agenda. *Lancet*. 2013;1(6):e328–330. doi: 10.1016/S2214-109X(13)70120-7. [Review]
3. American College of Obstetricians and Gynecologists. *ACOG Practice Bulletin No. 31: Assessment of Risk Factors for Preterm Birth*. Washington, DC: ACOG, 2001. [Review]
4. American College of Obstetricians and Gynecologists. *ACOG Practice Bulletin No. 48: Cervical Insufficiency*. Washington, DC: ACOG, 2003. [Review]
5. WHO. Preterm birth. Born Too Soon: WHO Factsheet. Available at: http://www.who.int/mediacentre/factsheets/fs363/en/. Accessed February 8, 2015. [Internet]
6. Hamilton BE, Martin JA, Osterman MJK, et al. Birth: Preliminary Data for 2014. National Vital Statistics Reports, Vol. 64, No. 6. Hyatsville, MD: National Center for Health Statistics, 2015. [Epidemiologic data]
7. Suhag A, Berghella V. Short cervical length dilemma. *Obstet Gynecol Clin North Am*. 2015;42(2):241–254. [Review]
8. Schoen CN, Tabbah S, Iams JD, et al. Why the United States preterm birth rate is declining? *Am J Obstet Gynecol*. 2015;213(2):175–180. [Clinical opinion]
9. Parets SE, Knight AK, Smith AK. Insights into genetic susceptibility in the etiology of spontaneous preterm birth. *Appl Clin Genet*. 2015;8:283–290. [Review]
10. Mella M, Mackeen D, Gache D, et al. The utility of screening for historical risk factors for preterm birth in women with known second trimester cervical length. *J Matern Fetal Neonatal Med*. 2013;26(7):710–715. doi: 10.3109/14767058.2012.752809. [II-3]
11. Manuck TA, Rice MM, Bailit JL, et al. Preterm neonatal morbidity and mortality by gestational age: A contemporary cohort. *Am J Obstet Gynecol*. 2016;215(1):103.e1–103.e14. doi: 10.1016/j.ajog.2016.01.004. [Epub ahead of print] [II-2].
12. Simhan HN, Berghella V, Iams JD. Preterm labor and birth. In: *Creasy and Resnik's Maternal-Fetal Medicine: Principles and Practice*. 40, 624–653.e9. [Review]
13. Simhan HN, Iams JD, Romero R. Preterm birth. In: *Obstetrics: Normal and Problem Pregnancies*. Chapter 28, 627–658.e12. [Review]
14. Platt MJ. Outcomes in preterm birth. *Public Health*. 2014;128:399–403. [Review]
15. Drassinower D, Obican SG, Siddiq Z, et al. Does the clinical presentation of a prior preterm birth predict risk in a subsequent pregnancy? *Am J Obstet Gynecol*. 2015;213:686.e1–686.e7. [II-2]
16. Davey MA, Watson L, Rayner JA, et al. Risk-scoring systems for predicting preterm birth with the aim of reducing associated adverse outcomes. *Cochrane Database Syst Rev*. 2015;(10):CD004902. doi: 10.1002/14651858.CD004902.pub5. [Review]
17. Urquhart C, Currell R, Harlow F, et al. Home uterine monitoring for detecting preterm labour. *Cochrane Database Syst Rev*. 2015;(1):CD006172. doi: 10.1002/14651858.CD006172.pub3. (15 Randomized trials, $n = 6{,}008$)
18. Carey JC, Klebanoff MA, Hauth JC, et al. Metronidazole to prevent preterm delivery in pregnant women with asymptomatic bacterial vaginosis. National Institute of Child Health and Human Development Network of Maternal-Fetal Medicine Units. *N Engl J Med*. 2000;342:534–540. [RCT, $n = 1{,}953$].
19. Zhu B-P, Rolfs RT, Nangle BE, et al. Effect of the interval between pregnancies on perinatal outcome. *N Engl J Med*. 1999;340:589–594. [II-2]
20. Conde-Agudelo A, Rosas-Bermudez A, Kafury-Goeta AC. Effects of birth spacing on maternal health: A systematic review. *Am J Obstet Gynecol*. 2007;196:297–308. [Systematic review; II-2]
21. Rodriguez MI, Chang R, Thiel de Bocanegra H. The impact of postpartum contraception on reducing preterm birth: Findings from California. *Am J Obstet Gynecol*. 2015;213(5):703.e1–703.e6. doi: 10.1016/j.ajog.2015.07.033. Epub 2015 Jul 26. [II-3]
22. Shah PS, Zao J. Knowledge synthesis group of determinants of preterm? LBW births. Induced termination of pregnancy and low birth weight and preterm birth: A systematic review and meta-analysis. *Br J Obstet Gynecol*. 2009;116:1425–1442. [Meta-analysis: II-1]
23. Lemmers M, Verschoor MA, Hooker AB, et al. Dilatation and curettage increases the risk of subsequent preterm birth: A systematic review and meta-analysis. *Hum Reprod*. 2016;31(1):34–45. doi: 10.1093/humrep/dev274. Epub 2015 Nov 2. [II-2]
24. Saccone G, Perriera L, Berghella V. Prior uterine evacuation of pregnancy as independent risk factor for preterm birth: A systematic review and meta-analysis. *Am J Obstet Gynecol*. 2016;214(5):572–91. doi: 10.1016/j.ajog.2015.12.044. [Epub ahead of print] [Meta-analysis: I]
25. Rodrigues T, Rocha L, Barros H. Physical abuse during pregnancy and preterm delivery. *Am J Obstet Gynecol*. 2008;198:171. [II-2]
26. Takser L. 'Pregnant pause': The need for an evidence-based approach for work leave in the prevention of preterm birth and low birthweight. *Br J Obstet Gynecol*. 2013;120:517–520. [Review]
27. Ota E, Hori H, Mori R, et al. Antenatal dietary education and supplementation to increase energy and protein intake. *Cochrane Database Syst Rev*. 2015;(6):CD000032. doi: 10.1002/14651858.CD000032.pub3. [Meta-analysis: 17 RCTs, $n = 9{,}030$]
28. Ota E, Hori H, Mori R, et al. Balanced energy and protein supplementation in pregnancy. *Cochrane Database Syst Rev*. 2015;(6):CD000032. doi: 10.1002/14651858.CD000032.pub3. [Meta-analysis: 12 RCTs, $n = 6{,}705$]
29. Ota E, Hori H, Mori R, et al. High protein supplementation in pregnancy. *Cochrane Database Syst Rev*. 2015;(6):CD000032. doi: 10.1002/14651858.CD000032.pub3. [Meta-analysis: 1 RCT, $n = 1{,}051$]

30. Linda EO, Lise BA, Verena S, et al. Maternal dietary patterns and preterm delivery: Results from large prospective cohort study. *BMJ*. 2014;348:g1446. [II-2]
31. Smuts CM, Huang M, Mundy D, et al. A randomized trial of docosahexaenoic acid supplementation during the third trimester of pregnancy. *Obstet Gynecol*. 2003;101:469–479. [RCT, $n = 291$] [Level I]
32. Makrides M, Duley L, Olsen SF. Marine oil, and other prostaglandin precursor, supplementation for pregnancy uncomplicated by pre-eclampsia or intrauterine growth restriction. *Cochrane Database Syst Rev*. 2006;(3):CD003402. [Meta-analysis: 6 RCTs, $n = 2783$]
33. Makrides M, Gibson RA, McPhee AJ, et al. Effect of DHA supplementation during pregnancy on maternal depression and neurodevelopment of young children. *JAMA*. 2010;304:1675–1683. [RCT, $n = 2399$] [Level I]
34. Saccone G, Berghella V. Omega-3 long chain polyunsaturated fatty acids to prevent preterm birth: A systematic review and meta-analysis. *Obstet Gynecol*. 2015;125(3):663. [Meta-analysis: 9 RCTs, $n = 3,854$].
35. Myhre R, Brantsater AL, Myking S, et al. Intake of probiotic food and risk of spontaneous preterm delivery. *Am J Clin Nutr*. 2011;93:151–157. [II-2]
36. Othman M, Alfirevic Z, Neilson JP. Probiotics for preventing preterm labour. *Cochrane Database Syst Rev*. 2007;(1):CD005941. [Meta-analysis: 3 RCTs, $n = 364$]
37. Rumbold A, Ota E, Nagata C, et al. Vitamin C supplementation in pregnancy. *Cochrane Database Syst Rev*. 2015;(9):CD004072. [Meta-analysis: 29 RCTs, $n = >24,000$].
38. Rumbold A, Ota E, Hori H, et al. Vitamin E supplementation in pregnancy. *Cochrane Database Syst Rev*. 2015;(9):CD004069. [Meta-analysis: 21 randomized or quasi-randomized trials, $n = 22,129$]
39. Hauth JC, Clifton RG, Robert JM, et al. Vitamin C and E supplementation to prevent spontaneous preterm bith—A randomized controlled trial. *Obstet Gynecol*. 2010;116:653–658. [RCT, $n = 9,968$]
40. Bodnar LM, Platt RW, Simhan HN. Early-pregnancy vitamin D deficiency and risk of preterm birth subtypes. *Obstet Gynecol*. 2015;125:439–447. [II-2]
41. Pranom B, Pisake L, Jadsada T, et al. Calcium supplementation (other than for preventing or treating hypertension) for improving pregnancy and infant outcomes. *Cochrane Database Syst Rev*. 2015;(2):CD007079. doi: 10.1002/14651858.CD007079.pub3. [Meta-analysis: 23 trials; $n = 17,842$]
42. Makrides M, Crosby DD, Bain E, et al. Magnesium supplementation in pregnancy. *Cochrane Database Syst Rev*. 2014;(4):CD000937. doi: 10.1002/14651858.CD000937.pub2. [Meta-analysis: 10 RCTs, $n = 9,090$]
43. Hauth JC, Gilstrap LC, Brekken AL, et al. The effect of 17P on pregnancy outcome in an active duty military population. *Am J Obstet Gynecol*. 1984;146:18790. [RCT, $n = 168$]
44. Tong VT, Dietz PM, Morrow B, et al. Trends in Smoking Before, During, and After Pregnancy—Pregnancy Risk Assessment Monitoring System, United States, 40 Sites, 2000–2010, November 8, 2013;62(SS06):1–19. Available at: http://www.cdc.gov/mmwr/preview/mmwrhtml/ss6206a1.htm?s_cid=ss6206a1_e. Accessed February 8, 2016. [Internet]
45. Coleman T, Chamberlain C, Davey MA, et al. Pharmacological interventions for promoting smoking cessation during pregnancy. *Cochrane Database Syst Rev*. 2015;(12):CD010078. doi: 10.1002/14651858.CD010078.pub2. [Meta-analysis: 9 randomized trials, $n = 2210$]
46. American College of Obstetricians and Gynecologists. *ACOG Educational Bulletin No. 260: Smoking Cessation During Pregnancy*. Washington, DC: ACOG, 2000. Available at: www.acog.org. [Review]
47. Sexton M, Hebel JR. A clinical trial of change in maternal smoking and its effect on birth weight. *JAMA*. 1984;251:911–915. [RCT, $n = 935$]
48. Donatelle RJ, Prows SL, Champeau D, et al. Randomised controlled trial using social support and financial incentives for high risk pregnant smokers: Significant Other Supporter (SOS) program. *Tob Control*. 2000;9(Suppl 3):iii67–iii69. [RCT, $n = 120$]
49. Wisborg K, Henriksen TB, Secher NJ. A prospective intervention study of stopping smoking in pregnancy in a routine antenatal care setting. *Br J Obstet Gynaecol*. 1998;105:1171–1176. [RCT, $n = 5,156$]
50. Kapur B, Hackman R, Selby P, et al. Randomized, double blind, placebo-controlled trial of nicotine replacement therapy in pregnancy. *Curr Therapeut Res*. 2001;62(4):274–278. [RCT, $n = 20$]
51. Hegaard H, Hjaergaard H, Moller L, et al. Multimodel intervention raises smoking cessation rate during pregnancy. *Acta Obstet Gynecol Scand*. 2003;82:813–819. [RCT, $n = 647$]
52. Cooper S, Lewis S, Thornton JG, et al. The SNAP trial: A randomised placebo-controlled trial of nicotine replacement therapy in pregnancy—Clinical effectiveness and safety until 2 years after delivery, with economic evaluation. *Health Technol Assess*. 2014;18(54):1–128. [RCT, $n = 1,050$]
53. Cooper S, Taggar J, Lewis S, et al. Effect of nicotine patches in pregnancy on infant and maternal outcomes at 2 years: Follow-up from the randomised, double-blind, placebo-controlled SNAP trial. *Lancet Respir Med*. 2014;2(9):728–737. [RCT, $n = 1,050$]
54. Ussher M, Lewis S, Aveyard P, et al. The London Exercise And Pregnant smokers (LEAP) trial: A randomised controlled trial of physical activity for smoking cessation in pregnancy with an economic evaluation. *Health Technol Assess*. 2015;19(84):1–136. [RCT, $n = 789$]
55. Kahr MK, Padgett S, Shope CD, et al. A qualitative assessment of the perceived risks of electronic cigarette and hookah use in pregnancy. *BMC Public Health*. 2015;15:1273. doi: 10.1186/s12889-015-2586-4. [II-3]
56. Action on Smoking and Health (ASH) Briefing on Electronic Cigarettes. *Annual Review 2014*. Available at: http://www.ash.org.uk/files/documents/ASH_945.pdf. Accessed February 8, 2016. [Internet]
57. Zhu SH, Sun JY, Bonnevie E, et al. Four hundred and sixty brands of e-cigarettes and counting: Implications for product regulation. *Tob Control*. 2014;23(Suppl 3):iii3–iii9. [III]
58. Goniewicz ML, Knysak J, Gawron M, et al. Levels of selected carcinogens and toxicants in vapour from electronic cigarettes. *Tob Control*. 2014;23(2):133–139. [II-3]
59. Grobman WA, Gilbert SA, Iams JD, et al. Activity restriction among women with a short cervix. *Obstet Gynecol*. 2013;121(6):1181–1186. [Secondary analysis, $n = 657$]
60. Grobman WA, Thom EA, Spong CY, et al. 17 Alpha-hydroxyprogesterone caproate to prevent prematurity in nulliparas with cervical length less than 30 mm. *Am J Obstet Gynecol*. 2012;207:390.e1–390.e8. [RCT, $n = 657$]
61. Keeler SM, Kiefer D, Rochon M, et al. A randomized trial of cerclage vs. 17 ∞--hydroxyprogesterone caproate for treatment of short cervix. *J Perinal Med*. 2009;37:473–479. [RCT, $n = 79$]
62. Fonseca EB, Celik E, Parra M, et al. Progesterone and the risk of preterm birth among women with a short cervix. *N Eng J Med*. 2007;357:462–469. [RCT, $n = 250$]
63. Hassan SS, Romero R, Vidyadhari D, et al.; for the pregnant trial. Vaginal progesterone reduces the rate of preterm birth in women with sonographic short cervix: A multicenter, randomized, double-blind, placebo-controlled trial. *Ultrasound Obstet Gynecol*. 2011;38:18–31. [RCT, $n = 458$]
64. Romero R, Nicolaides N, Conde-Agudelo A, et al. Vaginal progesterone in women with an asymptomatic sonographic short cervix in the midtrimester decreases preterm delivery and neonatal morbidity: A systematic review and meta-analysis of individual patient data. *Am J Obstet Gynecol*. 2012;206:124.e1–124.e19. [Meta-analysis: 5 RCTs, $n = 775$]
65. Cahill AG, Odibo AO, Caughey AB, et al. Universal cervical length screening and treatment with vaginal progesterone to

prevent preterm birth: A decision and economic analysis. *Am J Obstet Gynecol.* 2010;202(6):548.e1–548.e8. [Decision analysis]
66. Werner EF, Han CS, Pettker CM, et al. Universal cervical-length screening to prevent preterm birth: A cost-effectiveness analysis. *Ultrasound Obstet Gynecol.* 2011;38(1):32–37. [Decision analysis]
67. Khalifeh A, Berghella V. Universal cervical length screening in singleton gestations without a prior preterm birth: Ten reasons why it should be implemented. *Am J Obstet Gynecol.* 2016;214(5):603.e1–603.e5. doi: 10.1016/j.ajog.2015.12.017. [Epub ahead of print] [Review]
68. Werner EF, Hamel MS, Orzechowski K, et al. Cost-effectiveness of transvaginal ultrasound cervical length screening in singletons without a prior preterm birth: An update. *Am J Obstet Gynecol.* 2015;213(4):554.e1–554.e6. [Decision analysis]
69. Society for Maternal-Fetal Medicine, Berghella V. Progesterone and preterm birth prevention: Translating clinical trials data into clinical practice. *Am J Obstet Gynecol.* 2012;206:376–386. [Review]
70. American College of Obstetricians and Gynecologists. ACOG Practice Bulletin No. 130: Prediction and Prevention of Preterm Birth. Washington, DC: ACOG, October 2012. [Review]
71. FIGO Committee Report. Best practice in maternal-fetal medicine. *Int J Gynecol Obstet.* 2015;128:80–82. [Guideline]
72. Cervical Length Education and Review (CLEAR) program [Internet]. Available at: https://clear.perinatalquality.org. Accessed on August 30, 2016.
73. Fetal Medicine Foundation Cervical Assessment Certification [Internet]. Available at: https://fetalmedicine.org/cervical-assessment-1. Accessed on August 30, 2016.
74. Berghella V, Baxter J, Berghella M. Cervical insufficiency. In Apuzzio JJ, Vintzileos AM, Iffy L (eds.). *Operative Obstetrics.* 3rd ed. London, United Kingdom: Taylor and Francis, 2006:157–172. [Review chapter]
75. Berghella V, Obido AO, To MS, et al. Cerclage for short cervix on ultrasound: Meta-analysis of trials using individual patient-level data. *Obstet Gynecol.* 2005;106:181–189. [Meta-analysis: 4 RCTs, $n = 607$]
76. Goya M, Pratcorona L, Merced C, et al. Cervical pessary in pregnant women with a short cervix (PECEP): An open-label randomized controlled trial. *Lancet.* 2012;379(9828):1800–1806. [RCT, $n = 385$]
77. Hiu SYA, Chor CM, Lau TK, et al. Cerclage pessary for preventing preterm birth in women with a singleton pregnancy and a short cervix at 20 to 24 weeks: A randomized controlled trial. *Am J Perinatal.* 2012;30(4):283–288. [RCT, $n = 108$]
78. Nicolaides K, Syngelaki A, Poon L, et al. Randomized trial of cervical pessary for prevention of preterm birth in singleton pregnancies with short cervical length. *New Engl J Med.* 2016;374:1044–1052. [RCT, $n = 932$]
79. Berghella V, Rust OA, Althuisius SM. Short cervix on ultrasound: Does indomethacin prevent preterm birth? *Am J Obstet Gynecol.* 2006;195:809–813. [II-1]
80. Sosa CG, Althabe F, Belizán JM, et al. Bed rest in singleton pregnancies for preventing preterm birth. *Cochrane Database Syst Rev.* 2015;(3):CD003581. doi: 10.1002/14651858.CD003581.pub3. [Meta-analysis: 2 RCTs, n-1,266]
81. Elliott JP, Miller HS, Coleman S, et al. A randomized multicenter study to determine the efficacy of activity restriction for preterm labor management in patients testing negative for fetal fibronectin. *J Perinatol.* 2005;25:626–630. [RCT, $n = 73$]
82. American College of Obstetricians and Gynecologists. Practice Bulletin No. 127: Management of preterm labor. *Obstet Gynecol.* 2012, reaffirmed 2014;119:1308–1317. [Review]
83. Hobel CJ, Ross MG, Bemis RL, et al. The west Los Angeles preterm birth prevention project. I. Program impact on high-risk women. *Am J Obstet Gynecol.* 1994;170:54–62. [RCT, $n = >1500$]
84. Hegaard HK, Hedegaard M, Damm, et al. Leisure time physical activity is associated with a reduced risk of preterm delivery. *Am J Obstet Gynecol.* 2008;198:180. [II-2]
85. Hodnett ED, Fredericks S, Weston J. Support during pregnancy for women at increased risk of low birthweight babies. *Cochrane Database Syst Rev.* 2010;(6):CD000198. doi: 10.1002/14651858.CD000198.pub2. (17 RCTs, $n = 12,264$)
86. Mueller-Heubach E, Rddick D, Barnett B, et al. Preterm birth prevention: Evaluation of a prospective controlled trial. *Am J Obstet Gynecol.* 1989;160:1172–1178. [RCT, $n = <800$]
87. Main DM, Richardson DK, Hadley CB, et al. Controlled trial of a preterm labor detection program: Efficacy and costs. *Obstet Gynecol.* 1989;74:873–877. [RCT, $n = 376$]
88. Collaborative Group on Preterm Birth Prevention. Multicenter randomized controlled trial of a preterm birth prevention program. *Am J Obstet Gynecol.* 1993;169:352–366. [RCT; $n = 2395$ — includes Goldenberg RL, Davis RO, Copper RL, et al. The Alabama preterm birth prevention trial. *Obstet Gynecol.* 1990;75:933–939. [RCT, $n =$ about 1000]
89. Iams JD, Berghella V. Care for women with prior preterm birth. *Am J Obstet Gynecol.* 2010;203(2):89–100. [Review]
90. Silver RM, Ahrens K, Wong LF, et al. Low dose aspirin and preterm birth: A randomized controlled trial. *Obstet Gynecol.* 2015;125:876–884. [Secondary analysis, $n = 1,228$]
91. Klebanoff MA, Harper M, Lai Y, et al. Fish consumption, erythrocyte fatty acids, and preterm birth. *Obstet Gynecol.* 2011;117:1071–1077. [II-1]
92. Olsen SF, Secher NJ, Tabor A, et al. Randomized clinical trials of fish oil supplementation in high risk pregnancies. *Br J Obstet Gynecol.* 2000;107:382–395. [RCT; $n = 232$ for singletons; $n = 569$ for twins]
93. Harper M, Thom E, Klebanoff MA, et al. Omega-3 fatty acid supplementation to prevent recurrent PTB. A controlled trial. *Obstet Gynecol.* 2010;115:234–242. [RCT, $n = 852$]
94. Saccone G, Berghella V. Omega-3 supplementation to prevent recurrent preterm birth: A systematic review and meta-analysis of randomized controlled trials. *Am J Obstet Gynecol.* 2015;213(2):135–40. doi: 10.1016/j.ajog.2015.03.013. Epub 2015 Mar 7. [Meta-analysis: 2 RCTs, $n = 1,080$]
95. Andrews WW, Goldenberg RL, Hauth JC, et al. Interconceptional antibiotics to prevent spontaneous preterm birth: A randomized clinical trial. *Am J Obstet Gynecol.* 2006;194:617–623. [RCT, $n = 124$]
96. Vermeulen GM, Bruinse HW. Prophylactic administration of clindamycin 2% vaginal cream to reduce the incidence of spontaneous preterm birth in women with an increased recurrence risk: A randomized placebo-controlled double-blind trial. *Br J Obstet Gynecol.* 1999;106:652–657. [RCT, $n = 168$]
97. Gighangi PB, Ndinya-Achola JO, Ombete J, et al. Antimicrobial prophylaxis in pregnancy: A randomized, placebo-controlled trial with cefetamet-pivoxil in pregnant women with poor obstetrical history. *Am J Obstet Gynecol.* 1997;177:680–684. [RCT, $n = 253$]
98. Hauth JC, Goldenberg RL, Andrews WW, et al. Reduced incidence of preterm delivery with metronidazole and erythromycin in women with bacterial vaginosis. *N Engl J Med.* 1995;333:1732–1736. [RCT, $n = 358$ women with prior PTB or prepregnancy weight < 50 kg, and without BV; rx metro AND erythromycin]
99. Thinkhamrop J, Hofmeyr GJ, Adetoro O, et al. Antibiotic prophylaxis during the second and third trimester to reduce adverse pregnancy outcomes and morbidity. *Cochrane Database Syst Rev.* 2015;(6)CD002250. doi:10.1002/14651858.CD002250.pub3. [Meta-analysis: 8RCTs, n= 4300 both low and high risk women]
100. Johnson JW, Austin KL, Jones GS, et al. Efficacy of 17 alpha-hydroxyprogesterone caproate in the prevention of premature labor. *N Engl J Med.* 1975;293(14):675–680. [RCT, $n = 43$]
101. Meis PJ, Klebanoff M, Thom E, et al. Prevention of recurrent preterm delivery by 17 alpha-hydroxyprogesterone caproate. *N Engl J Med.* 2003;348:2379–2386. [RCT, $n =$ about 463]
102. American College of Obstetricians and Gynecologists. ACOG Committee Opinion No. 419: Use of progesterone to reduce preterm birth. *Obstet Gynecol.* 2008;112:963–965. [Review]

103. Kilpatrick S.J., Society for Maternal-Fetal Medicine Publication committee. Progesterone for prevention of prematurity. *Contemp Obstet Gynecol.* 2009;54:32–33. [Review]
104. Petrini JR, Callaghan WM, Klebanoff M, et al. Estimated effect of 17 alpha-hydroxyprogesterone caproate on preterm birth in the United States. *Obstet Gynecol.* 2005;105(2):267–272. [II-3]
105. da Fonseca EB, Bittar RE, Carvalho MH, et al. Prophylactic administration of progesterone by vaginal suppository to reduce the incidence of spontaneous preterm birth in women at increased risk: A randomized placebo-controlled double-blind study. *Am J Obstet Gynecol.* 2003;188:419–424. [RCT, n = 142]
106. O'Brien JM, Adair CD, Lewis DF, et al. Progesterone vaginal gel for the reduction of recurrent preterm birth: Primary results from a randomized, double-blind, placebo-controlled trial. *Ultrasound Obstet Gynecol.* 2007;30:687–696. [RCT, n = 659]
107. Maher MA, Abdelaziz A, Ellaithy M, et al. Prevention of preterm birth: A randomized trial of vaginal compared with intramuscular progesterone. *Acta Obstet Gynecol Scand.* 2013;92(2):215–222. doi: 10.1111/aogs.12017. [RCT, n = 518]
108. El-Gharib MN, El-Hawary. Matched sample comparison of intramuscular versus vaginal micronized progesterone for prevention of preterm birth. *J Matern Fetal Neonatal Med.* 2013;26(7):716–719. doi: 10.3109/14767058.2012.755165. Epub 2013 Jan 9. [Prospective clinical trial, n = 160] [II-2]
109. Bafghi AST, Bahrami E, Sekhavat L. Comparative study of vaginal versus intramuscular progesterone in the prevention of preterm delivery: A randomized clinical trial. *Electron Physician.* 2015;7(6):1301–1309. doi: 10.14661/1301. [Randomized trial, n = 78]
110. Rai P, Rajaram S, Goel N, et al. Oral micronized progesterone for prevention of preterm birth. *Int J Gynaecol Obstet.* 2009;104(1):40–43. [RCT, n = 150]
111. Glover MM, McKenna DS, Downing CM, et al. A randomized trial of micronized progesterone for the prevention of recurrent preterm birth. *Am J Perinat.* 2011;28:377–381. [RCT, n = 33]
112. Rush RW, Issacs S, McPherson K, et al. A randomized controlled trial of cervical cerclage in women at high risk of preterm delivery. *Br J Obstet Gynecol.* 1984;91:724–730. [RCT, n = 194]
113. Lazar P, Gueguen S, Dreyfus J, et al. Multicentre controlled trial of cervical cerclage in women at moderate risk of preterm delivery. *Br J Obstet Gynecol.* 1984;91:731–735. [RCT, n = 506]
114. MRC/RCOG Working Party on Cervical Cerclage. Final report of the Medical Research Council/Royal College of Obstetricians and Gynaecologists multicentre randomized trial of cervical cerclage. *Br J Obstet Gynecol.* 1993;100:516–523. [RCT, n = 1,292]
115. Davis G, Berghella V, Talucci M, et al. Patients with a prior failed transvaginal cerclage: A comparison of obstetric outcomes with either transabdominal or transvaginal cerclage. *Am J Obstet Gynecol.* 2000;183:836–839. [II-2]
116. Tulandi T, Alghanaim N, Hakeem G, et al. Pre and post-conceptional abdominal cerclage by laparoscopy or laparotomy. *J Minim Invasive Gynecol.* 2014;21(6):987–993. doi: 10.1016/j.jmig.2014.05.015. Epub 2014 Jun 4. [Review, n = 678 TA cerclages]
117. Berghella V, Mackeen AD. Cervical length screening with ultrasound-indicated cerclage compared with history-indicated cerclage for prevention of preterm birth: A meta-analysis. *Obstet Gynecol.* 2011;118(1):148–155. [Meta-analysis: 4 RCTs, n = 467]
118. Berghella V, Rafael TJ, Szychowski JM, et al. Cerclage for short cervix on ultrasonography in women with singleton gestations and previous preterm birth: A meta-analysis. *Obstet Gynecol.* 2011;117(3):663–671. [Meta-analysis: 5 RCTs, n = 504]
119. Berghella V, Ludmir J, Simonazzi G, et al. Transvaginal cervical cerclage: Evidence for perioperative management strategies. *Am J Obstet Gynecol.* 2013;209(3):181–192. [Review]
120. Tsai YL, Lin YH, Chong KM, et al. Effectiveness of double cervical cerclage in women with at least one previous pregnancy loss in the second trimester: A randomized controlled trial. *J. Obstet. Gynaecol. Res.* 2009;35(4):666–671. [RCT, n = 51]
121. Brix N, Secher NJ, McCormack CD, et al. Randomized trial of cervical cerclage, with and without occlusion, for the prevention of preterm birth in women suspected for cervical insufficiency. *Br J Obstet Gynecol.* 2013;120(5):613–620. [RCT, n = 309]
122. Mathews DD, Friend JB, Michael CA. A double-blind trial of oral isoxuprine in the prevention of premature labour. *J Obstet Gynaecol Br Commonw.* 1967;74:68–70. [RCT, n = 64]
123. DeFranco EA, O'Brien JM, Adair CD, et al. Vaginal progesterone is associated with a decrease in risk for early preterm birth and improved neonatal outcome in women with a short cervix: A secondary analysis from a randomized, double-blind, placebo-controlled trial. *Obstet Gynecol.* 2007;30:697–705. [Secondary analysis of RCT; n = 46]
124. Winer N, Bretelle F, Senat MV, et al. 17 Alpha-hydroxyprogesterone caproate does not prolong pregnancy or reduce the rate of preterm birth in women at high risk for preterm delivery and a short cervix: A randomized controlled trial. *Am J Obstet Gynecol.* 2015;212:485.e1–485.e10. [RCT, n = 105]
125. Owen J, Szychowski J. Can the optimal cervical length for placing ultrasound-indicated cerclage be identified? *Am J Obstet Gynecol.* 2011;204:s198–s199. [II-1]
126. Berghella V, Keeler SM, To MS, et al. Effectiveness of cerclage according to severity of cervical length shortening: A meta-analysis. *Ultrasound Obstet Gynecol.* 2010;35:468–473. [II-1]
127. Romero R, Yeo L, Chaemsaithong P, et al. Progesterone to prevent spontaneous preterm birth. *Semin Fetal Neonatal Med.* 2014;19(1):15–26. doi: 10.1016/j.siny.2013.10.004. Epub 2013 Dec 5. [Review]
128. Suhag A, Reina J, Sanapo L, et al. Prior ultrasound-indicated cerclage: Comparison of cervical length screening or history-indicated cerclage in the next pregnancy. *Obstet Gynecol.* 2015;126(5):962–968. [II-2]
129. Vousden N, Hezelgrave N, Carter J, et al. Prior ultrasound indicated cerclage: How should we manage the next pregnancy. *Eur J Obstet Gynecol Reprod Biol.* 2015;188:129–132. [II-2]
130. Baxter JK, Airoldi J, Berghella V. Short cervical length after history-indicated cerclage: Is a reinforcing cerclage beneficial? *Am J Obstet Gynecol.* 2005;193(3 Pt 2):1204–1207. [II-1]
131. Contag SA, Woo J, Schwartz DB, et al. Reinforcing cerclage for a short cervix at follow-up after the primary cerclage procedure. *J Matern Fetal Neonatal Med.* 2016;29(15):2422–2427. [II-2]
132. Conde-Agudelo A, Romero R, Nicolaides K, et al. Vaginal progesterone vs cervical cerclage for the prevention of preterm birth in women with a sonographic short cervix, previous preterm birth, and singleton gestation: A systematic review and indirect comparison meta-analysis. *Am J Obstet Gynecol.* 2013;208:42.e1–42.e18. [Meta-analysis: 9 RCTs, n = 662]
133. Rafael TJ, Mackeen AD, Berghella V. The effect of 17 alpha hydroxyprogesterone caproate on preterm birth in women with an ultrasound indicated cerclage. *Am J Perinatol.* 2011;28(5):389–394. [II-2]
134. Berghella V, Figueroa D, Szychowski JM, et al. Vaginal Ultrasound Trial Consortium. 17-Alpha-hydroxyprogesterone caproate for the prevention of preterm birth in women with prior preterm birth and a short cervical length. *Am J Obstet Gynecol.* 2010;202(4):351.e1–351.e6. doi: 10.1016/j.ajog.2010.02.019. [Secondary analysis of RCT, n = 300]
135. Szychowski JM, Berghella V, Owen J, et al. Vaginal Ultrasound Trial Consortium. Cerclage for the prevention of preterm birth in high risk women receiving intramuscular 17-α-hydroxyprogesterone caproate. *J Matern Fetal Neonatal Med.* 2012;25(12):2686–2689. doi: 10.3109/14767058.2012.717128. [Secondary analysis of RCT, n = 99]
136. Althuisius SM, Dekker GA, van Geijn HP, et al. Cervical incompetence prevention randomized cerclage trial (CIPRACT): Study design and preliminary results. *Am J Obstet Gynecol.* 2000;183:823–829. [RCT, n = 67]
137. Mackeen AD, Rafael TJ, Zavodnick J, et al. Effectiveness of 17 α-hydroxyprogesterone caproate on preterm birth prevention in women with history-indicated cerclage. *Am J Perinatol.* 2013;30(9):755–758. [II-2]

138. Pritts EA, Atwood AK. Luteal phase support in infertility treatment: A meta-analysis of the randomized trials. *Hum Reprod.* 2002;17:2287–2299. [Meta-analysis: *n* = about 200]
139. Corrado F, Dugo C, Cannata ML, et al. A randomized trial of progesterone prophylaxis after midtrimester amniocentesis. *Eur J Obstet Gynecol Reprod Biol.* 2002;188:196–198. [RCT, *n* = 584]
140. Morrison JC, Martin JN, Martin RW, et al. Prevention of preterm birth by ambulatory assessment of uterine activity: A randomized study. *Am J Obstet Gynecol.* 1987;156:536–543. [RCT; *n* = 67 (18 twins); cannot differentiate populations]
141. Iams JD, Johnson FF, O'shaunessy RW. A prospective random trial of home uterine activity monitoring in pregnancies at increased risk of preterm labor. *Am J Obstet Gynecol.* 1987;157:638–643. [RCT; *n* = 142 (40 twins); cannot differentiate]; Iams JD, Johnson FF, O'shaunessy RW. A prospective random trial of home uterine activity monitoring in pregnancies at increased risk of preterm labor. Part II. *Am J Obstet Gynecol.* 1988;159:595–603. [RCT, *n* = 266]
142. Hill WC, Fleming WC, Martin RW, et al. Home uterine activity monitoring is associated with a reduction in preterm birth. *Obstet Gynecol.* 1990;76:13–18. [RCT, *n* = 245; ?twins]
143. Dyson DC, Crites YM, Ray DA, et al. Prevention of preterm birth in high-risk patients: A role of education and provider contact versus home uterine monitoring. *Am J Obstet Gynecol.* 1991;164:756–762. [RCT; *n* = 247 (109 twins); CAN differentiate populations]
144. Mou SM, Sunderji SG, Gall S, et al. Multicenter randomized clinical trial of home uterine activity monitoring for detection of preterm labor. *Am J Obstet Gynecol.* 1991;165:858–866. [RCT; first report—see Corwin et al.]
145. Corwin MJ, Mou SM, Sunderji SG, et al. Multicenter randomized clinical trial of home uterine activity monitoring: Pregnancy outcomes for all women randomized. *Am J Obstet Gynecol.* 1996;175:1281–1285. [RCT; reports PTB outcomes of Mou et al. 1991 RCT—same RCT; *n* = 339; no twins]
146. Blondel B, Breart G, Berthoux Y, et al. Home uterine activity monitoring in France: A randomized, controlled trial. *Am J Obstet Gynecol.* 1992;167:424–429. [RCT; *n* = 52; cannot distinguish populations of high-risk singletons vs. twins vs. PTL pts]
147. Wapner RJ, Cotton DB, Artal R, et al. A randomized multicenter trial assessing a home uterine activity monitoring devise used in the absence of daily nursing contact. *Am J Obstet Gynecol.* 1995;172:1026–1034. [RCT; *n* = 187; ?twins—PTB outcomes not reported]
148. The Collaborative Home Uterine Monitoring Study Group. A multicenter randomized trial of home uterine monitoring: Active versus sham device. *Am J Obstet Gynecol.* 1995;173:1120–1127. [RCT (Devoe PI); *n* = about 1125; about 215 twins. Cannot differentiate populations]
149. Dyson DC, Danbe KH, Bamber JA, et al. Monitoring women at risk for preterm labor. *N Engl J Med.* 1998;338:15–19. [RCT; *n* = 2422 (844 twins) can differentiate populations; data reported in %, not actual #]
150. Althuisius SM, Dekker GA, Hummel P, et al. Cervical incompetence prevention randomized cerclage trial: Emergency cerclage with bed rest versus bed rest alone. *Am J Obstet Gynecol.* 2003;189:907. [RCT, *n* = 23]
151. Pereira L, Cotter A, Gomez R, et al. Expectant management compared with physical-examination indicated cerclage (EMPEC) in selected women with a dilated cervix at 14–25 weeks: Results from the EMPEC international cohort study. *Am J Obstet Gynecol.* 2007;197:483. [II-1]
152. Ehsanipoor RM, Seligman NS, Saccone G, et al. Physical examination indicated cerclage: A systematic review and meta-analysis. *Obstet Gynecol.* 2015;126(1):125–35. [Meta-analysis of 10 studies - 1 RCT, 2 prospective cohort studies, remaining 7 retrospective studies; *n* = 757]
153. Miller ES, Grobman WA, Fonseca L, et al. Indomethacin and antibiotics in examination-indicated cerclage: A randomized controlled trial. *Obstet Gynecol.* 2014;123(6):1311–1316. doi: 10.1097/AOG.0000000000000228. [RCT, *n* = 50]
154. Berghella V, Prasertcharoensuk W, Cotter A, et al. Does indomethacin preterm preterm birth in women with cervical dilatation in the second trimester? *Am J Perinatol.* 2009;26:13–19. [II-1]
155. Andrews WW, Sibai BM, Thom EA, et al. Randomized clinical trial of metronidazole plus erythromycin to prevent spontaneous preterm delivery in fetal-fibronectin-positive women. *Obstet Gynecol.* 2003;101:847–855. [RCT, *n* = 703]
156. Shennan A, Crawshaw S, Briley A, et al. A randomized controlled trial of metronidazole for the prevention of preterm birth in women positive for cervicovaginal fetal fibronectin: The PREMET study. *Br J Obstet Gynecol.* 2006;113:65–74. [RCT, *n* = 100]
157. Bujold E, Roberge S, Tapp S, et al. Could early aspirin prophylaxis prevent against preterm birth? *J Mat Fet Neo Med.* 2011;24:966–967. [Meta-analysis: 4 RCTs, *n* = 387]
158. Duley L, Henderson-Smart DJ, Meher S, et al. Antiplatelet agents for preventing preeclampsia and its complications. *Cochrane Database Syst Rev.* 2007;(10):CD004659. doi: 10.1002/14651858.CD004659.pub2. [Meta-analysis: 29 RCTs, *n* = 31,151]
159. LeFevre ML. Low-dose aspirin use for the prevention of morbidity and mortality from preeclampsia: US Preventive Services Task Force recommendation statement. US Preventive Services Task Force. *Ann Intern Med.* 2014;161:819–26.
160. Jeffcoat MK, Hauth JC, Geurs NC, et al. Periodontal disease and preterm birth: Results of a pilot intervention study. *J Periodontol.* 2003;74:1214–1218. [RCT, *n* = 366. Screened and rx at 21–25 weeks 3 rx groups: Dental prophylaxis; SRP; SRP and metronidazole (placebo controlled)]
161. Lopez NJ, Da Silva I, Ipinza J, et al. Periodontal therapy reduces the rate of preterm low birth weight in women with pregnancy-associated gingivitis. *J Perodontol.* 2005;76:2144–2153. [RCT, *n* = 834]
162. Fampa Fogacci M, Vettore MV, Thome Leao AT. The effect of periodontal therapy on preterm low birth weight—A meta-analysis. *Obstet Gynecol.* 2011;117:153–165. [Meta-analysis: 10 RCTs]
163. Smaill FM, Vazquez JC. Antibiotics for asymptomatic bacteriuria in pregnancy. *Cochrane Database Syst Rev.* 2015;(8):CD000490. doi: 10.1002/14651858.CD000490.pub3. [14 RCTs, *n* = 2,000)
164. Widmer M, Lopez I, Gulmezoglu AM, et al. Duration of treatment for asymptomatic bacteriuria during pregnancy. *Cochrane Database Syst Rev.* 2015;(11):CD000491. doi: 10.1002/14651858.CD000491.pub3. [Meta-analysis: 13 RCTs, *n* = 1,622]
165. Thompsen AC, Morup L, Hansen KB. Antibiotic elimination of group B streptococci in urine in prevention of preterm labour. *Lancet.* 1987;1(8533):591–593. [RCT, *n* = 69]
166. Brocklehurst P, Gordon A, Heatley E, et al. Antibiotics for treating bacterial vaginosis in pregnancy. *Cochrane Database Syst Rev.* 2013;(1):CD000262. doi: 10.1002/14651858.CD000262.pub4. [21 Randomized trials, *n* = 7,847]
167. Okun N, Gronau KA, Hannah ME. Antibiotics for bacterial vaginosis or *Trichomonas vaginalis* in pregnancy: A systematic review. *Obstet Gynecol.* 2005;105:857–868. [Meta-analysis: 14 RCTs on BV; *n* = >5500. 2 RCTs on TV; *n* = 842]
168. Gülmezoglu AM, Azhar M. Interventions for trichomoniasis in pregnancy. *Cochrane Database Syst Rev.* 2011;(5):CD000220. doi: 10.1002/14651858.CD000220.pub2. [Meta-analysis: 2 RCTs, *n* = 842]
169. Ross SM, Van Middelkoop A. Trichomonas infection in pregnancy: Does it affect outcome? *S AfrMed J.* 1983;63:566–567. [RCT, *n* = 225. 2 g metronidazole × 1 to women and their partners]
170. Klebanoff MA, Carey JC, Hauth JC, et al. Failure of metronidazole to prevent preterm delivery among pregnant women with asymptomatic *Trichomonas vaginalis* infection. *N Engl J Med.* 2001;345:487–493. [RCT, *n* = 617; 2 g metronidazole q48 hours × 2 doses]
171. Kigozi GG, Brahmbhatt H, Wabwire-Mangen F, et al. Treatment of Trichomonas in pregnancy and adverse outcomes of pregnancy: A subanalysis of a randomized trial in Rakai, Uganda. *Am J Obstet Gynecol.* 2003;189:1398–1400. [RCT, *n* = 206 with TV (PTB < 37 weeks: RR 1.28, 95% CI 0.81–2.02)—subanalysis of larger trial]

172. Kiss H, Petricevic L, Husslein P. Prospective randomised controlled trial of an infection screening programme to reduce the rate of preterm delivery. *BMJ*. 2004;329:371. [RCT, $n = 4166$]
173. Klebanoff MA, Regan JA, Rao AV, et al. Outcome of the vaginal infections and prematurity study: Results of a clinical trial of erythromycin among pregnant women colonized with group B streptococci. *Am J Obstet Gynecol*. 1995;172:1540–1545. [RCT, $n = 938$; vaginal-cervical GBS at 23–26 weeks: Erythromycin 333 mg tid or placebo for 10 weeks or up to 35 6/7 weeks, whichever came first]
174. McCormack WM, Rosner B, Lee Y-H, et al. Effect of birth weight of erythromycin treatment of pregnant women. *Obstet Gynecol*. 1987;69:202–207. [RCT, $n = 1071$]
175. Crowther CA, Han S. Hospitalisation and bed rest for multiple pregnancy. *Cochrane Database Syst Rev*. 2010;(7):CD000110. doi: 10.1002/14651858.CD000110.pub2. [Meta-analysis: 7 RCTs, $n = 713$]
176. Crowther CA, Verkuyl DAA, Neilson JP, et al. The effects of hospitalization for rest on fetal growth, neonatal morbidity and length of gestation in twin pregnancy. *Br J Obstet Gynecol*, 1990;97:872–877. [RCT, $n = 118$]
177. Crowther CA, Verkuyl D, Ashworth M, et al. The effects of hospitalisation for bed rest on duration of gestation, fetal growth and neonatal morbidity in triplet pregnancy. *Acta Genet Med Gemellol*. 1991;40:63–68. [RCT, $n = 19$]
178. Hartikainen-Sorri AL, Jouppila P. Is routine hospitalization needed in antenatal care of twin pregnancy? *J Perinat Med*. 1984;12:31–34. [RCT, $n = 73$]
179. MacLennan AH, Green RC, O'shea R, et al. Routine hospital admission in twin pregnancy between 26 and 30 weeks' gestation. *Lancet*. 1990;335:267–269. [RCT, $n = 141$]
180. Saunders MC, Dick JS, Brown IM, et al. The effects of hospital admission for bed rest on the duration of twin pregnancy: A randomised trial. *Lancet*, 1985;2:793–795. [RCT, $n = 212$]
181. Crowther CA, Neilson JP, Verkuyl DA, et al. Preterm labour in twin pregnancies: Can it be prevented by hospital admission? *Br J Obstet Gynecol*. 1989;96:850–853. [RCT, $n = 139$]
182. Gordon MC, McKenna DS, Stewart TL, et al. Transvaginal cervical length scans to prevent prematurity in twins: A randomized controlled trial. *Am J Obstet Gynecol*. 2016;214(2):277.e1–277.e7. doi: 10.1016/j.ajog.2015.08.065. Epub 2015 Sep 9. [RCT, $n = 125$]
183. Hartikainen-Sorri AL, Kauppila A, Tuimala R. Inefficacy of 17 α-hydroxyprogestrone caproate in the prevention of prematurity in twin pregnancy. *Obstet Gynecol*. 1980;56(6):692–695. [RCT]
184. Rouse DJ, Caritis SN, Peaceman AM, et al. A trial of 17 alpha-hydroxyprogesterone caproate to prevent prematurity in twins. *N Engl J Med*. 2007;357:454–461. [RCT, $n = 661$]
185. Combs CA, Garite T, Maurel K, et al.; for the Obstetrix Collaborative Research Network. 17-Hydroxyprogesterone caproate for twin pregnancy: A double-blind, randomized clinical trial. *Am J Obstet Gynecol*. 2011;204:221.e1–221.e8. [RCT, $n = 240$]
186. Durnwald CP, Momirova V, Rouse DJ, et al.; for the Eunice Kennedy Shriver National Institute of Child Health and Human Development (NICHD), Maternal-Fetal Medicine Units Network (MFMU). Second trimester cervical length and risk of preterm birth in women with twin gestations treated with 17 α-hydroxyprogesterone caproate. *J Matern Fetal Neonatal Med*. 2010;23(12):1360–1364. doi: 10.3109/14767051003702786. Epub 2010 May 4. [Secondary analysis of RCT, $n = 221$]
187. Briery CM, Veillon EW, Klauser CK, et al. Progesterone does not prevent preterm births in women with twins. *Southern Med J*. 2009;102:900–904. [RCT, $n = 30$]
188. Awwad J, Usta IM, Ghazeeri, et al. A randomised controlled double-blind clinical trial of 17-hydroxyprogesterone caproate for the prevention of preterm birth in twin gestation (PROGESTWIN): Evidence for reduced neonatal morbidity. *Br J Obstet Gynecol*. 2015;122(1):71–79. doi: 10.1111/1471-0528.13031. Epub 2014 Aug 27. [RCT, $n = 288$]
189. Schuit E, Stock S, Rode L, et al. Effectiveness of progestogens to improve perinatal outcome in twin pregnancies: An individual participant data meta-analysis. *Br J Obstet Gynecol*. 2015;122(1):27–37. [Meta-analysis: 13 RCTs, $n = 3,768$]
190. Senat MV, Porcher R, Winer N, et al. Prevention of preterm delivery by 17 alpha-hydroxyprogesterone caproate in asymptomatic twin pregnancies with a short cervix: A randomized controlled trial. *Am J Obstet Gynecol*. 2013;208:194.e1–194.e8. [RCT, $n = 165$]
191. Caritis SN, Rouse DJ, Peaceman AM, et al.; for the Eunice Kennedy Shriver National Institute of Child Health and Human Development (NICHD), Maternal-Fetal Medicine Units Network (MFMU). Prevention of preterm birth in triplets using 17 alpha-hydroxyprogesterone caproate: A randomized controlled trial. *Obstet Gynecol*. 2009;113(2):285–292. [RCT, $n = 134$]
192. Combs CA, Garite T, Maurel K, et al.; for the Obstetrix Collaborative Research Network. Failure of 17-hydroxyprogesterone to reduce neonatal morbidity or prolong triplet pregnancy: A double-blind, randomized clinical trial. *Am J Obstet Gynecol*. 2010;203(3):248.e1–248.e9. [RCT, $n = 81$]
193. Norman JE, Mackenzie F, Owen P, et al. Progesterone for the prevention of preterm birth in twin pregnancy (STOPPIT): A randomized, double-blind, placebo-controlled study and meta-analysis. *Lancet*. 2009;373:2034–2040. [RCT, $n = 494$]
194. Wood S, Ross S, Tang S, et al. Vaginal progesterone to prevent preterm birth in multiple pregnancy: A randomized controlled trial. *J Perinat Med*. 2012;40(6):593–599. [RCT, $n = 84$]
195. Rode L, Klein K, Nicolaides KH, et al. Prevention of preterm delivery in twin gestations (PREDICT): A multicentre randomised placebo-controlled trial on the effect of vaginal micronised progesterone. *Ultrasound Obstet Gynecol*. 2011;38(3):272–280. [RCT, $n = 675$]
196. Brizot ML, Hernandez W, Liao AW, et al. Vaginal progesterone for the prevention of preterm birth in twin gestations: A randomized placebo-controlled double-blind study. *Am J Obstet Gynecol*. 2015;213:82.e1–82.e9. [RCT, $n = 390$]
197. Serra V, Perales A, Meseguer J, et al. Increased doses of vaginal progesterone for the prevention of preterm birth in twin pregnancies: A randomized controlled double-blind multicentre trial. *Br J Obstet Gynecol*. 2013;120(1):50–57. [RCT, $n = 290$]
198. Dor J, Shalev J, Mashiach S, et al. Elective cervical suture of twin pregnancies diagnosed ultrasonically in the first trimester following induced ovulation. *Gynecol Obstet Invest*. 1982;13:55–60. [RCT, $n = 100$]
199. Saccone G, Rust O, Althuisius S, et al. Cerclage for short cervix in twin pregnancies: Systematic review and meta-analysis of randomized trials using indivisual patient-level data. *Acta Obstet Gynecol Scand*. 2015;94(4):352–358. [Meta-analysis: 3 randomized trials, $n = 49$]
200. Rafael TJ, Berghella V, Alfirevic Z. Cervical stitch (cerclage) for preventing preterm birth in multiple pregnancy. *Cochrane Database Syst Rev*. 2014;(9):CD009166. doi: 10.1002/14651858. CD009166.pub2. [Meta-analysis: 5 RCTs, $n = 128$ (122 twins, 6 triplets)]
201. Roman A, Rochelson B, Fox NS, et al. Efficacy of ultrasound-indicated cerclage in twin pregnancies. *Am J Obstet Gynecol*. 2015;212:788.e1–788.e6. [II-2]
202. Nicolaides KH, Syngelaki A, Poon LC, et al. Cervical pessary placement for prevention of preterm birth in unselected twin pregnancies: A randomized controlled trial. *Am J Obstet Gynecol*. 2016;214(1):3.e1–3.e9. [RCT, $n = 1080$ twins, of which 214 with short CL]
203. Goya M, de la Calle M, Pratcorona L, et al. Cervical pessary to prevent preterm birth in women with twin gestation and sonographic short cervix: A multicenter randomized controlled trial (PECEP-Twins). *Am J Obstet Gynecol*. 2016;214(2):145–152. [RCT, $n = 134$]
204. Liem S, Schuit E, Hegeman M, et al. Cervical pessaries for prevention of preterm birth in women with a multiple pregnancy (ProTWIN): A multicentre, open-label randomised controlled trial. *Lancet*. 2013;382(9901):1341–1349. [RCT, N (twins with CL < 38 mm) = 143].

Preterm labor

B. Anthony Armson

KEY POINTS
- See Chapter 17 for primary and secondary prevention of preterm birth (PTB) in asymptomatic women, and for risk factors and complications.
- The diagnosis of preterm labor (PTL) is based on the clinical criteria of regular **uterine contractions (≥4/20 minutes or ≥8/hour)** at 20–36 6/7 weeks **with either:**
  - Manually detected cervical dilatation of ≥3 cm, or
  - Transvaginal ultrasound (TVU) cervical length (CL) <20 mm, or
  - TVU CL 20–29 mm and positive fetal fibronectin (FFN)
- Threatened PTL (regular uterine contractions (≥4/20 minutes or ≥8/hour) at 20–36 6/7 weeks) should be assessed and managed with knowledge of **TVU CL, and FFN** results (Figure 18.1).
- Women with threatened PTL but TVU CL ≥30 mm have a ≤2% chance of delivering within 1 week, and a >95% chance of delivering ≥35 weeks without therapy, and should therefore not receive any treatment.
- **Corticosteroids (e.g., betamethasone 12 mg intramuscular (IM) every 24 hours × 2 doses)** given to pregnant women between 24 and 33 6/7 weeks prior to PTB (either spontaneous or indicated) are **effective in preventing respiratory distress syndrome (RDS), intraventricular hemorrhage (IVH), necrotizing enterocolitis (NEC), and neonatal mortality.** Steroids may be also considered for decreasing respiratory morbidities and other neonatal outcomes in some women ≥34 weeks.
- **Single rescue course** of antenatal corticosteroids should only be considered if more than 2 weeks have elapsed since the initial course of corticosteroids and a new episode of PTL or preterm premature rupture of membranes (PPROM) or impending risk of PTB presents again at <33 weeks. A single rescue course of betamethasone, two 12-mg doses 24 hours apart, received before 33 weeks at least 14 or more days after the first course, which was administered before 30 weeks, is associated with decreased RDS, ventilatory support, surfactant use, and composite neonatal morbidity. More than two courses of corticosteroids for fetal maturity should be avoided.
- **Intravenous magnesium sulfate** (loading dose of 4–6 g infused for 20–30 minutes, followed by a maintenance infusion of 1–2 g/hour) given at 24–31 6/7 weeks immediately (within 12 hours) before PTB **is associated with a significant decrease in the incidence of cerebral palsy.**
- Other interventions studied to prevent PTB in women with PTL and intact membranes, including bed rest, hydration, sedation, and antibiotics, have not been shown to be beneficial in the management of PTL.
- No tocolytic agent has been shown to **reduce perinatal mortality**.
- Tocolytics should not be used without concomitant use of corticosteroids for fetal maturity.
- There is **no tocolytic** agent that has been shown to be superior in safety and effectiveness. **Cyclooxygenase (COX) inhibitors** are the only class of primary tocolytics shown to **decrease PTB <37 weeks** compared with placebo. COX inhibitors and oxytocin receptor antagonists (ORAs) have been shown to significantly **prolong pregnancy by 48 hours and by 7 days** compared with placebo. COX inhibitors, calcium channel blockers (CCBs), and ORA have significantly **less side effects than betamimetics. CCB and COX inhibitors are the tocolytic agents best supported by evidence for safety and effectiveness.**
- In general, **maintenance tocolysis has not been proven to prevent PTB or reduce perinatal morbidity/mortality, and therefore maintenance tocolysis should not be used**. An exception is vaginal progesterone, which has been shown to be beneficial for maintenance tocolysis in small randomized controlled trials (RCTs) and a meta-analysis of these, and deserves more study.
- There is insufficient evidence to evaluate multiple tocolytic agents for primary tocolysis, refractory (primary agent is failing, so another is started) tocolysis, or repeated (after successful primary tocolysis) tocolysis.
- **In preterm neonates, delayed cord clamping for 30–60 (maximum 120) seconds** is associated with **fewer transfusions for anemia, better circulatory stability, less IVH and lower risk of NEC** compared with early clamping at <30 seconds.

DIAGNOSIS
PTL was often defined in the past as regular uterine contractions (≥4/20 minutes or ≥8/hour) with either manually-detected cervical change, or cervical effacement ≥80 percent, or cervical dilatation ≥3 cm at 20–36 6/7 weeks [1]. A more evidence-based definition using current diagnostic technology is regular **uterine contractions (≥4/20 minutes or ≥8/hour) with TVU CL <20 mm, or positive FFN and TVU CL 20–29 mm,** at 20–36 6/7 weeks. Threatened PTL can be defined as regular uterine contractions (≥4/20 minute or ≥8/hour) between 20 and 36 6/7 weeks, before cervical dilatation and TVU CL has been assessed.

SYMPTOMS
Symptoms of PTL are often nonspecific and include menstrual-like cramps, abdominal "tightenings," mild irregular contractions, low backache, pelvic pressure, increased vaginal discharge, spotting or bleeding.

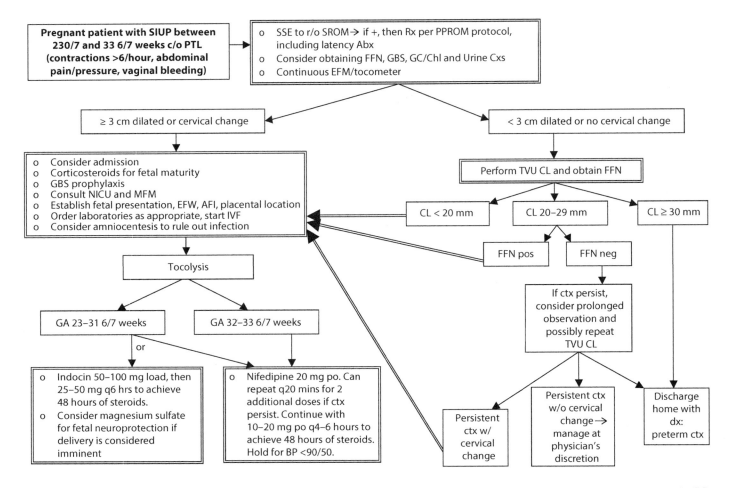

Figure 18.1 Suggested algorithm for the management of preterm labor (PTL). AFV, amniotic fluid volume; Amnio, amniocentesis; BP, blood pressure; Chl, chlamydia; c/o, complains of; CTX, contractions; dx, diagnosis; EFM, external fetal monitoring; EFW, estimated fetal weight; FFN, fetal fibronectin; GA, gestational age; GBS, group B streptococcus; GC, gonorrhea; IVF, intravenous fluids; MFM, maternal-fetal medicine specialist; NICU, neonatal intensive care unit; PPROM, preterm premature rupture of membranes; R/O, rule out; Rx, treat; SLIUP, single live intrauterine pregnancy; SROM, spontaneous rupture of membranes; SSE, sterile speculum examination; TVU CL, transvaginal ultrasound cervical length; w/, with.

For **epidemiology/incidence, genetics, etiology/basic pathophysiology, classification, risk factors/associations, and complications,** see Chapter 17.

WORKUP
- History: ensure correctness of gestational age (GA) estimation; evaluate signs and symptoms of PTL, and ALL risk factors for PTB (Table 17.1; Figure 17.1).
- Physical examination: maternal vital signs; frequency, intensity and duration of uterine contractions; fetal heart rate pattern; assess uterine tenderness, firmness, fetal position.
- Perform speculum examination:
  - Estimate cervical dilatation [2]
  - Assess presence/amount of uterine bleeding
  - Assess for PPROM (nitrazine, pooling, ferning)
  - Obtain swab for FFN testing
  - If no PPROM, perform digital cervical examination
  - If cervix <3 cm dilated, send FFN swab and perform TVU CL
  - If cervix ≥3 cm, discard FFN swab and manage PTL
- Laboratory tests: rectovaginal group B streptococcus (GBS) culture; gonorrhea and chlamydia; urinalysis and urine culture (Figure 18.1); FFN in women <34 weeks gestation with cervical dilation <3 cm and TVU CL 20–29 mm.

Transvaginal Ultrasound Cervical Length
Symptomatic women with CL ≥30 mm have a low risk (<5%) of delivering preterm, regardless of FFN result. For women with CL 20–29 mm, the PTB rate is somewhat increased but still <5% within 7 days if the FFN test is negative. A CL <20 mm is associated with a high risk (>25%) of PTB within 7 days. With this degree of cervical shortening, FFN testing does not improve the predictive accuracy of CL measurement alone [3,4].

Compared with no knowledge, **knowledge of TVU CL results** is associated with a nonsignificant **decrease in PTB <37 weeks** (22.3% vs. 34.7%, respectively; relative risk [RR] 0.59, 95% confidence interval [CI] 0.26–1.32). Delivery occurred at a later GA (by about 4–5 days) in the knowledge versus no knowledge groups [5]. Given the clinical and cost-effectiveness of TVU CL in the assessment of suspected PTL,

TVU CL should be used in the management of women with threatened PTL (Figure 18.1).

Fetal Fibronectin

FFN testing has been shown to predict PTB with moderate accuracy in symptomatic women resulting in health care cost benefits by identifying women who do not require intervention [6]. In a meta-analysis of six RCTs, compared with no knowledge, **knowledge of FFN results in women with threatened PTL had no effect on the incidence of PTB <37 weeks or any other outcome**, maternal or neonatal, including time in triage, PTB <34, 32, or 28 weeks; GA at delivery; birth weight less than 2500 g; perinatal death; maternal hospitalization; tocolysis; steroids for fetal lung maturity [7]. The benefit in knowledge of FFN was seen only in one RCT, in which TVU CL was the main screening test, with FFN used only for "indeterminate" results [8] (Figure 18.1).

MANAGEMENT
Principles of Management

Before treatment is considered, the diagnosis and risk of PTB must be established. **Women with preterm uterine contractions but negative FFN and TVU CL ≥30 mm have a <2% chance of delivering within 1 week, and a >95% chance of delivering ≥35 weeks without therapy, and should therefore not receive any treatment** [4] (Figure 18.1).

Women with **preterm uterine contractions and cervical dilatation ≥3 cm, TVU CL <20 mm or TVU CL 20 – 29 mm and positive FFN have a moderate to high risk of PTB within 7 days, are those with true PTL**, and should be managed with strong consideration for admission, steroids, magnesium for neuroprophylaxis, and possibly tocolysis, depending on GA.

If PTL is diagnosed without using TVU CL, about 70%–80% of women diagnosed with PTL deliver at term. Women without cervical change do not have PTL and should not receive tocolysis. Women with multiple gestations should not be treated differently than those with singletons, except that their risk of pulmonary edema is greater when exposed to betamimetics or magnesium sulfate [9].

Referral to a tertiary care center should be considered if the neonatal ICU is not adequate for GA of potential neonate. There is insufficient evidence to justify the use of steroids for fetal maturity and tocolysis before 23 weeks. Amniocentesis may be considered to assess intra-amniotic infection (IAI) (incidence about 5%–15%) and fetal lung maturity (especially between 33 and 35 weeks). IAI (documented by amniotic fluid culture) rates can be estimated by pregnancy status (Table 18.1). IAI rates can also be estimated by TVU CL [10].

Counseling regarding morbidity and mortality for preterm infant, using recent and ideally national or institutional data should be provided [11]. (Table 18.2). Neonatal consult at 22–34 weeks is indicated for counseling regarding prognosis and neonatal management. Current **neonatal survival** in the USA is *0% at 21 weeks, 5%–15% at 22 weeks, 15%–40% at 23 weeks, 60%–75% at 25 weeks, 75%–95% at 26–28 weeks and >95% at 29–30 weeks*, whereas intact survival at 18 months is about 50% after 25 weeks [12]. Disabilities in mental and psychomotor development, neuromotor function (including cerebral palsy), or sensory and communication function are present in at least 50% of fetuses born ≤25 weeks' gestation [13].

Table 18.1 Estimated Incidences of Intra-Amniotic Infection in Women in Different Clinical Scenarios

Condition	Percent
GA <37 weeks	
Asymptomatic second trimester	0.5
PTL (intact membranes)	13
PPROM, no labor	25
PPROM, labor	39
Cervix ≥2 cm/80% in second trimester	50
GA ≥37 weeks	
Labor	19
PROM	34

Abbreviations: GA, gestational age; PPROM, preterm premature rupture of membranes; PTL, preterm labor.

Table 18.2 General Guidance Regarding Obstetric Interventions for Periviable Birth[a]

	20⁰–21⁶ Weeks	22⁰–22⁶ Weeks	23⁰–23⁶ Weeks	24⁰–24⁶ Weeks
Neonatal assessment for resuscitation	Not recommended	Consider	Consider	Recommend
Antenatal steroids	Not recommended	Not recommended	Consider	Recommend
Tocolytics to allow steroids	Not recommended	Not recommended	Consider	Recommend
Magnesium sulfate for neuroprotection	Not recommended	Not recommended	Recommended	Recommend
Antibiotics for PROM to prolong latency	Consider	Consider	Consider	Recommend
Antibiotics for GBS prophylaxis	Not recommended	Not recommended	Consider	Recommend
Continuous intrapartum electronic fetal monitoring	Not recommended	Not recommended	Consider	Recommend
Cesarean delivery for fetal indication[b]	Not recommended	Not recommended	Consider	Recommend

Source: Adapted from Rogue TN, et al., *Obstet Gynecol*, 123:1083–1096, 2014.
Abbreviation: GBS, group B streptococcus.
[a]Survival of infants born in the periviable period is dependent on resuscitation and support. Several factors (e.g., intrauterine growth restriction, small fetal size, the presence of fetal malformations or aneuploidy, and pulmonary hypoplasia due to prolonged membrane rupture) can impact the potential for survival and the determination of viability. Personal and family values should be extensively discussed, allowing individual decisions.
[b]Persistently abnormal fetal heart rate patterns or biophysical testing (category II–III), malpresentation.

Pregnancies at risk for **periviable** PTB are particularly challenging to counsel and manage. The periviability period varies according to several factors, including by level of care provided in the hospital and the country where the care is being provided. In many developed countries, this period, in 2015, is between 22 and 24 weeks. Table 18.2 provides some guidance for care, but should be adjusted according to local capabilities [13]. Patients with an intrauterine demise or undergoing pregnancy termination are not to be included in this group. For patients in whom the GA has not been clearly established, plans for intervention and information provided to the patient should be based on the best estimate of GA. Several algorithms have been developed to provide patient-specific mortality and morbidity information [14], as well as an online calculator [15]. Status can be reevaluated with each additional gestational week.

Prophylaxis to Prevent Neonatal Morbidity/Mortality from PTB (Fetal Maturation)

Corticosteroids
Betamethasone, dexamethasone (only two corticosteroids that cross the placenta reliably).

Dose: One course: Betamethasone 12 mg SQ every 24 hours × 2 doses or dexamethasone 6 mg SQ q12h × 4 doses.

Mechanism of action: Enhanced maturational changes in lung architecture and induction of lung enzymes resulting in biochemical maturation.

Evidence for effectiveness: Corticosteroids given prior to PTB (either spontaneous or indicated) are effective in preventing RDS, IVH, NEC, and neonatal mortality [16]. Antenatal administration of 24 mg of **betamethasone (12 mg intramuscularly q24h)**, or of 24 mg of **dexamethasone (6 mg intramuscularly q12h)**, to women expected to give birth preterm is associated with significant **31% reduction in neonatal mortality, 34% reduction in RDS and respiratory support, 46% reduction in IVH, 54% reduction in NEC, 20% reduction in intensive care admissions, and 44% reduction in systemic infections in the first 48 hours of life** in preterm infants. There are also decreased needs for surfactant, oxygen, and mechanical ventilation in the neonatal period. Treatment with antenatal corticosteroids does not increase risk to the mother of death, chorioamnionitis, or puerperal sepsis.

These benefits apply to **GAs of at least 24–33 6/7 weeks**, and are not limited by gender or race. There is insufficient data to assess effectiveness before or after these GAs. At 22–25 weeks, cohort studies have shown benefit in decreasing neonatal death [17]. The **effects are optimal at 48 hours to 7 days from first dose** [17], but treatment should not be withheld even if delivery appears imminent. Antenatal corticosteroids should be administered when PTB is considered imminent within seven days, the GA estimate is accurate, adequate neonatal care is available and there is no clinical evidence of maternal infection.

There is new evidence that **steroids are associated with neonatal benefits also ≥34 weeks**, as three RCTs have been done on steroids 34–36 6/7 weeks in women at risk of PTB, and two RCTs in women at ≥37 weeks [18]. Women who received antenatal corticosteroids ≥34 weeks had a significantly lower incidence of RDS (RR 0.76, 95% CI 0.62–0.93), mild RDS (RR 0.40, 95% CI 0.23–0.69), moderate RDS (RR 0.39, 95% CI 0.18–0.89), transient tachypnea of the newborn (RR 0.62, 95% CI 0.50 to 0.77), severe RDS (RR 0.66, 95% CI 0.53–0.82), use of surfactant (RR 0.61, 95% CI 0.38–0.99), mechanical ventilation (RR 0.62, 95% CI 0.41–0.94), significantly lower time on oxygen (mean difference [MD] –2.06 hours, 95% CI –2.17 to –1.95), lower maximum inspired oxygen concentration (MD –0.66%, 95% CI –0.69 to –0.63), lower LOS in NICU (MD –7.64 days, 95% CI –7.65 to –7.64), higher APGAR score at 1 and at 5 minutes (MD 0.06, 95% CI 0.05–0.07) compared with those who did not [18]. **Steroids should be considered for decreasing respiratory morbidities and other neonatal outcomes in women ≥34 weeks** [19].

Type of steroid: There is **no clear evidence of superiority between betamethasone and dexamethasone**. Based on a recent Cochrane review, dexamethasone was associated with a reduced risk of IVH compared with betamethasone (RR 0.44, 95% CI 0.21–0.92) [20]. There were no statistically significant differences in other perinatal outcomes including perinatal death, RDS, NICU admissions, however. In one study, infants exposed to dexamethasone had a significantly shorter stay in the NICU. Results for biophysical parameters were inconsistent, but no important differences were seen for these or other secondary outcomes. Indirect comparisons of betamethasone and dexamethasone suggested that betamethasone is more effective in reducing RDS risk than dexamethasone, while chorioamnionitis and puerperal sepsis was more likely with dexamethasone [20].

Oral dexamethasone significantly increased the incidence of neonatal sepsis (RR 8.48, 95% CI 1.11–64.93) compared with intramuscular dexamethasone in one trial of 183 newborns [20].

Betamethasone administered at 12-hourly compared with 24-hourly intervals has been associated with reduced maternal length of stay, but no other differences in maternal or neonatal outcomes [20].

In a recent international cluster randomized trial designed to increase the use of antenatal corticosteroid therapy in low-resource settings, involving almost 100,000 pregnant women, identification of women at risk for PTB and increased use of antenatal corticosteroids increased overall newborn mortality by 12% (RR 1.2, 95% CI 1.01–1.22), perinatal mortality by 11% (RR 1.11, 95% CI 1.04–1.19) and suspected maternal infection rate by 45% (OR 1.45, 95% CI 1.33–1.58) [21]. Possible explanations for these unexpected findings in low-resource settings include unreliable dating criteria to establish GA, the reliance on birth weight rather than estimated GA to define PTB and evaluate other important outcomes, and the coding of suspected maternal infection by treatment rather than diagnosis. Inconsistent access and limited resources to provide optimal neonatal intensive care and potential targeting of term, low birth weight infants for antepartum corticosteroid treatment may have also contributed to these results. As recently reaffirmed by the World Health Organization, the study's findings should not alter current recommendations regarding the use of antenatal corticosteroids to improve newborn outcomes [22].

Weekly repeat courses of antenatal corticosteroids: Evidence for repeating antenatal corticosteroids weekly is provided by a recent Cochrane systematic review of 10 trials (4738 women/5700 babies) [23]. Administration of repeat dose(s) to women who remained at risk for PTB seven or more days after the initial dose was associated with a reduction in the risk of RDS (RR 0.83, 95% CI 0.75–0.91) and the risk of serious neonatal adverse outcome (RR 0.84, 95% CI 0.75–0.94). In the largest international multicenter RCT, multiple repeat doses were associated with decreased birth weight, length and head circumference at birth [24]. At early childhood follow-up, no statistically significant differences were seen for infants exposed to repeat prenatal corticosteroids compared with unexposed infants for the primary outcomes (total deaths; survival free of any disability or major disability; disability; or serious outcome) or in the secondary outcome growth assessments [23].

Single repeat (rescue) course of antenatal corticosteroids: Given the potential short and long term adverse effects of multiple doses of corticosteroids, combined with the optimal benefit 7 days following administration, **timing the first course is extremely important.** A single rescue course should only be considered if PTB has not occurred within 14 days of the initial dose, and subsequent clinical assessment demonstrates a new episode of PTL or PPROM and PTB appears highly likely within 7 days [25]. **A single rescue course of betamethasone, two 12-mg dose 24 hours apart, received before 33 weeks at least 14 or more days after the first course, that was administered before 30 weeks, is associated with decreased RDS, ventilatory support, surfactant use, and composite neonatal morbidity (RR 0.65, 95% CI 0.44–0.97)** [25,26]. Given the concerns regarding multiple courses of corticosteroids, **more than two courses should be avoided.**

Contraindications: None.

Side effects: When used for only 1 course, no significant side effects are seen, except for **transient maternal hyperglycemia** from 12 hours to about 5–7 days after the dose. This effect results in false-positive glucose screening tests or difficulty in managing diabetes. There is no significant increase in maternal or fetal/neonatal infection. If ≥4 courses are used, there is an association with birth weight <10th percentile and probably with small (<10th percentile) neonatal head circumference, with evidence of later "catch-up" [23,24]. No adverse consequences of prophylactic corticosteroids for PTB in either mothers or infants, even at 10+ years follow-up, have been identified, but long-term follow-up data is limited.

Thyrotropin-Releasing Hormone

Prenatal thyrotropin-releasing hormone (TRH), in addition to corticosteroids, given to women at risk of very PTB, does not improve infant outcomes and can cause maternal side effects [27]. Overall, prenatal TRH, in addition to corticosteroids, does not reduce the risk of neonatal respiratory disease or chronic oxygen dependence, and does not improve any of the fetal, neonatal, or childhood outcomes. Prenatal TRH may actually have adverse effects for women and their infants. Side effects (nausea, vomiting, lightheadedness, urgency, flushing) are more likely to occur in women receiving TRH. Among infants, prenatal TRH increases 16% the risk of needing ventilation, 48% having a low Apgar score at 5 minutes, and was associated with poorer childhood outcomes at follow-up [24].

Phenobarbital

The use of prophylactic maternal phenobarbital administration prior to preterm delivery does not prevent periventricular hemorrhage (PVH) or protect from neurological disability in preterm infants [28]. Prenatal maternal phenobarbital is associated with a significant 35% reduction in the rates of all grades of PVH and 59% reduction in severe grades PVH (3 and 4) in the infants. The results were influenced by poor quality trials that excessively influence the analysis due to their higher rates of severe PVH. When only higher quality trials were included, phenobarbital is not associated with any beneficial effects, including similar incidences of all grades of PVH and severe grades of PVH to placebo. No difference in the incidence of neurodevelopmental abnormalities at childhood follow-up assessed between 18 and 36 months of age was observed. Maternal sedation is a common side effect in women receiving phenobarbital [28].

Vitamin K

Vitamin K administered to women prior to very PTB has not been shown to significantly prevent PVHs or other neurodevelopmental abnormalities in preterm infants. Antenatal vitamin K is associated with a nonsignificant reduction in all grades of PVH (RR 0.76, 95% CI 0.54–1.06) and a significant reduction in severe PVH (grades 3 and 4) (RR 0.58, 95% CI 0.3–0.91) [29]. When the two quasi-randomized trials are excluded, antenatal vitamin K is not associated with a reduction in all grades of PVH (RR 0.87, 95% CI 0.60–1.26) or severe PVH (RR 0.82, 95% CI 0.49–1.36). Treatment with vitamin K results in a significant reduction in the Bayley Mental Development Index at 2 years of age; but, these results are derived from one trial with a high lost to follow-up rate. No difference is found in the incidence of other neurodevelopmental abnormalities at childhood follow-up at 18–24 months or 7 years of age between children exposed to vitamin K and children not exposed [29].

Ambroxol

Giving ambroxol to women at risk of PTB to prevent neonatal RDS is not supported by available evidence. Prenatal administration of ambroxol to reduce the risk of RDS in preterm infants has not been shown to reduce the incidence of RDS or perinatal mortality when compared with betamethasone or placebo. Maternal adverse effects were similar in ambroxol and betamethasone-treated women. Since the trials included in the Cochrane systematic review were of very low to moderate quality, there is insufficient evidence to support or refute this intervention [30].

Magnesium Sulfate for Neuroprotection

Antenatal magnesium sulfate therapy given to women at risk of PTB significantly reduces the risk of cerebral palsy in their child (RR 0.68, 95% CI 0.54–0.87). There was also a significant **reduction in the rate of substantial gross motor dysfunction** (RR 0.61, 95% CI 0.44–0.85). No statistically significant effect of antenatal magnesium sulfate therapy is detected on pediatric mortality (RR 1.04, 95% CI 0.92–1.17), or on other neurological impairments or disabilities in the first few years of life. There are higher rates of minor maternal side effects in the magnesium groups, but no significant effects on major maternal complications [31].

Magnesium sulfate should be administered to women with singleton or twin pregnancies 23 0/7–31 6/7 weeks for neuroprotection when PTB is imminent. Imminent PTB is defined as a high likelihood of birth due to active labor with ≥4 cm cervical dilatation with or without PPROM or planned PTB for maternal or fetal indications. Women with an indicated PTB anticipated within 2–24 hours (e.g., for severe preeclampsia) are candidates for magnesium sulfate.

Intravenous magnesium sulfate is administered with a loading dose of 4–6 g infused for 20–30 minutes, followed by a maintenance infusion of 1–2 g/hour [22]. If delivery has not occurred after 12 hours and is no longer considered imminent (e.g., if the patient is not having regular uterine contractions), the infusion should be discontinued and resumed when delivery is deemed imminent again (e.g., when contractions develop). If at least 6 hours have passed since the discontinuation of the magnesium sulfate, another loading dose should be given. Administration of magnesium sulfate for prevention of cerebral palsy **should not delay the delivery.**

Nontocolytic Interventions for PTL

Bed Rest

Bed rest in hospital or at home in **singleton gestations** complicated by PTL or PPROM has been evaluated in one multi-intervention RCT [32]. Bed rest offered *no benefit* over no treatment or placebo in preventing PTB. In multiple pregnancies, bed rest in the hospital **did not reduce the risk of PTB or** perinatal mortality whether uncomplicated **twin pregnancy, or twin or triplet pregnancy with cervical dilatation** [33].

Hydration
There is **no benefit** of intravenous hydration in preventing PTB. Intravenous hydration does not seem to be beneficial, even during the period of evaluation soon after admission, in women with PTL. Women with evidence of dehydration may, however, benefit from the intervention. **Compared with bed rest alone, hydration is associated with similar incidences of PTB <37 weeks, <34 weeks, or <32 weeks, and of admission to neonatal intensive care unit (NICU)** [34]. Cost of treatment was slightly higher (US$39) in the hydration group for hospital costs during a visit of less than 24 hours. Women studied were at low risk, as only 30% of women required tocolysis, and <30% had PTB. No studies evaluated oral hydration [34].

Screen for Infections
Several infections are associated with a higher risk of PTL and PTB. These include chlamydia, gonorrhea, syphilis, trichomoniasis, and others, as well as bacterial vaginosis (see Chapter 17) There is **insufficient evidence** to assess the effect of screening and treating for genitourinary infections in women with PTL, as no RCTs have been performed.

Antibiotics
There is **no evidence of benefit** with the use of prophylactic antibiotic treatment for PTL with intact membranes on important neonatal outcomes [35]. PTB <36 or 37 weeks was similar in antibiotics and placebo groups. There is **a trend for a 52% increase in neonatal mortality for those who received antibiotics** (RR 1.52, 95% CI 0.99–2.34), with similar overall perinatal mortality (RR 1.22, 95% CI 0.88–1.70) [30]. The only benefit is a 26% reduction in maternal infection with the use of prophylactic antibiotics. Follow-up at 7 years of the largest RCT showed **increased incidence of functional impairment associated with erythromycin, and increased incidence of cerebral palsy associated with either antibiotic studied (erythromycin or co-amoxiclav)** [36]. Given these data, **antibiotics should not be used for prevention of PTB in women with PTL and intact membranes.**

Tocolysis

Principles
Tocolytic therapy may provide short-term prolongation of pregnancy, allowing antenatal corticosteroid administration, magnesium sulfate for neuroprotection and/or maternal transport to a tertiary care facility. There is no evidence that treatment of PTL with tocolytic agents improves perinatal outcomes, however [22]. CCB and COX inhibitors are the agents best supported by evidence of safety and effectiveness (see Table 18.3).

Contraindications
See Table 18.4.

Primary Tocolysis—Single Agent

Betamimetics
Types: Ritodrine, terbutaline.
  Dose: Ritodrine: 50–100 mg/min intravenous (IV) initial dose, increase 50 mg/min q10minute (max 350 mg/min) (orally [po]: 1–20 mg po q2–4h). Terbutaline: 0.25 mg subcutaneously (SQ) q20minute at first, then 2–3 hours; or 5–10 mg/min IV, max 80 mg/min; or 2.5–5 mg po q2–4h (hold for maternal hazards ratio [HR] >120/min).
  Mechanism of action: Stimulate B2 receptor through cyclic adenosine monophosphate (AMP), so no free calcium for myometrial contraction.

Table 18.3 Principles of Tocolytic Therapy

- *At 24–33 6/7 week, steroids for fetal maturation should always be given if tocolysis is initiated.* Tocolytics should not be used without concomitant use of steroids for fetal maturation.
- Tocolysis is typically used for 48 hours to allow steroid effect. Given side effects, consider stopping tocolytic therapy at 48 hours after steroids given if PTL under control.
- *No tocolytic agent has been shown to improve perinatal mortality.*
- There is no tocolytic agent that is more safe and efficacious. *COX inhibitors* are the only class of primary tocolytics shown to decrease PTB <37 weeks compared with placebo. COX inhibitors and *ORA* have been shown to significantly prolong pregnancy at 48 hours and 7 days compared with placebo. COX inhibitors, *CCB*, and ORA, properly used, have significantly less side effects than betamimetics. Currently, *CCB and COX inhibitors are the tocolytic agents best supported by evidence for safety and effectiveness.*
- There is no maintenance tocolytic that prevents PTB or perinatal morbidity/mortality, and therefore *maintenance tocolysis should in general not be used.* One possible exception is vaginal progesterone, with more data needed. There is insufficient evidence to evaluate multiple tocolytic agents for primary tocolysis, refractory (primary agent is failing, so another is started) tocolysis, or repeated (after successful primary tocolysis) tocolysis.

Abbreviations: CCB, calcium channel blockers; COX, cyclooxygenase; ORA, oxytocin receptor antagonists; PTB preterm birth.

Table 18.4 Contraindications to Tocolytic Therapy

Maternal
  Chorioamnionitis
  Severe vaginal bleeding/abruption
  Preeclampsia
  Medical contraindications to specific tocolytic agent
  Other maternal medical condition that makes continuing the pregnancy inadvisable
Fetal
  Death
  Major (especially if lethal) fetal anomaly or chromosome abnormality
  Other fetal conditions in which prolongation of pregnancy is inadvisable
  Documented fetal maturity

Evidence for effectiveness (Table 18.5): **Compared with placebo, betamimetics are associated with a decrease in the number of women in PTL giving birth within 48 hours** (RR 0.68, 95% CI 0.53–0.88), and *a decrease in the number of births within 7 days* (RR 0.80, 95% CI 0.65–0.98) but there was no reduction in PTB <37 weeks [37]. No benefit is demonstrated for betamimetics on perinatal or neonatal death, and on RDS. A few trials reported the following outcomes, with no difference detected: cerebral palsy, infant death, and NEC. Betamimetics are significantly associated with the following side effects (see below): **withdrawal from treatment due to adverse effects, chest pain, dyspnea, tachycardia, palpitation, tremor, headaches, hypokalemia, hyperglycemia, nausea/vomiting, nasal stuffiness, and fetal tachycardia** [34]. There is insufficient evidence to assess which of the studied betamimetics is most effective and/or associated with fewer side effects, with most data reported for ritodrine. For comparison with

Table 18.5 Summary of the Evidence for Tocolytic Therapy

Tocolytics	<48 Hours	<7 Days	<34 Weeks	<37 Weeks	Perinatal Mortality
		Primary—single agent vs. placebo			
Betamimetics	**0.68 (0.53–0.88)** (n = 1209)	0.84 (0.46–1.55) (n = 1332)	NC	0.95 (0.88–1.03) (n = 1212)	0.90 (0.27–3.00) (n = 1174)
CCB	**0.30 (0.21–0.43)** (n = 173)	NC	NC	NC	NC
COX	0.20 (0.03–1.28) (n = 70)	0.41 (0.10–1.66) (n = 70)	NC	**0.21 (0.07–0.62)** (n = 36)	0.80 (0.25–2.58) (n = 106) (NND)
Mg	0.56 (0.27–1.14) (n = 182)	NC	NC	**0.62 (0.46–0.83)** (n = 265)	4.56 (1.00–20.86) (n = 257)
ORA	1.05 (1.15–7.43) (n = 152)	**0.74 (0.61–0.91)** (n = 302)[a]	1.33 (0.84–2.14) (n = 287)[a]	1.17 (0.99–1.37) (n = 501)	2.25 (0.79–6.30) (n = 566)
NOD	1.19 (0.74–1.90) (n = 186)	NC	0.93 (0.61–1.41) (n = 153)	NC	0.43 (0.06–2.89) (n = 186) (NND)
Progesterone	NC	NC	0.62 (0.30–1.27) (n = 62)	**0.62 (0.39–0.98)** (n = 293)	0.31 (0.01–7.41) (n = 83)
		Comparisons			
CCB vs. betamimetics	0.86 (0.67–1.10) (n = 1505)	**0.76 (0.59–0.99)** (n = 242)	**0.78 (0.66–0.93)** (n = 1505)	0.89 (0.76–1.05) (n = 389)	0.80 (0.53–1.22) (n = 630)
COX vs. betamimetics	**0.27 (0.08–0.96)** (n = 100)	0.88 (0.52–1.46) (n = 146)	NC	**0.53 (0.28–0.99)** (n = 80)	0.99 (0.27–3.57) (n = 237)(NND)
COX vs. CCB	1.08 (0.59–2.01) (n = 230)	0.26 (0.52–1.46) (n = 146)	0.92 (0.70–1.21) (n = 148)	1.08 (0.94–1.25) (n = 148)	2.81 (0.82–9.62) (n = 249)(NND)
COX vs. Mg	0.87 (0.59–1.29) (n = 547)	NC	0.84 (0.64–1.11) (n = 128)	0.88 (0.52–1.47) (n = 216)	1.59 (0.59–4.29) (n = 570)
Mg vs. betamimetics	1.09 (0.72–1.65) (n = 503)	NC	NC	1.03 (0.77–1.39) (n = 473)	0.49 (0.05–5.12) (n = 263)
Mg vs. CCB	1.19 (0.86–1.65) (n = 588)	NC	0.89 (0.55–1.45) (n = 88)	1.06 (0.87–1.29) (n = 362)	0.27 (0.03–2.29) (n = 292)
Tocolytics	<48 hours	<7 days	<34 weeks	<37 weeks	Perinatal mortality
Mg vs. COX	1.08 (0.91–1.27) (n = 318)	NC	NC	NC	0.98 (0.06–15.35) (n = 117)
ORA vs. betamimetics	0.89 (0.66–1.22) (n = 1389)	0.91 (0.69–1.20) (n = 731)	NC	NC	0.55 (0.21–1.48) (n = 816)
ORA vs. CCB	1.09 (0.44–2.73) (n = 225)	NC	NC	NC	NC
NOD vs. betamimetics	0.96 (0.87–1.05) (n = 420)	1.03 (0.92–1.15) (n = 679)	0.71 (0.36–1.42) (n = 365)	0.73 (0.50–1.05) (n = 679)	2.06 (0.19–22.38) (n = 191)
NOD vs. CCB	0.97 (0.77–1.21) (n = 50)	NC	NC	NC	NC
	Maintenance therapy after treatment of PTL (vs. placebo or no treatment)				
Betamimetics	NC	NC	2.41 (0.86–6.74) (n = 681)	1.11 (0.91–1.35) (n = 644)	2.96 (0.72–12.14) (n = 467)
CCB	0.46 (0.07–3.00) (n = 128)	NC	1.07 (0.88–1.30) (n = 540)	0.97 (0.87–1.09) (n = 681)	1.48 (0.45–4.86) (n = 466)
COX	NC	NC	NC	NC	NC
Mg	NC	NC	NC	1.05 (0.80–1.40) (n = 99)	5.00 (0.25–99.16) (n = 50)
ORA	NC	NC	0.85 (0.47–1.55) (n = 285)	0.89 (0.71–1.12) (n = 510)	0.77 (0.21–2.83) (n = 512)
Progesterone					
17P	NC	NC	0.60 (0.28–1.12) (n = 233)	0.78 (0.50–1.22) (n = 293)	0.15 (0.01–2.73) (n = 233)
Vaginal	NC	NC	0.71 (0.57–0.90) (298)	0.75 (0.36–1.57) (n = 215)	0.43 (0.12–1.54 (298)

Abbreviations: NC, not calculable from the available reports; NOD, nitric oxide donors; NND, neonatal death; Mg, magnesium sulfate; Rx, therapy; excl. cong. anom, excluding congenital anomalies.
Note: Data are shown as relative risk (95% confidence intervals). Significant results are shown in bold.
[a]Data courtesy of Vincenzo Berghella.

other tocolytics, RCTs are too small and varied to make meaningful comparisons [37].

Specific contraindications: Cardiac arrhythmia or other significant cardiac disease, DM, poorly controlled thyroid disease (for ritodrine).

Side effects:
Maternal: Hyperglycemia (glucose 140–200 mg/dL in 20%–50%; mechanism: decreased peripheral insulin sensitivity and increased endogenous glucose production); hyperinsulinemia; hypokalemia (K <3 mEq/L in 50%); tremors,

nervousness, shortness of breath (10%), chest pain (5%–10%), tachycardia/palpitations, arrhythmia (3%); electrocardiogram (EKG) changes (2%–3%); hypotension (2%–3%); pulmonary edema ([<1%–5%]; mechanism: reduced sodium excretion—sodium and therefore fluid retention). Ritodrine: altered thyroid function, antidiuresis.

Fetal/Neonatal: Ritodrine: Neonatal tachycardia, hypoglycemia, hypocalcemia, hyperbilirubinemia, hypotension, IVH. Terbutaline: tachycardia, hyperinsulinemia, hyperglycemia, myocardial and septal hypertrophy, myocardial ischemia.

Calcium Channel Blockers

Types: Nifedipine, nicardipine.

Dose: Nifedipine 20–30 mg × 1, then 10–20 mg q4–8h (max 90 mg/day) (nicardipine similar dosing).

Mechanism of action: Impair calcium channels, so inhibit influx of calcium into cell, and therefore myometrial contraction.

Evidence for effectiveness (Table 18.5): Two small RCTs comparing CCB with placebo showed a **reduction in PTB <48 hours (RR 0.30, 95% CI 0.21–0.43) and an increase in maternal adverse effects**, with insufficient evidence to assess effect on PTB within 7 days, and <37 weeks [38].

When compared with other tocolytic agents [betamimetics, nonsteroidal anti-inflammatory drugs (NSAIDs), glyceryl trinitrate (GTN), magnesium sulfate, and ORAs] **CCB increased the interval from initiation of treatment to delivery, increased GA at birth and decreased preterm and very PTB. RDS, NEC, IVH, hyperbilirubinemia and admission to the NICU were also decreased** [38]. **CCB also reduced the requirement for women to have treatment ceased for adverse drug reaction.** There are insufficient data regarding the effects of different dosage regimens and formulations of CCB on maternal and neonatal outcomes; the most studied is nifedipine, at dosage shown above. **CCB should be preferred to betamimetics for tocolysis.**

Specific contraindications: Cardiac disease; hypotension (<90/50); concomitant use of magnesium; caution in renal disease.

Side effects:
Maternal: Flushing, headache, dizziness, nausea, transient hypotension. Caution in women with hypotension and renal disease, as well as women on magnesium (cardiovascular collapse).
Fetal/Neonatal: None.

COX Inhibitors

Types: Nonselective COX inhibitors: indomethacin (indocin). Selective COX inhibitors (preferential COX-2 inhibitor): sulindac, rofecoxib (Vioxx), celecoxib, nimesulide.

Dose: Indomethacin: 50–100 mg loading dose (rectal or vaginal route preferred, oral otherwise), then 25–50 mg q6h **for 48 hours max,** and **always <32 weeks.** Sulindac 200 mg po q12h × 48 hours. Ketorolac: 60 mg IM, then 30 mg IM q6h × 48 hours.

Mechanism of action: Inhibit prostaglandin synthesis, therefore inhibit myometrial contraction.

Evidence for effectiveness (Table 18.5): The nonselective COX inhibitor, indomethacin, was used in most trials. When compared with placebo, COX inhibition (indomethacin only) results in a **79% reduction in PTB <37 weeks** in a small trial, an increase in GA of 3.5 weeks and a >700 g increase in birth weight [39]. No difference was shown in birth within 48 hours of initiation of treatment (RR 0.20, 95% CI 0.03–1.28). No differences were detected in neonatal morbidity or mortality.

Compared with other betamimetics, COX inhibition resulted in a 47% reduction in PTB <37 weeks' gestation and a 73% reduction in PTB within 48h [39]. No differences detected in the fetal or neonatal outcomes such as perinatal mortality, RDS, IVH, NEC, premature closure of the ductus, persistent pulmonary hypertension of the newborn (PPHN). No differences were found when COX inhibitors were compared with magnesium sulfate or CCBS [39].

A comparison of nonselective COX inhibitors versus selective COX-2 inhibitors did not demonstrate any differences in maternal or neonatal outcomes [39]. Due to small numbers, all estimates of effect are imprecise and need to be interpreted with caution.

Specific contraindications: Renal or hepatic disease, active peptic ulcer disease, poorly controlled hypertension, NSAID-sensitive asthma, coagulation disorders/thrombocytopenia.

Side effects: When used for only 48 hours, no serious maternal and fetal/neonatal side effects occur, and fetal surveillance is not indicated. Usually COX inhibitors are better tolerated by mother than other tocolytics such as magnesium and betamimetics.

Maternal: As with any NSAIDs, mild gastrointestinal (GI) upset—nausea, heartburn (take with some food/milk) (COX-1). GI bleeding (COX-1), coagulation, and platelet abnormalities (COX-1), asthma if ASA-sensitive. May obscure elevation in temperature. Long-term rofecoxib (Vioxx) use in adults has been associated with stroke, so this drug is now not available in many countries.

Fetal/neonatal: In trials, 403 women received short-term tocolysis (up to 48 hours) with COX inhibitors (mainly indomethacin) and there was only one case of antenatal **closure of the ductus arteriosus.** There was no increase in the incidence of patent ductus arteriosus (PDA) postnatally (eight treated with COX inhibitors versus eight treated with placebo or other tocolytics) [40]. No difference in incidences of IVH, BPD, PDA, NEC, or perinatal mortality was noted in a review of trials aimed at evaluating safety [41]. Use for **>48 hours,** especially ≥32 weeks, is associated with significant fetal effects such as constriction of the ductus arteriosus, which can lead to hydrops, pulmonary hypertension and death, and **renal insufficiency,** manifested in utero by oligohydramnios. Other effects with prolonged use such as hyperbilirubinemia, NEC, IVH have not been shown with <72 use. Selective COX-2 inhibitors have not been shown consistently to be any safer for the fetus/neonate than nonselective COX inhibitors such as indomethacin. Therefore, **continuous use of COX inhibitors for >48 hours and ≥32 weeks is contraindicated.**

Magnesium Sulfate (MgSO$_4$)

Dose: 40 g MgSO$_4$ in 1 L 1/2 normal saline. Initial: 4–6 g/30 minute, then 2–4 g/hour. A dose of 5 g/hour has not been shown beneficial in perinatal outcome compared with a dose of 2 g/hour, and is associated with significant side effects [42]. Weaning MgSO$_4$ tocolysis has no benefits and a few harmful side effects compared with stopping MgSO$_4$ abruptly [43].

Mechanism of action: Intracellular calcium antagonist.

Evidence for effectiveness (Table 18.5): Compared with placebo, there is **insufficient evidence** to show if MgSO$_4$ reduces the incidence of PTB or perinatal morbidity and mortality [44].

Compared with all controls (including other tocolytics), MgSO₄ did not prevent PTB at 48 hours, PTB <37 weeks or <32 weeks. Perinatal death was higher (only two perinatal deaths), while perinatal morbidities were similar. Dose of magnesium did not affect efficacy. Given these results, there is **no convincing evidence for recommending magnesium for tocolysis** [45].

Management: Aim for 4–7 MgSO₄ level. Monitor urinary output. Follow deep tendon reflexes: ↓ at level ≥8, absent ≥10. At ≥10, respiratory depression; at ≥15, risk of cardiac arrest.

Specific contraindications: Myasthenia gravis.

Side effects:

Maternal: Flushing, lethargy, headache, muscle weakness, diplopia, dry mouth, pulmonary edema (1%; mechanism: intravenous overhydration), cardiac arrest.

Fetal/neonatal: Lethargy, hypotonia, hypocalcemia, respiratory depression. Prolonged use: demineralization.

Oxytocin Receptor Antagonists

Types: Atosiban (Tractocile); barusiban.

Dose: Atosiban 6.75 mg bolus, then 300 mg/min IV × 3 hours, then 100 mg/min (max 45 hours).

Mechanism of action: Competitive inhibitor of oxytocin via blockade of oxytocin receptor.

Evidence for effectiveness (Table 18.5): **Compared with placebo, atosiban does not reduce incidence of PTB or improve neonatal outcome** [46]. In one trial, atosiban was associated with an increase in extreme PTB <28 weeks and infant deaths at 12 months of age compared with placebo [46]. However, this trial randomized significantly more women to atosiban before 26 weeks' gestation. Compared with placebo, use of atosiban results in about 140 g lower infant birth weight and milder maternal adverse drug reactions [46]. Compared with betamimetics, atosiban is associated with similar incidences of PTB and perinatal morbidity/mortality, and with fewer maternal drug reactions requiring treatment cessation [46]. There is insufficient evidence to assess the effectiveness of a different ORA, barusiban, as only one RCT has tested it against placebo at 34–35 weeks, with no changes in recorded outcomes [47]. Therefore, **as per magnesium, the only evidence supporting use of oxytocin receptor agonists for primary tocolysis is that they have less side effects than the (effective) betamimetics.**

Side effects: Minimal to none.

Nitric Oxide Donors

Type: Nitroglycerine.

Dose: Nitroglycerine transdermal patch 0.4 mg/hour.

Mechanism of action: Direct relaxation of uterine muscle.

Evidence for effectiveness (Table 18.5): There is currently **insufficient evidence** to support the routine administration of nitric oxide donors (NOD) for prevention of PTB in women with PTL [48]. Compared with placebo, there was no evidence that NOD prolonged pregnancy beyond 48 hours or improved neonatal outcomes. When compared with other tocolytic agents (betamimetics, magnesium sulfate, CCBS or combination of tocolytics), there was no evidence that NOD perform better than other tocolytics. Nitroglycerine has been the only NOD used in trials.

Specific contraindications: NOD should not be used in women with hypotension or with preload dependent cardiac lesions, such as aortic insufficiency.

Side effects:

Maternal: NOD cause dilatation of arterial smooth muscle and commonly cause headache and may result in hypotension. Other side effects include dizziness, flushing and palpitations.

Fetal/neonatal: Although maternal hypotension could compromise utero-placental blood flow, no adverse fetal or neonatal effects have been reported.

Progesterone

There is **insufficient data** to assess the efficacy for progesterone as primary tocolysis. There are some data suggesting that progesterone may reduce PTB and increase birth weight and that progesterone may reduce uterine contractility, prolong pregnancy and attenuate cervical shortening. However, current evidence does not support a role for progesterone as a tocolytic agent [49].

Primary Tocolysis—Multiple Agents Simultaneously

Indomethacin, Ampicillin-Sulbactam, and Magnesium versus Magnesium Alone

Compared with placebos, indomethacin and ampicillin-sulbactam did not prevent PTB in women in PTL already receiving magnesium sulfate tocolysis [50].

Primary Tocolysis—Additional Agents versus One Agent Only

Progesterone versus Placebo, in Addition to Ritodrine

Compared with placebo, in women receiving ritodrine tocolysis, the addition of progesterone was not associated with a significant reduction in PTB <37 weeks (16% vs. 33% in placebo) in a very small trial [51]. In this RCT, 44 women with mostly (>90%) singleton gestations and threatened PTL at less than 35 weeks treated with ritodrine, natural progesterone 400 mg orally q6h × 24 hours (then 400 mg q8h for next 24 hours, and then 300 mg q8h onward) was associated with similar incidence of PTB, with less quantity of ritodrine administered and shorter maternal hospital stay compared with placebo [51].

Refractory Tocolysis—Primary Agent Is Failing

Indomethacin was similar to sulindac in prevention of PTB in women failing primary magnesium sulfate tocolysis in a small trial [52].

Maintenance Tocolysis—After Successful Primary Tocolysis

Betamimetics (Oral)

Dose: Ritodrine: 1–20 mg po q2–4h. Terbutaline: 2.5–5 mg po q2–4h.

Evidence for effectiveness: Compared with **placebo**, oral betamimetic therapy for maintenance tocolysis **does not prevent PTB, recurrent PTL, recurrent hospitalizations, or perinatal morbidity and mortality** [53]. Some adverse effects such as tachycardia are more frequent in the betamimetics group. Given this ample evidence from 13 trials, there is **absolutely no evidence** to support the use of oral betamimetics after PTL has resolved.

Terbutaline Pump

Dose: 0.05 mg/hour.

Evidence for effectiveness: Compared with *placebo*, terbutaline pump does not prevent PTB or improve perinatal morbidity and mortality. Side effects and costs associated with this therapy further **advice against its use** [54].

Calcium Channel Blockers
There is insufficient evidence to assess the efficacy of CCB maintenance therapy after successful tocolysis. In three small RCTs, the incidence of PTB <37 weeks was similar to placebo, or no treatment [55].

COX Inhibitors
Compared with **placebo,** after successful tocolysis, oral sulindac either 200 mg q12h × 7 days or 100 mg q12h until 34 weeks does not reduce PTB compared with placebo [56]. Given the association with fetal/neonatal complications with COX inhibitor use for >48 hours, COX inhibitors should not be used for maintenance tocolysis.

Compared with oral **terbutaline,** oral indomethacin is associated with a similar incidence of PTB when used for maintenance tocolysis after successful IV tocolysis, but indomethacin is associated with significant constriction of ductus arteriosus and oligohydramnios when used for >48 hours [57]. Therefore, indomethacin should not be used for maintenance tocolysis, especially after 26 weeks.

Magnesium Sulfate
Compared with **placebo,** or **no treatment,** magnesium maintenance therapy **does not prevent PTB** (RR 1.05, 95% CI 0.80–1.40) **or affect perinatal morbidity and mortality** (mortality, RR 5.00, 95% CI 0.25–99.16) [58]. It has also similar effect on PTB as alternative tocolytic drugs (RR 0.99, 95% CI 0.57–1.72) (i.e., it is equally ineffective). Therefore, magnesium sulfate should not be used as a maintenance tocolytic.

Oxytocin Receptor Antagonists
Compared with **placebo,** ORA (atosiban) maintenance therapy (30 µg/min) via pump up to 36 weeks does not prevent PTB or affect perinatal morbidity and mortality, with a 5 days (32.6 vs. 27.6, p = .02) longer interval to delivery in one trial [59]. There are no side effects compared with placebo except for injection-site reactions. ORA are not available in oral form for maintenance.

Progesterone
Women with a singleton gestation who received **17P maintenance tocolysis** for arrested PTL had a **similar rate of PTB** <37 weeks (42% vs. 51%; RR 0.78; 95% CI 0.50–1.22) and PTB <34 weeks (25% vs. 34%; RR 0.60; 95% CI 0.28–1.12) compared with controls [62,63]. Women who received 17P had significantly later GA at delivery (MD 2.28 weeks; 95% CI 1.46–13.51), longer latency (MD 8.36 days; 95% CI, 3.20–13.51), and higher birth weight (MD 224 g; 95% CI, 71–378) as compared with controls. As 17P for maintenance tocolysis is associated with a significant prolongation of pregnancy, and significantly higher birth weight [60,61], further research is suggested.

Maintenance tocolysis with **vaginal progesterone** for arrested PTL is associated with a **significantly lower rate of PTB** <37 weeks (42% vs. 58%; RR 0.71; 95% CI 0.57–0.90), significantly longer latency (MD 14 days), later GA at delivery (MD 1.3 weeks), lower rate of recurrent PTL (24% vs. 46%; RR 0.51; 95% CI 0.31–0.84), and lower rate of neonatal sepsis (2% vs. 7%; RR 0.34; 95% CI 0.12–0.98) compared with placebo or no treatment [62]. However, due to the poor quality of the trials, maintenance therapy with vaginal progesterone should be studied further before a strong recommendation can be made.

In summary, **there is insufficient evidence to recommend progesterone for prevention of PTB in women who remain pregnant after an episode of PTL, but recent evidence about vaginal progesterone for maintenance tocolysis is encouraging.**

PTL RESOLVED: HOME VERSUS IN-HOSPITAL CARE

After PTL has resolved (and cervical dilatation has not progressed ≥4 cm), **home management is associated with similar incidences of reaching ≥36 weeks compared with hospital management** [63,64]. Hospitalization may increase maternal stress, vaginal examinations, time in recumbent position (and its consequences), and decreased plasma volume. **For the many women with arrested PTL, continued hospitalization after steroids administration is unnecessary.** Women sent home with a diagnosis of false PTL are not at increased risk for early (<34 weeks) PTB or neonatal mortality, but they are at risk for later (≥34 weeks) PTB [1].

PRECONCEPTION COUNSELING

Given its major impact of perinatal morbidity and mortality, it is important to **review risk factors for PTB in every pregnant woman.** In the woman with a risk factor (e.g., prior PTB), it is important to review prognosis, possible complications, and management of a future pregnancy (see above).

PRENATAL CARE

Preconception counseling as above, if not already done. Management should follow recommendations as above (Table 18.3) (see also Chapter 2).

ANTEPARTUM TESTING

No specific fetal testing is indicated. Home uterine activity monitoring (HUAM), discussed in Chapter 17, is not effective in preventing any complication.

MODE OF DELIVERY

There is **insufficient evidence** to evaluate the use of a policy for uniform planned cesarean delivery (CD) compared with expectant management and selective CD for preterm (24–36 weeks) infants [65]. Mothers in the planned CD group had more morbidity. There was no significant difference between planned CD and expectant management in perinatal morbidity or mortality or in abnormal childhood follow-up. Differentiation of data between breech and vertex presentations is difficult, with numbers too small for definite conclusions.

Delayed Cord Clamping

In preterm neonates, delayed cord clamping by about 30–60 seconds (120 maximum) is associated with **fewer transfusions for anemia, less hypotension, and less IVH** than early clamping at less than 30 seconds [66].

Milking of cord has been evaluated in two small RCTs in preterm neonates, so there is insufficient evidence for recommendation, even if it appears as beneficial as delayed cord clamping. Compared with no milking, milking of cord has been associated with less need for blood transfusions and less need for circulatory and respiratory support [67]. Compared with 30-second delayed cord clamping, milking of cord four times achieved a similar amount of placento-fetal blood transfusion [68].

ANALGESIA/ANESTHESIA

No specific changes from term intrapartum management (see Chapter 11).

POSTPARTUM/BREAST-FEEDING/COUNSELING

As in other pregnancies, breast-feeding is encouraged as tolerated for the preterm infant. Milk expression using breast pump is also encouraged. Extensive counseling should be provided regarding rate of recurrence of PTB, and future management in pregnancy. Treatment with antibiotics before pregnancy does not prevent recurrent PTB. **In women with a prior spontaneous PTB <34 weeks, oral azythromycin and metronidazole every 4 months after the PTB and before the next conception does not significantly reduce subsequent PTB** [69]. Vaginal and IM progesterone has been shown to reduce the risk of recurrent PTB and adverse perinatal outcomes in women with a history of spontaneous singleton PTB. Following spontaneous singleton PTB, women should be counseled about the benefits of progesterone prophylaxis in subsequent pregnancies [70] (see also Chapter 17).

REFERENCES

1. Chao TT, Bloom SL, Mitchell JS, et al. The diagnosis and natural history of false preterm labor. *Obstet Gynecol*. 2011;118:1301. [II-2]
2. Pereira L, Gould R, Pelham J, et al. Correlation between visual examination of the cervix and digital examination. *J Matern Fetal Neonatal Med*. 2005;17:223–227. [II-2].
3. Melamed N, Hiersch L, Dommiz N, et al. Predictive value of cervical length in women with threatened preterm labor. *Obstet Gynecol*. 2013;122:1279. [II-1]
4. Van Baaren GJ, Vis JY, Wilms FF, et al. Predictive value of cervical length measurement and fetal fibronectin testing in threatened preterm labor. *Obstet Gynecol*. 2014;123:1185. [II-1]
5. Berghella V, Baxter JK, Hendrix NW. Cervical assessment by ultrasound for preventing preterm delivery. *Cochrane Database of Syst Rev*. 2013;(1):CD007235. [Meta-analysis: 3 RCTs, n = 290].
6. Deshpande SN, van Asselt AD, Tomini F, et al. Rapid fetal fibronectin testing to predict preterm birth in women with symptoms of premature labour: A systematic review and cost analysis. *Health Technol Assess*. 2013;17:1. [Review]
7. Berghella V, Hayes E, Visintine J, et al. Fetal fibronectin testing for reducing the risk of preterm birth. *Cochrane Database of Syst Rev*. 2008;(4):CD006843. [Meta-analysis: 5 RCTs, n = 474].
8. Ness A, Visintine J, Ricci E, et al. Does knowledge of cervical length and fetal fibronectin affect management of women with preterm labor? A randomized trial. *Am J Obstet Gynecol*. 2007;197(4):426.el–426.e7. [RCT]
9. American College of Obstetricians and Gynecologists. *ACOG Practice Bulletin No. 127: Management of Preterm Labor*. Washington, DC: ACOG, 2012. [Review]
10. Gomez R, Romero R, Nien JK, et al. A short cervix in women with preterm labor and intact membranes: A risk factor for microbial invasion of the amniotic cavity. *Am J Obstet Gynecol*. 2005;192:678–689. [II-3]
11. Stoll BJ, Hansen NI, Bell EF, et al. Trends in care practices, morbidity, and mortality of extremely preterm neonates, 1993–2012. *JAMA*. 2015;314:1039–1051. [II-2]
12. National Center for Health Statistics. *National Vital Statistics System*. Available at: http://www.cdc.gov/nchs/nvss.htm. Accessed February 16, 2016. [Epidemiologic data]
13. Rogue TN, Mercer BM, Burchfield DJ, Jospeh GF. Previable birth: Executive summary of a joint workshop by the Eunice Kennedy Shriver National Institute of Child Health and Human Development, Society of Maternal Fetal Medicine, American Academy of Pediatrics, and American College of Obstetricians and Gynecologists. *Obstet Gynecol*. 2014;123:1083–1096. [Guideline]
14. Vincer MJ, Armson BA, Allen VM, et al. An algorithm for predicting neonatal mortality in threatened very preterm birth. *J Obstet Gynaecol Can*. 2015;37(11):958–965. [Algorithm; II-3]
15. *NICHD Neonatal Research Network (NRN): Extremely Preterm Birth Outcome Data*. Available at: https://www.nichd.nih.gov/about/org/der/branches/ppb/programs/epbo/pages/epbo_case.aspx. Accessed November 30, 2012. [Calculator on Website]
16. Roberts D, Dalziel SR. Antenatal corticosteroids for accelerating fetal lung maturation for women at risk of preterm birth. *Cochrane Database Syst Rev*. 2006;(3):CD004454. [Meta-analysis: 18 RCTs, n >3885]
17. Melamed N, Shah J, Soraisham A, et al. Association between antenatal corticosteroids administration-to-birth interval and outcomes for preterm neonates. *Obstet Gynecol*. 2015;125:1377–1384. [II-1]
18. Saccone G, Berghella V. Antenatal corticosteroids for term or near-term fetal maturity: A systematic review and meta-analysis of randomized controlled trials. *BMJ*. 2016;355:i5044. [Meta-analysis: 6 RCTs, n = 5,698].
19. Ahmed MR, Sayed Ahmed WA, Mohammed TY. Antenatal steroids at 37 weeks, does it reduce neonatal respiratory morbidity? A randomized trial. *J Matern Fetal Neonatal Med*. 2015;28(12):1486–1490. Epub 2014 Sep 22. [RCT]
20. Brownfoot FC, Gagliardi DI, Bain E, et al. Different corticosteroids and regimens for accelerating fetal lung maturation for women at risk of preterm birth. *Cochrane Database Syst Rev*. 2013;(8):CD006764. [Meta-analysis: 12 RCTs, n = 1557]
21. Althabe F, Belizán JM, McClure EM, et al. A population-based, multifaceted strategy to implement antenatal corticosteroid treatment versus standard care for the reduction of neonatal mortality due to preterm birth in low-income and middle-income countries: The ACT cluster-randomised trial. *Lancet*. 2015;385:629–639. [RCT]
22. World Health Organization. *WHO Recommendations on Interventions to Improve Preterm Birth Outcomes*. Geneva, Switzerland: World Health Organization, 2015. Available at: http://www.who.int/reproductivehealth/publications/maternal_perinatal_health/preterm-birth-guideline/en/. [Guideline]
23. Crowther CA, McKinlay CJD, Middleton P, et al. Repeat doses of prenatal corticosteroids for women at risk of preterm birth for improving neonatal health outcomes. *Cochrane Database Syst Rev*. 2015;(7):CD003935. [Meta-analysis: 10 RCTs, n = 4730]
24. Murphy KE, Hannah ME, Willan AR, et al. Multiple courses of antenatal corticosteroids for preterm birth (MACS): A randomized controlled trial. *Lancet*. 2008;372:2143–2151. [RCT, n = 1858]
25. Garite TJ, Kurtzman J, Maurel K, et al. Impact of a 'rescue course' of antenatal corticosteroids: A multicenter randomized placebo-controlled trial. *Am J Obstet Gynecol*. 2009;200:248. [RCT, n = 437]
26. McEvoy C, Schilling D, Peters D, et al. Respiratory compliance in preterm infants after a single rescue course of antenatal steroids: A randomized controlled trial. *Am J Obstet Gynecol*. 2010;202:544. [RCT, n = 44]
27. Crowther CA, Alfirevic Z, Han S, Haslam RR. Thyrotropin-releasing hormone added to corticosteroids for women at risk of preterm birth for preventing neonatal respiratory disease. *Cochrane Database Syst Rev*. 2013;(11):CD00019. [Meta-analysis: 13 RCTs, n = >4600].
28. Crowther CA, Henderson-Smart DJ. Phenobarbital prior to preterm birth for preventing neonatal periventricular haemorrhage. *Cochrane Database Syst Rev*. 2010;(1):CD000164. [Meta-analysis: 9 RCTs, n = 1750]
29. Crowther CA, Crosby DD. Vitamin K prior to preterm birth for preventing neonatal periventricular haemorrhage. *Cochrane Database Syst Rev*. 2010;(1):CD000229. [Meta-analysis: 8 RCTs, n = 843]
30. Gonzalez Garay AG, Reveiz L, Velasco Hidalgo L, Solis Galicia C. Ambroxol for women at risk of preterm birth for preventing

31. Doyle LW, Crowther CA, Middleton P, et al. Magnesium sulphate for women at risk of preterm birth for neuroprotection of the fetus. *Cochrane Database Syst Rev.* 2009;(1):CD004661. [Meta-analysis: 5 RCTs, $n = 6145$]
    neonatal respiratory distress syndrome. *Cochrane Database Syst Rev.* 2014;(10):CD009708. (Meta-analysis 14 RCTs, n = 1047]
32. Sosa CG, Althabe F, Belizán JM, Bergel E. Bed rest in singleton pregnancies for preventing preterm birth. *Cochrane Database Syst Rev.* 2015;(3):CD003581. [Meta-analysis: 1 RCT, $n = 1266$]
33. Crowther CA, Neilson JP, Verkuyl DAA, et al. Preterm labour in twin pregnancies: Can it be prevented by hospital admission? *BJOG.* 1989;96:850–853. [RCT, $n = 139$]
34. Stan C, Boulvain M, Hirsbrunner-Amagbaly P, et al. Hydration for treatment of preterm labour. *Cochrane Database Syst Rev.* 2013;(11):CD003096. [2 RCTs, $n = 228$]
35. Flenady V, Hawley G, Stock OM, et al. Prophylactic antibiotics for inhibiting preterm labour with intact membranes. *Cochrane Database Syst Rev.* 2013;(12):CD000246. [14 RCTs, $n = 7437$]
36. Kenyon S, Pike K, Jones DR, et al. Childhood outcomes after prescription of antibiotics to pregnant women with spontaneous preterm labor: 7-Year follow-up of the ORACLE II trial. *Lancet.* 2008;372:1319–1327. [RCT, $n = 3196$]
37. Neilson JP, West HM, Dowswell T, et al. Betamimetics for inhibiting preterm labour. *Cochrane Database Syst Rev.* 2014;(2):CD004352. [Meta-analysis: 20 RCTs, $n = 2655$]
38. Flenady VJ, Wojcieszek AM, Papatsonis DNM, et al. Calcium channel blockers for inhibiting preterm labour. *Cochrane Database Syst Rev.* 2014;(6):CD002255. [Meta-analysis: 38 RCTs, $n = 3550$]
39. Reinebrant HE, Pileggo-Castro C, Romero CLT, et al. Cyclooxygenase (COX) inhibitors for treating preterm labour. *Cochrane Database Syst Rev.* 2015;(6):CD001992. [Meta-analysis: 20 RCTs, $n = 1509$]
40. Sawdy RJ, Lye S, Fisk NM, et al. A double-blind randomized study of fetal side effects during and after the short-term maternal administration of indomethacin, sulindac, and nimesulide for the treatment of preterm labor. *Am J Obstet Gynecol.* 2003;188:1046–1051. [RCT, n = 30. Sulindac 200 mg orally and a placebo suppository every 12 hours; vs. nimesulide 200 mg rectally and a placebo capsule orally every 12 hours; vs. indomethacin 100 mg rectally and a placebo capsule orally every 12 hours]
41. Loe SM, Sanchez-Ramos L, Kaunitz A. Assessing the neonatal safety of indomethacon tocolysis: A systematic review with meta-analysis. *Obstet Gynecol.* 2005;106:173–179. [Meta-analysis of safety of indomethacin: $n = 1621$ fetuses exposed to indomethacin in RCTs and observational studies]
42. Terrone DA, Rinehart BK, Kimmel ES, et al. A prospective randomized controlled trial of high and low maintenance doses of magnesium sulfate for acute tocolysis. *Am J Obstet Gynecol.* 2000;182:1477–1482. [RCT, n = 160. All pts: MgSO4 4-g load, then RCT to 2 g vs. 5 g/hr]
43. Lewis DF, Bergstedt S, Edwards MS, et al. Successful magnesium sulfate tocolysis: Is "weaning" the drug necessary? *Am J Obstet Gynecol.* 1997;177:742–745. [RCT, n = 140. Stop MgSO4 abruptly vs. wean approx. 1 g q4h]
44. Crowther CA, Brown J, McKinlay CJ, et al. Magnesium sulfate for preventing preterm birth in threatened preterm labour. *Cochrane Database Syst Rev.* 2014;(8):CD001060. [Meta-analysis: 237 RCTs, $n = 3571$]
45. Mercer BM, Merlino AA, SMFM. Magnesium sulfate for preterm labor and preterm birth. *Obstet Gynecol.* 2009;114:650668. [Meta-analysis: 19 RCTs]
46. Flenady V, Reinebrant HE, Liley HG, et al. Oxytocin receptor antagonists for inhibiting preterm labour. *Cochrane Database Syst Rev.* 2014;(6):CD004452. [14 RCTs, $n = 2485$]
47. Thornton S, Goodwin TM, Greisen G, et al. The effect of barusiban, a selective oxytocin antagonist, in threatened preterm labor at late gestational age: A randomized, double-blind, placebo-controlled trial. *Am J Obstet Gynecol.* 2009;200:627. [RCT, $n = 163$]
48. Durckitt K, Thornton S, O'Donovan OP, et al. Nitric oxide donors for the treatment of preterm labour. *Cochrane Database Syst Rev.* 2014;(5):CD002860. [Meta-analysis: 12 RCTs, $n = 1227$]
49. Su LL, Samuel M, Chong YS. Progestational agents for treating threatened or established preterm labour. *Cochrane Database Syst Rev.* 2014;(1):CD006770. [7 RCTs, $n = 5387$]
50. Newton ER, Shields L, Rigway LE, et al. Combination antibiotics and indomethacin in idiopathic preterm labor: A randomized double-blind study. *Am J Obstet Gynecol.* 1991;165:1753–1759. [RCT, $n = 86$]
51. Noblot G, Audra P, Dargent D, et al. The use of micronized progesterone in the treatment of menace of preterm delivery. *Eur J Obstet Gynecol Reprod Biol.* 1991;40:203–209. [RCT, $n = 40$ singletons]
52. Carlan S, O'Brien WF, O'Leary TD, et al. Randomized comparative trial of indomethacin and sulindac for the treatment of refractory preterm labor. *Obstet Gynecol.* 1992;79:223–228. [RCT, $n = 36$]
53. Dodd JM, Crowther CA, Middleton P, et al. Oral betamimetics for maintenance therapy after threatened preterm labour. *Cochrane Database Syst Rev.* 2012;(12):CD003927. [Meta-analysis: 13 RCTs, $n = 1551$]
54. Chawanpaiboon S, Laopaiboon M, Lumbiganon P, et al. Terbutaline pump maintenance therapy after threatened preterm labour for reducing adverse neonatal outcomes. *Cochrane Database Syst Rev.* 2014;(3):CD010800. [Meta-analysis: 2 RCTs, $n = 94$]
55. Naik Gaunekar N, Raman P, Bain E, et al. Maintenance therapy with calcium channel blockers for preventing preterm birth after threatened preterm labour. *Cochrane Database Syst Rev.* 2013;(10):CD004071. [Meta-analysis]
56. Humprey RG, Bartfield MC, Carlan SJ, et al. Sulindac to prevent recurrent preterm labor: A randomized controlled trial. *Obstet Gynecol.* 2001;98:555–562. [RCT, $n = 95$. Sulindac 100 mg until 34 w vs. placebo]
57. Bivins HA, Newman RB, Fyfe DA, et al. Randomized trial of oral indomethacin and terbutaline for the long-term suppression of preterm labor. *Am J Obstet Gynecol.* 1993;169:1065–1070. [RCT, $n = 71$]
58. Han S, Crowther CA, Moore V. Magnesium maintenance therapy for preventing preterm birth after threatened preterm labour. *Cochrane Database Syst Rev.* 2013;(5):CD000940. [4 RCTs, $n = 422$]
59. Papatsonis DN, Flenady V, Liley HG. Maintenance therapy with oxytocin antagonists for inhibiting preterm birth after threatened preterm labour. *Cochrane Database Syst Rev.* 2013;(10):CD005938. [Meta-analysis: 1 RCT, $n = 512$]
60. Saccone G, Suhag A, Berghella V. 17-alpha-hydroxyprogesterone caproate for maintenance tocolysis: A systematic review and metaanalysis of randomized trials. *Am J Obstet Gynecol.* 2015;213(1):16–22. [Meta-analysis: 5 RCTs, $n = 426$]
61. Facchinetti F, Paganelli S, Comitini G, et al. Cervical length changes during preterm cervical ripening: Effects of 17-alpha-hydroxyprogesterone caproate. *Am J Obstet Gynecol.* 2007;196:453. [RCT, $n = 60$]
62. Suhag A, Saccone G, Berghella V. Vaginal progesterone for maintenance tocolysis: A systematic review and meta-analysis of randomized trials. *Am J Obstet Gynecol.* 2015;213(4):479–87. doi: 10.1016/j.ajog.2015.03.031. Epub 2015 Mar 19. [Meta-analysis: 5 trials, $n = 441$].
63. Yost NP, Bloom SL, McIntire DD, et al. Hospitalization for women with arrested preterm labor. *Obstet Gynecol.* 2005;106:14–18. [RCT, $n = 101$]
64. Goulet C, Gevry H, Lemay M, et al. A randomized clinical trial of care for women with preterm labour: Home management versus hospital management. *CMAJ.* 2001;164:985–991. [RCT, $n = 250$]
65. Alfirevic Z, Milan SJ, Livio S. Caesarean section versus vaginal delivery for preterm birth in singletons. *Cochrane Database Syst Rev.* 2013;(9):CD000078. [Meta-analysis: 4 RCTs, $n = 116$]

66. Rabe H, Diaz-Rossello JL, Duley L, et al. Effect of timing of umbilical cord clamping and other strategies to influence placental transfusion at preterm birth on maternal and infant outcomes. *Cochrane Database Syst Rev.* 2012;(8):CD003248. [7 RCTs, $n = 297$. All are small trials]
67. Hosono S, Mugishima H, Fijita H, et al. Umbilical cord milking reduces the need for red blood cell transfusions and improves neonatal adaptation in infants born at less than 29 weeks' gestation: A randomized controlled trial. *Arch Dis Child Fetal Neonatal Ed.* 2008;93:F14–F19. [RCT, $n = 40$]
68. Rabe H, Jewison A, Alvarez RF, et al. Milking compared to delayed cord clamping to increase placental transfusion in preterm neonates. *Obstet Gynecol.* 2011;117:205–211. [RCT, $n = 58$]
69. Andrews WW, Goldenberg RL, Hauth JC, et al. Interconceptional antibiotics to prevent spontaneous preterm birth: A randomized clinical trial. *Am J Obstet Gynecol.* 2006;194:617–623. [RCT, $n = 241$]
70. Dodd JM, Jones L, Flenady V, et al. Prenatal administration of progesterone for preventing preterm birth in women considered to be at risk of preterm birth. *Cochrane Database Syst Rev.* 2013;(7):CD004947. [Meta-analysis: 36 RCTs, $n = 8523$]

Preterm premature rupture of membranes

Anna Locatelli and Sara Consonni

KEY POINTS

- Definite diagnosis is by direct visualization of fluid (**pooling**), with **nitrazine** cervicovaginal swab and **ferning** as usual confirmatory tests. In dubious cases, additional biochemical tests may aid in the diagnosis.
- **Complications** of preterm premature rupture of membranes (PPROM) include **premature labor/delivery** with related complications of prematurity such as **respiratory distress syndrome (RDS), intraventricular hemorrhage (IVH) and periventricular leukomalacia (PVL), infection and necrotizing enterocolitis (NEC)**; maternal or neonatal infections **(chorioamnionitis, endometritis, and sepsis); abruptio placentae, cord prolapse**, and, especially for PPROM <24 weeks, **perinatal death, pulmonary hypoplasia (PH), compression deformities, long-term infant morbidities, increased need for cesarean delivery (CD)**, and **retained placenta**.
- **Corticosteroids** should be administered in women with PPROM at 23 0/7–33 6/7 weeks, as this intervention is associated with **lower** incidences of **RDS, IVH, NEC**, and a trend for a lower **neonatal death rate.**
- **Antibiotics** (in particular **ampicillin and erythromycin** or **erythromycin alone**) are associated with less **chorioamnionitis, preterm birth (PTB) within 48 hours, PTB within 7 days, neonatal infection, surfactant use, oxygen therapy,** and **abnormal cerebral ultrasound scan** (including IVH). **RDS** and **NEC** are also decreased with ampicillin and erythromycin treatment.
- **Tocolytic therapy in women with PPROM is not associated with maternal or perinatal benefits** and should, in general, be avoided.
- **Expectant management of PPROM in women with cerclage in place is associated with increased maternal and fetal/neonatal infection risks. Therefore, the cerclage should, in general, be removed when the diagnosis of PPROM is made.** At maximum, cerclage might be left in place for about 48 hours to allow steroid therapy.
- **Before 34 weeks**, conservative management of PPROM is usually indicated, if possible. **Delivery is indicated for NRFHT, preterm labor (PTL), chorioamnionitis, or ≥34 weeks** (Figure 19.1). In women with PPROM between 34 and 36 6/7 weeks, in the absence of overt signs of infection or fetal compromise, a policy of cautious expectant management can be considered.
- There are no strong published data to assess the benefit of interventions for PPROM <23 weeks. Series have reported live birth rates from 20% to 90% associated with expectant management, with high rates of perinatal morbidity.
- The management of PPROM in twin pregnancies should not differ from that of singletons.

DEFINITION

PPROM refers to chorioamniotic membrane rupture before the onset of labor in pregnancies at <37 weeks of gestation.

DIAGNOSIS

Definite diagnosis is by direct visualization of fluid (**pooling**) in the posterior vaginal fornix at sterile speculum examination. History of persistent leakage of fluid and ultrasonographic diagnosis of oligohydramnios are two other confirmatory but not diagnostic findings. Statistical measures (sensitivity, specificity, positive predictive value, negative predictive value) of the main PROM diagnostic tests are reported in Table 19.1 [1–5].

Traditional confirmatory tests:

- **Nitrazine test:** Evaluation of vaginal pH by a cervical–vaginal swab collected in a sterile way from the posterior vaginal fornix. Vaginal pH generally varies from 4.5 to 6. In presence of amniotic fluid it becomes >7. A nitrazine paper veers from yellow to blue if pH is >7. False positive results in presence of blood, seminal fluid, alkaline antiseptics, cervical–vaginal infections or alkaline urines. False negative results in case of prolonged rupture of membranes.
- **Ferning test:** The presence of arborization on a slide of amniotic fluid collected in a sterile way from posterior vaginal fornix. Arborization represents the crystallization of amniotic fluid due to its high contents of salts and proteins. False positive results for contamination by cervical–vaginal mucus, seminal fluid, fingerprints, and urine crystals. False negative results for blood or meconium contamination or inadequacy in slide preparation.

Main biochemical tests:

- **Placental alpha-microglobulin test** (AmniSure™): Placental alpha-microglobulin-1 (PAMG-1) is a glycoprotein of amniotic fluid (2,000–25,000 ng/mL); it can be detected also in lower concentrations in maternal blood (5–25 ng/mL) and in cervical–vaginal secretions (0.05–0.2 ng/mL) if fetal membranes are intact. PAMG-1 is a good marker for PROM diagnosis due to this different concentration between amniotic fluid and cervical–vaginal secretions. PAMG-1 is dosed by an immune-chromatographic test able to detect also little concentrations of this glycoprotein in cervical–vaginal secretions (Amnisure™ PROM test). It is an easy, rapid (5–10 minutes), noninvasive test (speculum examination is not necessary). This test can be performed from 11 to 42 weeks of pregnancy. The result is not influenced by the presence of seminal fluid, urine, blood or vaginal infections.
- **Insulin-like growth factor binding protein (IGFBP)-1 (PROM test):** Immune-chromatographic test that detects amniotic fluid in the vaginal secretions. Monoclonal antibodies identify IGFBP-1, whose concentration is elevated

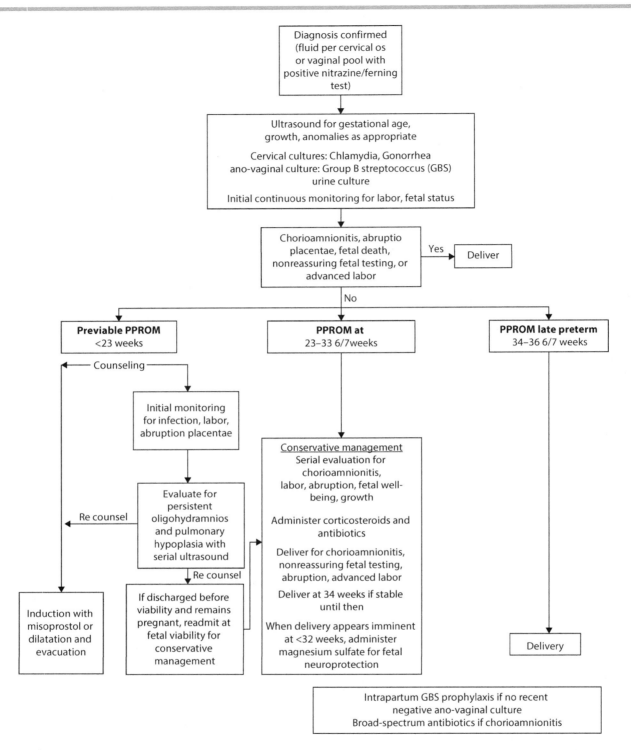

Figure 19.1 Management of preterm premature rupture of membrane (PPROM). (Adapted from Blumenfeld YJ et al., *Obstet Gynecol*, 116, 1381–1386, 2010.)

in amniotic fluid (IGFBP-1 ≥10 μg/L: positive test). Actim™ PROM test is easy and rapid. The result is not influenced by the presence of urine or seminal fluid, while it can be altered by contamination with blood.
- **Diagnostic panty liner with polymer-embedded strip**: A pad with a reactive strip put in contact with external genitalia detects the presence of amniotic fluid.

- **Fetal fibronectin**: This test is sensitive but not specific for PROM: a negative result suggests the absence of PROM with high accuracy, while a positive result is not diagnostic for PROM. Fetal fibronectin test is not recommended in case of PROM.

Transabdominal amnioinfusion of dye (indigo carmine, Evans blue, fluorescein) can be used as a confirmatory test in

Table 19.1 Predictive Accuracy of PROM Diagnostic Tests

	Sensitivity (%)	Specificity (%)	Positive Predictive Value (%)	Negative Predictive Value (%)
Nitrazine test	85	39.7	49.3	79.3
Ferning test	84	78.7	79.7	83.1
Placental alpha microglobulin test (AmniSure)	92.7	100	100	95.2
Insulin-like growth factor binding protein-1 (PROM test)	87.5	94.4	92.1	91.1
Diagnostic panty liner	95.4	80	82.4	94.7
Fetal fibronectin	94.5	89.1	89.7	94.2

Sources: Adapted from Abdelazim IA et al., *Arch Gynecol. Obstet*, 290, 457–464, 2014; Tagore S and Kwek K, *J Perinat Med*, 38, 609–612, 2010; Abdelazim IA, *J Obstet Gynaecol Res*, 40, 961–967, 2014; Bornstein J et al., *Am J Perinatol*, 26, 45–50, 2009; Ramsauer B et al., *J Perinatol Med*, 41, 233–240, 2013.
Abbreviation: PROM, premature rupture of membrane.

doubtful cases at low gestational ages (GAs). Methylene blue must be avoided as it can cause fetal meta-hemoglobinemia [6,7].

SYMPTOMS

Over 90% of women with PPROM report a history of "gush of fluid."

INCIDENCE

PPROM occurs in <1% at <24 weeks, and about 1%–3% at 24–33 weeks, 3%–5% at 34–36 weeks compared with about 8%–10% for PROM at term. PPROM is associated with about 25%–30% of all PTBs.

ETIOLOGY/BASIC PATHOPHYSIOLOGXY

Etiology is complex and multifactorial (see Chapter 17). Possible mechanisms leading to PPROM are choriodecidual infection, collagen degradation, decreased membrane collagen content, localized membrane defects, uterine overdistention, and programmed amniotic cell death [8]. Evidence that supports a causal association between PPROM and infection is vast and includes the fact that microorganisms in the amniotic fluid are more frequently present and the rate of histological chorioamnionitis is higher in PPROM than in intact membranes preterm delivery and the frequency of PPROM is significantly higher in women with lower genital tract infections (e.g., group B streptococcus [GBS] and bacterial vaginosis). Microorganisms that colonize the lower genital tract produce phospholipases, which can stimulate the production of prostaglandins and lead to uterine contractions; the immune response in endocervix and/or fetal membranes leads to the production of multiple inflammatory mediators (particularly matrix metalloproteinases) that can weaken membranes and result in PPROM [9]. Invasive uterine procedures performed during pregnancy (such as amniocentesis, chorionic villus sampling, fetoscopy, and cervical cerclage) can damage the membranes, causing them to leak.

CLASSIFICATION

PPROM can be classified into **PPROM <23 weeks** (usually 16–22 6/7 weeks, and called also previable or midtrimester or very early PPROM—see also the section "PPROM <23 WEEKS") and PPROM at 23 0/7–36 6/7 weeks. PPROM at 23–36 weeks can be further subdivided into **PPROM at 23–33 6/7 weeks** (early PPROM) and **PPROM at 34–36 6/7 weeks** (late preterm PPROM—for management, see also Chapter 20).

RISK FACTORS

Main risk factors for spontaneous PPROM are listed in Table 19.2 [10]. However, most cases of preterm PROM occur in otherwise healthy women without identifiable risk factors. See also Chapter 17.

COMPLICATIONS

Complications are inversely correlated with GA at PPROM and at delivery.

- **PTL/delivery:** In 50% of PPROM, labor occurs within 24 hours, and in 80%–90% within 7 days. Median latency to delivery after PPROM is similar from 24 to 28 weeks' gestation (about 9 days), and shortens with PPROM ≥29 weeks [11]. The latency with PPROM >30 weeks is usually only 2–4 days. **Preterm delivery** and complications of prematurity are the most important causes of **perinatal mortality** and morbidity; complications decrease with advancing GA. Infective/inflammatory factors involved in PPROM etiopathogenesis may enhance the risk of fetal white matter damage [12].
- Most common neonatal morbidities are *RDS, IVH, PVL, and NEC*.
- **Infections: Mother** is at risk of **chorioamnionitis, endometritis, and sepsis**. Serious maternal consequences are uncommon. Mean incidence of chorioamnionitis is about 3%–15%. Major **neonatal infections** occur in 5% of PPROM and 15%–20% of cases developing chorioamnionitis. Fetal infection can precede clinically evident chorioamnionitis, resulting in neonatal pulmonary and cerebral morbidities.
- Other complications such as **abruptio placentae, cord prolapse, perinatal death, PH, compression syndrome, long-term infant morbidities, increased need for CD**, and **retained placenta** are most common at very early PPROM and are discussed more in detail for PPROM <23 weeks.

MANAGEMENT
Prevention
See Chapter 17 (Figure 19.1) [13].

Preconception Counseling
Women with prior PPROM have a 20%–30% chance of PTB, including a 15%–20% chance of recurrent PPROM in the next pregnancy. Recurrence is higher in black race. These incidences are inversely related with GA at PPROM (the earlier the GA at PPROM, the higher the recurrence rate) and interpregnancy interval (shorter than 6 months particularly associated with higher recurrence) (see Chapters 1 and 17).

Counseling should also review all risk factors for PTB (Table 19.2). Several risk factors, such as smoking, low body mass index (BMI <20 kg/m²), inadequate maternal weight gain, exposure to infections, illicit drug use, nutritional deficiencies of copper and ascorbic acid, young or advanced maternal age, anemia, occupational factors such as prolonged walking or standing, strenuous working conditions, and long weekly work hours, psychological factors such as depression, anxiety, and chronic stress can be modified and best addressed preconception see also Chapter 17). The woman with a history of PPROM should also be made aware that interventions in pregnancy, such as for example progesterone and cerclage, can further decrease her chance of recurrence (see Chapter 17).

Prenatal Counseling

Counseling regarding prognosis, possible complications, management, and expectations for neonatal outcome should be provided. Prognosis depends mostly on GA at PPROM and GA at delivery. Latency is inversely related with GA at PPROM (Table 19.3) [14] and can be prolonged by some interventions. Fetal maturity depends on GA and is probably not enhanced or delayed by PPROM.

Workup

The current gold standard for the **diagnosis** of PROM is based on three traditional tests: visual pooling of clear fluid in the posterior fornix of the vagina or leakage of fluid from the cervical os at speculum examination; ferning test and nitrazine test tests (Figure 19.1). Such tests become progressively less accurate when more than 1 hour has elapsed after the membranes have ruptured. We still perform these three tests initially, with no need for additional tests in diagnosis in about 99% of women with possible PPROM. Alternative tests have been introduced, which are particularly helpful when traditional tests are indeterminate. See Table 19.1 for accuracy of diagnosis of PPROM with different.

Screening for **gonorrhea and chlamydia** is indicated, especially in high-risk groups. **GBS** culture should be sent from anorectal and vaginal areas. **Avoid manual/digital examination of the cervix** in any woman with suspected PPROM, and also after PPROM is diagnosed by speculum examination. Digital examination is associated with shorter latency and higher incidences of infection [15,16].

Ultrasound should evaluate at least presentation, biometry for GA, anatomy, placenta and cord location, and amniotic fluid. The lower is the amniotic fluid volume (usually measured by amniotic fluid index [AFI] in most studies, but maximum vertical pocket (MVP) is preferred currently), the higher is the incidence of perinatal infection and the shorter is the latency period [17,18].

Fifty to seventy percent of PPROM have low amniotic fluid volume on initial sonography. Low amniotic fluid volume is associated with an increased risk of umbilical cord compression and shorter latency but the predictive value is low [19]. Patients with nonvertex presentations have higher risk for prolapsed umbilical cord and of an unintended vaginal delivery when compared with vertex presentations [20].

See also Chapter 17.

Infection Precautions

Women with active herpes simplex virus (HSV) infection or human immunodeficiency virus (HIV) with viral loads >1000

Table 19.2 Selected Risk Factors for Spontaneous PPROM

Maternal Factors
- PPROM in a prior pregnancy (recurrence risk is 16%–32% as compared with 4% in women with a prior uncomplicated term delivery)
- Antepartum vaginal bleeding
- Chronic steroid therapy
- Collagen vascular disorders (such as Ehlers–Danlos syndrome, systemic lupus erythematosus)
- Direct abdominal trauma
- Preterm labor
- Exposure to infections
- Cigarette smoking
- Illicit drugs (cocaine)
- Anemia
- Low body mass index (<20 kg/m²)
- Inadequate maternal weight gain
- Nutritional deficiencies of copper and ascorbic acid
- Low socioeconomic status
- Unmarried status
- Young or advanced maternal age
- Occupational factors (strenuous working conditions, long weekly work hours)
- Psychological factors

Uteroplacental Factors
- Uterine anomalies (such as uterine septum)
- Placental abruption (may account for 10%–15% of preterm PROM)
- Advanced cervical dilatation (cervical insufficiency)
- Prior cervical conization
- Cervical shortening in the second trimester (<2.5 cm)
- Uterine overdistension (polyhydramnios, multiple pregnancy)
- Intra-amniotic infection (chorioamnionitis)
- Multiple bimanual vaginal examinations (but not sterile speculum or transvaginalultrasound examinations)

Fetal Factors
- Multiple pregnancy (preterm PROM complicates 7%–10% of twin pregnancies)
- Fetal anomalies (malformations, aneuploidies)

Source: Adapted from Caughey AB et al., *Rev Obstet Gynecol*, 1, 11–22, 2008.

Table 19.3 Latency Depending on GA at PPROM

GA at PPROM (weeks)	Mean Latency	Delivery		
		<48 Hours	<7 Days	<14 Days
<24	7 days	20%	40%–50%	70%
24–33 6/7	3–6 days	50%	70%–80%	90%
34–36 6/7	24 hours	70%–80%	90%	>95%

Source: Adapted from Schucker JL and Mercer BM, *Semin Perinatol*, 20, 389–400, 1996.
Abbreviation: GA, gestational age.

are **not**, in general, expectantly managed, especially if PPROM has occurred after 32 weeks (see Chapters 32 and 50 in *Maternal-Fetal Evidence Based Guidelines*). Management needs to be individualized with PPROM 23–31 6/7 weeks in the presence of these infections.

Amniocentesis
Amniocentesis can be of use for the evaluation of the following:
- The **diagnosis**. If diagnosis is in doubt, 1 mL of indigo carmine (not currently available in the United States; alternatives are Evans blue or fluorescein) in 9 mL of normal saline can be injected into the amniotic cavity under continuous ultrasound guidance. Presence of blue on a pad worn on the perineum for 2–4 hours confirms the diagnosis.
- The **infectious** state of the amniotic cavity. Send amniotic fluid glucose (<15 mg/dL associated with positive culture), Gram stain, and culture.
- The fetal **maturity**. Results of similar accuracy to amniocentesis can be obtained noninvasively by collecting vaginal fluid using a bedpan [21]. Despite oligohydramnios, there is a 90% rate of success for transabdominal amniocentesis in PROM. There are insufficient data to assess the effect of amniocentesis on outcomes in PPROM. A recent Cochrane review [22] reported no benefits for amniocentesis on perinatal outcomes in a single randomized study with 47 patients.

Fetal Maturity Assessment
Assessment of fetal maturity can be obtained from amniotic fluid by amniocentesis or from the vaginal pool (see Chapter 58 in *Maternal-Fetal Medicine Evidence Based Guidelines*). The predictive value of lung maturity tests is not modified by PPROM. Phosphatidylglycerol (PG), surfactant/albumin ratio (TDx/FLM), and lamellar body counts (LBC) are accurate when tested in the vaginal pool. PG is not accurate in the presence of meconium or blood, LBC is not accurate in the presence of meconium, while the **TDx/FLM is accurate with blood and/or meconium in the vaginal pool**, yielding results similar to those observed with samples obtained with amniocentesis.

Meconium
Meconium-stained amniotic fluid is associated with clinical chorioamnionitis and positive amniotic fluid cultures. In the absence of symptoms and signs of chorioamnionitis, meconium alone is not an indication for intervention.

Hospitalization
There is **insufficient evidence** to compare hospital versus home management for PPROM.

A Cochrane review [23] including only two small trials shows no significant differences between home management and hospitalization in pPROM. Home management can be offered only to consenting, reliable patients with the following: absence of infection, dependable transportation, living near hospital, evaluation in hospital before discharge, vertex presentation, vertical pocket of amniotic fluid >2 cm, recording of temperature and pulse every 6 hours, fetal movements count, twice-weekly nonstress tests (NST), and weekly ultrasound. **Only 18% of patients with PPROM meet these criteria**, so that **most are managed in the hospital**. Eleven percent of women with PPROM managed at home **delivered unexpectedly at outside hospitals** [24]. Women were **monitored for 48–72 hours** before randomization to hospitalization versus no hospitalization in the two randomized controlled trials (RCTs) on this subject [23]. Compared with hospitalization, no hospitalization was associated with similar incidences of perinatal mortality (relative risk [RR] 1.93, 95% confidence interval [CI] 0.19–20.05), serious neonatal morbidity, chorioamnionitis, GA at delivery, birth weight and admission to neonatal intensive care unit, as well as CD (RR 0.28, 95% CI 0.07–1.15). There was no information on serious maternal morbidity or mortality. Mothers randomized to care at home spent approximately 10 fewer days as inpatients and were more satisfied with their care. Furthermore, home care was associated with reduced costs [23].

Maternal Surveillance
All women with PPROM should be monitored for signs of infection by assessment of clinical parameters (e.g., fever, maternal/fetal tachycardia, uterine tenderness, and purulent vaginal discharge). A diagnosis of chorioamnionitis is usually made by the presence of two or more of these criteria. The presence of a fever of unknown origin in the presence of PPROM is highly suspicious for chorioamnionitis, so that an amniocentesis should be considered if expectant management is still being considered (Chapter 22).

There is no clear evidence to support the use of C-reactive protein (CRP) for the early diagnosis of chorioamnionitis (specificity 38%–55%). CRP has also a low sensitivity to identify intrauterine infection [25,26]. Maternal leukocytosis at admission is associated with higher adverse infant neurodevelopmental outcomes at 2 years of age in a study [27].

Fetal Surveillance (Antepartum Testing)
The two most common types of fetal surveillance are NST and biophysical profile score (BPS) [28]. Abnormalities of these tests can be somewhat predictive of fetal infection and umbilical cord compression related to oligohydramnios. There is **insufficient evidence to assess the optimal type or frequency of testing**. The NST or BPS performed daily have poor sensitivity (39% and 25%, respectively) and similar predictive values for predicting infection [29]. **No improvement in perinatal outcome has been reported in one trial** [30]. Given lower cost, the NST is usually suggested for daily to twice-a-week fetal surveillance. Monitoring may be more frequent with oligohydramnios, because it is associated with an increased risk of umbilical cord compression and shorter latency, with a preference for BPS as a backup if the NST is nonreassuring [19]. One non-RCT study supports continuous fetal monitoring (CFM) in the management of PPROM [31], but there is insufficient evidence for a recommendation, and most practitioners and patients adopt intermittent (e.g., 1 hour every 8 hours) fetal monitoring for inpatient management of PPROM. Moreover, continuous prolonged external fetal monitoring may not be practically feasible [32].

Amnioinfusion for Prolonging Latency
Transabdominal amnioinfusion is associated with a **reduction in neonatal death** (RR 0.30), **neonatal sepsis** (RR 0.26), **PH** (RR 0.22), **puerperal sepsis** (RR 0.20) and **less likelihood to deliver within seven days** of membrane rupture (RR 0.18) [33]. These results are encouraging but limited by the sparse data and low methodological robustness. Transcervical amnioinfusion to prevent NRFHT is discussed below, under section "Delivery."

Corticosteroids for Fetal/Neonatal Maturation and Benefit
A **single course of corticosteroids is recommended for pregnant women between 24 0/7 weeks and 33 6/7 weeks of gestation**

who are at risk of PTB [34]. Antenatal corticosteroid therapy in case of PPROM is associated with **lower combined fetal and neonatal death** (RR 0.62, 95% CI 0.46–0.82), RDS (RR 0.67, 95% CI 0.55–0.82), **cerebroventricular hemorrhage** (RR 0.47, 95% CI 0.28–0.79), and **NEC** (RR 0.39, 95% CI 0.18–0.86). There are no statistically significant differences for maternal death, chorioamnionitis, puerperal sepsis or neonatal infection with or without antenatal corticosteroids administration in the setting of PPROM [35]. A course of antenatal steroid therapy (*24 mg of betamethasone*—**12 mg intramuscular (IM) every 24 hours**—or 24 mg of dexamethasone—6 mg IM every 12 hours) should not be repeated in patients with PPROM, since weekly courses do improve severe RDS, resulting in less composite neonatal morbidity among neonates delivered at 24–27 weeks, but are associated with shorter latency, higher risks of chorioamnionitis and neonatal sepsis, and no improvement in overall composite neonatal morbidity [36,37].

A single **rescue course** of antenatal corticosteroids may be considered **if the antecedent treatment was given more than 2 weeks prior, the GA is less than 32 6/7 weeks, and the women are judged to be likely to give birth within the next week** [38,39]. Prior to 26 weeks' gestation there is paucity of data on the efficacy of the current dosing regimens of corticosteroids in women with PPROM; moreover at low GAs there are only a few primitive alveoli on which the drug can exert an effect to improve lung function. A recent review does not support or refute the administration of antenatal corticosteroids to women at risk of PTB <26 weeks' gestation [40]. If the initial course was given at less than 26 weeks of gestation a single repeated course may be considered if the delivery is expected within 1 week [41]. A single rescue corticosteroid course in PPROM is not associated with an increased rate of neonatal sepsis [42], maternal chorioamnionitis or neonatal morbidity [43] (see also Chapter 17).

Antibiotics for Prolongation of Latency and Fetal/Neonatal Benefit

Compared with placebo, antibiotics for women with PPROM are associated with short-term **benefits** for both women and neonates and should be routinely given [44,45]. Benefits of maternal antibiotic therapy when there is PPROM are as follows:

- Maternal: 44% less **chorioamnionitis**
- Fetal/Neonatal:
  - 29% reduction in **PTB within 48 hours**
  - 21% reduction in **PTB within 7 days**
  - 33% reduction in **neonatal infection**
- 21% reduction in positive neonatal **blood culture**
- 17% reduction in use of **surfactant**
- 12% reduction in **oxygen therapy**
- 19% reduction in **abnormal cerebral ultrasound scan** (including IVH) prior to discharge from hospital
- A 10% prolongation of pregnancy
- Decreasing trend in perinatal mortality (RR 0.93, 95% CI 0.76–1.14)
- Decrease in RDS and NEC with ampicillin and erythromycin treatment [46]

A meta-analysis limited to PPROM before 34 weeks shows similar results [47]. The ORACLE study evaluated the children's health at **7 years of age** and found no difference in any functional impairment after prescription of erythromycin, with or without co-amoxiclav, compared with those born to mothers who received no erythromycin, or after prescription of coamoxiclav, with or without erythromycin, compared with those born to mothers who received no co-amoxiclav. **Long-term adverse effects** of antepartum prophylactic antibiotics for PPROM have **not been observed** in children followed to age 7 years [48]. This finding is in contrast to the observation from the same authors that in patients with spontaneous PTL and intact membranes, the rate of cerebral palsy was increased in children exposed to antibiotics in utero [49]. These results would suggest further caution should be used when considering the routine treatment of women with antibiotics if there is uncertainty about the diagnosis of PROM.

Benefits in short-term outcomes (prolongation of pregnancy, infection, need for respiratory therapy, less abnormal cerebral ultrasound before discharge from hospital, etc.) should be balanced against a lack of evidence of benefit for other outcomes, including perinatal mortality, and for long-term outcomes.

Type
There is insufficient evidence on the optimal antibiotic type (and regimen) in women with PPROM. **Ampicillin and erythromycin** [46] or **erythromycin alone** [44] are associated with significant benefits in neonatal outcomes and should be used routinely in women with PPROM 24–34 weeks [34,44,46,47,50–52] (Table 19.4). A combination of ampicillin and erythromycin—for example, ampicillin 2 g and erythromycin 250 mg both intravenous (IV) every 6 hours for 48 hours, followed by amoxicillin 250 mg and erythromycin base 333 mg both orally (PO) every 8 hours for 5 days, for a total of 7 days—in women with PPROM with no concomitant steroids use showed an improvement in

Table 19.4 Possible Antibiotic Regimens

Reference	Antibiotic	Dose
34, 46	Ampicillin	2 g IV every 6 hours and
	Erythromycin	250 mg IV every 6 hours for 48 hours followed by
	Amoxicillin	250 mg PO every 8 hours and
	Erythromycin	333 mg PO every 8 hours for 5 days.
44, 52	Erythromycin	250 mg PO every 6 hours for a maximum of 10 days
50	Cefazolin	1 g IV every 6 hours and
	Erythromycin	250 mg PO every 6 hours for 7 days
51	Ampicillin	2 g IV, then 1 g IV every 6 hours and
	Azithromycin	500 mg PO single dose every 24 hours for 3 days followed by
	Ampicillin	500 mg PO every 6 hours for 4 days

Sources: Adapted from American College of Obstetricians and Gynecologists, *Obstet Gynecol*, 122, 918–930, 2013; Kenyon SL et al., *Lancet.*, 357, 979–988, 2001; Mercer BM et al., *JAMA*, 278, 989–995, 1997; Kwak, HM et al., *Placenta*, 34, 346–352, 2013; Pierson RC et al., *Obstet Gynecol*, 124, 515–519, 2014; National Institute for Health and Care Excellence, *Preterm Labour and Birth*, NICE Guidelines 2015, London, United Kingdom, NICE, 2015.
Abbreviations: IV, intravenous; PO, by mouth.

neonatal health by significantly reducing the rates of infants with one or more major infant morbidity (composite morbidity: death, RDS, early sepsis, severe IVH, and severe NEC) from 53% to 44% [45]. Compared with placebo, erythromycin 250 mg PO four times a day for 10 days is associated with decreases in neonatal death, chronic lung disease, major cerebral abnormalities, and prolongation of pregnancy in women with PPROM <37 weeks who received steroids in >75% of cases [44].

Azithromycin can be used instead of erythromycin, but there are less data on its efficacy in women with PPROM. A retrospective comparison between azithromycin and erythromycin in addition to ampicillin in preterm PROM shows no differences in latency or maternal or fetal outcomes [51]. Cephalosporins are also commonly used in pregnancy, and have few side effects and a broad-spectrum antibacterial effect [53]. A randomized trial comparing cefazolin plus macrolide (erythromycin or clarithromycin) versus cefazolin alone in PPROM showed no difference among the three antibiotic regimens in term of newborn outcome [50]. In a large trial, amoxicillin/clavulanate was associated with an increased risk of neonatal NEC, although there is no consistent trend toward a positive or negative effect of broad-spectrum antibiotics for NEC in the literature [28,44]. According to Cochrane review, **co-amoxiclav should be avoided** in women at risk of PTB due to increased risk of neonatal NEC (RR 4.72, 95% CI 1.57–14.23). Possible antibiotic regimens are listed in Table 19.4.

The mechanism of action of single antibiotic drugs should also be considered when selecting the best antibiotic regimens. Macrolides may be considered a good choice as they diffuse slowly in the tissues and act mainly on gram + and chlamydia; moreover, the microorganism disruption in the phagocyte prevents prostaglandins release and the consequent inflammatory cascade activation.

Detection of specific cervicovaginal pathogens should be appropriately treated (see Chapters 32 through 37 of *Maternal-Fetal Evidence Based Guidelines*) but the routine cervicovaginal swab analysis is not indicated.

Clinical chorioamnionitis requires therapeutic antibiotics. For example, ampicillin (2 g IV every 6 hours) or cefazolin (1 g IV every 6 hours), plus gentamicin (3–5 mg/kg single dose IV every 24 hours). If CD is performed, prophylactic antibiotics are indicated (see Chapter 13). Intrapartum GBS prophylaxis should be given until culture results are available, and to carriers. There are insufficient data to assess the need for this intervention in women with PPROM in whom GBS is sensitive to antibiotics—like ampicillin—already given for PPROM. The suggested regimen is penicillin (5 million units IV, and then 2.5 million units every 4 hours), or (if unavailable) ampicillin (2 g IV, then 1 g every 4 hours).

Tocolysis for Prolongation of Latency and Fetal/Neonatal Benefit

In a Cochrane review tocolysis was associated with **longer latency** (mean difference 73.12 hours; 95% CI 20.21–126.03) and **fewer births within 48 hours** (average RR 0.55; 95% CI 0.32–0.95). However, tocolysis was associated with **increased incidence of 5-minute Apgar of less than seven** (RR 6.05; 95% CI 1.65–22.23) and *increased need for ventilation of the neonate* (RR 2.46; 95% CI 1.14–5.34), while it was not associated with a significant effect on perinatal mortality. For women with PPROM before 34 weeks, there was a **significantly increased risk of chorioamnionitis**; neonatal outcomes were not significantly different. There were no significant differences in maternal/neonatal outcomes in subgroup analyses of different classes of tocolytics, antibiotic, corticosteroid or combined antibiotic/corticosteroid.

The review suggests **there is insufficient evidence to support tocolytic therapy for women with PPROM, as there was an increase in maternal chorioamnionitis without significant benefits to the infant**. However, studies did not consistently administer antibiotics and corticosteroids, both of which are now considered standard of care [54].

Compared with short-term tocolysis to allow steroid effect, **long-term tocolysis >48 hours** is associated with a nonsignificant prolongation of pregnancy, no differences in neonatal complications, but increases in chorioamnionitis and postpartum endometritis. It **should** therefore **be avoided** [55].

Magnesium Sulfate for Fetal Neuroprotection

A protective role of magnesium sulfate against the risk of cerebral palsy in preterm infants born before 32 weeks has been demonstrated by randomized trials (cumulative absolute risk reduction of 1.7) [56–60]. Results in PPROM cases were not reported separately in any study but constituted almost the 90% of the population in the largest study [60]. In the absence of evidence for an optimal dose of magnesium sulfate, scientific societies suggest adopting the minimum dosage used in the published trials and when delivery appears imminent at <32 weeks [61–63]. According to our Institution's protocol, we administer magnesium sulfate 4 g load over 20 minutes, followed by 1 g/hour for a maximum duration of treatment of 12 hours (see Chapter 18).

Progesterone

17 alpha-hydroxyprogesterone caproate (17P) is **not associated with increased latency** versus placebo in women with PPROM [64]. In women with singleton gestations and PPROM at 24–30 weeks, 17P 250 mg IM is associated with no effect on interval to delivery, GA at delivery, or neonatal mortality and morbidity in a small RCT [65]. In a recent RCT, weekly 17OHP-C injections did not prolong pregnancy or reduce perinatal morbidity in patients with PPROM [66]. In summary, there is **insufficient evidence** to recommend the use of progesterone in women with PPROM. In a woman who has been receiving 17P for prior spontaneous PTB, in the absence of evidence to the contrary, it is reasonable to continue 17P once membranes have ruptured [67].

Vitamin C and E

There is **insufficient evidence** to assess the effect of vitamin supplementation in women with PPROM. In one small trial, compared with placebo, vitamin C 500 mg and vitamin E 400 IU daily in women with PPROM at 26–34 weeks were associated with 7-day prolongation in latency, but no other effects on maternal or neonatal morbidity and mortality [68]. In a recent RCT, the use of vitamins C 1000 mg and E 400 IU in women with PPROM was associated with a longer latency period before delivery. Adverse neonatal and maternal outcomes, which are often associated with prolonged latency periods, were similar between the groups [69].

Cerclage Removal

PPROM occurs in about 38% of women with cerclage in place [70]. The benefit of a retained cerclage to prolong latency and decrease complications related to prematurity has to be weighed against the risk of adverse maternal and neonatal outcomes. Compared with immediate cerclage removal, leaving the cerclage in place in women with PPROM is associated with longer latency between PPROM and delivery, but higher incidence of maternal (chorioamnionitis, endometritis) and neonatal (sepsis) infections [71,72]. **Leaving the cerclage in place >24 hours is associated with a longer latency >48 hours** (94% vs. 51%; OR

16.1, 95% CI 3.7–71.3), but also **significantly increased maternal and fetal/neonatal infection risks, such as chorioamnionitis** (43% vs. 20%; OR 2.9, 95% CI 1.7–5.0) **and neonatal mortality from sepsis** (12% vs. 1%; OR 13.2, 95% CI 1.6–108.3), and **a trend for more neonatal sepsis** (13% vs. 6%; OR 2.4, 95% CI 0.9–6.0) and **neonatal mortality** (17% vs. 10%; OR 2.0, 95% CI 0.9–4.3) [39,42–44,70]. A recent small randomized trial, terminated after an interim analysis, showed no differences between the two managements in terms of latency, infection and composite neonatal outcomes. However, there was a **numerical trend in the direction of less infectious morbidity with immediate removal of cerclage** [73]. In a recent meta-analysis, cerclage retention after PPROM did not significantly prolong the gestational latency period, but it increased the rates of delivery after the first 48 hours. It did not significantly increase the rates of neonatal sepsis or neonatal death. Maternal chorioamnionitis was more prevalent among women with cerclage retention (OR 1.78) [74]. Therefore, **in most cases, cerclage should be removed in women upon diagnosis of PPROM.**

Delivery

Timing
Once PPROM occurs, and steroids for fetal maturity have been administered, **the options for management include early delivery versus expectant management** until later in pregnancy. In the absence of **clear indications for expeditious delivery, such as nonreassuring fetal status, clinical chorioamnionitis, and abruptio placentae,** the optimal GA for delivery is less clear. A longer latency is associated with higher rate of chorioamnionitis, and a shorter latency with higher risk of severe prematurity. Delivery before 34 weeks is associated with risk of neonatal complications, including severe morbidity and death.

A meta-analysis of seven RCTs, including 690 women, concluded there was insufficient evidence to guide clinical practice regarding the risks and benefits of expectant management versus delivery in PPROM. In particular early delivery is associated with similar incidence of intrauterine deaths (RR 0.26, 95% CI 0.04–1.52), neonatal sepsis (RR 1.33, 95% CI 0.72–2.47), RDS (RR 0.98, 95% CI 0.74–1.29), cerebroventricular hemorrhage (RR 1.90 95% CI 0.52–6.92), NEC (RR 0.58, 95% CI 0.08–4.08), duration of neonatal hospitalization, neonatal deaths (RR 1.59, 95% CI 0.61–4.16), and perinatal mortality (RR 0.98, 95% CI 0.41–2.36), compared with expectant management. Regarding maternal outcomes, early delivery is associated with an increase in the incidence of CD (RR 1.51, 95% CI 1.08–2.10), endometritis (RR 2.32, 95% CI 1.33–4.07), and about 1 day less in duration of maternal hospital stay, but no effect on chorioamnionitis (RR 0.44, 95% CI 0.17–1.14) [75]. Unfortunately, most trials of this meta-analysis did not use steroids for fetal maturity, or antibiotics for pregnancy prolongation [76–79]. Because **steroids and antibiotics are associated with major perinatal benefits**, these RCTs therefore have limited clinical validity. According to most authorities based on the data reviewed above, **women with PROM before 34 0/7 weeks should be managed expectantly if no maternal or fetal contraindications exist** [34].

Recently PPROMEXIL 1–2 trials have compared immediate delivery after **PPROM in near term (34–37 weeks) gestation** versus expectant management. The studies conclude that the risk of neonatal sepsis after PPROM near term is low and induction of labor does not reduce this risk [80,81]. A recent secondary analysis of PPROMEXIL trials, with early onset neonatal sepsis as main outcome measure, suggests that **women with PROM between 34 and 37 weeks might benefit from immediate delivery if they have GBS vaginal colonization, while in GBS-negative women labor induction could be delayed until 37 weeks** [82]. Another recent RCT (PPROMT trial) has compared immediate delivery with expectant management after PPROM close to term (34–37 weeks) in the absence of overt signs of infection. The primary outcome, neonatal sepsis, did not differ between the study groups, just like the composite secondary outcome of neonatal morbidity and mortality. However, neonates born to mothers in the immediate delivery group had increased rates of respiratory distress (RR 1.6) and any mechanical ventilation (RR 1.4) and spent more time in intensive care (median 4.0 days). The study concludes that, in the absence of overt signs of infection or fetal compromise, a policy of expectant management with appropriate surveillance of maternal and fetal wellbeing should be followed in pregnant women who present with ruptured membranes close to term [83].

At ≥34 0/7 weeks, American College of Obstetricians and Gynecologists (ACOG) recommendations still suggest delivery in women with PPROM [34], but recent evidence suggest a cautious expectant management policy even ≥34 0/7 weeks as a viable alternative, especially if GBS negative.

Amnioinfusion for Preventing NRFHT
There is **insufficient evidence** to assess the effect of routine amnioinfusion in all women with PPROM, for prophylaxis either before labor or during labor. Compared with no amnioinfusion, **transcervical amnioinfusion** (warmed saline at 10 mL/minute for 1 hour, then 3 mL/minute—total volume infused mean 1160 mL) at the time of labor for women with PPROM at 26–35 weeks is associated with statistically similar but more favorable incidences of CD, low Apgar scores, and neonatal death in one small trial [84]. In the amnioinfusion group, the number of severe fetal heart rate decelerations per hour during the first stage of labor was reduced by just about one in this small trial. Fetal umbilical artery pH at delivery was higher. These outcomes are consistent with the benefits found for amnioinfusion for cord compression. Transcervical amnioinfusion reduced persistent variable decelerations during labor (RR 0.52) also in a trial with 86 participants [85].

In conclusion, to date, routine intrapartum amnioinfusion cannot be recommended for all women with PPROM given the limited data (see Chapter 10).

Mode and Site of Delivery
Mode of delivery should not be altered solely for the presence of PPROM. Malpresentation is more common with PTB, with the incidence of malpresentation being indirectly related to weeks of GA (see Chapter 22). Early preterm delivery should occur in a facility and by personnel capable of providing all the necessary support to the mother and fetus/neonate born preterm. **Transferring women** at risk of very PTB to perinatal centers for delivery **decreases the neonatal mortality and morbidity rate considerably** [86,87]. Predicting the time of delivery in PPROM is often impossible.

Anesthesia
No specific precautions.

Postpartum
See Chapter 17. Women with PPROM are at high risk of recurrence in subsequent pregnancies, with an association between GA at the time of PPROM, latency period, interval between pregnancies, and PPROM recurrence. Patients with a history of cervical insufficiency and fetal loss/miscarriage should be

considered at increased risk of midtrimester PPROM in the following pregnancy. See the section "Prevention."

Special considerations must be given when PPROM occurs before fetal viability, after invasive procedures, and in twin gestation.

PPROM <23 WEEKS
Definition
PROM <23 weeks or "previable PPROM" (arbitrary definition that varies among investigators and from year to year because of advances in neonatal intensive care) is a relevant and unique nosological entity because of its significant association with fetal and neonatal morbidity and mortality.

Incidence
The incidence is about 0.6% of pregnancies.

Etiology/Basic Pathophysiology
There are two different categories: spontaneous and iatrogenic. **Risk factors for spontaneous PPROM <23 weeks are similar to those for PTL and for PPROM later in pregnancy** (see Table 19.2 and 17.1 in Chapter 17). Fluid leakage or PPROM occurs in about 1% of genetic amniocenteses [88], 3%–5% of diagnostic fetoscopies, and 10% of invasive fetoscopies [89], see below.

Complications
Incidences of most complications are **inversely proportional to GA at PPROM, latency, residual amniotic fluid volume, and GA at delivery.**

Fetal/Neonatal

Neonatal death. Published data on **neonatal survival after early PPROM varies widely (20%–68%)** [90–94]. The mortality rates may be underestimated by selection bias due to the high rate of elective termination prior to viability and consequent inclusion of only patients continuing pregnancy or who have experienced initial latency. A study was performed to investigate if, in settings where elective termination of pregnancy (TOP) is frequent, perinatal outcomes could be better (assuming that patients with a poorer prognosis opted more frequently for TOP). Perinatal outcomes (mean GA at delivery, latency, birthweight and survival) were better in the centers with lower TOP rate; in particular survival among live births was 95.8% in the center with lower TOP and 65% in center with higher TOP [93]. A retrospective study on 58 women with prolonged PPROM at less than 24 weeks reported a survival rate in newborns of 90%. Pulmonary morbidities were common in the neonates [95]. The most recent reports on perinatal survival in PROM <24 weeks involve patients routinely managed with antibiotics, antenatal steroids, postnatal surfactant, and high-frequency ventilation. A comparison between PPROM less than 25.0 weeks and 25.0–31.9 weeks showed higher rate of severe composite neonatal morbidity and composite severe childhood morbidity in case of early PPROM. Neonatal death occurred in nearly 17% of early PPROM [94]. Neonatal mortality is comparable to that in preterm deliveries matched for GA without PPROM.

Chorioamnionitis. Antenatal infection is the major complication limiting the latency interval. **If clinical infection occurs at any time during the latency period, delivery is indicated.** Chorioamnionitis complicates about 40% of midtrimester PPROM [96,97]. The occurrence of chorioamnionitis is higher early in the latency period; **more than 50% of cases occur within the first 7 days after rupture**, with the maximum clinical occurrence on 2–5 days [98,99]. After the first week of latency, the incidence falls, suggesting that subclinical uterine or chorioamniotic infection that weakens membranes and causes rupture infection was probably present prior to membrane rupture, whereas bacteria migration is a less important component. The risk of chorioamnionitis is inversely proportional to residual amniotic fluid volume [100].

Placental abruption. Abruptio placentae is more frequent in pregnancies with midtrimester PPROM, occurring up to **44%** of cases compared with 0.8% of the general obstetric population [101]. The risk is highest with lower GA at PPROM and with vaginal bleeding occurring prior to or after membrane rupture [101,102].

Cord prolapse. The incidence of cord prolapsed is about **2%**. The risk is higher (11% in one study) in the setting of nonvertex fetal presentations [20].

Gestational age (weeks)	Stage of lung development	Description
4 to 6	EMBRIONIC	Lung bud arises
7 to 16	PSEUDOGLANDULAR	Non respiratory bronchi and bronchioles develop
17 to 24	CANALICULAR	First gas exchanging acini and pulmonary capillaries are forming
25 to 37	TERMINAL SAC	Subsaccules and alveoli develop with extensive capillary invasion and expansion of the alveolar blood barrier surface area
38 to age 3 years	ALVEOLAR	Subsaccules become alveoli

Figure 19.2 Phases of lung development.

Fetal death. Fetal demise is primarily related to abruption, cord prolapse and compression, or infection. The average risk of fetal death after midtrimester PPROM is about **10%**, and is inversely related to GA at PPROM and residual amniotic fluid volume [102].

Pulmonary hypoplasia. PH is a decrease in the number of lung cells, airways, and alveoli, mainly due in PPROM to alterations of normal amniotic fluid pressure and egress of lung fluid during the canalicular stage of lung development (ending at nearly 24 weeks) (Figure 19.2). The gold standard for the diagnosis of PH is lung weight by autopsy. The incidence of PH resulting from midtrimester PPROM varies from **13% to 28%** [102–106]. The mortality rate in neonates with this condition is 50% to 95% [84, 88, 89]. The main independent reported risk factors for development of PH are as follows: (a) early GA at membrane rupture [103, 105, 106–109]; a risk of 50%–60% was reported when PPROM occurs at 20 weeks or less; and (b) low residual amniotic fluid volume [89,110,104,106]. PH is more common among pregnancies with maximum pocket <2 cm or AFI <5, after controlling for GA at rupture [106,108]. Incidences of PH with severe, moderate, and absent-to-mild oligohydramnios are 43%, 21%, and 7%, respectively [103].

Tests proposed to identify PH prenatally are ultrasound measurement of amniotic fluid, fetal breathing movements, fetal chest circumference, lung length, lung volume, Doppler studies of pulmonary vessels, and O_2 tests. In general, the predictive accuracy is poor and may be improved by combining tests [105,109,111].

Fetal compression syndrome. In early PPROM, asymmetric intrauterine pressure and restriction in fetal movement can lead to limb position deformities and craniofacial defects of variable severity, originally described in the context of renal agenesis. The mean frequency of skeletal deformities is **7%**. Duration of latency and severity of oligohydramnios independently increase the risk of skeletal abnormalities and act synergistically [107]. The GA at PPROM is not a significant determinant due to the progressive and continuous development of the axial skeleton.

Increased likelihood of skeletal deformities observed among infants diagnosed with PH suggests that the two disorders share common risk factors. Surgical correction is not generally required as they resolve with postnatal growth and physiotherapy.

Other morbidities. Other neonatal morbidities are similar to that in PTB and are related to GA at PPROM. These include *RDS*, **bronchopulmonary dysplasia (BPD), IVH, NEC, sepsis, and retinopathy of prematurity**. The incidence of neonatal IVH and cystic PVL increases in cases complicated by clinical chorioamnionitis [112]. Since midtrimester PPROM is associated with early delivery and infections, it constitutes a potential risk factor for long-term neurological morbidities. There may be a higher risk of PVL in infants born after prolonged PPROM compared with other types of prematurity [113]. Prolonged latency in midtrimester PROM patients is not associated with an increasing frequency of abnormal neonatal cranial ultrasound examination [99].

Long-term morbidities. About 63%–84% of survivors after midtrimester PPROM will be neurologically intact [104]. **Cerebral palsy** rate in a group of 275 pregnancies complicated by early PPROM was **9.8%** [94].

Maternal
Cesarean delivery. The CD rate increases secondary to more common fetal heart rate abnormalities (related to oligohydramnios and chorioamnionitis), malpresentation, and abruptio. A classical uterine incision may be required to reduce fetal trauma at early GA (oligohydramnios, fetal malpresentation, and lower uterine segment characteristics constitute risk factors).

Retained placenta. The risk of undergoing either uterine exploration or curettage is **9%–18%**, and more likely if rupture occurs prior to 20 weeks of gestation.

Postpartum endometritis. This condition occurs in about **13%** of cases. Postpartum maternal **sepsis** (about 0.8%) and **death** (about 1/1000) are uncommon. The risk of maternal infection is inversely proportional to the latency period.

Management
Counseling
Parents should be counseled regarding the prognosis, complications, and management of PPROM <23 weeks. The **options** are **expectant management** or **delivery**. The impact of immediate delivery on neonatal outcome, and potential benefits and risks of conservative management, should be reviewed. PPROM related to genetic amniocentesis is associated with favorable outcomes even with expectant management (91%–99% perinatal survival), which is very different than the prognosis with spontaneous PPROM <23 weeks.

Incidences of most complications are inversely proportional to **GA at PPROM, latency, residual amniotic fluid volume,** and **GA at delivery**.

The *latency* period between membrane rupture and delivery is critical in determining perinatal outcome.

Latency is indirectly correlated with GA at PPROM (Table 19.3) [14]. While the mean latency is about 7 days, the median latency may be up to about 10–21 days because of the few pregnancies that gain a lot more than 14 days. **Up to 14% of women with midtrimester PPROM stop amniotic fluid loss,** presumably due to resealing of membranes [98,114]. This subgroup of cases has outcomes similar to pregnancies uncomplicated by membrane rupture. In 10%–20% of patients, amniotic fluid loss continues, but a partial reaccumulation during expectant management is observed [17,105].

Oligohydramnios (AFI <5 or MVP <2 cm) on admission, during latency period, or at the last ultrasonographic examination is associated with shorter latency, and higher occurrences of PH, chorioamnionitis, and perinatal mortality [108,115,116]. Conversely, adequate residual amniotic fluid volume identifies cases with elevated odds of perinatal survival (85%–93%) and better long-term neurological outcomes [102,115].

In a retrospective cohort of 92 cases of PPROM under 24 weeks, the overall neonatal survival rate at discharge was 85%; the survival rate was lower and the developmental delay more frequent in patients with persistent oligohydramnios compared with those with normal amniotic fluid volume [117].

Workup
Similar to PROM >23 weeks.

Therapy
See Figure 19.1.

Delivery in previable PPROM is *indicated in* the presence of

- **Intrauterine death**
- Spontaneous onset of **labor**
- Evidence of **maternal and/or or fetal infections**
- Any other obstetric **medical condition necessitating delivery** (e.g., abruptio placentae and preeclampsia)
- **Pregnancy termination request**

Delivery (termination) can be carried out usually by induction or by dilatation and extraction (D&X) by experienced operators, with no trials comparing these two modalities.

For management of women who elect **expectant management,** unfortunately there **are no trials on any interventions** (e.g., **steroids, antibiotics, and magnesium sulfate) for previable PPROM**. Data for any benefit of most interventions are available only for PPROM diagnosed at ≥23 weeks, so these interventions should be used with caution before this GA, with the patients understanding these limitations in medical knowledge. If pregnancy continues, patients need to be counseled on clinical variables and complications that may affect outcome and treatment serially at diagnosis, during the latency period, and at delivery. Given the high incidence of infection, cerclage should be removed in women with cerclage in place at the time of PPROM.

Transabdominal Amnioinfusion

Serial transabdominal amnioinfusions in the second trimester aim to enhance amniotic fluid volume, reduce lung hypoplasia, prolong latency and improve pregnancy outcomes. Data come mainly from nonrandomized perspective or retrospective trials. A meta-analysis on this topic, not including PPROM <23 weeks, reports a perinatal mortality reduction and a longer latency period after amnioinfusion [118], while the Cochrane review doesn't identify any randomized study about transabdominal amnioinfusion before 26 weeks [119]. A recent randomized study on 56 women (serial weekly transabdominal or expectant management) shows no major differences in maternal, perinatal or pregnancy outcomes. It is considered a pilot study, but it demonstrates that such a study is feasible [120]. **Because amnioinfusion in previable PPROM has not been validated in large randomized studies, it can be proposed only in research programs after informed consent of the patient.**

Resealing Techniques

Resealing techniques as amniopatch (see section PPROM Following Invasive Procedures (Iatrogenic PPROM) and Strategies to Repair) has been proposed, but their efficacy in spontaneous PROM is low.

Proposed Management
In women desiring expectant management with PPROM <23 weeks, there is no data to support benefit of hospitalization, optimal GA for corticosteroids, antibiotics, or other interventions (Figure 19.1). Some consider hospital bed rest during the first few days, but this is not supported by level 1 or other data. Some administer an initial course of broad-spectrum antibiotic prophylaxis (7 days or until culture results), but again this is not supported by any RCT or other data. **Avoid vaginal examination until labor or delivery**. During expectant management, monitor for the onset of infectious complications, observing temperature, maternal or fetal tachycardia, uterine contractions or tenderness, or purulent vaginal discharge. As outpatient, instruct to avoid intercourse, check temperature, and refer to hospital for vaginal bleeding and contractions. **At 23 0/7 weeks, suggest (re)admission to the hospital** and active expectant management, including administration of at least one course of steroids and antibiotics, assuming not already given.

PPROM FOLLOWING INVASIVE PROCEDURES (IATROGENIC PPROM) AND STRATEGIES TO REPAIR

Iatrogenic PPROM (iPPROM) and spontaneous PPROM have different pathophysiologies. In iPPROM the medical instrument creates the hole in the membranes, which subsequently fails to close.

In studies of women undergoing **second-trimester amniocentesis** for prenatal diagnosis, the risk of PROM is approximately 1% [88]. When leakage of amniotic fluid occurs after amniocentesis, the outcome is better than after spontaneous preterm PROM and reaccumulation of normal amniotic fluid volume is more probable [10,121]. In one series of 11 patients with PROM after genetic amniocentesis, there was one previable pregnancy loss, reaccumulation of normal amniotic fluid occurred within 1 month in 72% of patients, and the perinatal survival rate was 91% [88]. After appropriate counseling, patients with PROM after genetic amniocentesis typically are managed expectantly as outpatients.

PPROM may also occur following **fetoscopy** for fetal surgical procedures (e.g., laser therapy for twin–twin transfusion syndrome [TTTS] or for twin-reversed arterial perfusion [TRAP sequence], or tracheal occlusion for congenital diaphragmatic hernia) or other minimally invasive fetal surgery (e.g., intrauterine blood sampling and transfusion or fetal shunting for lower urinary tract obstructions and pleural effusions). The incidence of iPPROM after these procedures varies significantly in the literature. iPPROM occurred in about 30% of cases treated by minimally invasive fetal surgery in one report [122]. Parameters that have been suggested to impact iPPROM rates are the diameter of the surgical instrument and the number of entries to the uterine cavity [123]. Other possible risk factors are duration and difficulty of the procedure, operator experience, membrane friction due to instrument manipulation, type of anesthesia, GA at intervention, number of interventions and placental location. In one review the maximum diameter of the instrument predicted iPPROM rate, GA at birth and fetal survival [122].

Several techniques have been developed in an **attempt to artificially reseal the fetal membranes** and prevent leakage of amniotic fluid. These include intra-amniotic injection of platelets and cryoprecipitate (amniopatch), sealing the cervical canal, and fetoscopic laser coagulation [89,124–126]. Compared with spontaneous PPROM, iPPROM is not only a different entity etiologically, but also in its better response to therapeutic measures. One report demonstrated successful membrane sealing for persistent oligohydramnios after amniocentesis and fetoscopy in seven women, using intraamniotic injection of platelets and cryoprecipitate through a 22-gauge needle [89]. Other case reports include successful membrane sealing with intrauterine injection of gelatin sponge, fibrinogen and thrombin combinations, and with fibrin glue with powdered collagen [126–129]. Another study reported cessation of leakage and restoration of normal amniotic fluid volume in twelve women with intracervical instillation of fibrin sealants [124].

According to a review of cases of iPPROM, amniopatch effectively seals the fetal membranes in over two-thirds of cases [130]. A retrospective analysis of 24 amniopatch procedures performed for PPROM after a needle-based procedure or after fetoscopic intervention reported a success rate of 58% [131]. Unfortunately, **the safety of these approaches has not been evaluated in large studies**, and there are several anecdotal reports of maternal and perinatal morbidity and mortality. Even if such practices have not yet been incorporated into clinical practice, current experience suggests that, in cases of fluid leakage following an invasive fetal procedure, the use of sealing techniques is a therapeutic option that should be researched further.

PPROM IN TWIN GESTATIONS

Overall, PPROM complicates 7%–8% of twin pregnancies at a mean GA of 30–32 weeks (see also Chapter 44, in *Maternal-Fetal Evidence Based Guidelines*). PPROM occurs at an earlier GA among multiple gestations with 36% of twin PPROM cases occurring at less than 28 weeks. PPROM in singleton pregnancies is related mainly to infection/inflammation, while PPROM in twin gestation may probably be more related to uterine overdistension. **The latency period seems to be shorter in twins** compared with singleton pregnancies. Most studies report a median latency of less than 24 hours with only 16%–50% of twin pregnancies remaining undelivered at 48 hours, decreasing to 7%–22% at 7 days. Latency tends to be longer when PPROM occurs before 30 weeks of gestation [132]. The membrane rupture usually occurs in the **lower sac (90% of cases)** [133].

Studies comparing **obstetric outcome between singleton and twin pregnancies with PPROM reported no difference in neonatal outcome** [134,135]. A retrospective cohort of 23 multifetal pregnancies complicated by PPROM before 26 0/7 weeks showed a median latency of 11 days with expectant management. Of the 46 newborns, 20 (43%) survived to hospital discharge. Of these, 12 (60%) experienced severe neonatal morbidity. The multiple with ruptured membranes was more likely to experience intrauterine fetal demise, but all other outcomes did not differ by membrane status [136]. In 48 multiple pregnancies complicated by PPROM and delivering at a median GA of 31 weeks, neonatal morbidity and mortality were not different between the presenting and nonpresenting twin and no difference was found between fetuses with or without ruptured sac. The outcomes were not affected by duration of the latency period [137]. These data suggest that **rupture of membranes per se probably do not worsen the outcomes, and support a conservative management of twin pregnancies with PPROM**. The incidence of both clinical and subclinical chorioamnionitis has been reported as significantly higher in singleton pregnancies compared with twin pregnancies complicated by PPROM [133,138]. A study evaluating neonatal and infant outcomes in 151 twin gestations with PPROM at 24–31 weeks reported a neonatal mortality rate of 9.0% and an overall cerebral palsy rate of 7.3% [139].

The management of PPROM in twin pregnancies does not differ significantly from that of singletons. Antenatal **steroids, antibiotics to prolong latency, magnesium sulfate for neuroprotection** with delivery no later than 34 weeks of gestation are all recommended in twins with PPROM.

REFERENCES

1. Abdelazim IA, Abdelrazak KM, Al-Kadi M, et al. Fetal fibronectin (Quick Check fFN test) versus placental alpha microglobulin-1 (AmniSure test) for detection of premature rupture of fetal membranes. *Arch Gynecol Obstet*. 2014;290:457–464. [II-2]
2. Tagore S, Kwek K. Comparative analysis of insulin-like growth factor binding protein-1 (IGFBP-1), placental alpha-microglobulin-1 (PAMG-1) and nitrazine test to diagnose premature rupture of membranes in pregnancy. *J Perinat Med*. 2010;38:609–612. [II-2]
3. Abdelazim IA. Insulin-like growth factor binding protein-1 (Actim PROM test) for detection of premature rupture of fetal membranes. *J Obstet Gynaecol Res*. 2014;40:961–967. [II-2]
4. Bornstein J, Ohel G, Sorokin Y, et al. Effectiveness of a novel home-based testing device for the detection of rupture of membranes. *Am J Perinatol*. 2009;26:45–50. [II-2]
5. Ramsauer B, Vidaeff AC, Hosli I, et al. The diagnosis of rupture of fetal membranes (ROM): A meta-analysis. *J Perinatal Med*. 2013;41:233–240. [Meta-analysis of observational studies]
6. McEnerney JK, McEnerney LN. Unfavorable neonatal outcome after intraamniotic injection of methylene blue. *Obstet Gynecol*. 1983;61(3 Suppl):35S–37S. [III]
7. Spahr RC, Salsburey DJ, Krissberg A, et al. Intraamniotic injection of methylene blue leading to methemoglobinemia in one of twins. *Int J Gynaecol Obstet*. 1980;17:477–478. [III]
8. Lee SE, Park JS, Norwitz ER, et al. Measurement of placental alpha-microglobulin-1 in cervicovaginal discharge to diagnose rupture of membranes. *Obstet Gynecol*. 2007;109:634–640. [II-3]
9. Canavan TP, Simhan HN, Caritis S. An evidence-based approach to the evaluation and treatment of premature rupture of membranes: Part I. Obstet Gynecol Surv. 2004;59:669–677. [Review]
10. Caughey AB, Robinson JN, Norwitz ER. Contemporary diagnosis and management of preterm premature rupture of membranes. *Rev Obstet Gynecol*. 2008;1:11–22. [Review]
11. Peaceman AM, Lai Y, Rouse DJ, et al. Length of latency with preterm premature rupture of membranes before 32 weeks' gestation. *Am J Perinatol*. 2015;32:57–62. [II-2]
12. Melamed N, Ben-Haroush A, Pardo J, et al. Expectant management of preterm premature rupture of membranes: Is it all about gestational age? *Am J Obstet Gynecol*. 2011;204:48.e1–48.e8. [II-2]
13. Blumenfeld YJ, Lee HC, Gould JB, et al. The effect of preterm premature rupture of membranes on neonatal mortality rates. *Obstet Gynecol*. 2010;116:1381–1386. [II-2]
14. Schucker JL, Mercer BM. Midtrimester premature rupture of the membranes. *Semin Perinatol*. 1996;20:389–400. [Review]
15. Alexander JM, Mercer BM, Miodovnik M, et al. The impact of digital cervical examination on expectantly managed preterm rupture of membranes. *Am J Obstet Gynecol*. 2000;183:1003–1007. [II-2]
16. Munson LA, Graham A, Koos BJ, et al. Is there a need for digital examination in patients with spontaneous rupture of the membranes? *Am J Obstet Gynecol*. 1985;153:562–563. [II-3]
17. Hadi HA, Hodson CA, Strickland D. Premature rupture of the membranes between 20 and 25 weeks' gestation: Role of amniotic fluid volume in perinatal outcome. *Am J Obstet Gynecol*. 1994;170:1139–1144. [II-2]
18. Park JS, Yoon BH, Romero R, et al. The relationship between oligohydramnios and the onset of preterm labor in preterm premature rupture of membranes. *Am J Obstet Gynecol*. 2001;184:459–462. [II-2]
19. Mercer BM, Rabello YA, Thurnau GR, et al. The NICHD-MFMU antibiotic treatment of preterm PROM study: Impact

of initial amniotic fluid volume on pregnancy outcome. *Am J Obstet Gynecol.* 2006;194:438. [II-2]
20. Lewis DF, Robichaux AG, Jaekle RK, et al. Expectant management of preterm premature rupture of membranes and non-vertex presentation: What are the risks? *Am J Obstet Gynecol.* 2007;196:566. [III]
21. Edwards RK, Duff P, Ross KC. Amniotic fluid indices of fetal pulmonary maturity with preterm premature rupture of membranes. *Obstet Gynecol.* 2000;96:102–105. [II-3]
22. Sharp GC, Stock SJ, Norman JE. Fetal assessment methods for improving neonatal and maternal outcomes in preterm prelabour rupture of membranes. *Cochrane Database Syst Rev.* 2014;(10):CD010209. [Meta-analysis: 3 RCTs, *n* = 275]
23. Abou El Senoun G, Dowswell T, Mousa HA. Planned home versus hospital care for preterm prelabour rupture of the membranes (PPROM) prior to 37 weeks' gestation. *Cochrane Database Syst Rev.* 2014;(4):CD008053. [Meta-analysis: 2 RCTs, *n* = 116]
24. Carlan SJ, O'Brien WF, Parsons MT, et al. Preterm premature rupture of membranes: A randomized study of home versus hospital management. *Obstet Gynecol.* 1993;81:61–64. [RCT, *n* = 67]
25. Ismail MA, Zinaman MJ, Lowensohn RI, et al. The significance of C-reactive protein levels in women with premature rupture of membranes. *Am J Obstet Gynecol.* 1985;151:541–544. [II-2]
26. Romem Y, Artal R. C-reactive protein as a predictor for chorioamnionitis in cases of premature rupture of the membranes. *Am J Obstet Gynecol.* 1984;150:546–550. [II-3]
27. Pasquier JC, Picaud JC, Rabilloud M, et al. Maternal leukocytosis after preterm premature rupture of membranes and infant neurodevelopmental outcome: A prospective, population-based study (DOMINOS Study). *J Obstet Gynaecol Can.* 2007;29:20–26. [Prospective cohort of 394 PPROM between 24 weeks and 33.6 weeks. II-2]
28. Mercer BM. Preterm premature rupture of membranes. *Obstet Gynecol.* 2003;101:178–193. [Review]
29. Pasquier JC, Bujold E, Rabilloud M, et al. Effect of latency period after premature rupture of membranes on 2 years infant mortality (DOMINOS study). *Eur J Obstet Gynecol Reprod Biol.* 2007;135:21–27. [II-2]
30. Lewis DF, Adair CD, Weeks JW, et al. A randomized clinical trial of daily nonstress testing versus biophysical profile in the management of preterm premature rupture of membranes. *Am J Obstet Gynecol.* 1999;181:1495–1499. [RCT, *n* = 135]
31. Davis JM, Krew MA, Gill P, et al. The role of continuous fetal monitoring in the management of preterm premature rupture of membranes. *J Matern Fetal Neonatal Med.* 2008;21:301–304. [II-3]
32. Li Y, Gonik B. Continuous fetal heart rate monitoring in patients with preterm premature rupture of membranes undergoing expectant management. *J Matern Fetal Neonatal Med.* 2009;22:589–592. [II-3]
33. Hofmeyr GJ, Eke AC, Lawrie TA. Amnioinfusion for third trimester preterm premature rupture of membranes. *Cochrane Database Syst Rev.* 2014;(3):CD000942. [Meta-analysis: 4 RCTs, *n* = 241]
34. American College of Obstetricians and Gynecologists. ACOG practice bulletin 2013: Premature rupture of membranes. *Obstet Gynecol.* 2013;122:918–930. [Guideline]
35. Roberts D, Dalziel S. Antenatal corticosteroids for accelerating fetal lung maturation for women at risk of preterm birth. *Cochrane Database Syst Rev.* 2006;(3):CD004454. [Meta-analysis: 21 RCTs, *n* = 3885]
36. Harding JE, Pang JM, Knight DB, et al. Do antenatal corticosteroids help in the setting of preterm rupture of membranes? *Am J Obstet Gynecol.* 2001;184:131–139. [Meta-analysis: 15 RCTs, *n* = >1400]
37. Lee MJ, Davies J, Guinn D, et al. Single versus weekly courses of antenatal corticosteroids in preterm premature rupture of membranes. *Obstet Gynecol.* 2004;103:274–281. [RCT, *n* = 161 with PPROM]
38. American College of Obstetricians and Gynecologists. ACOG Committee Opinion. Antenatal corticosteroid therapy for fetal maturation. *Obstet Gynecol.* 2011;117:422–424. [Guideline]
39. Garite TJ, Kurtzman J, Maurel K, et al. Impact of a "rescue course" of antenatal corticosteroids: A multicenter randomized placebo-controlled trial. *Am J Obstet Gynecol.* 2009;200:248. e1–248.e9. [RCT, *n* = 437]
40. Onland W, de Laat MW, Mol BW, Offringa M. Effects of antenatal corticosteroids given prior to 26 weeks' gestation: A systematic review of randomized controlled trials. *Am J Perinatol.* 2011;28:33–44. [Meta-analysis: 9 RCTs]
41. Royal College of Obstetricians. *Green Top Guideline No. 7: Antenatal Corticosteroids to Reduce Neonatal Morbidity and Mortality*. London, United Kingdom: Royal College of Obstetricians, 2010.
42. Gyamfi-Bannerman C, Son M. Preterm premature rupture of membranes and the rate of neonatal sepsis after two courses of antenatal corticosteroids. *Obstet Gynecol.* 2014;124:999–1003. [II-2]
43. Brookfield KF, El-Sayed YY, Chao L, et al. Antenatal corticosteroids for preterm premature rupture of membranes: Single or repeat course? *Am J Perinatol.* 2015;32:537–544. [II-2]
44. Kenyon SL, Taylor DJ, Tarnow-Mordi W et al. Broad-spectrum antibiotics for preterm, prelabour rupture of fetal membranes: The ORACLE I randomised trial. *Lancet.* 2001;357:979–988. [RCT, *n* = 4826]
45. Kenyon S, Boulvain M, Neilson JP. Antibiotics for preterm rupture of membranes. *Cochrane Database Syst Rev.* 2013;(12):CD001058. [Meta-analysis: 22 RCTs, *n* = 6872]
46. Mercer BM, Miodovnik M, Thurnau GR, et al. Antibiotic therapy for reduction of infant morbidity after preterm premature rupture of the membranes: A randomized controlled trial. *JAMA.* 1997;278:989–995. [RCT, *n* = 614]
47. Hutzal CE, Boyle EM, Kenyon SL, et al. Use of antibiotics for the treatment of preterm parturition and prevention of neonatal morbidity: A metaanalysis. *Am J Obstet Gynecol.* 2008;199:620. [Meta-analysis: 21 RCTs, *n* = >4000]
48. Kenyon S, Pike K, Jones DR, et al. Childhood outcomes after prescription of antibiotics to pregnant women with preterm rupture of the membranes: 7-Year follow-up of the ORACLE I trial. *Lancet.* 2008;372:1310. [RCT, *n* = 3298]
49. Kenyon S, Pike K, Jones DR, et al. Childhood outcomes after prescription of antibiotics to pregnant women with spontaneous preterm labour: 7-year follow-up of the ORACLE II trial. *Lancet.* 2008;372:1319. [RCT, *n* = 3196]
50. Kwak HM, Shin MY, Cha HH, et al. The efficacy of cefazolin plus macrolide (erythromycin or clarithromycin) versus cefazolin alone in neonatal morbidity and placental inflammation for women with preterm premature rupture of membranes. *Placenta.* 2013;34:346–352. [RCT, *n* = 102]
51. Pierson RC, Gordon SS, Haas DM. A retrospective comparison of antibiotic regimens for preterm premature rupture of membranes. *Obstet Gynecol.* 2014;124:515–519. [II-2]
52. National Institute for Health and Care Excellence. Preterm Labour and Birth. *NICE Guidelines 2015.* London, United Kingdom: NICE, 2015. [Guideline]
53. Singh K, Mercer B. Antibiotics after preterm premature rupture of the membranes. *Clin Obstet Gynecol.* 2011;54:344–350. [Review]
54. Mackeen AD, Seibel-Seamon J, Muhammad J, et al. Tocolytics for preterm premature rupture of membranes. *Cochrane Database Syst Rev.* 2014;(2):CD007062. [Meta-analysis: 8 RCTs, *n* = 408]
55. Decavalas G, Mastrogiannis D, Papadopoulos U, et al. Short term versus long-term prophylactic tocolysis in patient with preterm premature rupture of membranes. *Eur J Obstet Gynecol Reprod Biol.* 1995;59:143–147. [RCT, *n* = 241]
56. Doyle LW, Crowther CA, Middleton P, et al. Magnesium sulphate for women at risk of preterm birth for neuroprotection of the fetus. *Cochrane Database Syst Rev.* 2009;(1):CD004661. [Meta-analysis: 5 RCTs, *n* = 6145]
57. Mittendorf R, Dambrosia J, Pryde PG, et al. Association between the use of antenatal magnesium sulfate in preterm labor

and adverse health outcomes in infants. *Am J Obstet Gynecol.* 2002;186:1111–1118. [RCT, n = 149]
58. Crowther CA, Hiller JE, Doyle LW, et al. Effect of magnesium sulfate given for neuroprotection before preterm birth: A randomized controlled trial. *JAMA.* 2003;290:2669–2676. [RCT, n = 1062]
59. Marret S, Marpeau L, Zupan-Simunek V, et al. Magnesium sulfate given before very-preterm birth to protect infant brain: The randomized controlled PREMAG trial. *BJOG.* 2007;114:310–318. [RCT, n = 688]
60. Rouse DJ, Hirtz DG, Thom E, et al. A randomized controlled trial of magnesium sulfate for the prevention of cerebral palsy. *NEJM.* 2008;359:895–905. [RCT, n = 2241]
61. Bain E, Middleton P, Crowther CA. Different magnesium sulphate regimens for neuroprotection of the fetus for women at risk of preterm birth. *Cochrane Database Syst Rev.* 2012;(2):CD009302. [No eligible completed trials identified]
62. Magee L, Sawchuck D, Synnes A, et al. SOGC Clinical Practice Guideline. Magnesium sulphate for fetal neuroprotection. *J Obstet Gynaecol Can.* 2011;33:516–529. [Guideline]
63. Australian Government National Health and Medical Research Council. *Clinical Practice Guidelines on Antenatal Magnesium Sulphate Prior to Preterm Birth for Neuroprotection of the Fetus, Infant and Child.* Canberra, Australia: NHMRC, 2010. [Guideline]
64. How HY, Cook CR, Cook VD, et al. Preterm premature rupture of membranes: Aggressive tocolysis versus expectant management. *J Matern Fetal Med.* 1998;7:8–12. [RCT, n = 145]
65. Briery CM, Veillon EW, Klauser CK, et al. Women with preterm premature rupture of the membranes do not benefit from weekly progesterone. *Am J Obstet Gynecol.* 2011;204:54.e1–54.e5. [RCT, n = 69 (17P, n = 33; placebo, n = 36)]
66. Combs CA, Garite TJ, Maurel K, et al. 17-Hydroxyprogesterone caproate for preterm rupture of the membranes: A multicenter, randomized, double-blind, placebo-controlled trial. *Am J Obstet Gynecol.* 2015;213:364.e1–364.e12. [RCT, n = 152]
67. Meis PJ, Society for Maternal-Fetal Medicine. 17-Hydroxyprogesterone for the prevention of preterm delivery. *Obstet Gynecol.* 2005;105(5 Pt 1):1128–1135. [Review]
68. Borna S, Borna H, Daneshbodie B. Vitamins C and E in the latency period in women with preterm premature rupture of membranes. *Int J Gynaecol Obstet.* 2005;90:16–20. [RCT, n = 60]
69. Gungorduk K, Asicioglu O, Gungorduk OC, et al. Does vitamin C and vitamin E supplementation prolong the latency period before delivery following the preterm premature rupture of the membranes? A randomized controlled study. *Am J Perinatol.* 2014;31:195–202. [RCT, n = 229]
70. Giraldo-Isaza MA, Berghella V. Cervical cerclage and preterm PPROM. *Clin Obstet Gynecol.* 2011;54:313–320. [Review]
71. Yeast JD, Garite TR. The role of cervical cerclage in the management of preterm premature rupture of membranes. *Am J Obstet Gynecol.* 1988;158:106–110. [II-2]
72. Blickstein I, Katz Z, Lancet M, et al. The outcome of pregnancies complicated by preterm rupture of the membranes with and without cerclage. *Int J Gynaecol Obstet.* 1989;28:237–242. [II-2]
73. Galyean A, Garite TJ, Maurel K, et al. Removal versus retention of cerclage in preterm premature rupture of membranes: A randomized controlled trial. *Am J Obstet Gynecol.* 2014;211:399. e1–399.e7. [RCT, n = 56]
74. Pergialiotis V, Gkioka E, Bakoyiannis I, et al. Retention of cervical cerclage after preterm premature rupture of the membranes: A critical appraisal. *Arch Gynecol Obstet.* 2015;291:745–753. [Meta-analysis: 6 studies, n = 293]
75. Buchanan SL, Crowther CA, Levett KM, et al. Planned early birth versus expectant management for women with preterm prelabour rupture of membranes prior to 37 weeks' gestation for improving pregnancy outcome. *Cochrane Database Syst Rev.* 2010;(3):CD004735. [Meta-analysis: 7 RCTs, n = 690]
76. Spinnato JA, Shaver DC, Bray EM, et al. Preterm premature rupture of the membranes with fetal pulmonary maturity present: A prospective study. *Obstet Gynecol.* 1987;69:196–201. [RCT, n = 47. PPROM at 25–36 weeks with L/S >2 or foam stability index >46. Tocolytics, steroids, or antibiotics were not used]
77. Mercer BM, Crocker LG, Boe NM, et al. Induction versus expectant management in premature rupture of the membranes with mature amniotic fluid at 32 to 36 weeks: A randomized trial. *Am J Obstet Gynecol.* 1993;169:775. [RCT, n = 93 women with PPROM at 32–36 6/7 weeks of gestation and a mature fetal lung profile. Tocolytics, steroids, or antibiotics were not used]
78. Cox SM, Leveno KJ. Intentional delivery versus expectant management with preterm ruptured membranes at 30–34 weeks' gestation. *Obstet Gynecol.* 1995;86:875. [RCT, n = 129 women with PPROM at 30–34 weeks of gestation. Tocolytics, steroids, or antibiotics were not used. 3/62 (5%) neonatal death in intentional delivery, vs 1/69 (1.4%) fetal death in induction groups]
79. Naef RW III, Allbert JR, Ross EL, et al. Premature rupture of membranes at 34 to 37 weeks' gestation: Aggressive versus conservative management. *Am J Obstet Gynecol.* 1998;178:126. [RCT, n = 120 women with PPROM at 34–36 weeks of gestation: chorioamnionitis 2% in induction vs. 16% in expectantly managed group. Tocolytics, steroids were not used; penicillin to all women for GBS prophylaxis]
80. van der Ham DP, Vijgen SM, Nijhuis JG, et al. Induction of labor versus expectant management in women with preterm prelabor rupture of membranes between 34 and 37 weeks: A randomized controlled trial. *PLoS Med.* 2012;9:e1001208. [RCT, n = 536]
81. van der Ham DP, van der Heyden JL, Opmeer BC, et al. Management of late-preterm premature rupture of membranes: The PPROMEXIL-2 trial. *Am J Obstet Gynecol.* 2012;207:276.e1–276.e10. [RCT, n = 195]
82. Tajik P, van der Ham DP, Zafarmand MH, et al. Using vaginal group B streptococcus colonisation in women with preterm premature rupture of membranes to guide the decision for immediate delivery: A secondary analysis of the PPROMEXIL trials. *BJOG.* 2014;121:1263–1272; discussion 1273. [Secondary analysis of the PPROMEXIL trials]
83. Morris JM, Roberts CL, Bowen JR, et al. Immediate delivery compared with expectant management after preterm prelabour rupture of the membranes close to term (PPROMT trial): A randomised controlled trial. *Lancet.* 2016;387:—444–452. [RCT, n = 1839]
84. Nageotte MP, Freeman RK, Garite TJ, et al. Prophylactic intrapartum amnioinfusion in patients with preterm premature rupture of membranes. *Am J Obstet Gynecol.* 1985;153:557–562. [RCT, n = 61]
85. Puertas A, Tirado P, Pérez I, et al. Transcervical intrapartum amnioinfusion for preterm premature rupture of the membranes. *Eur J Obstet Gynecol Reprod Biol.* 2007;131:40–44. [RCT, n = 86]
86. Lorch SA, Baiocchi M, Ahlberg CE, et al. The differential impact of delivery hospital on the outcomes of premature infants. *Pediatrics.* 2012;130:270–278. [II-2]
87. Chien LY, Whyte R, Aziz K, et al. Improved outcome of preterm infants when delivered in tertiary care centers. *Obstet Gynecol.* 2001;98:247–252. [II-2]
88. Borgida AF, Mills AA, Feldman DM, et al. Outcome of pregnancies complicated by ruptured membranes after genetic amniocentesis. *Am J Obstet Gynecol.* 2000;183:937–939. [II-3]
89. Quintero RA, Morales WJ, Allen M, et al. Treatment of iatrogenic previable premature rupture of membranes with intra-amniotic injection of platelets and cryoprecipitate (amniopatch): Preliminary experience. *Am J Obstet Gynecol.* 1999;181:744–749. [III]
90. Dinsmoor MJ, Bachman R, Haney EI, et al. Outcomes after expectant management of extremely preterm premature rupture of the membranes. *Am J Obstet Gynecol.* 2004;190:183–187. [II-3]
91. Waters TP, Mercer BM. The management of preterm premature rupture of the membranes near the limit of fetal viability. *Am J Obstet Gynecol.* 2009;201:230–240. [Review]

92. Manuck TA, Eller AG, Esplin MS, et al. Outcomes of expectantly managed preterm premature rupture of membranes occurring before 24 weeks of gestation. *Obstet Gynecol.* 2009;114:29–37. [II-2]
93. Azria E, Anselem O, Schmitz T, et al. Comparison of perinatal outcome after pre-viable preterm prelabour rupture of membranes in two centres with different rates of termination of pregnancy. *BJOG.* 2012;119:449–457. [II-2]
94. Manuck TA, Varner MW. Neonatal and early childhood outcomes following early vs later preterm premature rupture of membranes. *Am J Obstet Gynecol.* 2014;211:308.e1–308.e6. [Secondary analysis of RCT, 275 early PPROM cases]
95. Brumbaugh JE, Colaizy TT, Nuangchamnong N, et al. Neonatal survival after prolonged preterm premature rupture of membranes before 24 weeks of gestation. *Obstet Gynecol.* 2014;124:992–998. [II-3]
96. Taylor J, Garite J. Premature rupture of membranes before fetal viability. *Obstet Gynecol.* 1984;64:615–620. [III]
97. Dowd J, Permezel M. Pregnancy outcome following preterm premature rupture of the membranes at less than 26 weeks' gestation. *Aust NZ J Obstet Gynaecol.* 1992;32:120–124. [III]
98. Beydoun SN, Yasin SY. Premature rupture of the membranes before 28 weeks: Conservative management. *Am J Obstet Gynecol.* 1986;155:471–479. [II-3]
99. McElrath TF, Allred EN, Leviton A. Prolonged latency after preterm premature rupture of membranes: An evaluation of histologic condition and intracranial ultrasonic abnormality in the neonate born at <28 weeks of gestation. *Am J Obstet Gynecol.* 2003;189:794–798. [II-2]
100. Hadi HA, Hodson CA, Strickland D. Premature rupture of the membranes between 20 and 25 weeks' gestation: Role of amniotic fluid volume in perinatal outcome. *Am J Obstet Gynecol.* 1994;170:1139–1144. [II-2]
101. Holmgren PA, Olofsson JI. Preterm premature rupture of membranes and the associated risk for placental abruption. Inverse correlation to gestational length. *Acta Obstet Gynecol Scand.* 1997;76:743–747. [II-2]
102. Farooqi A, Holmgren PA, Engberg S, et al. Survival and 2-year outcome with expectant management of second-trimester rupture of membranes. *Obstet Gynecol.* 1998;92:895–901. [II-3]
103. Kilbride HW, Yeast J, Thibeault DW. Defining limits of survival: Lethal pulmonary hypoplasia after midtrimester premature rupture of membranes. *Am J Obstet Gynecol.* 1996;175:675–681. [II-2]
104. Canavan TP, Simhan HN, Caritis S. An evidence based approach to the evaluation and treatment of premature rupture of membranes: Part II. *Obstet Gynecol Surv.* 2004;59:678–689. [Review]
105. Winn HN, Chen M, Amon E, et al. Neonatal pulmonary hypoplasia and perinatal mortality in patients with midtrimester rupture of amniotic membranes—a critical analysis. *Am J Obstet Gynecol.* 2000;182:1638–1644. [II-3]
106. Vergani P, Ghidini A, Locatelli A, et al. Risk factors of pulmonary hypoplasia in second trimester premature rupture of membranes. *Am J Obstet Gynecol.* 1994;170:1359–1364. [II-2]
107. Rotschild A, Ling EW, Puterman ML, et al. Neonatal outcome after prolonged preterm rupture of the membranes. *Am J Obstet Gynecol.* 1990;162:46–52. [II-2]
108. Shumway JB, Al-Malt A, Amon E, et al. Impact of oligohydramnios on maternal and perinatal outcomes of spontaneous premature rupture of the membranes at 18–28 weeks. *J Matern Fetal Med.* 1999;8:20–23. [II-3]
109. Vergani P, Andreani M, Greco M, et al. Two- or three-dimensional ultrasonography: Which is the best predictor of pulmonary hypoplasia? *Prenat Diagn.* 2010;30:834–838. [II-2]
110. Falk SJ, Campbell LJ, Lee-Parritz A, et al. Expectant management in spontaneous preterm premature rupture of membranes between 14 and 24 weeks' gestation. *J Perinatol.* 2004;24:611–616. [II-3]
111. van Teeffelen AS, Van Der Heijden J, Oei SG, et al. Accuracy of imaging parameters in the prediction of lethal pulmonary hypoplasia secondary to mid-trimester prelabor rupture of fetal membranes: A systematic review and meta-analysis. *Ultrasound Obstet Gynecol.* 2012;39:495–499. [Meta-analysis, 13 studies]
112. Verma U, Tejani N, Klein S, et al. Obstetric antecedents of intraventricular hemorrhage and periventricular leukomalacia in the lowbirth—eight neonate. *Am J Obstet Gynecol.* 1997;176:275–281. [II-2]
113. Perlman JM, Risser R, Broyles S. Bilateral cystic periventricular leukomalacia in the premature infant: Associated risk factors. *Pediatrics.* 1996;97:822–827. [II-2]
114. Fortunato SJ, Welt SI, Eggleston MK Jr., et al. Active expectant management in very early gestations complicated by premature rupture of the fetal membranes. *J Reprod Med.* 1994;39:13–16. [II-3]
115. Locatelli A, Vergani P, Di Pirro G, et al. Role of amnioinfusion in the management of premature preterm rupture of membranes at <26 weeks gestation. *Am J Obstet Gynecol.* 2000;183:878–882. [II-2]
116. Vintzileos AM, Campbell WA, Nochimson DJ, et al. Degree of oligohydramnios and pregnancy outcome in patients with premature rupture of the membranes. *Obstet Gynecol.* 1985;66:162–167. [II-2]
117. Lee JY, Ahn TG, Jun JK. Short-term and long-term postnatal outcomes of expectant management after previable preterm premature rupture of membranes with and without persistent oligohydramnios. *Obstet Gynecol.* 2015;126:947–953. [II-2]
118. Porat S, Amsalem H, Shah PS, et al. Transabdominal amnioinfusion for preterm premature rupture of membranes: A systematic review and meta-analysis of randomized and observational studies. *Am J Obstet Gynecol.* 2012;207:393.e1–393.e11. [Meta-analysis, 7 studies]
119. Van Teeffelen S, Pajkrt E, Willekes C, et al. Transabdominal amnioinfusion for improving fetal outcomes after oligohydramnios secondary to preterm prelabour rupture of membranes before 26 weeks. *Cochrane Database Syst Rev.* 2013;(8):CD009952. [No eligible trials identified]
120. Roberts D, Vause S, Martin W, et al. Amnioinfusion in very early preterm prelabor rupture of membranes (AMIPROM): Pregnancy, neonatal and maternal outcomes in a randomized controlled pilot study. *Ultrasound Obstet Gynecol.* 2014;43:490–499. [RCT, *n* = 56]
121. Gold RB, Goyert GL, Schwartz DB, et al. Conservative management of second-trimester postamniocentesis fluid leakage. *Obstet Gynecol.* 1989;74:745–747. [II-3]
122. Beck V, Lewi P, Gucciardo L, et al. Preterm prelabor rupture of membranes and fetal survival after minimally invasive fetal surgery: A systematic review of the literature. *Fetal Diagn Ther.* 2012;31:1–9. [Review]
123. Gratacos E, Sanin-Blair J, Lewi L, et al. A histological study of fetoscopic membrane defects to document membrane healing. *Placenta.* 2006;27:452–456. [III]
124. Sciscione AC, Manley JS, Pollock M, et al. Intracervical fibrin sealants: A potential treatment for early preterm premature rupture of the membranes. *Am J Obstet Gynecol.* 2001;184:368–373. [III]
125. Reddy UM, Shah SS, Nemiroff RL, et al. In vitro sealing of punctured fetal membranes: Potential treatment for midtrimester premature rupture of membranes. *Am J Obstet Gynecol.* 2001;185:1090–1093. [III]
126. Lewi L, Van Schoubroeck D, Van Ranst M, et al. Successful patching of iatrogenic rupture of the fetal membranes. *Placenta.* 2004;25:352–356. [III]
127. O'Brien JM, Barton JR, Milligan DA. An aggressive interventional protocol for early midtrimester premature rupture of the membranes using gelatin sponge for cervical plugging. *Am J Obstet Gynecol.* 2002;187:1143–1146. [III]
128. Young BK, Roque H, Abdelhak YE, et al. Minimally invasive endoscopy in the treatment of preterm premature rupture of membranes by application of fibrin sealant. *J Perinat Med.* 2000;28:326–330. [III]

129. Young BK, Roman AS, MacKenzie AP, et al. The closure of iatrogenic membrane defects after amniocentesis and endoscopic intrauterine procedures. *Fetal Diagn Ther.* 2004;19:296–300. [III]
130. Deprest J, Emonds MP, Richter J, et al. Amniopatch for iatrogenic rupture of the fetal membranes. *Prenat Diagn.* 2011;31:661–666. [Review]
131. Richter J, Henry A, Ryan G, et al. Amniopatch procedure after previable iatrogenic rupture of the membranes: A two-center review. *Prenat Diagn.* 2013;33:391–396. [III]
132. Sela HY, Simpson LL. Preterm premature rupture of membranes complicating twin pregnancy: Management considerations. *Clin Obstet Gynecol.* 2011;54:321–329. [Review]
133. Ehsanipoor RM, Arora N, Lagrew DC, et al. Twin versus singleton pregnancies complicated by preterm premature rupture of membranes. *J Matern Fetal Neonatal Med.* 2012;25:658–661. [II-3]
134. Hsieh YY, Chang CC, Tsai HD, et al. Twin vs. singleton pregnancy. Clinical characteristics and latency periods in preterm premature rupture of membranes. *J Reprod Med.* 1999;44:616–620. [II-3]
135. Myles TD, Espinoza R, Meyer W, Bieniarz A. Preterm premature rupture of membranes: Comparison between twin and singleton gestations. *J Matern Fetal Med.* 1997;6:159–163. [II-3]
136. Wong L, Holmgren C, Silver R, et al. Outcomes of expectantly managed pregnancies with multiple gestations and preterm premature rupture of membranes prior to 26 weeks. *Am J Obstet Gynecol.* 2015;212:215.e1–215.e9. [II-3]
137. Cohen A, Skornick-Rapaport A, Cohen Y, et al. The influence of prolonged preterm premature rupture of the membranes on neonatal outcome of the presenting and non-presenting twin. *Eur J Obstet Gynecol Reprod Biol.* 2014;181:28–31. [II-3]
138. Trentacoste SV, Jean-Pierre C, Baergen R, Chasen ST. Outcomes of preterm premature rupture of membranes in twin pregnancies. *J Matern Fetal Neonatal Med.* 2008;21:555–557. [II-3]
139. Mendez-Figueroa H, Dahlke JD, Viteri OA, et al. Neonatal and infant outcomes in twin gestations with preterm premature rupture of membranes at 24–31 weeks of gestation. *Obstet Gynecol.* 2014;124(2 Pt 1):323–331. [II-2, secondary analysis of RCT]

Premature rupture of membranes at or near term

Kimberly Ma and Sally Segel

KEY POINTS

- **The diagnosis** of premature rupture of membranes (PROMs) at term is based on **pooling, ferning**, and **nitrazine tests** on speculum examination. Rapid bedside immunoassays such as placental alpha-microglobulin-1 or others may be helpful in cases in which the diagnosis of rupture of membrane (ROM) is suspected, but cannot be confirmed with pooling, ferning, and/or nitrazine tests. Initial digital examinations should be avoided, as it is associated with a higher risk of infection.
- **The main complication is intrauterine infection; this incidence** increases with duration of PROM, and, with longer latency, the risk of **neonatal infection** also increases.
- Women with PROM at term should be **hospitalized** and **induced** with **oxytocin** within 6 to 12 hours of PROM, or earlier as feasible. **Most women with PROM at term, if given a choice, prefer induction.** Oxytocin induction is safe, effective, and cost-effective. Misoprostol induction is an alternative that is just as effective when 25 mg every 4 hour dosing is used, but there is limited data regarding its safety. Foley catheter ripening is another safe and efficacious alternative, especially in cases of unfavorable cervical examination.
- Antibiotics are recommended if the patient is group B streptococcus (GBS) positive, or complications (chorioamnionitis, PROM >18 hours) develop during labor. In women expected to have a latency from PROM to delivery of over 12 hours, antibiotics are associated with significantly decreased chorioamnionitis and endometritis.

DEFINITION

Premature rupture of membranes (PROM) is rupture of fetal membranes prior to the onset of labor [1]. Preterm premature rupture of membranes (PPROM) is premature rupture of fetal membranes ≤37 weeks [1]. This chapter includes guidance for near-term (34–36 6/7 weeks) as well as term (≥37 weeks) PROM. For PPROM <34 weeks, see Chapter 19.

DIAGNOSIS

The diagnosis of PROM and PPROM is based on history and physical examination findings (see also Chapter 19). A maternal history suggestive of PROM includes a gush of fluid soaking clothes or a constant trickle of fluid that does not stop. Physical examination for PROM starts with a *sterile speculum* examination [1–3]. **Visualization of amniotic fluid passing from the cervical canal is diagnostic** of this condition [1–3].

Another helpful test is the **nitrazine test**. The pH of the vagina is usually 4.5 to 6.0, whereas amniotic fluid has a pH 7.0 to 7.7; nitrazine paper turns blue with pH >6.5 [1,2]. A false positive nitrazine test can be caused from blood, semen, alkaline antiseptic, or bacterial vaginosis. A false-negative nitrazine test can be caused by prolonged leaking of amniotic fluid or minimal residual fluid. The sensitivity of nitrazine is 90.2% (81.3%–100%) and the specificity is 79.3% (16%–100%) [2].

A third helpful test is called **"ferning."** A swab of vaginal fluid from the posterior fornix is placed on a slide and allowed to air dry. Arborization (ferning) under microscopic visualization suggests rupture of membranes. Cervical mucus can cause a false positive result. Ferning has a sensitivity of 90.8% (62.0%–98.5%) and a specificity of 95.3% (88.2%–100%) [2].

The combination of vaginal pool of fluid, nitrazine, and ferning has a sensitivity of 90.8% and a specificity of 95.6% [2]. These tests are more accurate when patients present in labor and less accurate when nonlaboring [3]. If these tests are equivocal, an ultrasound can be performed to evaluate for amniotic fluid, but oligohydramnios is not diagnostic of PROM, since it can be associated with other etiologies, such as placental insufficiency.

Placental alpha-microglobulin-1 is a 34-kDa glycoprotein abundant in amniotic fluid (2,000–25,000 ng/mL); there is a negligible amount of this glycoprotein in vaginal fluid with intact fetal membranes (0.05–2.0 ng/mL) [2,4,5]. AmniSure is a bedside immunoassay that uses the delta in concentration of placental alpha-microglobulin-1 for diagnostic accuracy. AmniSure has a sensitivity of 98.7% to 98.9% and a specificity of 87.5% to 100% [4,5].

Insulin-like growth factor–binding protein 1 (IGFBP-1) has a high concentration in the amniotic fluid compared with other body fluids such as vaginal secretions, urine, or semen [6]. An immunochromatography dipstick method (Actim PROM) is available to diagnose rupture of membranes. The test is more popular in Europe compared with the United States and is most accurate when the timing of the test is close to the timing of rupture of membranes. The sensitivity of the test is 95%–100% with a specificity of 93%–98%. [7–10].

A negative fetal fibronectin can be helpful in ruling out rupture of membranes, however a positive test cannot distinguish between intact and rupture of membranes [11]. Alpha-fetoprotein levels are higher in amniotic fluid compared with urine, semen, or normal vaginal discharge. A recent study showed a 96.2% sensitivity and 100% specificity, however may be falsely positive if a vaginal infection is present and requires further study in a larger cohort [12]. Further studies are needed to assess reliability with special attention paid to time of presumed membrane rupture [2,3]. **Placental alpha-microglobulin-1, IGFBP-1, and these other tests have limited clinical applicability** currently given the high accuracy of pooling, ferning, and nitrazine tests. Nonetheless, they **can be helpful in cases in which the diagnosis of ROM is suspected, but cannot be confirmed with pooling, ferning, and/or nitrazine tests.**

INCIDENCE

PROM occurs in approximately 8% of all term deliveries [1].

ETIOLOGY

The etiology of PROM without signs of infection or bleeding is often unknown, and this should be considered a physiologic, not pathologic, event.

RISK FACTORS

The risk factors associated with rupture of fetal membranes include low socioeconomic status, low body mass index (BMI) <19.8 kg/m^2, nutritional deficiencies of ascorbic acid and cooper, connective tissue disorders, smoking, cold knife cone biopsy, cervical cerclage, pulmonary disease, uterine overdistension, and amniocentesis [1]. In addition, pregnant women with a previous preterm birth, midtrimester short cervix, and preterm labor are at increased risk for PROM; however, the majority of cases have no identifiable cause [1].

COMPLICATIONS

The most common complications of PROM are **chorioamnionitis, endomyometritis, and postpartum hemorrhage.** With increasing time interval from rupture of membranes, there is a significant increase in these complications: about 12 hours for chorioamnionitis, 16 hours for endometritis, and 8 hours for postpartum hemorrhage [13]. As the latency from ROM to delivery increases, so does the risk for neonatal infection. Maternal GBS colonization also increases the risk for neonatal infection. Incidence of cesarean section is not affected by management with either induction or expectant management, but depends on other risk factors (e.g., nulliparity) [14].

MANAGEMENT
Initial Evaluation

Initial evaluation of PROM involves confirmation of the diagnosis. **Digital examination** can increase the risk of infection and as a result **should be avoided** [14]. The cervix can be visually assessed for dilation and effacement [15]. Fetal presentation should be confirmed by ultrasound. Fetal well-being and the presence of uterine contractions should be assessed by external monitoring.

Counseling

Risk factors, complications, and management of PROM should be reviewed with the patient. About 50% of women with PROM at term deliver within 6–12 hours and 95% of women will deliver within 28 hours of membrane rupture [1,14]. Principles of management can be reviewed (Table 20.1).

Hospitalization

Compared with management in the hospital, expectant management of PROM at term at **home** is associated with a 52% increase in **need for maternal antibiotics** for nulliparas and 97% more **neonatal infections** [16]. **PROM at term should be managed in hospital.**

Delivery versus Expectant Management

Women with PPROM ≥34 weeks should be delivered (see also Chapter 19). Induction of labor with oxytocin has been shown to **decrease the rate of maternal chorioamnionitis and postpartum fevers** without significantly affecting the rate of cesarean delivery, compared with expectant management [14]. In most randomized controlled trials (RCTs), induction was with oxytocin or prostaglandin, with one trial using homeopathic caulophyllum. Overall, no differences are detected for mode of birth between induced and expectant groups: cesarean (relative risk [RR] 0.94, 95% confidence interval [CI] 0.82–1.08); operative vaginal birth (RR 0.98, 95% 0.84–1.16). Significantly fewer women in the induced compared with expectant management groups have chorioamnionitis (RR 0.74, 95% CI 0.56–0.97) or endometritis (RR 0.30, 95% CI 0.12–0.74). No difference is seen for neonatal infection (RR 0.83, 95% CI 0.61–1.12). However, fewer infants under induced management went to neonatal intensive or special care compared with expectant management (RR 0.72, 95% CI 0.57–0.92, number needed to treat is 20) [17].

Compared with expectant management, induction of labor by **oxytocin** is associated with a 37% *decrease* in risk of **maternal infection,** 28% in **endometritis,** and 36% in **neonatal infection** [17]. Based on one trial, women were more likely to view their care positively if labor was induced with oxytocin [14]. Cesarean delivery rates are similar between groups. Oxytocin is associated with more frequent use of pain relief and internal fetal heart rate monitoring. Perinatal mortality rates are low and not significantly different between groups, although the **trend** is toward **fewer perinatal deaths** with induction of labor by oxytocin [17].

Compared with placebo or no treatment, both **vaginal prostaglandin E2 (PGE2) and F2a (PGF2a)** reduce the likelihood of vaginal delivery not being achieved within 24 hours, with no evidence of a difference in cesarean delivery [17]. Induction of labor by prostaglandins is associated with a decrease by 23% in risk of chorioamnionitis and by 21% in admission to neonatal intensive care. Induction by prostaglandins is associated with a more frequent maternal diarrhea and use of anesthesia and/or analgesia [17]. There is insufficient data to make meaningful conclusions for the comparison of vaginal PGE2 and PGF2a. PGE2 tablet, gel, and pessary appear to be as efficacious as each other. Lower-dose regimens appear as efficacious as higher dose regimens [17].

Medications for Induction

Immediate induction of labor with intravenous **oxytocin** has been shown to decrease the rate of maternal infection without increasing the rate of cesarean section [14]. Please see above data on individual agents for induction compared with placebo or no treatment.

Currently, there have been no studies that demonstrate misoprostol or PGE2 are superior to intravenous oxytocin even in women with an unfavorable cervix [18]. However, when misoprostol is compared with PGE2, length of labor is shorter but there is increased uterine tachysystole [18].

Table 20.1 Management of PPROM at ≥34 Weeks

- Deliver
- Manage in hospital
- There is insufficient evidence to recommend one induction agent over another, but oxytocin has been the best studied for safety and effectiveness. The balloon is also safe and effective, and can be considered especially when the cervix is <3 cm dilated
- Antibiotics are recommended if the patient is GBS positive, or complications (chorioamnionitis, PROM >18 hours) develop during labor. In women expected to have a latency from PROM to delivery of over 12 hours, antibiotics are associated with significantly decreased chorioamnionitis and endometritis

Abbreviations: GBS, group B streptococcus; PPROM, preterm premature rupture of membranes; PROM, premature rupture of membranes.

Compared with **prostaglandins,** induction with **oxytocin** is associated with **decrease** in maternal nausea and/or vomiting, numerous vaginal examinations, **chorioamnionitis** and **neonatal infections,** neonatal antibiotic therapy, and **admission to neonatal intensive care unit (NICU),** but increase in epidural analgesia and internal fetal heart rate monitoring. Cesarean delivery, endometritis, and perinatal mortality are not significantly different between the groups [17]. Cost is less with oxytocin induction.

Vaginal **misoprostol** in doses above 25 μg every 4 hours is more effective than PGE2, intracervical PGE2, and oxytocin (or obviously expectant management) in achieving vaginal delivery [17,19]. **Compared with oxytocin, misoprostol** was associated with a decrease in cesarean section from 51% to 20% in a small trial in women with an unfavorable cervix and from 14% to 11% in other women [17,19]. If a dose of 50 μg of vaginal misoprostol is used, in 85% of cases only one dose is needed for induction with term PROM, but this is associated with a higher rate of uterine tachysystole compared with oxytocin, with similar maternal and neonatal outcomes [20]. However, the studies reviewed were not large enough to exclude the possibility of serious adverse events with misoprostol including neonatal complications from uterine hyperstimulation. Lower doses of vaginal misoprostol were similar to other methods in effectiveness and risk. Oral misoprostol appears to be an effective means of labor induction comparable to oxytocin, but again the studies reviewed were not large enough to exclude the possibility of serious adverse events with misoprostol [21–23].

There is insufficient evidence to assess if the combination of dinoprostone (PGE2) together with oxytocin is superior to oxytocin alone [24].

The safety and efficacy of **Foley bulbs** or other mechanical means of induction in women with PROM have been evaluated, and Foley appears to be both **safe and efficacious** for cervical ripening of women with PROM and unfavorable cervical examination [25–27] (see also Chapter 21).

In summary, in patients with PROM at term, once the diagnosis has been confirmed, **induction of labor is recommended.** Induction should probably occur at least within 6–12 hours of PPROM, or earlier if feasible. If expectant management is performed, there is a significant increase in chorioamnionitis and neonatal infection and time duration increases [28–30]. **Currently, oxytocin is the recommended induction medication, as it is safe, effective, and cost-effective.** Foley bulb (or other balloon) is also a safe and effective intervention, especially if unfavorable cervical examination (e.g., cervix <3 cm dilated) [25–27]. Vaginal and oral misoprostol are also safe and effective but have not been proven to be superior to oxytocin when appropriate doses (e.g., 25 μg for vaginal misoprostol) are used [18]. With increasing latency from PROM to delivery, there is an increased risk for chorioamnionitis, endomyometritis, and postpartum hemorrhage [13]. Women should be counseled to initiate induction of labor in order to decrease the risk of these complications.

Antibiotics

GBS positive: In women with a positive GBS culture, antibiotics should be administered according to the CDC guideline [31] (see Chapter 37 in *Maternal-Fetal Evidence Based Guidelines*). **Women who are GBS positive with PROM at ≥34 weeks are treated with penicillin in labor.** Ampicillin is a reasonable alternative. If the patient is penicillin-allergic but not at high risk for anaphylaxis, cefazolin is the agent of choice. For women at high risk for anaphylaxis, GBS isolate should be tested for susceptibility to clindamycin and erythromycin. Vancomycin is recommended if isolate is resistant to either clindamycin or erythromycin. Intrapartum treatment for chorioamnionitis is recommended regardless of GBS maternal status.

In these revised recommendations, 4 hours of intravenous antibiotics are considered adequate treatment for a neonate; however, no medically necessary obstetric procedure should be delayed to achieve 4 hours of intravenous antibiotic therapy [31]. If a patient presents with PROM at term, antibiotics can be administered and induction of labor can begin concurrently. In addition, if a woman is scheduled for a repeat cesarean section and presents with PROM, GBS antibiotic prophylaxis should be administered while arranging for the repeat cesarean section [31].

GBS negative: There is **some evidence to recommend for antibiotics in GBS-negative women with PPROM at ≥34 weeks.** A recent meta-analysis evaluated the efficacy of antibiotic prophylaxis in women with term or near-term premature rupture of membranes and concluded antibiotic prophylaxis was not associated with maternal or neonatal benefits. However in women with latency greater than 12 hours, prophylactic antibiotics were associated with significantly lower rates of chorioamnionitis (2.9% vs. 6.1%, RR 0.49, 95% CI 0.27–0.91) and endometritis (0% vs. 2.2%, RR 0.12, 95% CI 0.02–0.62) [32].

GBS status unknown: If the patient has no risk factors (previous infant with GBS sepsis, <37 weeks, rupture of membranes >18 hours, chorioamnionitis), antibiotics can still be considered, especially in the woman expected to have a latency to delivery interval >12 hours [20]. Alternatively, in PPROM 34 to 36 6/7 weeks, if the patient has no GBS culture from the previous 5 weeks, antibiotics can be administered per protocol or a rapid GBS test can be performed. If the rapid GBS result is negative, antibiotics can be withheld unless other risk factors develop (chorioamnionitis or rupture of fetal membranes greater than 18 hours) [31].

In summary, for PROM at ≥34 weeks, antibiotics should be given if the woman is GBS+ or infectious complications develop during labor [33], and considered for all women with expected latency from PPROM to delivery >12 hours [32].

Special Considerations for PPROM at 34 to 36 Weeks' Gestation

Management of PPROM from 34 0/7 to 36 6/7 weeks is based on extrapolation from a few small studies [34–38], and therefore the scientific evidence is limited. These studies were performed before a standardized therapy for PPROM was developed, and corticosteroids and antibiotics were not routinely used. The current The American Congress of Obstetricians and Gynecologists (ACOG) Practice Bulletin states that "**At 34 0/7 weeks or greater of gestation, delivery is recommended for all women with ruptured membranes.** If expectant management is continued beyond 34 0/7 weeks of gestation, the balance between benefit and risk should be carefully considered and discussed with the patient, and expectant management should not extend beyond 37 0/7 weeks of gestation." [1].

Recent studies have called attention to the neonatal complications of late PTB, which include respiratory complications, sepsis evaluations, hyperbilirubinemia requiring phototherapy, and death. This combination of potential complications has led to an increase in NICU admissions, increasing length of stay (LOS), urgent hospital visits, and hospital readmissions [39–46]. The effort to decrease late-preterm birth in the United

States has been successful, with a decrease from 9.15% in 2006 to 7.99% in 2013 (a 13% decrease) [47].

The original research determining the best antenatal approach to PPROM including the late preterm period studied patients with documented fetal lung maturity [35,36]. Spinnato et al. randomized 47 nonlaboring PPROM patients to either delivery or expectant management with hospitalization and intensive antenatal surveillance. There was a statistically significant increase in chorioamnionitis or postpartum endometritis in expectant management group; however, neonatal morbidity and mortality were similar between groups [35]. Mercer et al. also randomized 93 PPROM patients from 32 to 36 weeks' gestation with fetal lung maturity to immediate induction of labor or expectant management. Women randomized to expectant management had a significant increase in chorioamnionitis and fetal heart rate abnormalities in labor [36]. In addition, neonates from the expectant management group had a significant increase in the initiation and length of antibiotic treatment for presumed neonatal infection [36]. These two trials had significant similarities in that the expectant management group was hospitalized with intensive surveillance and antibiotics were only administered for chorioamnionitis. Overall their results demonstrated that expectant management in PPROM patients, including the late preterm period and with fetal lung maturity, had longer latencies and increased maternal infection without significant neonatal benefit. Naef et al. also performed a randomized trial of 120 PPROM patients in the late preterm period. Women in the expectant management group received GBS prophylaxis during their hospitalization [37]. Even with the addition of GBS prophylaxis, women randomized to the expectant management group had a significant increase in chorioamnionitis and their neonates had a significant increase in NICU admission with a trend toward an increase in culture-proven sepsis [37]. Overall, these studies found that **expectant management produced longer latencies; however, there was a significant increase in maternal infection without demonstration of neonatal benefit** [35–37]. Unfortunately the meta-analysis of the seven RCTs on this issue is not clinically helpful as studies have been underpowered for significant neonatal and maternal outcomes [48].

Two international RCTs compared delivery versus expectant management in women with PPROM diagnosed at 34–36 6/7 weeks gestation. In the combined analysis of 736 women who were randomized, induction of labor reduced the risk of chorioamnionitis (1.6% vs. 5.3%, RR 0.31, 95% CI 0.1–0.8). There was no statistical difference in neonatal sepsis with (2.7% with induction of labor vs. 4.1% with expectant management; RR 0.66, 95% CI 0.30–1.5). The overall rate of neonatal sepsis was lower than expected, and therefore the studies did not have adequate power to show a statistical difference in neonatal sepsis [49–50].

A recent multicenter randomized controlled trial was performed at 65 centers in 11 countries with 1839 women [51]. Women with ruptured membranes between 34 0/7 and 36 6/7 weeks gestation were randomized to immediate delivery or expectant management looking at the primary outcome of neonatal sepsis. There was no statistical difference in neonatal sepsis (2% in immediate delivery versus 3% in expectant management, RR 0.8, 95% CI 0.5–1.3). The immediate delivery group had increased rates of respiratory distress (RR 1.6, 95% CI 1.1–2.3), mechanical ventilation (RR 1.4, 95% CI 1.0–1.8), and longer intensive care unit days (4 days vs. 2 days, $p < 0.01$) compared with the expectant management group. However, women in the immediate delivery group had a lower rate of antepartum or intrapartum hemorrhage (RR 0.6, 95% CI 0.4–0.9), intrapartum fever (RR 0.4, 95% CI 0.2–0.9), postpartum antibiotic use (RR 0.8, 95% CI 0.7–1.0), and longer hospital stay (5 days vs. 6 days, $p < 0.01$). Expectant management performed at this gestational age should weigh the potential neonatal benefits with the maternal risks with the consideration of the use of latency antibiotics.

With the additional information from these studies, ACOG continues to **recommend delivery for all women with ruptured membranes after 34 0/7 weeks or greater**. Although there is concern for neonatal risks associated with late preterm birth, neonates born to women with ruptured membranes have a higher rate of adverse outcomes when matched with controls for gestational age and higher complications when chorioamnionitis is present [52,53]. Delivery of all women with ruptured membranes after 34 0/7 weeks or greater should continue to be the standard of care until there is additional data.

There is new evidence that steroids are associated with neonatal benefits also ≥34 weeks, as three RCTs have been done on steroids 34–36 6/7 weeks in women at risk of PTB, and two RCTs in women at ≥37 weeks. Infants of women who received antenatal corticosteroids ≥34 weeks had a significantly lower incidence of respiratory distress syndrome (RDS) (RR 0.76, 95% CI 0.62–0.93), mild RDS (RR 0.40, 95% CI 0.23–0.69), moderate RDS (RR 0.39, 95% CI 0.18–0.89), transient tachypnea of the newborn (RR 0.62, 95% CI 0.50–0.77), severe RDS (RR 0.66, 95% CI 0.53–0.82), use of surfactant (RR 0.61, 95% CI 0.38–0.99), mechanical ventilation (RR 0.62, 95% CI 0.41 to 0.94), significantly lower time on oxygen (mean difference [MD] –2.06 hours, 95% CI –2.17 to –1.95), lower maximum inspired oxygen concentration (MD –0.66%, 95% CI –0.69 to –0.63), lower LOS in NICU (MD –7.64 days, 95% CI –7.65 to –7.64), higher Apgar score at 1 and at 5 minutes (MD 0.06, 95% CI 0.05–0.07) compared with those who did not. Steroids should be considered for decreasing respiratory morbidities and other neonatal outcomes in women ≥34 weeks [54,55]. See Chapter 19 for other details on management for women with PPROM <34 weeks [48].

REFERENCES

1. American College of Obstetricians and Gynecologists. *ACOG Practice Bulletin No. 139: Premature Rupture of Membranes.* Washington, DC: ACOG, 2013. [Review]
2. El-Messidi A, Cameron A. Diagnosis of premature rupture of membranes: Inspiration from the past and insights for the future. *J Obstet Gynaecol Can.* 2010;32(6):561–569. [Review]
3. Strevens H, Allen K, Thornton JG. Management of premature prelabor rupture of the membranes. *Ann N Y Acad Sci.* 2010;1205:123–129. [Review; 44 refs]
4. Lee SE, Park JS, Norwitz ER, et al. Measurement of placental alpha-microglobulin-1 in cervicovaginal discharge to diagnose rupture of membranes. *Obstet Gynecol.* 2007;109(3):634–640. [II-2]
5. Cousins LM, Smok DP, Lovett SM, et al. AmniSure placental alpha microglobulin-1 rapid immunoassay versus standard diagnostic methods for detection of rupture of membranes. *Am J Perinatol.* 2005;22(6):317–320. [II-3]
6. Darj E, Lyrenäs S. Insulin-like growth factor binding protein-1, a quick way to detect amniotic fluid. *Acta Obstet Gynecol Scand.* 1998;77:295. [II-3]
7. Gaucherand P, Salle B, Sergeant P, et al. Comparative study of three vaginal markers of the premature rupture of membranes. Insulin like growth factor binding protein 1 diamine-oxidase pH. *Acta Obstet Gynecol Scand.* 1997;76:536. [II-2]

8. Erdemoglu E, Mungan T. Significance of detecting insulin-like growth factor binding protein-1 in cervicovaginal secretions: Comparison with nitrazine test and amniotic fluid volume assessment. *Acta Obstet Gynecol Scand.* 2004;83:622. [II-3]
9. Akercan F, Cirpan T, Kazandi M, et al. The value of the insulin-like growth factor binding protein-1 in the cervical-vaginal secretion detected by immunochromatographic dipstick test in the prediction of delivery in women with clinically unconfirmed preterm premature rupture of membranes. *Eur J Obstet Gynecol Reprod Biol.* 2005;121:159. [II-2]
10. Marcellin L, Anselem O, Guibourdenche J, et al. Comparison of two bedside tests performed on cervicovaginal fluid to diagnose premature rupture of membranes. *J Gynecol Obstet Biol Reprod (Paris).* 2011;40:651. [II-2]
11. Eriksen NL, Parisi VM, Daoust S, et al. Fetal fibronectin: A method for detecting the presence of amniotic fluid. *Obstet Gynecol.* 1992;80:451. [II-2]
12. Mor A, Tal R, Haberman S, et al. Alpha-fetoprotein as a tool to distinguish amniotic fluid from urine, vaginal discharge, and semen. *Obstet Gynecol.* 2015;125:448. [II-2]
13. Tran SH, Cheng YW, Kaimal AJ, et al. Length of rupture of membranes in the setting of premature rupture of membranes at term and infectious maternal morbidity. *Am J Obstet Gynecol.* 2008;198(6):700.e1–700.e5. [II-2]
14. Hannah ME, Ohlsson A, Farine D, et al. Induction of labor compared with expectant management for prelabor rupture of the membranes at term. *N Engl J Med.* 1996;334:1005–1010. [RCT, n = 5041]
15. Pereira L, Gould R, Pelham J, et al. Correlation between visual examination of the cervix and digital examination. *J Matern Fetal Neonatal Med.* 2005;17(3):223–227. [II-2]
16. Hannah ME, Hodnett ED, Willan A, et al. Prelabor rupture of the membranes at term: Expectant management at home or in the hospital? Obstet Gynecol. 2000;96:533–538. [RCT secondary analysis, n = 1670]
17. Dare MR, Middleton P, Crowther CA, et al. Planned early birth versus expectant management (waiting) for prelabour rupture of membranes at term (37 weeks or more). *Cochrane Database Syst Rev.* 2006;(1):CD005302. [Meta-analysis: 12 RCTs, n = 6814]
18. Mozurkewich E. Prelabor rupture of membranes at term: Induction techniques. *Clin Obstet Gynecol.* 2006;49(3):672–683. [Review]
19. Hofmeyr GJ, Gülmezoglu AM, Pileggi C. Vaginal misoprostol for cervical ripening and induction of labour. *Cochrane Database Syst Rev.* 2010;(10):CD000941. [Meta-analysis]
20. Sanchez-Ramos L, Chen AH, Kaunitz AM, et al. Labor induction with intravaginal misoprostol in term premature rupture of membranes: A randomized study. *Obstet Gynecol.* 1997;89:909–912. [RCT, n = 141]
21. Butt KD, Bennett KA, Crane JMG, et al. Randomized comparison of oral misoprostol and oxytocin for labor induction in term prelabor membranes rupture. *Obstet Gynecol.* 1999;94:994–999. [RCT, n = 108]
22. Ngai SW, Chan YM, Lam SW, et al. Labour characteristics and uterine activity: Misoprostol compared to oxytocin in women at term with prelabour rupture of membranes. *Br J Obstet Gynecol.* 2000;107:222–227. [RCT, n = 80]
23. Mozurkewich E, Horrocks J, Daley S, et al.; MisoPROM study. The MisoPROM study: A multicenter randomized comparison of oral misoprostol and oxytocin for premature rupture of membranes at term. *Am J Obstet Gynecol.* 2003;189:1026–1030. [RCT, n = 305]
24. Tan PC, Daoud SA, Omar SZ. Concurrent dinoprostone and oxytocin for labor induction in term premature rupture of membranes. *Obstet Gynecol.* 2009;113:1059–1065. [RCT, n = 114]
25. Wolff K, Swahn ML, Westgren M. Balloon catheter for induction of labor in nulliparous women with prelabor rupture of the membranes at term. A preliminary report. *Gynecol Obstet Invest.* 1998;46(1):1–4. [II-3]
26. Mackeen AD, Walker L, Ruhstaller K, et al. Foley catheter vs prostaglandin as ripening agent in pregnant women with premature rupture of membranes. *J Am Osteopath Assoc.* 2014;114(9):686–692. [II-3]
27. Cabrera IB, Quiñones JN, Durie D, et al. Use of intracervical balloons and chorioamnionitis in term premature rupture of membranes. *J Matern Fetal Neonatal Med.* 2015:1–5. [Epub ahead of print] [II-3]
28. Seaward PG, Hannah ME, Myhr TL, et al. International Multicentre Term Prelabor Rupture of Membranes Study: Evaluation of predictors of clinical chorioamnionitis and postpartum fever in patients with prelabor rupture of membranes at term. *Am J Obstet Gynecol.* 1997;177(5):1024. [II-1]
29. Seaward PG, Hannah ME, Myhr TL, et al. International multicenter term PROM study: Evaluation of predictors of neonatal infection in infants born to patients with premature rupture of membranes at term. Premature rupture of the membranes. *Am J Obstet Gynecol.* 1998;179:635. [II-1]
30. Herbst A, Källén K. Time between membrane rupture and delivery and septicemia in term neonates. *Obstet Gynecol.* 2007;110:612.
31. CDC Revised Guidelines from CDC. Prevention of perinatal group B streptococcal disease. *MMWR Morb Mortal Wkly Rep.* 2010;59(RR10):1–32. [Epidemiologic data]
32. Saccone G, Berghella V. Antibiotic prophylaxis for term or near-term premature rupture of membranes: Meta-analysis of randomized trials. *Am J Obstet Gynecol.* 2015;212:627.e1–627.e9. [Meta-analysis: 5 RCTs, n = 2699]
33. Wojcieszek AM, Stock OM, Flenady V. Antibiotics for prelabour rupture of membranes at or near term. *Cochrane Database Syst Rev.* 2014;(10):CD001807. [Meta-analysis: 4 RCTs, n = 1801]
34. Buchanan SL, Crowther CA, Levett KM, et al. Planned early birth versus expectant management for women with preterm prelabour rupture of membranes prior to 37 weeks' gestation for improving pregnancy outcome. *Cochrane Database Syst Rev.* 2010;(3):CD004735. [Meta-analysis: 7 RCTs, n = 690]
35. Spinnato JA, Shaver DC, Bray EM, et al. Preterm premature rupture of the membranes with fetal pulmonary maturity present: A prospective study. *Obstet Gynecol.* 1987;69(2):196–201. [RCT]
36. Mercer BM, Crocker LG, Boe NM, et al. Induction versus expectant management in premature rupture of the membranes with mature amniotic fluid at 32 to 36 weeks: A randomized trial. *Am J Obstet Gynecol.* 1993;169(4):775–782. [RCT]
37. Naef RW III, Allbert JR, Ross EL, et al. Premature rupture of membranes at 34 to 37 weeks' gestation: Aggressive versus conservative management. *Am J Obstet Gynecol.* 1998;178(1 Pt 1):126–130. [RCT]
38. Neerhof MG, Cravello C, Haney EI, et al. Timing of labor induction after premature rupture of membranes between 32 and 36 weeks' gestation. *Am J Obstet Gynecol.* 1999;180(2 pt 1):349–352. [RCT]
39. Bhutani VK, Johnson L. Kernicterus in late preterm infants cared for as term healthy infants. *Semin Perinatol.* 2006;30(2):89–97. [II-3]
40. Clark RH. The epidemiology of respiratory failure in neonates born at an estimated gestational age of 34 weeks or more. *J Perinatol,* 2005;25(4):251–257. [II-3]
41. Jain L, Eaton DC. Physiology of fetal lung fluid clearance and the effect of labor. *Semin Perinatol.* 2006;30(1):34–43. [II-3]
42. Laptook A, Jackson GL. Cold stress and hypoglycemia in the late preterm ("near-term") infant: Impact on nursery of admission. *Semin Perinatol.* 2006;30(1):24–27. [II-3]
43. McIntire DD, Leveno KJ. Neonatal mortality and morbidity rates in late preterm births compared with births at term. *Obstet Gynecol.* 2008;111(1):35–41. [II-2]
44. Shapiro-Mendoza CK, Tomashek KM, Kotelchuck M, et al. Risk factors for neonatal morbidity and mortality among "healthy," late preterm newborns. *Semin Perinatol.* 2006;30(2):54–60. [II-3]

45. Tomashek KM, Shapiro-Mendoza CK, Weiss J, et al. Early discharge among late preterm and term newborns and risk of neonatal morbidity. *Semin Perinatol*. 2006;30(2):61–68. [II-3]
46. Wang ML, Dorer DJ, Fleming MP, et al. Clinical outcomes of near-term infants. *Pediatrics*. 2004;114(2):372–376. [II-3]
47. Martin JA, Hamilton BE, Osterman MJK, et al. Births: Final Data for 2013. *National Vital Statistics Reports*, Vol. 64, No. 1. Hyattsville, MD: National Center for Health Statistics, 2015. [Epidemiologic data]
48. Buchanan SL, Crowther CA, Levett KM, et al. Planned early birth versus expectant management for women with preterm prelabour rupture of membranes prior to 37 weeks' gestation for improving pregnancy outcome. *Cochrane Pregnancy Childbirth Group Cochrane Database Syst Rev*. 2010;(6):CD004735. [Meta-analysis: 7 RCTs, $n = 690$]
49. van der Ham DP, Vijgen SMC, Nijhuis JG, et al. Induction of labor versus expectant management in women with preterm prelabor rupture of membranes between 34 and 37 weeks: A randomized controlled trial. *PLoS Med*. 2012;9(4):e1001208. [RCT]
50. van der Ham DP, van der Heyden JL, Opmeer BC, et al. Management of late-preterm premature rupture of membranes: The PPROMEXIL-2 trial. *Am J Obstet Gynecol*. 2012;207:276.e1–276.e10. [RCT]
51. Morris JM, Roberts CL, Bowen JR, et al. Immediate delivery compared with expectant management after preterm pre-labour rupture of the membranes close to term (PPROMT trial): A randomised controlled trial. *Lancet*. 2015;S0140–6736(15)00724-2. [RCT]
52. Melamed N, Ben-Haroush A, Pardo J, et al. Expectant management of preterm premature rupture of membranes: Is it all about gestational age? *Am J Obstet Gynecol*. 2011;204:48.e1–48.e8. [II-3]
53. Ramsey PS, Lieman JM, Brumfield CG, Carlo W. Chorioamnionitis increases neonatal morbidity in pregnancies complicated by preterm premature rupture of membranes. *Am J Obstet Gynecol*. 2005;192:1162–1166. [II-3]
54. Saccone G, Berghella V. Antenatal corticosteroids for term or near-term fetal maturity: A systematic review and meta-analysis of randomized controlled trials. *BMJ*. 2016;355:i5044. [Meta-analysis: 6 RCTs, $n = 5698$]
55. Gyamfi-Bannerman C, Thom EA, Blackwell SC, et al. Antenatal betamethasone for women at risk for late preterm delivery. *NEJM* 2016;374:1311–1320. [RCT]

Induction of labor

Corina N. Schoen and Anthony C. Sciscione

KEY POINTS

- **Complications** of induction of labor at term include **prolonged first stage of labor, operative delivery** and their risks.
- An **early (e.g., <20 weeks) ultrasound examination** helps determine accurate gestational age and is associated with a **reduction in the rates of induction of labor for post-term pregnancy**.
- **Gestational age** should be **documented accurately** before considering induction.
- **Possible indications** for induction of labor, and suggested best gestational age for induction, are listed in Table 21.1.
- **Without indications, induction before 39 weeks should be avoided**. An induction based solely on maternal request should be designated as such (induction for maternal request).
- **Contraindications** to induction of labor include transverse or oblique fetal lie, umbilical cord prolapse, previous classical uterine incision or transfundal uterine surgery (e.g., from myomectomy), placenta or vasa previa, active genital herpes infection, and any contraindications to vaginal delivery, or indication for cesarean delivery (CD) (Table 21.2).
- **Misoprostol should not be used for cervical ripening or labor induction in women with prior uterine incisions, given the >5% risk of uterine rupture**. In women with prior uterine incisions, **prostaglandin E2 (PGE2)** for cervical ripening is associated with approximately *1.4%–2.5%* **risk of rupture; oxytocin has a 1.1% risk**. Cervical ripening with the Foley catheter does not appear to be associated with any additional risk of uterine rupture in patients undergoing a trial of labor after cesarean section.
- A Bishop score of ≥9 is usually associated with the **probability of vaginal delivery** after labor induction **similar to that after spontaneous labor**.
- In women with **an unfavorable** (Bishop score <5, or even <9) cervical examination:
  - **Sweeping of membranes** at term doubles the rate of onset of labor (to approximately *36%) in the next 48 hours,* without major complications.
  - **The Foley balloon** is associated with **less hyperstimulation accompanied by fetal heart rate (FHR) changes, and increased use of oxytocin,** but results in the same number of vaginal deliveries and the same number of women delivered within 24 hours as all of the locally applied prostaglandins ([LAPG]; prostaglandin E1 [PGE1] and PGE2). It is therefore **one of the preferred methods for labor induction** when the cervix is <3 cm dilated.
  - **Vaginal misoprostol 25 mg every 3–6 hours** is the preferred safe dosage, as effective as PGE2 or any other method; this is also a preferred method of labor induction.
  - PGE2 tablet, gel, and insert appear to be as safe and efficacious as each other in terms of tachysystole, CD rates, and neonatal outcomes.
  - Other cervical ripening or induction agents are either not sufficiently studied, unsafe, or not as effective as the agents already mentioned.
- In women with **favorable** cervical examination:
  - Oxytocin is safe and effective for induction of labor in these women.
  - There are insufficient safety data for **outpatient use** of pharmacologic cervical ripening or induction agents. However, there is emerging evidence that the Foley catheter may be an effective and safe method for outpatient cervical ripening.
  - Contraction pressures of **≥200 Montevideo units** should be targeted in induction or augmentation of laboring patients to achieve **adequate labor**. While the definition of a failed induction of labor is elusive, a **failed induction** should not be diagnosed until after **24 hours of oxytocin after membrane rupture in the active phase (usually ≥6 cm in nulliparous women),** assuming reassuring fetal heart pattern.
- **Induced labor should be managed, in general, as spontaneous labor.**

DEFINITIONS

Induction of labor is the stimulation of uterine contractions prior to spontaneous labor in order to achieve childbirth. **Cervical ripening** is a process that occurs prior to labor in which the cervix is softened, thinned, and dilated.

INCIDENCE/EPIDEMIOLOGY

In 2013, there were 3,932,181 total births in the United States, of which 903,638 were induced (23%) [1]. From 1990 to 2010, the induction rate has increased for all gestational ages [2]. However, the incidence of preterm inductions has decreased since 2005, and accounted for just 13.9% of all inductions in 2013 [2]. Although previous trends showed an increased rate of inductions without medical indication [3], there is now evidence for a decreasing rate of indicated preterm births (17% decline from 2005 through 2012) [4]. However, it has been shown that using birth certificate data overestimates the number of non-medically indicated inductions by 11-fold [5].

BASIC PATHOPHYSIOLOGY

The cervix functions as the gatekeeper to parturition maintaining a fine balance between the integrity of the pregnancy and delivery. Histologically, the cervix is composed of mostly collagen, with some smooth muscle; the stability of these components and the ability to become dynamic when stressed on

Table 21.1 Common Indications for Possible Induction of Labor or Cesarean Delivery (Suggested Timing of Delivery for Selected Conditions)

Placental and Uterine Issues	Gestational Age[a] for Delivery
• Placenta previa[b]	36–37 weeks
• Placenta accreta/increta/percreta with placenta previa	34–35 weeks
• Prior classical cesarean (upper segment uterine incision)	36–37 weeks
• Prior myomectomy requiring cesarean delivery	37–38 weeks (Situations with more extensive or complicated procedures may require earlier delivery, similar to prior classical cesarean)
• Prior uterine rupture	36–37 weeks
• Abruptio placentae	At detection (see Chapter 26)
• Intrauterine infection (e.g., chorioamnionitis)	At detection

Fetal Issues	Gestational Age[a] for Delivery
• FGR—singleton	38–39 weeks • Otherwise uncomplicated, no concurrent findings 34–37 weeks • Concurrent conditions (e.g., abnormal umbilical artery Dopplers) Expeditious delivery regardless of gestational age • Persistent abnormal fetal surveillance suggesting imminent fetal jeopardy
• FGR—twin gestation	• 36–37 weeks • Dichorionic-diamniotic twins with isolated FGR 32–34 weeks • Monochorionic-diamniotic twins with isolated fetal growth restriction • Concurrent conditions (e.g., abnormal umbilical artery Dopplers) Expeditious delivery regardless of gestational age • Persistent abnormal fetal surveillance suggesting imminent fetal jeopardy
• Fetal congenital malformations	• 34–39 weeks • Suspected worsening of fetal organ damage • Potential for fetal intracranial hemorrhage (e.g., Vein of Galen aneurysm and NAIT) • When delivery prior to labor is preferred (e.g., EXIT procedure) • Previous fetal intervention • Concurrent maternal disease (e.g., preeclampsia and chronic hypertension) • Potential for adverse maternal effect from fetal condition Expeditious delivery regardless of gestational age • When intervention is expected to be beneficial • Fetal complications develop (abnormal fetal surveillance, new onset hydrops fetalis, and progressive/new-onset organ injury) • Maternal complications develop (mirror syndrome)
• Multiple gestations: dichorionic/diamniotic[b]	38 weeks
• Multiple gestations: monochorionic/diamniotic[b]	34–37 weeks
• Multiple gestations: di/di or mono/di with single fetal death[b]	If occurs at or after 34 weeks, consider delivery If occurs before 34 weeks, individualize based on concurrent maternal/fetal conditions
• Multiple gestations: monochorionic/monoamniotic[b]	32–34 weeks
• Multiple gestations: monochorionic/monoamniotic with single fetal death[b]	Consider delivery; individualized according to gestational age and concurrent complications
• Oligohydramnios (MVP <2 cm)—isolated but persistent[b]	37 weeks
• Nonreassuring fetal heart testing (e.g., category III FHR tracing)	At detection (see Chapter 10)
• Fetal death	At detection (see Chapter 10)

Maternal Issues	Gestational Age[a] for Delivery
• Chronic hypertension—no medications[b]	38–39 weeks
• Chronic hypertension—controlled on medications[b]	37–39 weeks
• Chronic hypertension—difficult to control (requiring frequent medication adjustments)[b]	36–37 weeks
• Gestational hypertension[c]	38 weeks
• Preeclampsia—severe	At diagnosis (recommendations limited to pregnancies at or after 34 weeks)
• Preeclampsia—mild	37 weeks
• Eclampsia	At detection
• Diabetes—pregestational well-controlled[b]	39–40 weeks
• Diabetes—pregestational with vascular disease	37–39 weeks
• Diabetes—pregestational, poorly controlled	34–39 weeks (individualized to situation)
• Diabetes—gestational well-controlled on diet[b]	Induction before 40 weeks not recommended
• Diabetes—gestational well-controlled on medication[b]	39–40 weeks
• Diabetes—gestational poorly controlled on medication[b]	34–39 weeks individualized to situation
• Cardiac disease	39 weeks (individualize depending on type and severity)

(Continued)

Table 21.1 Common Indications for Possible Induction of Labor or Cesarean Delivery (Suggested Timing of Delivery for Selected Conditions) (*Continued*)

Obstetrical Issues	Gestational Age[a] for Delivery
• Prior stillbirth—unexplained	39 weeks Consider amniocentesis for fetal pulmonary maturity if delivery planned before 38 weeks
• Spontaneous PPROM	34 weeks
• Spontaneous preterm labor	Delivery at 34–36 weeks if progressive labor or additional maternal/fetal
Prolonged pregnancy	≥41 weeks

Source: Modified from Wood S et al., *BJOG*, 121, 674–685, 2014.
Abbreviations: EXIT, ex utero intrapartum treatment; FHR, fetal heart rate; FGR, fetal growth restriction; MVP, maximum vertical pocket; NAIT, neonatal alloimmune thrombocytopenia; PPROM, preterm premature rupture of membranes.
[a]Gestational age is in completed weeks, thus "34 weeks" includes 34 weeks and 0 days through 34 weeks and 6 days.
[b]Uncomplicated, thus no FGR, superimposed preeclampsia, etc. If these are present, then the complicating conditions take precedence and earlier delivery may be indicated.
[c]Maintenance antihypertensive therapy should in general not be used to treat gestational hypertension.

Table 21.2 Contraindications to Induction of Labor

- Transverse or oblique fetal lie
- Umbilical cord prolapse
- Previous classical uterine incision or transfundal uterine surgery (e.g., from myomectomy)
- Placenta or vasa previa
- Active genital herpes infection
- Any contraindications to vaginal delivery, or indication for cesarean delivery

a physical and molecular level are what changes the cervical status. This cervical status prior to induction is predictive of induction success, as described below [6].

RISK FACTORS/ASSOCIATIONS

Factors that may increase the risk for complications associated with induction are nulliparity, no prior vaginal delivery, unfavorable cervical examination, postterm, obesity, and a large fetus.

COMPLICATIONS

Complications of inductions include prolonged first stage of labor, especially in the latent phase [7], leading to increased risk of postpartum hemorrhage, chorioamnionitis and endometritis [8,9]. CD risk is not increased with induction of labor [10,11]. Preterm (<37 weeks) induction is associated with prematurity risks, and should only be performed for appropriate maternal or fetal indications. The safety of the induced patient can be enhanced through the use of safety checklists, available through American Congress of Obstetricians and Gynecologist (ACOG) [12].

PREGNANCY CONSIDERATIONS

The risks and complications of induction of labor should be weighed against the possible benefits. A **successful induction** has been defined in many different ways but usually is one that achieves an uncomplicated vaginal delivery within 24 hours. If active phase is not achieved within 24 hours, this is not a reason per se for CD. Compared with a shorter induction-to-delivery interval, an induction lasting greater than 24 hours is associated with a higher risk for adverse outcomes, with a higher (e.g., 50%) risk of CD [13]. Neonatal outcomes including intensive care unit (ICU) admission, Apgar <7, and arterial cord pH <7 do not appear to increase with a prolonged latent stage as long as fetal status is reassuring [8,9]. A minimum of 24 hours should be allowed *after* cervical ripening *and* oxytocin administration (optimally with membranes ruptured) prior to diagnosing a failed induction [13–15]. After appropriate counseling, this time period may be extended assuming a reassuring fetal status.

PREVENTION

A routine (i.e., performed on every pregnant woman) early (e.g., before 20 weeks) ultrasound examination is associated with a 39% **reduction in the incidence of postterm pregnancies and rates of induction of labor for postterm pregnancy**, by allowing a more precise estimation of exact gestational age. An ultrasound performed in the first trimester (6–14 weeks) provides the best estimate of gestational age and the most benefit in terms of avoiding induction for postterm pregnancy [16] (see also Chapter 4).

CRITERIA FOR INDUCTION
Workup/Counseling

Gestational age should be **documented accurately** before considering induction, to avoid inadvertent postterm and preterm deliveries. Indications and contraindications need to be carefully reviewed. Counseling with the patient should include discussion of specific indications, risks (possible complications), and benefits of induction.

Indications

Once a term gestation has been confirmed, possible **indications for induction and suggested best timing** are shown in Table 21.1 [17,18].

For more details on the indications, see each specific guideline (e.g., Chapter 27 "Postterm Pregnancy," Chapter 19 "Preterm Premature Rupture of Membranes," Chapter 14 "Trial of Labor After Cesarean" in this volume; and Chapter 4 "Pregestational Diabetes," Chapter 5 "Gestational Diabetes," Chapter 46 "Fetal Macrosomia," Chapter 44 "Multiple Gestations," and Chapter 10 "Intrahepatic Cholestasis of Pregnancy" in *Maternal-Fetal Evidence Based Guidelines*). The term *elective* induction should be avoided, as an induction should be performed upon a precise and accepted indication [19]. An induction based solely on maternal request should be designated as such.

Gestational Age of Induction

The gestational age at which the induction is being considered is very important. There are some indications for induction before 39 weeks (Table 21.1), but **without indications induction before 39 weeks should be avoided** [20]. In this chapter, induction and ripening in the third trimester, and usually at or near term, is reviewed. For second-trimester induction and ripening, see Chapter 55 in *Maternal-Fetal Evidence Based Guidelines*. For induction for gestational age ≥41 weeks, see Chapter 27.

Induction without Medical Indication

Some have advocated induction at 39 0/7–40 6/7 weeks, even without medical indications. In a meta-analysis including 11 randomized controlled trials (RCTs) and 25 observational studies evaluating pregnancies at **37 0/7–41 6/7 weeks, compared with "elective" induction, expectant management was associated with higher incidence of CD** (odds ratio [OR] 1.22, 95% CI 1.07–1.39), and **higher incidence of meconium** (OR 2.04, 95% CI 1.34–3.09), but otherwise similar maternal and perinatal outcomes [11]. These results are driven mostly by data at 41 weeks or more, when induction is indicated (see Chapter 27). Another meta-analysis of 31 trials including 6248 women randomized to induction of labor between 37 0/7 and 41 6/7 weeks confirmed these results, with a reduced risk of CD (OR 0.83, 95% CI 0.76–0.92) and no difference in neonatal outcomes of 5 minute Apgar score <7, neonatal intensive care unit (NICU) admission, or perinatal death [10]. A meta-analysis restricted to five trials including women randomized to induction or expectant management from 39 0/7 to 40 6/7 showed no difference in CD or perinatal outcomes [21]. Another individual patient data (IPD) meta-analysis of advanced maternal age (AMA) women also showed no difference in CD rate, though the number of patients included was low ($n = 367$) [22]. A RCT of nulliparous women without medical indication for delivery were randomized to induction or expectant management with a primary outcome of increase in CD rate by 50%. Although this increase was not statistically significant, the rate of CD was higher in the induction group (30.5% vs. 17.7%) (relative risk [RR] 1.72, 95% confidence interval [CI] 0.97–3.06) [23]. **There are insufficient data to evaluate the safety and effectiveness of induction without a medical indication at 39–40 6/7 weeks,** though the data from these meta-analyses [21,22] are useful when counseling women considering induction by maternal request. The Maternal-Fetal Medicine Units Network is currently conducting a study randomizing nulliparous women to induction or expectant management at 39 weeks (ARRIVE) (NCT01990612) [24]. Results from this trial may have significant effects on management of these women at term.

Contraindications

Induction of labor is **contraindicated** in the situations shown in Table 21.2 [20]. The attending physician should use his or her own discretion in the event of multifetal pregnancy, maternal heart disease, prior low-transverse CD, severe hypertension, and abnormal fetal heart rate (FHR) patterns not necessitating emergent delivery.

Induction of Labor after Cesarean

The **risk of uterine rupture** after induction in **women with a prior CD** deserves special attention (see Chapter 14). Misoprostol induction in women with a prior CD was associated with a 5.6% risk of uterine rupture in one of the largest series [25]. **Therefore, misoprostol should not be used for cervical ripening or labor induction in women with prior uterine incisions except under very unusual circumstances or management of stillbirth in the second trimester** (see Chapter 55 in *Maternal-Fetal Evidenced Based Guidelines*). According to retrospective studies, using PGE2 for cervical ripening in women who have a history of previous cesarean also increases the risk of uterine rupture [26–29]. Risk of uterine rupture is approximately **1.4–2.5 with PGE2 use (with or without oxytocin)** [28,29], and about **1.1 with oxytocin alone** [29]. Alternatively, **cervical ripening with the Foley catheter is not associated with any additional risk of uterine rupture in patients undergoing a trial of labor after cesarean section** [30]. A patient who has a prior CD, no previous vaginal delivery, and an unfavorable Bishop score up to 39–40 weeks has more risks (e.g., septicemia, uterine rupture, and hysterectomy) from induction of labor; these women may elect for repeat CD after counseling [26–29] (Chapter 14). However, in a prospective observational trial of 12,676 women undergoing either induction of labor or expectant management after a prior CD, induction at 39 weeks remained associated with a significantly higher chance of vaginal birth after cesarean (VBAC) as well as uterine rupture (OR 1.31, 95% CI 1.03–1.67; and OR 2.73, 95% CI 1.22–6.12, respectively) [31]. Uterine rupture was not statistically different in those women induced at 40 completed weeks compared with expectantly managed women, however there was also no increase in VBAC odds [31].

Time of Day for Induction

Spontaneous labor has been shown to have a circadian rhythm with a higher occurrence at night due to a higher concentration of myometrial oxytocin receptors and maternal oxytocin concentrations. A meta-analysis of three RCTs was performed, however results were not pooled secondary to substantial heterogeneity between studies [32]. One RCT comparing morning and evening oxytocin inductions showed no difference in outcomes for women induced in the morning versus the evening, except for slightly increased neonatal admission to the maternity ward, medium care neonatal unit, or ICU (RR 1.48, 95% CI 1.02–2.14) in the morning group, though the authors could not explain a reason for this effect [33]. The remaining two RCTs compared prostaglandin induction timing, and showed no differences in neonatal outcomes or CD, but higher maternal satisfaction in morning inductions [32]. There were less operative vaginal delivery in the morning nulliparas group in one trial, and less multiparas delivered during the evening, without an effect on nighttime deliveries [34].

PREDICTION OF SUCCESSFUL INDUCTION
Maternal Characteristics

There are certain maternal characteristics that have been shown to favorably predict successful induction of labor. A secondary analysis of a study investigating vaginal misoprostol versus vaginal dinoprostone showed that prior vaginal delivery, lower maternal BMI, tall maternal stature, and neonatal birth weight <4000 g were associated with a higher likelihood of a vaginal delivery, independent of method. Race was also predictive, with Hispanic race being a positive predictor of successful induction and African-American race being associated with a lower likelihood of successful induction of labor [35].

Bishop Score

In 1964, Bishop reported that his pelvic score (Table 21.3) is inversely proportional to the time from examination to time at which spontaneous labor begins [6]. **Unfavorable (<5) Bishop scores at admission for induction of labor are associated with two- to threefold increased risk of CD** when compared with spontaneous onset of labor [6,7,36]. Data show a score of ≥9 to predict a short time until onset of spontaneous labor and, therefore, indicate favorability for induction [35]. A simplified Bishop score might also be considered [37]. In a meta-analysis of mostly cohort studies aimed primarily to assess Bishop score as a predictor of cesarean, scores of 4, 5, or 6 were not predictive. A Bishop score of 8 or 9 had a negative predictive value of 96% for cesarean [38]. An additional meta-analysis that included a larger sample of studies and randomized trials, higher Bishop scores were associated with a higher rate of vaginal delivery. A Bishop score of 4 had an OR of 2 for vaginal delivery, where a Bishop of 8 increased the odds of vaginal delivery by 5.5 [39]. A Bishop score of ≥9 is usually associated with a **probability of vaginal delivery** after labor induction similar to that after spontaneous labor [20].

Transvaginal Cervical Length

Compared with using a Bishop score <5 for defining an unfavorable cervix, using a transvaginal ultrasound (TVU) cervical length (CL) >27 mm is associated with a reduced need for prostaglandins without affecting the outcome of the induction in one RCT [40]. However, in a systematic review of mostly observational studies, a CL of <30 mm did not predict vaginal delivery; a CL >30 mm did not predict cesarean section [41]. When compared with Bishop score, there was no significant difference in prediction of successful labor induction, mode of delivery, vaginal delivery within 24 hours of starting induction, or achievement of the active stage of labor [40,42]. Cervical wedging/funneling has been investigated in eight studies including 1139 patients and has a low sensitivity to predict a failed induction [42]. In nulliparas, a CL cut-off of 30 mm had a sensitivity of 70% and specificity of 74% for predicting cesarean [42].

Fetal Fibronectin

Of five prospective observational trials [43–47], only one showed an association with positive fetal fibronectin and successful induction [43]. As such, **fetal fibronectin is not recommended to predict which patient's labor induction will result in a successful vaginal delivery.**

INDUCTION/RIPENING METHODS

Induction of labor is one of the most-studied interventions in obstetrics, with hundreds of trials reported. Cervical ripening/induction agents can be functionally divided into two methods: **mechanical** and **pharmacologic**. Mechanical methods have been utilized since the days of Hippocrates, 460–360 BC. Many methods have been compared not only to placebo or no treatment but also among themselves, in different populations and clinical settings, making for an extensive experience.

Mechanical Methods

Mechanical methods include the following: hygroscopic dilators (laminaria, lamicel, or dilapan); balloon (e.g., Foley catheter); and balloon with extra-amniotic infusion. Other methods reviewed under this category are membrane stripping and amniotomy.

Hygroscopic (Osmotic) Dilators (Laminaria, Lamicel, or Dilapan)
Hygroscopic devices are made either from synthetic or from organic material. The **laminaria** are the organic hygroscopic devices, which are made from cold water seaweed. Under direct visualization facilitated by a vaginal speculum, laminaria are placed in the cervical canal. Once in the cervix, the device absorbs water from surrounding tissues causing it to slowly swell, dilating the cervix. Generally the laminaria are left in place for 6–12 hours.

Currently, **no evidence exists to support using laminaria to decrease either the interval from induction to delivery or the rate of CD**. However, their use may cause an increase in maternal endometritis and neonatal sepsis likely due to the inability to reliably ensure sterility in this organic product [48]. In attempt to avoid problems associated with lack of sterility, polyvinyl alcohol polymer–magnesium sulfate (**lamicel**) and polyacrylonitrile (**dilapan**) were developed as synthetic hygroscopic devices. Like the laminaria, they are inserted in the same manner and function by attracting water from the surrounding tissue to achieve cervical softening, effacement, and dilation. However, lamicel and dilapan may be delivered sterilely.

Compared with placebo/no treatment, laminaria are associated with similar incidence of CD [48]. Similarly, no differences were noted between lack of treatment and dilapan in one trial [49].

Compared with any prostaglandins (vaginal PGE2, intracervical PGE2, or misoprostol), laminaria are also associated with similar incidence of CD, but less tachysystole with FHR changes. Serious maternal or perinatal morbidity is infrequent [48].

Compared with oxytocin, laminaria are associated with similar incidence of CD [48].

Compared with extra-amniotic induction, laminaria are associated with similar outcomes [48].

Compared with prostaglandin alone, the addition of laminaria is not associated with significant benefit [48].

Compared with oxytocin alone, there is insufficient evidence (one trial only) but no evidence of benefit from the addition of laminaria [48].

Balloon Catheter
In 1853, Kraus first described a balloon device for preinduction cervical ripening. Much like the placement of laminaria, a vaginal speculum is often utilized to insert the Foley catheter in the cervical os; however, placement via a digital examination is becoming more common. Optimally, the catheter is placed at a level above the internal cervical os sometimes with the assistance of forceps or a clamp to guide the catheter. The

Table 21.3 Bishop Score for Cervical Favorability

Score	Dilation (cm)	Effacement (%)	Station	Cervical Consistency	Position of Cervix
0	Closed	0–3	−3	Firm	Posterior
1	1–2	40–50	−2	Medium	Midposition
2	3–4	60–70	−1,0	Soft	Anterior
3	5–6	80	+1,+2	–	–

Source: Modified from Gyamfi-Bannerman C and Ananth CV, *Obstet Gynecol*, 124, 1069–1074, 2014.

Foley catheter affects cervical ripening in two ways: (1) gradual mechanical dilation and (2) separation of the decidua from the amnion, stimulating prostaglandin release. Many studies have demonstrated the Foley catheter to be an effective tool for achieving a favorable cervix [48,50–55].

There is some evidence to assess the type of Foley catheter to use. Various sizes and balloon capacities have been investigated and used; these include a range from 25- to 80-mL balloons with 14- to 18-F catheters. **Filling the balloon to 80 mL versus 30 mL resulted in an increased rate of delivery within 24 hours, increase in vaginal delivery rate, decreased need for oxytocin, and higher rate of postripening dilation of 3 cm or more** [56–58].

Once placed above the internal os, the operator uses sterile saline or water to inflate the catheter's balloon. Correct placement is verified by gentle traction on the catheter until the inflated balloon meets the resistance of the internal os. Once the location is verified, gentle traction is applied by taping the distal end of the catheter to the patient's inner thigh. Adding weighted traction has not been shown to increase vaginal delivery overall, vaginal delivery within 24 hours, or decrease CD rate [59]. The cervix dilates as the balloon is expelled. After expulsion, a favorable Bishop score is most often achieved and induction may begin. If the Foley is not expulsed within 12 hours, consideration should be given to removing it, as leaving it in 24 hours is associated with longer inductions [60].

Compared with no treatment, one trial reported Foley catheters to have no effect in the risk of CD [48].

Compared with all LAPG, including PGE2 and misoprostol, the rate of CDs is the same in a meta-analysis of 21 studies ($n = 3202$) [48]. There was no significant difference in vaginal delivery in 24 hours in the Foley catheter group [48]. LAPG were associated with a higher rate of excessive uterine activity and Foley catheter was associated with an increased need for oxytocin augmentation in labor, according to a meta-analysis of nine trials [48]. Obviously this analysis is not very clinically helpful, as comparison group should not mix PGE1 and PGE2.

Compared with vaginal misoprostol, transcervical Foley catheter has been demonstrated to be **equivalent** for cervical ripening. There is a **similar risk of CD, chorioamnionitis and other maternal and perinatal outcomes, except a higher incidence of tachysystole associated with misoprostol** (RR 2.9, 95% CI 1.39–5.81) [55,61–63]. Foley was associated with a longer time to from induction-to-delivery in two meta-analyses [62,64]. In a network meta-analyses of 51 RCTs, vaginal misoprostol reduced the risk of vaginal delivery not achieved in 24 hours (RR 0.43, CI 95% 0.35–0.67) and cesarean section (RR 0.84, 95% CI 0.71–0.99), but Foley catheter reduced the risk of hyperstimulation (RR 0.15, 95% CI 0.07–0.3) [64].

Compared with dinoprostone (intracervical and vaginal), Foley catheter had similar rates of vaginal delivery not achieved in 24 hours and CD. Foley catheter was significantly less likely to cause hyperstimulation than vaginal dinoprostone (RR 0.27, 95% CI 0.12–0.52), but not intracervical dinoprostone [64].

Compared with use with oxytocin for cervical ripening, Foley use without oxytocin was associated with a lower rate of CD (RR 0.57, 95% CI 0.38–0.88) [48]. There was no difference in tachysystole with or without FHR changes between groups [48]. There is insufficient evidence to support concurrent use of Foley catheter with oxytocin [48,65].

Compared with prostaglandin alone, the addition of a Foley catheter to locally applied PGE1 and PGE2 increases the likelihood of vaginal delivery within 24 hours, in three trials, with a lower likelihood of observing no cervical change when a balloon catheter is used [48]. There was no difference in CD between the groups in a meta-analysis of eight trials [48]. Additional RCTs performed after the previous meta-analysis [48] again showed shorter time to delivery, but again no difference in mode of delivery [66,67].

Foley bulbs were equally effective ripening agents in both **outpatient** and inpatient settings per the results of one trial [68], but data is insufficient to fully assess outpatient Foley balloon safety and effectiveness.

In women with a singleton gestation who undergo term induction with the intracervical Foley catheter, **two trials showed conflicting results regarding length of labor and risk of CD after early amniotomy. There is insufficient evidence to support early amniotomy after Foley induction** [69,70].

Theoretical risks associated with Foley catheter use include bleeding, fever, displacement of the presenting part, and premature rupture of membranes (PROM); however **no randomized trial has shown an increase in these complications** in comparison to other methods. Foley should not be used in women with low-lying placentas. Overall, **the Foley catheter is an inexpensive, safe, well-tolerated, and easy tool for cervical dilation** [50–54]. In a recent review of over 1200 low-risk women who received the intracervical Foley catheter for cervical ripening, there were no adverse events necessitating delivery in the preinduction ripening period [71]. In a meta-analysis of 26 trials including 5563 women, there was no increased risk of infectious morbidity with Foley catheter use [72]. **Foley is as effective as other methods, including misoprostol, and possibly safer than pharmaceutical methods, and should be considered as first line in all inductions (Figure 21.1), including those with PROM** (see Chapter 20).

Extra-Amniotic Saline Infusion (EASI)
EASI involves, as the term states, infusing usually saline through the cervix by a Foley balloon. For infusion of PGE2, see section "Extra-Amniotic Prostaglandins."

Compared with LAPG, EASI showed no difference in risk to delivery >24 hours, CD, or tachysystole (six studies, $n = 747$) [48].

Compared with PGE2, EASI with an intracervical Foley balloon is associated with *shorter time intervals to yield a favorable Bishop score,* and similar incidence of CD [48,73–75].

Compared with vaginal misoprostol, EASI with an intracervical Foley balloon and oxytocin is associated with shorter induction-to-delivery interval in one trial, but no difference in another [76]. There was similar incidence of CD in both trials [48,76,77].

Compared with laminaria, EASI with an intracervical Foley balloon is associated with *shorter induction-to-delivery interval* and less *CD for failed induction* in one trial [77].

Compared with Foley only, EASI with Foley catheters has been associated with shorter induction-to-delivery interval in one RCT [78] but not in another larger RCT [79].

In summary, **there is insufficient evidence to use EASI instead of Foley balloon for cervical ripening.**

Double-Balloon Foley Catheters
Double-balloon Foley catheters (Cook® Catheter or Atad catheters) have become more frequently used for mechanical labor

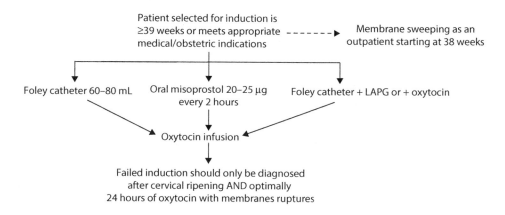

Figure 21.1 Induction algorithm to reduce the risk of cesarean delivery (CD) and time to delivery. LAPG, locally applied prostaglandins.

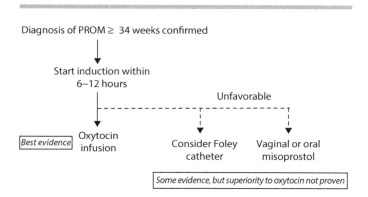

Figure 21.2 Induction for premature rupture of membrane (PROM) (see Chapter 20).

induction. The catheter is designed specifically for labor induction, providing an intra-cervical and vaginal balloon to compress the cervix in addition to membrane separation to ripen the cervix. Both balloons in the Cook catheter are approved to fill to a volume of 80 mL in each balloon.

Compared with PGE2, no difference in CD rates were reported in five RCTs [80–83]; one RCT of 126 women found a higher rate of CD in the dinoprostone group [84]. Time to vaginal delivery was shorter in the double-balloon group in two of four RCTs reporting on the outcome [81–84] and delivery within 24 hours was increased for the double-balloon group in two of three trials reporting the outcome [82–84]. Overall maternal and neonatal morbidity was similar in both groups, with the exception of tachysystole being more common with PGE2 [84]. **There is insufficient evidence to support the use of double-balloon catheter over PGE2 for labor induction.**

Compared with single-balloon Foley catheter, there was no difference in vaginal delivery within 24 hours, CD rate in two trials [81, 85]. Time from induction to delivery was longer in the double-balloon group in one trial [81]. There were more operative deliveries in the double-balloon group in one RCT [79] but not the other [81]. There is a significant cost difference between the catheters: single-balloon Foley catheters may cost up to $12–14 (the United States) for large balloon catheters (75 mL), but are cheaper when 30 mL balloons are used. The double-balloon catheter costs Labor and Delivery units $45-$200 in the United States per unit. **There is currently insufficient evidence to support the use of double-balloon catheters over single-balloon catheters for the induction of labor. Until further information is available, a Foley catheter should be used over double-balloon catheter for both efficacy and economic concerns.**

Membrane Stripping (or Sweeping)
Membrane stripping is the practice of inserting a finger through the internal os and sweeping to separate the membranes from the lower uterine segment. This technique stimulates prostaglandin release as plasma prostaglandin levels have been observed to increase poststripping. Sweeping the membranes promotes the onset of labor.

Compared with no sweeping, **sweeping of the membranes**, performed as a general policy in women at term (e.g., weekly starting at 38 weeks), **is associated with reduced duration of pregnancy and reduced frequency of pregnancy continuing beyond 41 weeks** (RR 0.59, 95% CI 0.46–0.74) *and 42 weeks* (RR 0.28, 95% CI 0.15–0.50) [86–90]. To avoid one formal induction of labor, sweeping of membranes must be performed in eight women. **Rate of CD and maternal or neonatal infection are similar.** Discomfort during vaginal examination and other adverse effects (bleeding and irregular contractions) are more frequently reported by women allocated to sweeping, but not associated with complications. Studies comparing sweeping with prostaglandin administration are of limited sample size and do not provide evidence of benefit.

When used as a means for induction of labor, the woman should be counseled that her chance of going to spontaneous labor after one sweeping at term is about **36% in the next 48 hours,** versus 17% without sweeping (so doubling the rate of onset of labor) [86,87]. Possible complications such as bleeding, infection, and ruptured membranes are not found to be increased with stripping [86,87].

In nulliparas being induced with PGE2 and oxytocin, **the addition of membrane sweeping** is associated with **shorter induction-to-delivery interval and increased vaginal delivery rates** in one trial [88]. There were no differences noted in nulliparas with favorable cervices or in multiparas.

In women attempting trial of labor after cesarean (TOLAC), weekly membrane sweeping had no effect on duration of pregnancy, spontaneous labor, or CD rate [91].

Amniotomy
Amniotomy—artificial rupture of the membranes—is another technique used in labor induction. There is **insufficient evidence** to assess the effectiveness of amniotomy alone [92]. No trials compared amniotomy alone with intracervical prostaglandins. If performed without cervical ripening or achieving a favorable cervix, amniotomy may be followed by long intervals before onset of labor. **In induced patients, early amniotomy is associated with shorter duration of labor and no increase in CD rates in most studies** [65–93-95]. One RCT of 168 patients showed longer duration of labor and CD rate in early amniotomy group [96], but this is contrary to findings in the aforementioned RCTs. The rate of intrapartum fever is mixed in RCTs and warrants additional research [93–97].

Compared with **placebo**, amniotomy and intravenous (IV) oxytocin are associated with significantly fewer instrumental vaginal deliveries than placebo. Compared with **vaginal prostaglandins,** amniotomy and IV oxytocin result in **more postpartum hemorrhage** and **more dissatisfaction in women** [65,92-97].

Pharmacologic Methods

Pharmacologic methods include the prostaglandins—E1: misoprostol; E2: dinoprostone; and F2a—as well as mifepristone, estrogen, relaxin, oxytocin, etc.

Misoprostol
Misoprostol (Cytotec™) is PGE1, which is an endogenously produced hormone that acts locally on surrounding tissues. Through complex molecular actions, PGE1 stimulates uterine contractions and cervical dilation in a manner akin to the onset of spontaneous labor. More specifically, PGE1 potentiates calcium ion transport across the cellular membrane and regulates cyclic adenosine monophosphate (AMP) within the uterine smooth muscle cells to trigger contractions. Additionally PGE1 facilitates cervical ripening by stimulating the pathway leading to the activation of collagenases. Collagenases, in turn, break down the structural collagen network of the cervix yielding a softer, thinner cervix.

Although it is currently on the market as a 100-mg tablet **to prevent peptic ulcers, misoprostol is available and widely** used in an "off label" form for preinduction cervical ripening and induction. **Misoprostol should not be used for cervical ripening or labor induction in women with prior uterine incisions** (e.g., prior CD) **after 28 weeks** [20–25]. For use of misoprostol for induction in the second trimester, see Chapter 55 in *Maternal-Fetal Evidence Based Guidelines*. Misoprostol can be administered vaginally, orally (buccal), or sublingually.

Vaginal misoprostol suppository. Vaginal misoprostol is most commonly administered by placing a tablet in the **posterior fornix of the vagina.** Several studies have focused on the dose administered. **Vaginal misoprostol in doses above 25 µg every 4 hour is more effective** (higher success rate for vaginal delivery within 24 hours of induction, decrease need for oxytocin, and decrease induction-to-delivery intervals) **than conventional methods of labor induction, but with more uterine hyperstimulation. Lower doses (25 µg) are similar to conventional methods in effectiveness and risks.** Lower doses of misoprostol compared with higher doses were associated with more need for oxytocin augmentation and less uterine tachysystole, with and without FHR changes, and less meconium aspiration, and less CD for NRFHT [72,98,99]. Therefore, **25 µg of misoprostol** (one-quarter of a 100-µg tablet) **given not more frequently than every 3–6 hours has been recommended** by the American College of Obstetricians and Gynecologists [20].

Compared with placebo, misoprostol is associated with reduced failure to achieve vaginal delivery within 24 hours (RR 0.51, 95% CI 0.37–0.71), and with increased uterine tachysystole without FHR changes (RR 3.52, 95% CI 1.78–6.99) [98,99].

Compared with vaginal PGE2, intracervical PGE2, and oxytocin, vaginal misoprostol is associated with less epidural analgesia use, **fewer failures to achieve vaginal delivery within 24 hours,** and **more uterine tachysystole** [64,98].

Compared with vaginal or intracervical PGE2, oxytocin augmentation was less common with misoprostol, and meconium-stained liquor more common [97,98]. **Compared with vaginal PGE2 only,** a meta-analysis of 11 RCTs showed that vaginal misoprostol was associated with a higher likelihood of vaginal delivery within 12 and 24 hours and lower use of oxytocin augmentation. There was no difference between the groups in relation to rate of CD, or incidence of tachysystole. A second meta-analysis including only singleton pregnancies confirmed these results [98,100]. A network meta-analysis comparing **intracervical PGE2** and vaginal misoprostol showed a reduction in hyperstimulation, decreased number of failed vaginal deliveries in 24 hours, and reduced risk of CD [64]. Additionally, the cost of a 25-mg pill of misoprostol is approximately $2 compared with the dinoprostone vaginal insert at approximately $168 [98].

Compared with oral misoprostol solution and all formulation of PGE2, a network meta-analysis including over 48,000 women showed that oral misoprostol solution had higher vaginal delivery rate in 24 hours and reduced risk of CD. High-dose vaginal misoprostol, then low-dose misoprostol, followed as the most effective treatments [99].

In summary, **vaginal misoprostol 25 µg every 4–6 hours is a safe, effective means for cervical ripening, more effective than PGE2.**

Vaginal misoprostol insert. A phase III clinical trial of a 50 and 100 µg vaginal insert (which is equivalent to a 25 µg tablet fragment being inserted every 6 hours) showed that the 100 µg vaginal insert had equal median times to vaginal delivery as the 10 mg dinoprostone vaginal insert. The 50 and 100 µg misoprostol inserts and the 10 mg dinoprostone insert all had comparable rates of CD and safety profile [101]. Misoprostol inserts of 50, 100, and 200 µg have similar rates of vaginal delivery within 24 hours, but higher rate of NRFHT requiring CD and tachysystole in the 200 µg group [102]. A more recent RCT by the same authors compared misoprostol insert 200 µg to dinoprostone 10 mg insert, and showed shorter time to delivery without an increase in CD rate. However, **tachysystole was more common in the misoprostol insert group** [103]. In a secondary analysis, there was a higher rate of NRFHT and CD secondary to NRFHT in the high-dose misoprostol insert groups [103,104]. In summary, **there is still insufficient evidence for clinical use of misoprostol vaginal insert.**

Oral misoprostol. Studies that examine patient satisfaction have shown a definite preference toward oral administration [103,104].

Compared with placebo in women with PROM, women who received oral misoprostol had a higher likelihood to deliver vaginally within 24 hours (RR 0.16, 95% CI 0.05–0.49), needed less oxytocin (RR 0.42, 95% CI 0.37–0.49), and had a lower cesarean section rate (RR 0.72, 95% CI 0.54–0.95) [105] (see Chapter 20).

Compared with vaginal PGE2 prostaglandins, low-dose oral misoprostol (e.g., 20 µg) administered every 2 hours had the same rate of vaginal delivery in 24 hours and a significantly lower rate of CD [105,106]. Women given oral misoprostol were also less likely to need a cesarean section (RR 0.88, 95% CI 0.78–0.99). There was some evidence that they had slower inductions, but there were no other significant differences [105].

Compared with oxytocin, oral misoprostol was associated with an increase in meconium-stained liquor in women with ruptured membranes (RR 1.65, 95% CI 1.04–2.6) but lower CD rate (RR 0.77, 95% CI 1.04–2.6) [105].

Compared with vaginal misoprostol, oral misoprostol had similar outcomes in regards to vaginal delivery in 24 hours and CD in a meta-analysis of 37 RCTs [105]. There were fewer babies with low Apgar score, postpartum hemorrhage in the oral misoprostol group, but higher rate of meconium-stained fluid [105]. A network meta-analysis, which allows for ranking treatments across studies through indirect comparisons, found that vaginal misoprostol had the highest probability of performing best among all prostaglandins to achieve vaginal delivery in 24 hours, but oral misoprostol avoided the most CD [99]. When the informal analysis of both achieving vaginal delivery in 24 hours and avoid CD was combined, low-dose (<50 µg) oral misoprostol performed best, followed by high-dose, then low-dose vaginal misoprostol [99]. A later network meta-analysis showed again that vaginal misoprostol avoided failed vaginal delivery in 24 hours the most, but was not different from oral misoprosol for reduced chance of CD [64]. Compared with vaginal misoprostol, **low-dose titrated oral misoprostol (20–25 µg) given every 2 hours** was shown in a review of two trials to cause fewer incidences of uterine tachysystole with FHR changes and a higher rate of vaginal delivery in 24 hours [106].

Sublingual misoprostol. Based on only three small trials, **sublingual** misoprostol appears to be at least as effective as when the same dose is administered orally [107].

Compared with vaginal misoprostol, a meta-analysis of five trials found no difference was found in vaginal delivery within 24 hours, tachysystole (when grouped according to dose), or CD [108]. There is **inadequate data** to assess safety, optimal dose, and side effects.

Prostaglandin E2 (Dinoprostone). PGE2 is an endogenously produced hormone that acts locally on surrounding tissues. Such effect is manifested in the smooth muscle of the uterus and gastrointestinal tract.

PGE2 can be used for induction of labor via different routes of administration, such as vaginal, extra-amniotic, oral, and IV. The vaginal route is the most common route of administration of PGE2 for labor induction. It can be given in different forms, such as tablet, gel, and insert.

All PGE2 vaginal forms. **Compared with placebo or no treatment, vaginal PGE2 (all forms)** is associated with a **higher likelihood of vaginal delivery within 24 hours** (RR 0.32, 95% CI 0.02–4.83), no difference in CD rates, and an increase in the risk of uterine tachysystole with FHR changes (4.4% vs. 0.5%; RR 3.16, 95% CI 1.67–5.98) [109]. PGE2 tablet, gel, and pessary appear to be as efficacious as each other [109].

PGE2 vaginal gel. Dinoprostone gel (Prepidil) is packaged as a 0.5-mg dose in a 2.5-mL syringe. A shielded catheter is added to the syringe end to facilitate safe injection, usually intracervical. Under direct visualization using a speculum, the syringe contents should be injected into the endocervical canal using sterile technique. The patient should remain supine for 30 minutes to minimize leakage from the canal. An alternative method for administering the gel is to inject into the posterior fornix or intravaginal administration. Until achieving a favorable cervix, dinoprostone 0.5 mg may be repeated every 6 hours up to a maximum dose of 1.5 mg in a 24-hour period. Once the cervix is favorable, oxytocin may be initiated for induction 6 hours after the last dose.

Compared with placebo, intracervical PGE2 is associated with decreased risk of not achieving vaginal delivery within 24 hours (RR 0.61, 95% CI 0.47–0.79). There was a small, and statistically nonsignificant, reduction of the risk of cesarean section when PGE2 was used (RR 0.88, 95% CI 0.77–1.0). The finding was statistically significant in a subgroup of women with intact membranes and unfavorable cervix only (RR 0.82, 95% CI 0.68–0.98). The risk of tachysystole with FHR changes was not significantly increased (RR 1.21, 95% CI 0.72–2.05). However, the risk of tachysystole without FHR changes was significantly increased (RR 1.59, 95% CI 1.09–2.33) [109,110].

Compared with PGE2 tablets, PGE2 gel has similar rate of vaginal delivery not achieved in 24 hours, CD, hyperstimulation causing FHR changes, and oxytocin use [109].

PGE2 vaginal insert. PGE2 vaginal insert (Cervidil) (also called slow-release pessary) is a thin, vaginal insert containing 10 mg of dinoprostone and delivers roughly 0.3 mg of dinoprostone each hour over a 24-hour period. The insert is placed in the posterior fornix of the vagina and left in place until the desired ripening has occurred when the insert is removed. Removal should occur at least 30 minutes prior to starting oxytocin. Cervidil use is indicated for cervical ripening and induction of labor in patients who have a medical indication for induction at or near term.

Compared with PGE2 gel, a PGE2 insert is associated with an increased risk of not achieving a vaginal delivery within 24 hours (RR 1.26, 95% CI 1.12–1.41). There was no change in the risk of cesarean section (RR 1.07, 95% CI 0.93–1.22). The risks of tachysystole with FHR changes (RR 0.76, 95% CI 0.39–1.49) and without FHR changes (RR 0.80, 95% CI 0.56–1.15) were nonsignificantly different with the two methods of PGE2 administration. Only one trial with a small sample size reported on women's views, with no difference between groups [109–113]. The use of sustained-release PGE2 inserts is associated with a reduction in instrumental vaginal delivery rates (RR 0.47, 95% CI 0.32–0.68) when compared with vaginal PGE2 gel or tablet [109]. Compared with intracervical PGE2 low dose, intracervical PGE2 high dose has higher rate of hyperstimulation with FHR changes but no change in CD rate [109].

Compared with Cervidil followed by oxytocin, Cervidil started concurrently with oxytocin is associated with a shorter induction-to-delivery interval and higher incidence of vaginal deliveries within 24 hours in one small trial [114].

Extra-amniotic prostaglandins. There is **insufficient evidence** to fully assess the effectiveness of extra-amniotic prostaglandins for induction of labor, with enough evidence to discourage its use compared with other methods (see also the section "Extra-Amniotic Saline Infusion"). Extra-amniotic placement of prostaglandins was first undertaken in the early 1970s and has been largely replaced with cervical or vaginal placement. Most of the studies used PGE2 (the minority prostaglandin F2a [PGF2a]) and gel preparations. Of the primary outcomes, there were significantly fewer women delivered vaginally within 24 hours among those induced with extra-amniotic PGF2a compared with vaginal misoprostol (RR 2.43, 95% CI 1.42–4.15). No other differences between groups for primary outcomes were found to be statistically significant. Oxytocin was used to initiate or augment labor significantly less frequently with extra-amniotic prostaglandins when compared with placebo (RR 0.51, 95% CI 0.39–0.67) but significantly more frequently when compared with vaginal misoprostol (RR 1.73, 95% CI 1.20–2.49). When extra-amniotic PGE2 was compared with Foley catheter only, the only difference between groups was that there were fewer cases of unfavorable cervix at 12–24 hours following treatment (RR 0.59, 95% CI 0.41–0.86). Women receiving extra-amniotic prostaglandin were more likely to be satisfied by the treatment compared with vaginal PGE2. There were no other significant differences when extra-amniotic prostaglandins were compared with other methods of cervical ripening or induction of labor. Although this could suggest that extra-amniotic prostaglandins are as effective as other agents, the findings are difficult to interpret because they are based on very small numbers and may lack the power to show a real difference [115].

Oral prostaglandins. Compared with placebo or no treatment, PGE2 is associated with a 54% decrease in CD. Otherwise, there were no significant differences between PGE2 and other interventions for this outcome [116].

Compared with vaginal prostaglandins, there is insufficient evidence, but no gross differences in three small trials [116].

Compared with all oxytocin treatments, oral PGE2 is associated with a trend for a lower incidence of vaginal delivery not achieved within 24 hours (RR 1.97, 95% CI 0.86–4.48).

Oral prostaglandin was associated with **vomiting** across all comparison groups. There are **no clear advantages** to oral prostaglandin over other methods of induction of labor.

IV prostaglandins. IV prostaglandins **should not be used** for induction or cervical ripening, as they are no more efficient than IV oxytocin for the induction of labor, but their use is associated with higher rates of maternal side effects and uterine tachysystole. Compared with oxytocin, IV prostaglandins are associated with **higher rates of uterine tachysystole** both with and without changes in the FHR, and similar incidence of vaginal delivery [117]. Use of IV prostaglandins is also associated with significantly **more maternal side effects** (gastrointestinal, thrombophlebitis, and pyrexia). No significant differences emerged from subgroup analysis or from the trials comparing combination oxytocin/PGF2a and oxytocin or extra-amniotic versus IV PGE2 [117]. There is insufficient information to assess a combination of PGF2a and oxytocin compared with oxytocin alone or extra-amniotic and IV PGE2.

Oxytocin
In 1948, the posterior pituitary extract, oxytocin, was first used for labor induction via IV drip. Oxytocin was then synthesized by du Vigneaud and associates in 1953; this accomplishment won the Nobel Prize in chemistry in 1955. Oxytocin is now widely utilized worldwide. Oxytocin is routinely utilized as it is the drug of choice also for augmentation of labor. While induction of labor is the stimulation of contractions before the spontaneous onset of labor, augmentation is the stimulation of contractions in the face of inadequate contractions following the spontaneous onset of labor.

By increasing intracellular calcium concentration, oxytocin stimulates the smooth muscle cells of breast, vessels, and, moreover, the uterus. Receptors for oxytocin are expressed in cells of the endometrium, liver, pancreas, and breast tissue. After the 13th week of gestation, myometrial cells express oxytocin receptors as well. Peak expression by the myometrium and endometrium occurs at term. Oxytocin increases both the amplitude and frequency of contractions, making labor effective. When continuously administered IV, oxytocin affects uterine response within 1 minute. Steady-state plasma concentrations are obtained within 40 minutes.

Overall, comparison of oxytocin with either intravaginal or intracervical PGE2 reveals that the **prostaglandin agents probably increase the chances of achieving vaginal birth within 24 hours.** Oxytocin induction may increase the rate of interventions in labor. In women with ruptured membranes induction can be recommended by either method, and in women with intact membranes there is insufficient information to make firm recommendations [108].

Compared with expectant management, oxytocin alone inductions are associated with fewer women failing to deliver vaginally within 24 hours (8% vs. 54%; RR 0.16, 95% CI 0.10–0.25), with the CD rate slightly increased (RR 1.17, 95% CI 1.01–1.35). There is a significant increase in the number of women requiring epidural analgesia (RR 1.10, 95% CI 1.04–1.17) [119].

Compared with vaginal prostaglandins, oxytocin alone is associated with an **increase in unsuccessful vaginal delivery within 24 hours** (70% vs. 21%; RR 3.33, 95% CI 1.61–6.89), irrespective of membrane status, but there was no difference in cesarean section rates [118].

There was a small increase in epidurals when oxytocin alone was used (RR 1.09, 95% CI 1.01–1.17). Most of the studies included women with ruptured membranes, and there was some evidence that oxytocin decreased infection in mothers (chorioamnionitis; RR 0.66, 95% CI 0.47–0.92) and babies (use of antibiotics; RR 0.68, 95% CI 0.53–0.87). These data should be interpreted cautiously as infection was not prespecified in the original review protocol [118].

Compared with intracervical PGE2 prostaglandins, oxytocin alone is associated with an **increase in unsuccessful vaginal delivery within 24 hours** (50% vs. 35%; RR 1.47, 95% CI 1.10–1.96). For all women with an unfavorable cervix regardless of membrane status, the cesarean section rate is increased (19% vs. 13%; RR 1.37, 95% CI 1.08–1.74) [118].

Compared with vaginal prostaglandin F2a, there was no difference in CD rate (RR 1.19, 95% CI 0.65–2.18). The outcome of failing to delivery vaginally in 24 hours was not reported in any of the three RCTs included in the meta-analysis [118].

Oxytocin seems to be as effective as prostaglandins in women with PROM [118] (see Chapter 20).

Compared with low-dose oxytocin regimens (<100 mU in the first 40 minutes and <600 mU in the first 2 hours), there were no differences in rates of vaginal delivery not achieved within 24 hours (RR 0.94, 95% CI 0.78–1.14) or CD (RR 0.96, 95% CI 0.81–1.14). There was no difference in serious maternal or neonatal morbidity. No trials reported on the number of women who had uterine hyperstimulation with fetal heart rate changes. When high bias studies were removed from the meta-analysis, there was a significant reduction of induction to delivery interval and increase in hyperstimulation without specifying fetal heart rate changes. Table 21.4 shows examples of each regimen (see also Chapter 7). **There is insufficient evidence to support the use of high-dose oxytocin over low-dose protocols** [119].

Prostaglandin F2α
Compared with placebo, vaginal PGF2α has a similar CD rate (RR 0.59, 95% CI 0.31–1.14). Vaginal delivery within 24 hours was not reported in the three trials included in a meta-analysis [109]. There were insufficient data to make meaningful conclusions for the comparison of vaginal PGE2 and PGF2α [109]. There is therefore *insufficient data* to assess the safety and efficacy of PGF2α for induction.

Mifepristone
Compared with placebo, mifepristone-treated women were more likely to be in labor or to have a favorable cervix at 48 hours (RR 2.41, 95% CI 1.70–3.42), were less likely to need augmentation with oxytocin (RR 0.80, 95% CI 0.66–0.97), and less likely to undergo cesarean section (RR 0.74, 95% CI 0.60–0.92), but more likely to have an instrumental delivery (RR 1.43, 95% CI 1.04–1.96) [120].

Compared with oxytocin, women treated with mifepristone for PROM after 36 weeks were less likely to have a vaginal delivery within 24 hours (RR 0.30, 95% CI 0.1–0.88) and their babies had an increased likelihood of neonatal adverse outcomes with more NICU admissions (RR 4.83, 95% CI 1.20–19.44), and abnormal fetal heart rate patterns (RR 5.63, 95% CI 1.11–28.52) in one trial [120].

There is insufficient information available from clinical trials to support the use of mifepristone to induce labor.

Estrogen
Several studies have shown that estradiol given via a variety of routes has the ability to achieve some degree of improved cervical ripening with minimal myometrial stimulation [121]. However, on a whole there were **insufficient data** to draw any conclusions regarding the efficacy of estrogen as an induction agent, given small, differing trials with different controls and different outcomes reported [122].

Relaxin
There is **insufficient evidence** to assess the safety and efficacy of relaxin as an intervention for induction of labor. There are no reported cases of uterine tachysystole with NRFHT in any of the four small trials [93]. Compared with placebo, relaxin is not associated with differences in CD [124].

Dehydroepiandrosterone Sulfate
Dehydroepiandrosterone sulfate (DHEAS) is converted to estrogen by the fetoplacental unit, and it was investigated as a possible mechanism for cervical ripening without myometrial contractions. There is **insufficient evidence** on its efficacy as one trial that investigated its use showed poor results when compared with placebo [123].

Dexamethasone Sulfate
There is **insufficient evidence** to assess the safety and efficacy of steroids as inductions agents. Compared with oxytocin alone, dexamethasone IM and oxytocin are not associated with significant effects in maternal and perinatal outcomes in one small RCT [124]. Compared with Foley catheter, Foley catheter plus extra-amniotic infusion of dexamethasone solution had a significantly shorter time from induction to delivery in one small RCT (11.9 ± 3 hours vs. 14.5 ± 4.8 hours, $p < .01$ [125]).

Hyaluronidase
There is **insufficient evidence** to assess the safety and efficacy of intracervical injections of hyaluronidase for cervical ripening. It is not common practice, and it is an invasive procedure that women may find unacceptable in the presence of less invasive methods. In one RCT, when compared with placebo for cervical ripening, intracervical injections of hyaluronidase resulted in women receiving significantly fewer cesarean sections (RR 0.37, 95% CI 0.22–0.61), less need for oxytocin augmentation (10% vs. 47%; RR 0.20, 95% CI 0.10–0.41), and increased cervical favorability after 24 hours (60% vs. 98%; RR 0.62, 95% CI 0.52–0.74). No side effects for mother or baby were reported in this trial [126]. Compared with Foley catheter, hyaluronidase was associated with a higher CD rate, and no difference in oxytocin use [127].

Nitric Oxide Donors
Nitric oxide (NO) donors **do not appear currently to be a useful tool** in the process of induction of labor. A meta-analysis including 10 studies compared NO donors with placebo, vaginal PGE2, intracervical PGE2, and vaginal misoprostol. There are very limited data available to compare NO donors to any other induction agent. There is no evidence of any difference between failed vaginal delivery within 24 hours, CD, or hyperstimulation [128]. There was an increase in nonserious maternal side effects (nausea, headache) [128].

Other Methods

Acupuncture
There is insufficient and conflicting evidence to assess the efficacy of acupuncture for induction of labor. Compared with a sham procedure, **the use of acupuncture prior to a scheduled induction is not associated with any difference in the need for induction agents, CD, but had greater cervical change** [129].

Breast Stimulation
Compared with no intervention, breast stimulation is associated with a significant **reduction in the number of women not in labor at 72 hours** (63% vs. 94%; RR 0.67, 95% CI 0.6–0.74). This result is not significant in women with an unfavorable cervix.

Table 21.4 Labor Stimulation with Oxytocin: Examples of Low- and High-Dose Oxytocin Protocols

Regimen	Starting Dose	Incremental Increase (mU/minute)	Dosage Interval (Minutes)
Low dose	0.5–1	1	30–40
	1–2	2	15
High dose	~6	~6	15
	6	6[a], 3, 1	20–40

[a]The incremental increase is reduced to 3 mU/minute in presence of tachysystole and reduced to 1 mU/minute with recurrent tachysystole.

The rate of postpartum hemorrhage is reduced (0.7% vs. 6%; RR 0.16, 95% CI 0.03–0.87). There is no significant difference in the cesarean section rate, in the rate of meconium staining or uterine tachysystole. The three perinatal deaths were associated just with breast stimulation (1.8% vs. 0%; RR 8.17, 95% CI 0.45–147.77) [130].

Compared with oxytocin alone, breast stimulation had similar rates of women not in labor after 72 hours, cesarean section rates, and meconium staining. Three of the four perinatal deaths were in high-risk women in the breast stimulation group (17.6% vs. 5%; RR 3.53, 95% CI 0.40–30.88) [130]. Until **safety issues** have been fully evaluated, breast stimulation should not be used in high-risk women [130].

Castor Oil
Castor oil **should not be used for induction of labor** [131]. There was no evidence of differences in caesarean section rates in the two trials reporting this outcome (RR 2.04, 95% CI 0.92–4.55). There were no data presented on neonatal or maternal mortality or morbidity. All women who ingested castor oil felt nauseous [131].

Enemas and Baths
There are no trials on enemas or baths for induction of labor.

Homeopathy
There is insufficient evidence to recommend the use of homeopathy (e.g., with caulophyllum) as a method of induction. **No benefits** were seen in the two small, poor-quality trials [132].

Sexual Intercourse
There is **insufficient evidence** to assess the efficacy of sexual intercourse for induction of labor. A "coital diary" prospective study showed no difference in the incidence of spontaneous labor in the "advised-coitus" group despite 1.5 times as many participants in that group reporting intercourse. There was also no difference in the rate of cesarean section or adverse outcomes [133]. One RCT is too small for meaningful guidance [134]. In another RCT, compared with no such advice, advice for coitus was associated with more coital activity (60% vs. 40%; RR 1.5, 95% CI 1.1–2.0), but similar rates of spontaneous labor (56% vs. 52%; RR 1.1, 95% CI 0.8–1.4) [135]. In a trial of 1175 women randomized to coitus-advised versus no advice, there were no differences in intervention to delivery, gestational age at delivery, or need for induction [136]. A limitation is that only 144 women returned their coital diary.

ANTEPARTUM TESTING DURING CERVICAL RIPENING

Fetal heart monitoring during cervical ripening depends on the agent used. There are no trials to assess the effectiveness and best modality for monitoring. In general, a nonstress test (NST) should be obtained before any induction or cervical ripening agent is used to assure fetal well-being. After administration of **PGE2 gel or tablet,** the fetal heart can be monitored continuously for about 0.5–2 hours, although the proper amount of time for monitoring is unclear. After administration of **PGE2 insert,** the fetal heart can be monitored continuously for the duration of the insertion [137]. After administration of **misoprostol,** the fetal heart should be monitored continuously, given the higher chance of contractions, and uterine tachysystole with related NRFHT.

OUTPATIENT VERSUS INPATIENT

Induction of labor in outpatient settings appears **feasible, but the evidence is still insufficient for routine use.** Important **adverse events are rare** [138]. There is **insufficient evidence to know which induction agents are most effective and safe to use in outpatient setting.** Studies examined **vaginal and intracervical PGE2, isosorbide mononitrate** (for these three agents there is most evidence of safety, n ≥500 each), Foley [71], vaginal and oral misoprostol, mifepristone, estrogens, and acupuncture (very limited evidence for these other agents) [139]. There *is insufficient evidence to assess the safety of outpatient misoprostol* for induction of labor. While effective in decreasing the length of gestation and induction-to-delivery interval, the safety of this approach, even at low (25 mg) doses, is still unproven in the three small trials [139–141]. There **is insufficient data to assess the safety of outpatient dinosprostone for induction of labor.** In a RCT including 827 women, the outpatient dinoprostone group has more NRFHT and was unable to be discharged home. Over half of the randomized women did not receive the allocated intervention secondary to labor or not requiring ripening [142].

There was no strong evidence that agents used to induce labor in outpatient settings had an impact (positive or negative) on maternal or neonatal health. There was some evidence that, compared with placebo or no treatment, **induction agents reduced the need for further interventions to induce labor and shortened the interval from intervention to birth.** There was no evidence that induction agents increased interventions in labor such as operative deliveries. In one cost analysis performed alongside a prospective RCT, inpatient prostaglandin gel did not have a significantly increased cost compared with outpatient Foley catheter, although outpatient Foley catheter was associated with fewer prelabor hours spent on the birthing unit [143]. A survey conducted along with an outpatient induction RCT found that women were willing to accept an extra 1.42 trips to hospital (2.42 trips total) and a travel time of 30.6 minutes per trip (73.3 minutes total) to be able to return to their own home while waiting for the priming to work, and overall preferred outpatient priming when the option was to return to their own home (OR 1.8, 95% CI 1.4–2.1, $p < .0001$) [144].

Labor Management with Induction
The patterns by which labor progresses in spontaneous labor and electively induced labor are significantly different [36]. **Latent and early active phases proceed slower than a spontaneous labor in induced labor** in which cervical ripening was necessary. Induction not requiring cervical ripening may be associated with a quicker labor course from 4 to 10 cm [36]. The risk of CD is increased during the first stage of labor of an induction needing cervical ripening, mainly because of dystocia. Induction without need for cervical ripening may have no or only a minor effect on the risk of cesarean [36]. Applying the same standards of spontaneous labor curves (e.g., Friedman's curve) to induced patients may lead to an increase cesarean section rate in induction (see Chapters 7 and 8).

When administering oxytocin, the target is to stimulate uterine activity that is sufficient to effect cervical change as well as fetal descent without compromising the fetus. Minimal criteria for effective uterine activity are 3 contractions per 10 minutes averaging greater than 25 mmHg above baseline, with 5 contractions in 10 minutes. The Montevideo unit was created in 1957 to describe the summation of the amplitudes of all contractions in a 10-minute window. Uterine tachysystole is defined as >5 contractions in 10 minutes. During induction with oxytocin, 91% of patients delivered vaginally achieved 200 Montevideo units without neonatal morbidity in one retrospective study [145]. Contraction pressures of ≥200 Montevideo units should be targeted in induction or augmentation of laboring patients to achieve adequate labor [145,146]. **Induced labor should be managed, in general, as for spontaneous labor** (see Chapters 7 and 8). If active phase is not achieved within 24 hours, this is not a reason per se for CD. A **failed induction** should not be diagnosed until after **24 hours of oxytocin after membrane rupture in the active phase** (usually 6 cm in a nulliparous patient), assuming reassuring fetal heart pattern [14,15,36].

REFERENCES

1. Martin JA, Hamilton BE, Osterman MJ, et al. Births: Final data for 2013. *Natl Vital Stat Rep.* 2015;64:1–65. [III, Epidemiologic data report]
2. National Center for Health Statistics. Available at: VitalStats. /nchs/vitalstats.htm. Accessed March 9, 2015. [III, Epidemiologic data report]
3. Glantz JC. Labor induction rate variation in upstate New York: What is the difference? *Birth.* 2003;30(3):168–174. [II-2]
4. Gyamfi-Bannerman C and Ananth CV. Trends in spontaneous and indicated preterm delivery among singleton gestations in the United States, 2005-2012. *Obstet Gynecol.* 2014;124:1069–1074. [III, Epidemiologic data report]
5. Bailit JL, Gregory KD, Reddy UM, et al. Maternal and neonatal outcomes by labor onset type and gestational age. *Am J Obstet Gynecol.* 2010;202(3):245.e1–245.e12. [II-2]
6. Bishop EH. Pelvic scoring for elective induction. *Obstet Gynecol.* 1964;24:266–268. [II-3]
7. Vrouenraets FP, Roumen FJ, Dehing CJ, et al. Bishop score and risk of cesarean delivery after induction of labor in nulliparous women. *Obstet Gynecol.* 2005;105:690–697. [II-2, $n = 765$]
8. Simon CE, Grobman WA. When has an induction failed? *Obstet Gynecol.* 2005;105:705–9. [II-2]
9. Rouse DJ, Weiner SJ, Bloom SL, et al. Failed labor induction: Toward an objective diagnosis. *Obstet Gynecol.* 2011;117:267–72. [III]
10. Wood S, Cooper S, Ross S. Does induction of labour increase the risk of caesarean section? A systematic review and meta-analysis of trials in women with intact membranes. *BJOG.* 2014;121:674–685. [I, Meta-analysis: 31 RCTs, $n = 6248$]
11. Caughey AB, Sundaram V, Kaimal AJ, et al. Systematic review: Elective induction of labor versus expectant management of pregnancy. *Ann Intern Med.* 2009;151:252–263. [II-2]
12. American Congress of Obstetricians and Gynecologists (ACOG). *Patient Safety Checklists. American Congress of Obstetricians and Gynecologists [Internet].* Washington, DC: ACOG. Available at: http://www.acog.org/Resources-And-Publications/Patient-Safety-Checklists. Accessed January 12, 2016.
13. Sciscione AC, Zhang J, Laughon K, et al. The duration of labor induction and maternal and neonatal outcomes. Poster Presentation. SMFM Annual Meeting, San Francisco, CA, February 2011. [II-2]
14. Spong CY, Berghella V, Wenstrom KD, et al. Preventing the first cesarean delivery: Summary of a joint Eunice Kennedy Shriver National Institute of Child Health and Human Development, Society for Maternal-Fetal Medicine, and American College of Obstetricians and Gynecologists Workshop. *Obstet Gynecol.* 2012;120:1181–1193. [III]
15. Rouse DJ, Owen J, Hauth JC. Criteria for failed labor induction: Prospective evaluation of a standardized protocol. *Obstet Gynecol.* 2000;96:671–677. [II-3, $n = 509$]
16. Neilson JP. Ultrasound for fetal assessment in early pregnancy. *Cochrane Database Syst Rev.* [I, Meta-analysis: 9 RCTs, $n = >24,000$]
17. Mozurkewich E, Chilimigras J, Koepke E, et al. Indications for induction of labour: a best evidence review. *BJOG.* 2009;116:626–636. [III, Review]
18. Spong CY, Mercer BM, D'Alton M, et al. Timing of indicated late-preterm and early-term birth. *Obstet Gynecol.* 2011;118(2 Pt 1): 323–333. [III, Review]
19. Berghella V, Blackwell SC, Ramin SM, et al. Use and misuse of the term "elective" in obstetrics. *Obstet Gynecol.* 2011;117(2 Pt 1): 372–376. [III, Review]
20. American College of Obstetricians and Gynecologists. ACOG Practice Bulletin No. 107: Induction of labor. *Obstet Gynecol.* 2009;114:386–397. [III, Review]
21. Saccone G, Berghella V. Induction of labor at full term in uncomplicated singleton gestations: A systematic review and meta-analysis of randomized controlled trials. *Am J Obstet Gynecol.* 2015;213(5):629–636. (Epub ahead of print) [I, Meta-analysis: 5 RCTs, $n = 884$]
22. Walker KF, Malin G, Wilson P, Thornto JG. Induction of labour versus expectant management at term by subgroups of maternal age: An individual patient data meta-analysis. *Eur J Obstet Gynecol Reprod Biol.* 2015;197:1–5. doi 10.1016/j.ejogrb.2015.11.004. [Epub ahead of print]
23. Miller NR, Cypher RL, Foglia LM, et al. Elective induction of labor compared with expectant management of nulliparous women at 39 weeks of gestation. *Obstet Gynecol.* 2015;126(6):1258–1264. [RCT, $n = 162$]
24. U.S. National Institutes of Health (NIH) ClinicalTrials. gov. A Randomized Trial of Induction versus Expectant Management (ARRIVE) [Internet]. Washington, DC: NIH. Available at: https://www.clinicaltrials.gov/ct2/show/NCT01990612?term<=arrive&rank=4. Accessed January 15, 2016
25. Plaut MM, Schwartz ML, Lubarsky SL. Uterine rupture associated with the use of misoprostol in the gravid patient with a previous cesarean section. *Am J Obstet Gynecol.* 1999;180:1535–1542. [II-2, $n = 512$]
26. Hoffman MK, Sciscione AC, Srinivasana M, et al. Uterine rupture in patients with a prior cesarean delivery: The impact of cervical ripening. *Am J Perinatol.* 2004;21:217–222. [II-2, $n = 972$]
27. Bujold E, Blackwell SC, Hendler I, et al. Modified Bishop's score and induction of labor in patients with previous cesarean delivery. *Am J Obstet Gynecol.* 2004;191:1644–1648. [II-2, $n = 685$]
28. Landon MB, Hauth JC, Leveno KJ, et al. Maternal and perinatal outcomes associated with a trial of labor after prior cesarean delivery. *N Engl J Med.* 2004;351(25):2581–2589. [II-2; prospective; $n = 33,699$]
29. Lyndon-Rochelle M, Holt VL, Easterling TR, et al. Risk of uterine rupture during labor among women with a prior cesarean delivery. *N Engl J Med.* 2001;345(1):3–8. [II-2, $n = 20,095$]
30. Bujold E, Blackwell SC, Gauthier RJ. Cervical ripening with transcervical Foley catheter and the risk of uterine rupture. *Obstet Gynecol.* 2004;103:18–23. [II-2, $n = 2479$]
31. Palatnik A, Grobman WA. Induction of labor versus expectant management for women with a prior cesarean delivery. *Am J Obstet Gynecol.* 2015;212:358.e1–358.e6. [II-2]
32. Bakker JJ, van der Goes BY, Pel M, Mol BW, et al. Morning versus evening induction of labour for improving outcomes. *Cochrane Database Syst Rev.* 2013;2:CD007707. [I, Meta-analysis: 3 RCTs, $n = 1150$]
33. Bakker JJ, De Vos R, Pel M, et al. Start of Induction of labour with oxytocin in the morning or in the evening. A randomized controlled trial. *BJOG.* 2009;116:562–568. [I, RCT, $n = 371$]
34. Dodd JM, Crowther CA, Robinson JS. Morning compared with evening induction of labor—A nested randomized controlled trial. *Obstet Gynecol.* 2006;108:350–360. [I, RCT, $n = 620$]
35. Pevzner L, Rayburn WF, Rumney P, et al. Factors predicting successful labor and induction with dinoprostone and misoprostol vaginal inserts. *Obstet Gynecol.* 2009;114:261–267. [II-2, $n = 1274$]
36. Vahration A, Zhang J, Troendle JF, et al. Labor progression and risk of cesarean delivery in electively induced nulliparas. *Obstet Gynecol.* 2005;105:698–704. [II-2, $n = 429$]
37. Laughton SK, Zhang J, Troendle J, et al. Using a simplified Bishop score to predict vaginal delivery. *Obstet Gynecol.* 2011;117(4):805–811. [II-2]

38. Kolkman DG, Verhoeven CJ, Brinkhorst SJ, et al. The bishop score as a predictor of labor induction success: A systematic review. *Am J Perinatol.* 2013;30:625–630. [III]
39. Teixeira C, Lunet N, Rodrigues T, Barros H. The bishop score as a determinant of labour induction success: A systematic review and meta-analysis. *Arch Gynecol Obstet.* 2012;286:739–753. [III, Review]
40. Park KH, Kim SN, Lee SY, et al. Comparison between sonographic cervical length and Bishop score in preinduction cervical assessment: A randomized trial. *Ultrasound Obstet Gynecol.* 2011;38:198–204. [RCT, n = 154]
41. Hatfield AS, Sanchez-Ramos L, Kaunitz AM. Sonographic cervical assessment to predict the success of labor induction: A systematic review with meta-analysis. *Am J Obstet Gynecol.* 2007;197:186–192. [III, Review]
42. Verhoeven CJ, Opmeer BC, Oei SG, et al. Transvaginal sonographic assessment of cervical length and wedging for predicting outcome of labor induction at term: A systematic review and meta-analysis. *Ultrasound Obstet Gynecol.* 2013;42:500–508. [III, Review]
43. Garite TJ, Carcia-Alonso A, Kreaden U, et al. Fetal fibronectin: A new tool for the prediction of successful induction of labor. *Am J Obstet Gynecol.* 1996;175:1516–1521. [II-2]
44. Sciscione AC, Hoffman MK, DeLuca S, et al. Fetal fibronectin as a predictor of vaginal birth in nulliparas undergoing preinduction cervical ripening. *Obstet Gynecol.* 2005;106:980–985. [II-2, n = 241]
45. Droulez A, Girard R, Dumas AM, et al. Prediction of successful induction of labor: A comparison between fetal fibronectin assay and the Bishop score. *J Gynecol Obstet Biol Reprod (Paris).* 2008;37:691–696. [II-2]
46. Reis FM, Gervasi MT, Florio P, et al. Prediction of successful induction of labor at term: Role of clinical history, digital examination, ultrasound assessment of the cervix, and fetal fibronectin assay. *Am J Obstet Gynecol.* 2003;189:1361–1367. [II-2]
47. Ojutiku D, Jones G, Bewley S. Quantitative foetal fibronectin as a predictor of successful induction of labour in post-date pregnancies. *Eur J Obstet Gynecol Reprod Biol.* 2002;101:143–146. [II-2, n = 33]
48. Jozwiak M, Bloemenkamp KWM, Kelly AJ, et al. Mechanical methods for induction of labour. *Cochrane Database Syst Rev.* 2012;(3):CD001233. [I, Meta-analysis: 71 RCTs, n = >9000]
49. Gilson GJ, Russell DJ, Izquierdo LA, et al. A prospective, randomized evaluation of a hygroscopic cervical dilator, Dilapan, in the preinduction ripening of patients undergoing induction of labor. *Am J Obstet Gynecol.* 1996;175:145–149. [I, RCT, n = 240]
50. Sciscione AC, McCullough H, Manley JS, et al. A prospective, randomized comparison of Foley catheter insertion versus intracervical prostaglandin E2 gel for preinduction cervical ripening. *Am J Obstet Gynecol.* 1999;180:55–59. [I, RCT, n = 149]
51. Thomas IL, Chenowith JN, Tronc GN, et al. Preparation for induction of labour of the unfavourable cervix with Foley catheter compared with vaginal prostaglandin. *Aust NZ J Obstet Gynaecol.* 1986;26:30–35. [I, RCT, n = 57]
52. Orhue A. Induction of labour at term in primigravidae with low Bishop's score: A comparison of three methods. *Eur J Obstet Gynecol Reprod Biol.* 1995;58:119–125. [I, RCT, n = 90]
53. St. Onge RD, Conners GT. Preinduction cervical ripening: A comparison of intracervical prostaglandin E2 gel versus the Foley catheter. *Am J Obstet Gynecol.* 1995;172:687–690. [I, RCT, n = 66]
54. Lieberman JR, Piura B, Choim W, et al. The cervical balloon method for induction of labor. *Acta Obstet Gynecol Scand.* 1977;56:499–503. [RCT, n = 194]
55. Sciscione AC, Ngyuen L, Manley J, et al. A randomized comparison of transcervical Foley catheter to intravaginal misoprostol for preinduction cervical ripening. *Obstet Gynecol.* 2001;97:603–607. [I, RCT, n = 111]
56. Delaney S, Shaffer BL, Yvonne CW, et al. Labor induction with a Foley balloon inflated to 30 mL compared with 60 mL. *Obstet Gynecol.* 2010;115:1239–1245. [I, RCT, n = 192]
57. Levy R, Kanengiser B, Furman B, et al. A randomized trial comparing a 30-mL and an 80-mL Foley catheter balloon for preinduction cervical ripening. *Am J Obstet Gynecol.* 2004;191:1632–1636. [I, RCT, n = 203]
58. Kashanian M, Nazemi M, Malakzadegan A. Comparison of 30-mL and 80-mL Foley catheter balloons and oxytocin for pre-induction cervical ripening. *Int J Gynaecol Obstet.* 2009;105:174–175. [I, RCT, n = 270]
59. Gibson KS, Mercer BM, Louis JM. Inner thigh taping vs traction for cervical ripening with a Foley catheter: A randomized controlled trial. *Am J Obstet Gynecol.* 2013;209:272.e1–272.e7. [I, RCT, n = 191]
60. Cromi A, Ghezzi F, Agosti M, et al. Is transcervical Foley catheter actually slower than prostaglandins in ripening the cervix? A randomized study. *Am J Obstet Gynecol.* 2011;204:338.e1–338.e7. [I, RCT, n = 397]
61. Fox NS, Saltzman DH, Roman AS, et al. Intravaginal misoprostol versus Foley catheter for labour induction: A meta-analysis. *BJOG.* 2011;118(6):647–654. [I, Meta-analysis: 9 RCTs, n = 1603]
62. Jozwiak M, ten Eikelder M, Oude Rengerink K, et al. Foley catheter versus vaginal misoprostol: Randomized controlled trial (PROBAAT-M study) and systematic review and meta-analysis of literature. *Am J Perinatol.* 2014;31:145–156. [I, Meta-analysis, 10 RCTs, n = 1520]
63. Vaknin Z, Kurzweil Y, Sherman D. Foley catheter balloon vs locally applied prostaglandins for cervical ripening and labor induction: A systematic review and metaanalysis. *Am J Obstet Gynecol.* 2010;204:418–429. [I, Meta-analysis: 27 RCTs, n = 3470]
64. Chen W, Xue J, Peprah MK, Wen SW. A systemic review and network meta-analysis comparing the use of Foley catheters, misoprostol, and dinoprostone for cervical ripening in the induction of labour. *BJOG.* 2016;123(3):346–354. doi: 10.1111/1471-0528.13456. [Epub ahead of print] [I, Meta-analysis n = 17,387]
65. Pettker C, Pocock SB, Smok DB, et al. Transcervical Foley catheter with and without oxytocin for cervical ripening: A randomized controlled trial. *Obstet Gynecol.* 2008;111:1320–1326. [I, RCT, n = 183]
66. Carbone JF, Tuuli MG, Fogertey PJ, et al. Combination of Foley bulb and vaginal misoprostol compared with vaginal misoprostol alone for cervical ripening and labor induction: A randomized controlled trial. *Obstet Gynecol.* 2013;121:247–252. [I, RCT n = 123]
67. Chen W, Xue J, Gaudet L, et al. Meta-analysis of Foley catheter plus misoprostol versus misoprostol alone for cervical ripening. *Int J Gynaecol Obstet.* 2015;129(3):193–198 [I, Meta-analysis n = 1153]
68. Sciscione AC, Muench M, Pollock M, et al. Transcervical Foley catheter for preinduction cervical ripening in an outpatient versus inpatient setting. *Obstet Gynecol.* 2001;98:5(1):751–756. [I, RCT, n = 111]
69. Gagnon-Gervais K, Bujold E, Iglesias MH, et al. Early versus late amniotomy for labour induction: A randomized controlled trial. *J Matern Fetal Neonatal Med.* 2012;25:2326–2329. [I RCT, n = 143]
70. Levy R, Ferber A, Ben-Arie A, et al. A randomised comparison of early versus late amniotomy following cervical ripening with a foley catheter. *BJOG.* 2002;109:168–172. [I, RCT, n = 148]
71. Sciscione AC, Hoffman MK, Bedder CL, et al. The timing of adverse events with Foley catheter preinduction cervical ripening; implications for outpatient use. *Am J Perinatol.* 2014;31:781–786. [II-1]
72. McMaster K, Sanchez-Ramos L, Kaunitz AM. Evaluation of a transcervical foley catheter as a source of infection: A systematic review and meta-analysis. *Obstet Gynecol.* 2015;126:539–551. [I, Meta-analysis, 26 RCTs, n = 5563]
73. Schreyer P, Sherman DJ, Ariely S, et al. Ripening the highly unfavorable cervix with extra-amniotic saline instillation or vaginal prostaglandin E2 application. *Obstet Gynecol.* 1989;73:938–941. [I, RCT, n = 106]
74. Rouben D, Arias F. A randomized trial of extra-amniotic saline infusion plus intracervical Foley catheter balloon versus

prostaglandin E2 vaginal gel for ripening the cervix and inducing labor in patients with unfavorable cervices. *Obstet Gynecol.* 1993;82:290–294. [I, RCT, n = 112]
75. Goldman JB, Wigton TR. A randomized comparison of extra-amniotic saline infusion and intracervical dinoprostone gel for cervical ripening. *Obstet Gynecol.* 1999;93:271–274. [I, RCT, n = 52]
76. Vengalil SR, Guinn DA, Olabi NF, et al. A randomized trial of misoprostol and extra-amniotic saline infusion for cervical ripening and labor induction. *Obstet Gynecol.* 1998;91:774–779. [I, RCT, n = 248]
77. Mullin PM, House M, Paul RH, et al. A comparison of vaginally administered misoprostol with extra-amniotic saline infusion for cervical ripening and labor induction. *Am J Obstet Gynecol.* 2002;187:847–852. [I, RCT, n = 200]
78. Karyane NW, Brock EL, Walsh SW. Induction of labor using a Foley balloon, with and without extra-amniotic saline infusion. *Obstet Gynecol.* 2006;107:234–239. [I, RCT, n = 120]
79. Lin MG, Reid KJ, Treaster MR, et al. Transcervical Foley catheter with and without extraamniotic saline infusion for labor induction. *Obstet Gynecol.* 2007;110:558–565. [I, RCT, n = 188]
80. Atad J, Hallak M, Auslender R, et al. A randomized comparison of prostaglandin E2, oxytocin, and the double-balloon device in inducing labor. *Obstet Gynecol.* 1996;87:223–227. [I, RCT, n = 95]
81. Pennell CE, Henderson JJ, O'Neill MJ, et al. Induction of labour in nulliparous women with an unfavourable cervix: A randomised controlled trial comparing double and single balloon catheters and PGE2 gel. *BJOG.* 2009;116:1443–1452. [I, RCT, n = 330]
82. Cromi A, Ghezzi F, Uccella S, et al. A randomized trial of pre-induction cervical ripening: Dinoprostone vaginal insert versus double-balloon catheter. *Am J Obstet Gynecol.* 2012;207:125.e1,125.e7. [I, RCT, n = 210]
83. Suffecool K, Rosenn BM, Kam S, et al. Labor induction in nulliparous women with an unfavorable cervix: Double balloon catheter versus dinoprostone. *J Perinat Med.* 2014;42:213–218. [I, RCT, n = 62]
84. Wang W, Zheng J, Fu J, et al. Which is the safer method of labor induction for oligohydramnios women? transcervical double balloon catheter or dinoprostone vaginal insert. *J Matern Fetal Neonatal Med.* 2014;27:1805–1808 [I, RCT, n = 126]
85. Salim R, Zafran N, Nachum Z, et al. Single-balloon compared with double-balloon catheters for induction of labor: A randomized controlled trial. *Obstet Gynecol.* 2011;118:79–86. [I, RCT, n = 293]
86. Boulvain M, Stan CM, Irion O. Membrane sweeping for induction of labour. *Cochrane Database Syst Rev.* 2005;(1):CD000451. [I, Meta-analysis: 22 RCTs, n = 2797]
87. Berghella V, Rogers RA, Lescale K. Stripping of membranes as a safe method to reduce prolonged pregnancies. *Obstet Gynecol.* 1996;87(6):927–929. [I, RCT, n = 142]
88. Foong LC, Vanaja K, Tan G, et al. Membranes sweeping in conjunction with labor induction. *Obstet Gynecol.* 2000;96:539–542. [I, RCT, n = 248 (n = 130 nulliparas)]
89. Yildirim G, Gungorduk K, Karadag OI, et al. Membrane sweeping to induce labor in low-risk patients at term pregnancy: A randomised controlled trial. *J Matern Fetal Neonatal Med.* 2010;23:681–687. [I, RCT, n = 246]
90. de Miranda E, van der Bom JG, Bonsel GJ, et al. Membrane sweeping and prevention of post-term pregnancy in low-risk pregnancies: A randomised controlled trial. *BJOG.* 2006;113:402–408. [I, RCT, n = 742]
91. Hamdan M, Sidhu K, Sabir N, et al. Serial membrane sweeping at term in planned vaginal birth after cesarean: A randomized controlled trial. *Obstet Gynecol.* 2009;114:745–751. [I, RCT, n = 213]
92. Bricker L, Luckas M. Amniotomy alone for induction of labour. *Cochrane Database Syst Rev.* 2000;(4):CD002862. [I, Meta-analysis: 2 RCTs, n = 310]
93. Mercer BM, McNanley T, O'Brien JM, et al. Early versus late amniotomy for labor induction: A randomized trial. *Am J Obstet Gynecol.* 1995;173:1371. [I, RCT, n = 209]
94. Macones GA, Cahill A, Stamilio DM, Odibo AO. The efficacy of early amniotomy in nulliparous labor induction: A randomized controlled trial. *Am J Obstet Gynecol.* 2012;207(5):403.e1–403.e5 [I, RCT n = 585]
95. Makarem MH, Zahran KM, Abdellah MS, Karen MA. Early amniotomy after vaginal misoprostol for induction of labor: A randomized clinical trial. *Arch Gynecol Obstet.* 2013;288(2):261–265 [I, RCT n = 320]
96. Levy R, Ferber A, Ben-Arie A, et al. A randomised comparison of early versus late amniotomy following cervical ripening with a Foley catheter. *BJOG.* 2002;109(2): 168–172 [I, RCT n = 168]
97. Howarth G, Botha DJ. Amniotomy plus intravenous oxytocin for induction of labour. *Cochrane Database Syst Rev.* 2001 (3):CD003250. [I, Meta-analysis: 17 RCTs, n = 2566]
98. Austin SC, Sanchez-Ramos L, Adair CD. Labor Induction with intravaginal misoprostol compared with dinoprostone vaginal insert: A systematic review and meta-analysis. *Am J Obstet Gynecol.* 2010;202:624.e1–624.e9. [I, Meta-analysis: 11 RCTs, n = 1572]
99. Alfirevic Z, Keeney E, Dowswell T, et al. Labour induction with prostaglandins: A systematic review and network meta-analysis. *BMJ.* 2015;350:h217. [I, Meta-analysis: 280 RCTs, n>48,000]
100. Liu A, Lv J, Hu Y, et al. Efficacy and safety of intravaginal misoprostol versus intracervical dinoprostone for labor induction at term: A systematic review and meta-analysis. *J Obstet Gynaecol Res.* 2014;40:897–906. [I, Meta-analysis: 10 RCTs, n = 1061]
101. Wing DA. Misoprostol Vaginal Insert Consortium. Misoprostol vaginal insert compared with dinoprostone vaginal insert: A randomized controlled trial. *Obstet Gynecol.* 2008;112:801–812. [I, RCT, n = 1308]
102. Wing DA, Miller H, Parker L, et al. Misoprostol vaginal insert for successful labor induction—A randomized controlled trial. *Obstet Gynecol.* 2011;117:533–541. [I, RCT, n = 374]
103. Wing DA, Brown R, Plante LA, et al. Misoprostol vaginal insert and time to vaginal delivery: A randomized controlled trial. *Obstet Gynecol.* 2013;122:201–209. [I, RCT, n = 1358]
104. Stephenson ML, Powers BL, Wing DA. Fetal heart rate and cardiotocographic abnormalities with varying dose misoprostol vaginal inserts. *J Matern Fetal Neonatal Med.* 2013;26:127–131. [II-2]
105. Alfirevic Z, Aflaifel N, Weeks A. Oral misoprostol for induction of labour. *Cochrane Database Syst Rev.* 2014;(6):CD001338. [I, Meta-analysis: vs. placebo: 9 RCTs, n = 1109; vs. vaginal PGE2: 12 RCTs, n = 3859; IV oxytocin: 9 RCTs, n = 1282; vaginal misoprostol: 37 RCTs, n = 6417]
106. Kundodyiwa TW, Alfirevic Z, Weeks AD. Low-dose oral misoprostol for induction of labor: A systematic review. *Obstet Gynecol.* 2009;113:374–383. [I, Meta-analysis, n = 2937]
107. Muzonzini G, Hofmeyr GJ. Buccal or sublingual misoprostol for cervical ripening and induction of labour. *Cochrane Database Syst Rev.* 2004;(4):CD004221. [I, Meta-analysis: 3 RCTs, n = 502]
108. Souza AS, Amorim MM, Feitosa FE. Comparison of sublingual versus vaginal misoprostol for the induction of labour: A systematic review. *BJOG.* 2008;115:1340–1349. [I, Meta-analysis, n = 740]
109. Thomas J, Fairclough A, Kavanaugh J, et al. Vaginal prostaglandin (PGE2 and PGF2a) for induction of labour at term. *Cochrane Database Syst Rev.* 2014;(6):CD003101. [I, Meta-analysis: 70 RCTs, n = 11,487]
110. Boulvain M, Kelly AJ, Irion O. Intra-cervical prostaglandins for induction of labour. *Cochrane Database Syst Rev.* 2008;(1):CD006971. [I, Meta-analysis: 56 RCTs, n = 7738; intra-cervical PGE2 with placebo/no treatment: 28 trials, 3764 women; intra-cervical PGE2 with intravaginal PGE2: 29 trials, 3881 women]
111. Chyu J, Strassner HT. Prostaglandin E2 for cervical ripening: A randomized comparison of Cervidil versus Prepidil. *Am J Obstet Gynecol.* 1997;177:606–611. [I, RCT, n = 73]
112. Smith CV, Rayburn WF, Miller AM. Intravaginal prostaglandin E2 for cervical ripening and initiation of labor. Comparison of a multidose gel and single, controlled-release pessary. *J Reprod Med.* 1994;39(5):381–384. [I, RCT, n = 121]

113. Perryman D, Yeast J, Holst V. Cervical ripening: A randomized study comparing prostaglandin E2 gel to prostaglandin E2 suppositories. *Obstet Gynecol.* 1992;79:670–672. [I, RCT, n = 90]
114. Christensen FC, Tehranifar M, Gonzalez JL, et al. Randomized trial of concurrent oxytocin with a sustained-release dinoprostone vaginal insert for labor induction at term. *Am J Obstet Gynecol.* 2002;186:61–65. [I, RCT, n = 71]
115. Hutton EK, Mozurkewich EL. Extra-amniotic prostaglandin for induction of labour. *Cochrane Database Syst Rev.* 2001;(2):CD003092. [I, Meta-analysis: 12 RCTs]
116. French L. Oral prostaglandin E2 for induction of labour. *Cochrane Database Syst Rev.* 2001;(2):CD003098. [I, Meta-analysis: 15 RCTs, n = >500]
117. Luckas M, Bricker L. Intravenous prostaglandin for induction of labour. *Cochrane Database Syst Rev.* 2000;(4):CD002864. [I, Meta-analysis: 13 RCTs, n = 1165]
118. Alfirevic Z, Kelly AJ, Dowswell T. Intravenous oxytocin alone for cervical ripening and induction of labour. *Cochrane Database Syst Rev.* 2009;(4):CD003246. [I, Meta-analysis: 61 RCTs, n = 12,819]
119. Budden A, Chen LJ, Henry A. High-dose versus low-dose oxytocin infusion regimens for induction of labour at term. *Cochrane Database Syst Rev.* 2014;(10):CD009701. [I, Meta-analysis, 9 RCTs, n = 2391]
120. Hapangama D, Neilson JP. Mifepristone for induction of labour. *Cochrane Database Syst Rev.* 2009;(3):CD002865. [I, Meta-analysis: 10 RCTs, n = 1108]
121. MacKenzie IZ. Induction of labour at the start of the new millennium. *Reproduction.* 2006;131:989–998. [III, Review]
122. Thomas J, Kelly AJ, Kavanagh J. Oestrogens alone or with amniotomy for cervical ripening or induction of labour. *Cochrane Database Syst Rev.* 2001;(4):CD003393. [I, Meta-analysis: 8 RCTs, n = 421]
123. Kelly AJ, Kavanagh J, Thomas J. Relaxin for cervical ripening and induction of labour. *Cochrane Database Syst Rev.* 2001;(2):CD003103. [I, Meta-analysis: 4 RCTs, n = 267]
124. Ziaei S, Rosebehani N, Kazeminejad A, et al. The effects of intramuscular administration of corticosteroids on the induction of parturition. *J Perinat Med.* 2003;31:134–139. [I RCT, n = 66]
125. Barkai G, Cohen SB, Kees S, et al. Induction of labor with use of a foley catheter and extraamniotic corticosteroids. *Am J Obstet Gynecol.* 1997;177:1145–1148. [I, CT, n = 98]
126. Spallicci MDB, Bittar RE. Randomized double blind study of ripening of the cervix with hyaluronidase in term gestations [Estudo clinico aleatorizado com grupo controle e mascaramento duplo da maturacao do colo uterino pela hialuronidase em gestacoes a termo]. *Rev Bras Ginecol Obstet.* 2003;25:67. [I, RCT, n = 168]
127. Surita FG, Cecatti JG, Parpinelli MA, et al. Hyaluronidase versus foley catheter for cervical ripening in high-risk term and post term pregnancies. *Int J Gynaecol Obstet.* 2005;88:258–264. [I, RCT, n = 140]
128. Kelly AJ, Munson C, Minden L. Nitric oxide donors for cervical ripening and induction of labour. *Cochrane Database Syst Rev.* 2011;(6):CD006901. [I, Meta-analysis: 10 RCTs, n = 1889]
129. Smith CA, Crowther CA, Grant SJ. Acupuncture for induction of labour. *Cochrane Database Syst Rev.* 2013;(8):CD002962. [I, Meta-analysis: 14 RCTs, n = 2220]
130. Kavanagh J, Kelly AJ, Thomas J. Breast stimulation for cervical ripening and induction of labour. *Cochrane Database Syst Rev.* 2005;(3):CD003392. [I, Meta-analysis: 6 RCTs, n = 719]
131. Kelly AJ, Kavanagh J, Thomas J. Castor oil, bath and/or enema for cervical priming and induction of labour. *Cochrane Database Syst Rev.* 2013;(7):CD003099. [I, Meta-analysis: 3 RCTs, n = 233]
132. Smith CA. Homoeopathy for induction of labour. *Cochrane Database Syst Rev.* 2003;(4):CD003399. [I, Meta-analysis: 2 RCTs, n = 133]
133. Tan PC, Anggeriana M, Azmi N, et al. Effect of coitus at term on length of gestation, induction of labor and mode of delivery. *Obstet Gynecol.* 2006;134–140. [II-2]
134. Bendvold E. Coitus and induction of labour [Samleie og induksjon av fodsel]. *Tidsskrift for Jordmodre.* 1990;96:6–8. [I, RCT, n = 28]
135. Tan PC, Yow CM, Omar SZ. Effect of coital activity on onset of labor in women scheduled for labor induction. *Obstet Gynecol.* 2007;110:820–826. [I, RCT, n = 210]
136. Omar NS, Tan PC, Sabir N, et al. Coitus to expedite the onset of labour: A randomised trial. *BJOG.* 2013;120:338–345. [I, RCT, n = 1175]
137. American College of Obstetricians and Gynecologists. *ACOG Committee Opinion No. 209: Monitoring During Induction of Labor with Dinoprostone.* Washington, DC: ACOG, 1998. [III, Review]
138. Dowswell T, Kelly AJ, Livio S, et al. Different methods for the induction of labour in outpatient settings. *Cochrane Database Syst Rev.* 2010;(8):CD007701. [I, Meta-analysis: 28 RCTs, n = 2616]
139. McKenna DS, Ester JB, Proffitt M, et al. Misoprostol outpatient cervical ripening without subsequent induction of labor: A randomized trial. *Obstet Gynecol.* 2004;104:579–584. [I, RCT, n = 33]
140. Stitely ML, Browning J, Fowler M, et al. Outpatient cervical ripening with intravaginal misoprostol. *Obstet Gynecol.* 2000;96:684–688. [I, RCT, n = 60]
141. Incerpi MH, Fassett MJ, Kjos SL, et al. Vaginally administered misoprostol for outpatient cervical ripening in pregnancies complicated by diabetes mellitus. *Am J Obstet Gynecol.* 2001;185:916–919. [I, RCT, n = 120]
142. Wilkinson C, Bryce R, Adelson P, Turnbull D. A randomised controlled trial of outpatient compared with inpatient cervical ripening with prostaglandin E(2) (OPRA study). *BJOG.* 2015;122:94–104. [I, RCT, n = 827]
143. Austin K, Chambers GM, de Abreu Lourenco R, et al. Cost-effectiveness of term induction of labour using inpatient prostaglandin gel versus outpatient foley catheter. *Aust N Z J Obstet Gynaecol.* 2015;55(5):440–445. [III, cost-analysis]
144. Howard K, Gerard K, Adelson P, et al. Women's preferences for inpatient and outpatient priming for labour induction: A discrete choice experiment. *BMC Health Serv Res.* 2014;14:330. [III]
145. Hauth JC, Hankins GD, Gilstrap LC III, Strickland DM. Uterine contraction pressures with oxytocin induction/augmentation. *Obstet Gynecol.* 1986;68:305–309. [II-2, n = 109]
146. American College of Obstetricians and Gynecologists. *ACOG Practice Bulletin No. 49: Dystocia and Augmentation of Labor.* Washington, DC: ACOG, 2003. [III, Review]

Intra-amniotic infection

Elizabeth Liveright and Sara Campbell

KEY POINTS

- Intra-amniotic infection (IAI) is diagnosed by **maternal fever, and one or more other clinical criteria**: maternal tachycardia (>100 beats per minute), leukocytosis, fundal tenderness, foul-smelling amniotic fluid, and/or fetal tachycardia (>160 beats per minute), in the absence of other causes of fever.
- Rates of IAI increase with duration of labor and rupture of membranes (ROM) greater than 24 hours.
- Rates of cesarean delivery are higher in women with a diagnosis of IAI.
- The clinical diagnosis of IAI may not correlate with histologic findings in the placenta.
- IAI is associated with increased maternal and neonatal morbidity.
- **Antibiotics (e.g., ampicillin and single dose gentamicin) should be given at the time of intrapartum IAI diagnosis.**
- **Antibiotics treatment can in general be stopped with vaginal delivery. For cesarean, anaerobic coverage (clindamycin or metronidazole) should be added intrapartum, and one more dose of triple antibiotics given postpartum.**
- Neonates delivered after IAI should be evaluated and treated as per Centers for Disease Control and Prevention (CDC) and American Academy of Pediatrics (AAP) guidelines. In general, if IAI happens before the birth of a neonate <34 weeks, workup and antibiotic treatment are recommended. In neonates ≥34 weeks born to mothers with IAI, workup and treatment with antibiotics are recommended only for ill-appearing babies, while most can be instead closely observed in the nursery. Antibiotics are usually continued for about 48 hours, and stopped when culture results return as negative.
- There are several **preventive techniques** shown to decrease rates of IAI. Some of these include, among others, antibiotic prophylaxis in premature rupture of membranes, as well as limiting the length of labor and the number of vaginal examinations.

DEFINITIONS/DIAGNOSIS

A wide range of terminology is used in the literature to describe intrapartum infection. The term **"chorioamnionitis"** has traditionally been used to describe infection of the amniotic fluid, placenta, membranes, and/or umbilical cord; however **IAI** may be a more accurate representation of the clinical picture. The clinical and histological presentation of IAI is heterogeneous, and its association with maternal and neonatal morbidity varies widely. Most studies utilize a combination of maternal fever, tachycardia (>100 beats per minute), leukocytosis, fundal tenderness, foul-smelling amniotic fluid, and fetal tachycardia (>160 beats per minute) to diagnose IAI (Table 22.1). Maternal fever is the most important and identifiable sign [1]; however, isolated maternal fever may be from an extra-uterine source, or may not be infectious in etiology. A well accepted definition is **maternal fever (≥100.4°F) with at least one more of these criteria: maternal tachycardia (>100 beats per minute), leukocytosis, fundal tenderness, foul-smelling amniotic fluid, and/or fetal tachycardia (>160 beats per minute), in the absence of other causes of fever.**

Ancillary signs have been identified and quantified in a number of studies. The presence of maternal tachycardia is reported in 50%–80% of cases of IAI, and fetal tachycardia in 40%–70% of cases [1]. Uterine tenderness and foul-smelling amniotic fluid are present in 70%–90% of cases, but tenderness may be masked by epidural anesthesia [2].

Traditionally, the presence of one to three of these clinical features, in addition to fever, is used for diagnosis, but there have been no universally accepted diagnostic criteria published in the literature to date. In fact, studies report that these clinical criteria used for IAI diagnosis correlate poorly (accuracy of each or the combination of clinical signs was 47%–58%) with positive bacterial polymerase chain reaction (PCR) or culture by amniocentesis [3].

EPIDEMIOLOGY

This chapter focuses on IAI **at term** (≥37 weeks). The incidence of IAI in preterm births may be as high as 40% in deliveries under 27 weeks' gestation [2]. In term deliveries, however, the reported incidence is from **2% to 4%**. The rate is higher in cesarean section, with as many as 12% of cesarean deliveries having a clinical diagnosis of IAI [4].

In women with premature (or prelabor) rupture of membranes (PROM), the reported incidence is higher. The Term PROM study showed a rate overall of 7% in women with rupture of membranes prior to active labor [5]. In women with PROM greater than 24 hours, the rates of infection may be as high as 40% [6].

PATHOPHYSIOLOGY

IAI is largely considered to be an acute inflammation that is due to an ascending polymicrobial infection after membrane rupture. In this setting, the most common bacteria implicated are ureaplasma, urealyticum, and mycoplasma. Other bacteria often isolated in amniotic fluid cultures are *Gardnerella*, bacteroides, group B streptococcus, and *Escherichia coli* [7]. Rarely, hematogenous spread is the source, as in the case of Listeria infection [8].

IAI can be diagnosed histologically based on placental evaluation; however, a clinical diagnosis may not be confirmed by histological studies. It has been reported that **up to one-third of clinical diagnoses may not have corresponding histologic findings** [9]. A number of grading systems have been proposed to describe the histologic severity of chorioamnionitis,

Table 22.1 Definition/Diagnosis of IAI

Maternal fever plus at least one of the following:
- Maternal tachycardia (>100 beats per minute)
- Leukocytosis
- Fundal tenderness
- Foul-smelling amniotic fluid
- Fetal tachycardia (>160 beats per minute)

Abbreviation: IAI, intra-amniotic infection.

and they include depth and location of neutrophil infiltration of the placenta. There are a number of inflammatory markers that may be associated with the clinical syndrome and histologic diagnosis of IAI, including cytokines, such as interleukin-1 alpha (IL-1alpha), IL-1beta, IL-6, and IL-8, among others. It is suggested that microorganisms invading the amniotic space stimulate these inflammatory cytokines, which favors the migration of neutrophils and ultimately produces the histologic diagnosis of chorioamnionitis [10].

RISK FACTORS

Risk factors for developing IAI include: **longer duration of labor, prolonged rupture of membranes, meconium-stained amniotic fluid, use of internal fetal monitoring, group B strep colonization, nulliparity, bacterial vaginosis, and increased number of vaginal examinations** [2,5,11–18]. For example, the International Multicentre Term Prelabor Rupture of Membranes Study (Term PROM) demonstrated that increasing number of digital vaginal examinations, longer duration of labor, and meconium stained amniotic fluid were the most commonly identified risk factors for developing infection [5]. More recent studies suggest that some of these previously identified risk factors are eliminated by controlling for confounders. Additionally, a meta-analysis of several randomized controlled trials (RCTs) demonstrated that **the use of transcervical Foley catheters for induction of labor was not associated with increased infectious morbidity** [19].

COMPLICATIONS: MATERNAL

Intrauterine infection is associated with increased risk of **cesarean delivery and endomyometritis, as well as postpartum hemorrhage, need for blood transfusion, intensive care unit (ICU) admission, and need for hysterectomy** (Table 22.2). The duration of chorioamnionitis has been shown to be associated directly with blood transfusion and ICU admissions [4]. Fortunately, infection rarely lasts greater than 24 hours after delivery, particularly when given a dose of antibiotics postpartum (see "Management" section below). Treatment failure, defined as persistent fevers after receiving one postpartum dose of antibiotics, is reported to be from 2% to 6% [20].

The risk of cesarean section is approximately two- to threefold higher for a woman meeting clinical criteria for IAI [21,22]. The increased risk is thought to be due to decreased uterine contractility and subsequent dysfunctional labor. Decreased uterine contractility may also lead to higher rates of postpartum hemorrhage due to atony; risk of postpartum hemorrhage after vaginal delivery may be up to 80% more likely and 50% more likely after cesarean section [21,23].

COMPLICATIONS: NEONATAL

IAI is associated with increased rates of **bacteremia, sepsis, and mortality in neonates, as well as an increased risk of cerebral palsy** [4,24]. Intrapartum fever has been shown to increase transient neonatal adverse effects as well as neonatal

Table 22.2 Selected Possible Complications Associated with IAI

Maternal
- Cesarean delivery
- Endomyometritis
- Postpartum hemorrhage
- Need for blood transfusion
- ICU admission
- Need for hysterectomy

Neonatal
- Bacteremia
- Sepsis
- Mortality
- Risk of cerebral palsy

Abbreviation: ICU, intensive care unit.

seizures and encephalopathy [25–28]. These risks are present in both term and preterm infants, though the relative risk is greater in preterm neonates. The overall relative risk for cerebral palsy in term neonates born to mothers with IAI is reported as 4.7 [29]. It is thought that the fetal inflammatory response is a contributing factor to cerebral palsy in infants of mothers with IAI. Studies show that elevated levels of inflammatory cytokines were present in the amniotic fluid of mothers of children with cerebral palsy [30].

MANAGEMENT
Treatment of IAI

Initiation of antibiotics at the time of diagnosis is the standard of care for treatment of IAI (Table 22.3). This recommendation is supported by several studies demonstrating decreased maternal and fetal morbidity with administration of intrapartum antibiotics. These studies most consistently have shown decreased rates of neonatal bacteremia and sepsis, and also decreased rates of maternal febrile morbidity and length of postpartum stay [8,25,31,32]. These data are exclusively from cohort studies; there have been no RCTs to date comparing antibiotics to no treatment or placebo for women with IAI [33].

The source of IAI is thought to originate in the vaginal flora; coverage is therefore recommended to target beta-lactamase producing aerobes and anaerobes. **Ampicillin and gentamicin** are the antibiotics most commonly used when the diagnosis of IAI is made in labor, based largely on clinical consensus, in the absence of data supporting other regimens [33,34]. **Daily dosing of the aminoglycoside** is equally effective as 8-hour dosing with the advantages of increased bactericidal effects, decreased nephrotoxicity, as well as decreased cost [35]. The two RCTs identified in a Cochrane Review showed no statistically significant difference in maternal or neonatal outcomes when clindamycin was added to ampicillin and gentamicin [31,36].

For patients undergoing cesarean section, however, anaerobic coverage through antepartum **addition of clindamycin or metronidazole** to ampicillin and gentamicin is associated with fewer wound infections postpartum [37].

Antipyretics should be considered when maternal fever is present.

Delivery

IAI itself does not necessitate cesarean section, unless otherwise motivated by standard obstetric indications, though there is an increased rate of cesarean delivery in the setting of IAI, as described above. Time from initiation of antibiotic treatment to

Table 22.3 Antibiotic Treatment for IAI

Regimen
- Ampicillin and gentamicin
- Add clindamycin (or metronidazole) for cesarean section

Duration
- Initiate treatment at time of diagnosis, and continue intrapartum
- Vaginal delivery: stop postpartum
- Cesarean: single additional doses of antibiotics postpartum
- No indication for prolonged treatment in absence of clinical indications

Benefits
- Decreased neonatal bacteremia and sepsis
- Shorter maternal hospital stay
- Lower rates of persistent maternal fever

---

delivery has not been shown to affect outcomes; it is therefore **not recommended to expedite delivery for IAI alone** [4,31].

POSTPARTUM

For women who had a vaginal delivery, antibiotics do not need to be continued postpartum, as shown by RCTs comparing antibiotics versus placebo [33]. The cure in these cases is the delivery itself.

In women who had a **cesarean delivery**, at least **a single dose of antibiotics after delivery is recommended** to decrease postpartum maternal morbidity, but prolonged treatment has not been shown to improve outcomes [20,38,39].

NEONATAL MANAGEMENT

Maternal diagnosis of IAI can be associated serious implications even for well-appearing term infants. The Centers for Disease Control and American Academy of Pediatrics state that infants born to mothers with either suspected or clinically proven IAI require antibiotic treatment, as well as laboratory testing [40,41]. This often results in separation from mother, admission to neonatal intensive care units (NICU), and exposure to drug-resistant bacteria in the NICU setting. A "sepsis calculator" has been suggested as a tool to calculate need for treatment based on maternal risk factors (GBS status, intrapartum antibiotic treatment), as well as continuous variables (peak febrile temperature, duration of ruptured membranes) and infant's clinical appearance (clinically ill, equivocal, or well-appearing) [42,43]. This model reduced the proportion of unnecessary laboratory testing and antibiotic treatment, while not missing any cases of culture positive sepsis [43].

In general, if IAI happens before the birth of a **neonate <34 weeks, workup and antibiotic treatment are recommended**. In **neonates ≥34 weeks born to mothers with IAI, workup and treatment with antibiotics are recommended only for ill-appearing babies**, while most can be instead closely observed in the nursery. There is limited evidence regarding the length of neonatal antibiotic therapy. Antibiotics are usually continued for about 48 hours, and stopped when culture results return as negative.

PREVENTION

There are several interventions associated with prevention of IAI.

Antibiotics prophylaxis for prevention of IAI in preterm, premature rupture of membranes (**PPROM**) has been consistently shown to yield benefit for the neonate [44] (see Chapter 19). Even in women with **term PROM**, antibiotics prophylaxis, especially in women expected to have latency from PROM to delivery > 12 hours, has been associated with significant reduction in IAI and endometritis [44]. (Chapter 20)

Modifiable risk factors for IAI in term pregnancies present the opportunity for prevention, particularly length of ruptured membranes and length of labor. Techniques used to shorten active labor have been shown to decrease maternal infectious morbidity [45]. **Decreasing length of labor** inherently decreases other risk factors associated with IAI, such as increased **number of digital examinations** [11,18].

Perineal hygiene, in addition to prolonged supine positioning and digital examinations, are suggested to be contributing factors to IAI [46]. A Cochrane review, however, showed no evidence for the prevention of IAI and only a statistically insignificant trend toward a decrease in postpartum endometritis [47]. Prophylactic antibiotics to reduce vaginal infections have been shown to lower rates of bacterial vaginosis and trichomonas, without a decrease in risk of IAI or preterm birth [48]. Intrapartum antibiotic amnioinfusion has not been shown to provide consistent improvement in maternal or neonatal outcomes [49].

REFERENCES

1. Tita AT, Andrews WW. Diagnosis and management of clinical chorioamnionitis. *Clin Perinatol.* 2010;37(2):339–354. [Review]
2. Newton ER. Chorioamnionitis and intraamniotic infection. *Clin Obstet Gynecol.* 1993;36(4):795. [Review]
3. Romero R, Chaemsaithong P, Korzeniewski SJ, et al. Clinical chorioamnionitis at term III: How well do clinical criteria perform in the identification of proven intra-amniotic infection? *J Perinat Med.* 2016;44:23–32. [II-1]
4. Rouse DJ, Landon M, Leveno KJ, et al. The maternal-fetal medicine units cesarean registry: Chorioamnionitis at term and its duration—Relationship to outcomes. *Am J Obstet Gynecol.* 2004;191(1):211–216. [II-2]
5. Seaward PG, Hannah ME, Myhr TL, et al. International multicentre term prelabor rupture of membranes study: Evaluation of predictors of clinical chorioamnionitis and postpartum fever in patients with prelabor rupture of membranes at term. *Am J Obstet Gynecol.* 1997;177(5):1024–1029. [II-1]
6. Romero R, Ghidini A, Bahado-Singh R. Premature rupture of the membranes. In: Reece EA, Hobbins JC, Mahoney J, Petrie RH (eds.), *Medicine of the Fetus and Mother.* Philadelphia, PA: JB Lippincott, 1992:1430–1468. [Book chapter]
7. Sperling RS, Newton E, Gibbs RS. Intraamniotic infection in low-birth-weight infants. *J Infect Dis.* 1988;157(1):113–117. [II-2]
8. Gibbs RS, Duff P. Progress in pathogenesis and management of clinical intraamniotic infection. *Am J Obstet Gynecol.* 1991;164:1317. [Review]
9. Smulian JC, Shen-Schwarz S, Vintzileos AM, et al. Clinical chorioamnionitis and histologic placental inflammation. *Obstet Gynecol.* 1999;94(6):1000–1005. [II-2]
10. Kim CJ, Romero R, Chaemsaithong P, et al. Acute chorioamnionitis and funisitis: Definition, pathologic features, and clinical significance. *Am J Obstet Gynecol.* 2015; 213(4):S29–S52. [Review]
11. Soper DE, Mayhall CG, Dalton HP. Risk factors for intraamniotic infection: A prospective epidemiologic study. *Am J Obstet Gynecol.* 1989;161:562. [Epidemiologic data]
12. Newton ER, Prihoda TJ, Gibbs RS. Logistic regression analysis of risk factors for intra-amniotic infection. *Obstet Gynecol.* 1989;73(4):571–575. [II-2]
13. Piper JM, Newton ER, Berkus MD, Peairs WA. Meconium: A marker for peripartum infection. *Obstet Gynecol.* 1998;91:741. [II-2]
14. Tran SH, Caughey AB, Musci TJ. Meconium-stained amniotic fluid is associated with puerperal infections. *Am J Obstet Gynecol.* 2003:189(3);746–750. [II-2]

15. Rickert VI, Wiemann CM, Hankins GD. Prevalence and risk factors of chorioamnionitis among adolescents. *Obstet Gynecol.* 1998;92(2):254–257. [II-2]
16. Yancey MK, Duff P, Clark P, et al. Peripartum infection associated with vaginal group B streptococcal colonization. *Obstet Gynecol.* 1994;84(5):816–819. [II-2]
17. Newton ER, Piper J, Peairs W. Bacterial vaginosis and intraamniotic infection. *Am J Obstet Gynecol.* 1997:176(3):672–677. [II-2]
18. Cahill AG, Duffy CR, Odibo AO, et al. Number of cervical examinations and risk of intrapartum maternal fever. *Obstet Gynecol.* 2012;119(6):1096–1101. [II-2]
19. McMaster K, Sanchez-Ramos L, Kaunitz AM. Evaluation of a transcervical foley catheter as a source of infection: A systematic review and meta-analysis. *Obstet Gynecol.* 2015;126(3):539–551. [Meta-analysis of 26 RCTs]
20. Black LP, Hinson L, Duff P. Limited course of antibiotic treatment for chorioamnionitis. *Obstet Gynecol.* 2012;119(6):1102–1105. [II-3]
21. Mark SP, Croughan-Minihane MS, Kilpatrick SJ. Chorioamnionitis and uterine function. *Obstet Gynecol.* 2000;95(6 Pt 1):909–912. [II-2]
22. Satin AJ, Maberry MC, Leveno KJ, et al. Chorioamnionitis: A harbinger of dystocia. *Obstet Gynecol.* 1992;79(6):913–915. [II-2]
23. Duff P, Sanders R, Gibbs RS. The course of labor in term patients with chorioamnionitis. *Am J Obstet Gynecol.* 1983;147(4):391–395. [II-2]
24. Yoder PR, Gibbs RS, Blanco JD, et al. A prospective, controlled study of maternal and perinatal outcome after intra-amniotic infection at term. *Am J Obstet Gynecol.* 1983;145(6):695–701. [II-1]
25. Sperling RS, Ramamurthy RS, Gibbs RS. A comparison of intrapartum versus immediate postpartum treatment of intra-amniotic infection. *Obstet Gynecol.* 1987;70(6):861–865. [II-1]
26. Impey LW, Greenwood CE, Black RS, et al. The relationship between intrapartum maternal fever and neonatal acidosis as risk factors for neonatal encephalopathy. *Am J Obstet Gynecol.* 2008;198(1):49.e1–6. [II-2]
27. Impey L, Greenwood C, MacQuillan K, et al. Fever in labour and neonatal encephalopathy: A prospective cohort study. *BJOG.* 2001;108(6):594–597. [II-2]
28. Lieberman E, Lang J, Richardson DK, et al. Intrapartum maternal fever and neonatal outcome. *Pediatrics.* 2000;105(1):8–13. [II-2]
29. Wu YW, Colford JM Jr. Chorioamnionitis as a risk factor for cerebral palsy: A meta-analysis. *JAMA.* 2000;284(11):1417–1424. [Meta-analysis, no RCT]
30. Yoon BH, Jun JK, Romero R, et al. Amniotic fluid inflammatory cytokines (interleukin-6, interleukin-1β, and tumor necrosis factor-α), neonatal brain white matter lesions, and cerebral palsy. *Am J Obstet Gynecol.* 1997;177(1):19–26. [II-2]
31. Gibbs RS, Dinsmoor MJ, Newton ER, Ramamurthy RS. A randomized trial of intrapartum versus immediate postpartum treatment of women with intra-amniotic infection. *Obstet Gynecol.* 1988;72(6):823–828. [II-1]
32. Gilstrap LC III, Leveno KJ, Cox SM, et al. Intrapartum treatment of acute chorioamnionitis: Impact on neonatal sepsis. *Am J Obstet Gynecol.* 1988;159(3):579–583. [II-2]
33. Chapman E, Reveiz L, Illanes E, Bonfill Cosp X. Antibiotic regimens for management of intra-amniotic infection. *Cochrane Database Syst Rev.* 2014;(12):CD010976. [Meta-analysis, 11 RCTs]
34. Hopkins L, Smaill FM. Antibiotic regimens for management of intraamniotic infection. *Cochrane Database Syst Rev.* 2002;(3):CD003254. [Meta-analysis, 2 RCTs]
35. Lyell DJ, Pullen K, Fuh K, et al. Daily compared with 8-hour gentamicin for the treatment of intrapartum chorioamnionitis: A randomized controlled trial. *Obstet Gynecol.* 2010;115(2 Pt 1):344–349. [I]
36. Maberry MC, Gilstrap LC III, Bawdon R, et al. Anaerobic coverage for intra-amnionic infection: Maternal and perinatal impact. *Am J Perinatol.* 1991;8(5):338–341. [II-2]
37. Mackeen AD, et al. Antibiotic regimens for postpartum endometritis. *Cochrane Database Syst Rev.* 2015;(2):CD001067. [Meta-analysis, 42 RCTs]
38. Edwards RK, Duff P. Single additional dose postpartum therapy for women with chorioamnionitis. *Obstet Gynecol.* 2003;102(5 Pt 1):957–961. [I]
39. Dinsmoor MJ, Newton ER, Gibbs RS. A randomized, double-blind, placebo-controlled trial of oral antibiotic therapy following intravenous antibiotic therapy for postpartum endometritis. *Obstet Gynecol.* 1991;77(1):60–62. [I]
40. Verani JR, McGee L, Schrag SJ, Division of Bacterial Diseases, National Center for Immunization and Respiratory Diseases, Centers for Disease Control and Prevention (CDC). Prevention of perinatal group B streptococcal disease: Revised guidelines from CDC, 2010. *MMWR Recomm Rep.* 2010;59(RR-10):1–36. [Guidelines]
41. Polin RA, Committee on Fetus and Newborn. Management of neonates with suspected or proven early-onset bacterial sepsis. *Pediatrics.* 2012;129(5):1006–1015. [Review]
42. Puopolo KM, Draper D, Wi S, et al. Estimating the probability of neonatal early-onset infection on the basis of maternal risk factors. *Pediatrics.* 2011;128(5):e1155–e1163. [II-2]
43. Escobar GJ, Puopolo KM, Wi S, et al. Stratification of risk of early-onset sepsis in newborns ≥ 34 weeks' gestation. *Pediatrics.* 2014;133(1):30–36. [II-2]
44. Saccone G, Berghella V. Antibiotic prophylaxis for term or near-term premature rupture of membranes: Metaanalysis of randomized trials. *Am J Obstet Gynecol.* 2015;212(5):627.e1–627.e9. [Meta-analysis, 5 RCTs]
45. Lopez-Zeno JA, Peaceman AM, Adashek JA, Socol ML. A controlled trial of a program for the active management of labor. *N Engl J Med.* 1992;326(7):450–454. [II-1]
46. Hastings-Tolsma M, Bernard R, Brody MG, et al. Chorioamnionitis: Prevention and management. *MCN Am J Matern Child Nurs.* 2013;38(4):206–212. [Review]
47. Lumbiganon P, Thinkhamrop J, Thinkhamrop B, Tolosa JE. Vaginal chlorhexidine during labour for preventing maternal and neonatal infections (excluding group B streptococcal and HIV). *Cochrane Database Syst Rev.* 2004;(4):CD004070. [Meta-analysis, 3 RCTs]
48. Goldenberg RL, Mwatha A, Read JS, et al. The HPTN 024 Study: The efficacy of antibiotics to prevent chorioamnionitis and preterm birth. *Am J Obstet Gynecol.* 2006;194(3):650–661. [I]
49. Czikk MJ, McCarthy FP, Murphy KE. Chorioamnionitis: From pathogenesis to treatment. *Clin Microbiol Infect.* 2011;17(9):1304–1311. [Review]

Meconium

Alessandro Ghidini

KEY POINTS

- **Fetal passage of meconium is common (about 12%) at term and postterm, while rare (<1%) in the preterm period.**
  - Meconium-stained amniotic fluid (MSAF) is due to a combination of increased fetal bowel motility and decreased clearance of meconium by the fetus or placenta. In a minority of cases such effects are due to fetal hypoxia.
  - **Meconium aspiration syndrome (MAS) is frequently a misnomer, as the respiratory compromise in the fetus is often due to chronic processes (e.g. infection or hypoxia, acute or chronic) which also stimulate colonic activity and fetal gasping.**
- Prevention of meconium passage and of MAS may be accomplished by reducing the rate of postterm deliveries.
- **Amnioinfusion for MSAF is associated with improvements in perinatal outcome only in settings where facilities for perinatal surveillance are limited.** Under **standard perinatal surveillance**, compared with no amnioinfusion, **amnioinfusion** for MSAF is not associated with significant **reductions in MAS, perinatal mortality, or combined outcome perinatal death or severe morbidity.**
- **Oro- and nasopharyngeal suctioning** before delivery of the shoulder **does not decrease the incidence of MAS, need for mechanical ventilation for MAS, any other associated morbidities, or neonatal mortality.**
- **Routine endotracheal intubation** at birth in meconium-stained neonates who are otherwise vigorous **does not improve neonatal outcomes over routine resuscitation.**

HISTORIC NOTES

Meconium is a term derived from the Greek "mekoni," which means poppy juice or opium. Confirming previous clinical impressions, meconium passage was formally recognized to be associated with increased perinatal morbidity and mortality in the 1975 Collaborative Study of Cerebral Palsy.

DIAGNOSES/DEFINITIONS

Meconium is the intestinal content of the fetus and is variably composed of mucopolysaccharides, blood by-products, hair, and squamous cells. Diagnosis of MSAF is made clinically on the basis of appearance (greenish or brownish staining) or by histopathologic examination of the placenta. Particularly in the preterm (<33-week) gestation, a clinical impression of MSAF may be false and instead reflect staining by another mechanism (i.e., hemosiderin). The diagnosis of MAS is respiratory distress requiring supplemental oxygen usually in the first 4 hours of life in the presence of meconium in a neonate without other causes of respiratory distress, and classified as shown below.

EPIDEMIOLOGY/INCIDENCE

The incidence of MSAF increases with gestational age: It is <1% before 37 weeks, about 10% of 39- to 41-week gestations, 18% of >41-week gestations [1]. Meconium in placenta macrophages is documented in about 17%–19% of term placentas; clinical evidence of MASF is present in about **12%** (7%–22%) of term deliveries [1]. However there is a poor concordance between histologic and clinical evidence of meconium presence, probably due to persistence of old meconium in macrophages after its clearance from the amniotic fluid, as well new release of meconium by the fetus before uptake by placenta macrophages [2]. Moreover, there is discordance among histopathologists in the definition of presence of placental meconium [3]. **MAS occurs in about 5% of MSAF cases, and, of these, approximately 4% die** [4].

ETIOLOGY/BASIC PATHOPHYSIOLOGY

Although regular fetal bowel movements occur since the early second trimester [5], meconium does not become green (i.e., contains biliverdin pigments) until 22–24 weeks. In term and postterm fetuses, physiologic increased motilin levels or pathologic increases mediated by fetal stress from hypoxia, infection, or cord compression may lead to meconium passage. MSAF may also be caused by decreased clearance of meconium by the fetus or placenta in the presence of hypoxia [1].

Aspiration of meconium can lead to respiratory compromise by causing a chemical pneumonitis, associated with inhibition of surfactant function, inflammation, and obstruction. However, respiratory compromise in the presence of meconium (i.e., MAS) is more commonly due to other processes (such as chronic or acute asphyxia, or intrauterine infection) than damage from meconium aspiration itself [6]. For example, **hypoxia may stimulate colonic activity and fetal gasping, leading to meconium aspiration. In such cases, meconium is not causative of the respiratory compromise, but rather a manifestation of underlying chronic or acute processes leading to fetal compromise.**

SYMPTOMS

Symptoms of neonatal MAS include respiratory compromise, with tachypnea, cyanosis, and reduced pulmonary compliance. In some cases, pulmonary hypertension develops [4].

CLASSIFICATION (OF MECONIUM ASPIRATION SYNDROME)

- Mild: Supplemental oxygen <40% for <48 hours
- Moderate: Supplemental oxygen ≥40% or for ≥48 hours
- Severe: Need for intubation (or primary pulmonary hypertension)

RISK FACTORS

Postterm pregnancy; acute fetal acidemia; intrauterine infection (as suggested by higher rates of histologic acute chorioamnionitis, clinical chorioamnionitis and endometritis, and neonatal sepsis in the presence of MSAF); placental dysfunction leading to chronic fetal hypoxia (e.g., fetal growth restriction, preeclampsia, oligohydramnios); uterine hyperstimulation (e.g., with misoprostol); long labors (every 2-hour increase in duration of labor is associated with a 30% increase in risk of MSAF) [7,8].

The multiplicity of risk factors, and the possible coexistence of independent risk factors (e.g., meconium and oligohydramnios) may explain why MSAF has inconsistently been associated with lower umbilical artery pH at birth.

COMPLICATIONS

Because the intrauterine processes underlying accumulation of meconium can jeopardize the fetus, MSAF and MAS can be associated with **increased risk of fetal acidemia, neonatal seizures, neonatal intensive care unit (NICU) admission, neonatal sepsis, respiratory distress, neonatal encephalopathy, cerebral palsy, and neonatal death** [1,4,9–11].

PREGNANCY MANAGEMENT
Meconium at Genetic Amniocentesis

As discolored amniotic fluid before 24 weeks (i.e., at genetic amniocentesis) is not due to MSAF but rather to intra-amniotic bleed or infection, **evaluation for such causes of discolored amniotic fluid** may be considered. These may include for example microbiologic studies on amniotic fluid, Kleiheuer–Betke test on maternal blood, careful sonographic examination for evidence of retroplacental or intra-amniotic bleeds; assessment of placental implantation by evaluating placental thickness, dimensions, echotexture, and cord insertion.

Meconium in Late Preterm and Early Term Fetus <39 Weeks

MSAF in the later preterm and term fetus <39 weeks should prompt evaluation for **infection and fetal hypoxia** as the finding is quite uncommon and unlikely to be physiologic at this gestational ages.

Meconium at ≥39 Weeks

MSAF in the full-term or postterm fetus may reflect normal physiology and maturation of the gastrointestinal tract, but one should first exclude the possibilities of infection or hypoxia as etiologies. Progression in meconium consistency in labor from no/little meconium to presence of thick meconium, or occurrence of meconium in the setting of category II fetal heart rate tracings, should elicit particular concern as this is associated with higher rates of fetal acidemia and lower Apgar scores at 5 minutes [12–14].

PREVENTION

Prevention of meconium passage and of MAS may be accomplished by reducing the rate of postterm deliveries. Early ultrasound dating, stripping of membranes at ≥38 weeks, and induction of labor at 41 weeks decrease the incidence of postterm pregnancies (see Chapter 27).

MANAGEMENT TECHNIQUES USED IN THE SETTING OF MSAF
Fetal

Amnioinfusion

The efficacy of amnioinfusion to "dilute" meconium and reduce associated neonatal morbidity has historically been controversial. The most recent meta-analysis includes 14 total randomized controlled trials (RCTs) [15]. Results are reported separately for sites with standard versus those with limited perinatal surveillance. The main outcome in the RCTs was usually occurrence of MAS.

Under **standard perinatal surveillance**, compared with no amnioinfusion, **amnioinfusion** for MSAF was **not associated** with a reduction in MAS (relative risk [RR] 0.52, 95% confidence interval [CI] 0.26–1.06) or perinatal deaths (RR 1.00, 95% CI 0.29–3.45), or the combined outcome perinatal death or severe morbidity (RR 1.13, 95% CI 0.88–1.47). There was considerable heterogeneity among studies for several secondary outcomes, such as presence of heavy meconium staining, cesarean section for non-reassuring fetal testing, occurrence of fetal heart rate decelerations, 5-minute Apgar score less than 7, presence of meconium below the vocal cords, need for neonatal ventilation or NICU admission.

Under **limited perinatal surveillance**, compared with no amnioinfusion, **amnioinfusion** for MSAF was **associated with a significant reduction in MAS** (RR 0.17, 95% CI 0.05–0.52) and **perinatal mortality** (RR 0.24, 95% CI 0.11–0.53), as well as reductions in **cesarean section for non-reassuring fetal testing, 5-minute Apgar score less than seven, neonatal ventilation or neonatal intensive care unit admission, and neonatal encephalopathy**.

In summary, **amnioinfusion for MSAF is associated with improvements in perinatal outcome in settings where facilities for perinatal surveillance are limited, but not in settings with standard perinatal surveillance.** In general, amnioinfusion is offered at >34 weeks. There are many variations of the amnioinfusion technique, but a "typical" protocol calls for infusion via an intrauterine pressure catheter (obviously in a woman with dilated cervix and ruptured membranes) of **500 mL of normal saline over a period of 30 minutes**, see also Chapter 10. For amnioinfusion in presence of variable decelerations, see Chapter 10; for amnioinfusion for oligohydramnios without preterm premature rupture of membranes (PPROM), see Chapter 57 in *Maternal-Fetal Evidence Based Guidelines*; for amnioinfusion for PPROM, see Chapter 19.

Antibiotics

There is **insufficient evidence** to assess the effectiveness of antibiotics for women with meconium in labor. A meta-analysis on the subject (inclusive of two studies, both of which utilized ampicillin-sulbactam) has shown that compared with normal saline, antibiotic prophylaxis in women with MSAF is associated with no statistically significant reduction in the incidence of neonatal sepsis (RR 1.00, 95% CI 0.21–4.76), NICU admission (RR 0.83, 95% CI 0.39–1.78), and postpartum endometritis (RR 0.50, 95% CI 0.18–1.38), but a significant decrease in the risk of chorioamnionitis (RR 0.36, 95% CI 0.21–0.62) [16]. No serious adverse effects have been reported.

Oro- and Nasopharyngeal Suctioning

Suctioning of the oro- and nasopharynx before delivery of the shoulder or the "first cry" **does not decrease the incidence of MAS, need for mechanical ventilation for MAS, any other associated morbidities, or neonatal mortality** [17,18].

Neonatal

Endotracheal Intubation

A policy of routine endotracheal intubation at birth in meconium-stained babies who are otherwise vigorous **does not improve neonatal outcomes over routine resuscitation** [19]. For depressed or nonvigorous newborns, endotracheal intubation and suctioning may still be performed in infants born through MSAF [19].

REFERENCES

1. Caughey AB, Musci TJ. Complications of term pregnancies beyond 37 weeks of gestation. *Obstet Gynecol.* 2004;103(1):57–62. [II-2]
2. Incerti M, Locatelli A, Consonni S, et al. Can placental histology establish the timing of meconium passage during labor? *Acta Obstet Gynecol Scand.* 2011;90(8):863–868 [II-2]
3. Poggi SH, Salafia C, Paiva S, et al. Variability in pathologists' detection of placental meconium uptake. *Am J Perinatol.* 2009;26(3):207–210. [II-3]
4. Rossi EM, Philipson EH, Williams TG, et al. Meconium aspiration syndrome: Intrapartum and neonatal attributes. *Am J Obstet Gynecol.* 1989;161:1106–1110. [II-3]
5. López Ramón y Cajal C, Ocampo Martínez R. Defecation in utero: A physiologic fetal function. *Am J Obstet Gynecol.* 2003;188:153–156 [III]
6. Ghidini A, Spong C. Severe meconium aspiration is not caused by aspiration of meconium. *Obstet Gynecol.* 2001;185:931–938. [Review]
7. Lee KA, Mi Lee S, Jin Yang H, et al. The frequency of meconium-stained amniotic fluid increases as a function of the duration of labor. *J Matern Fetal Neonatal Med.* 2011;24(7):880–885. [II-2]
8. Tran SH, Caughey AB, Musci TJ. Meconium-stained amniotic fluid is associated with puerperal infections. *Am J Obstet Gynecol.* 2003;189(3):746–750. [II-2]
9. Hayes BC, McGarvey C, Mulvany S, et al. A case-control study of hypoxic-ischemic encephalopathy in newborn infants at >36 weeks gestation. *Am J Obstet Gynecol.* 2013;209(1):29.e1–29.e19. [II-2]
10. Gaffney G, Flavell V, Johnson A, et al. Cerebral palsy and neonatal encephalopathy. *Arch Dis Child Fetal Neonatal Ed.* 1994;70(3):F195–200. [II-2]
11. Walstab JE, Bell RJ, Reddihough DS, et al. Factors identified during the neonatal period associated with risk of cerebral palsy. *Aust N Z J Obstet Gynaecol.* 2004;44(4):342–346. [II-2]
12. Locatelli A, Regalia AL, Patregnani C, et al. Prognostic value of change in amniotic fluid color during labor. *Fetal Diagn Ther.* 2005;20(1):5–9. [II-2]
13. Greenwood C, Lalchandani S, MacQuillan K, et al. Meconium passed in labor: How reassuring is clear amniotic fluid? *Obstet Gynecol.* 2003;102(1):89–93. [II-2]
14. Frey HA, Tuuli MG, Shanks AL, et al. Interpreting category II fetal heart rate tracings: Does meconium matter? *Am J Obstet Gynecol.* 2014;211(6):644.e1–8. [II-2]
15. Hofmeyr GJ, Xu H, Eke AC. Amnioinfusion for meconium-stained liquor in labor. *Cochrane Database Syst Rev.* 2014;(1):CD000014. [Meta-analysis of RCTs]
16. Siriwachirachai T, Sangkomkamhang US, Lumbiganon P, et al. Antibiotics for meconium-stained amniotic fluid in labour for preventing maternal and neonatal infections. *Cochrane Cochrane Database Syst Rev.* 2014;Nov 6;(11):CD007772 [Meta-analysis; 2 RCTs, n = 362]
17. Falciglia HS, Henderschott C, Potter P, et al. Does DeLee suction at the perineum prevent meconium aspiration syndrome? *Am J Obstet Gynecol.* 1992;167(5):1243–1249. [II-2]
18. Vain NE, Szyld EG, Prudent LM, et al. Oropharyngeal and nasopharyngeal suctioning of meconium-stained neonates before delivery of their shoulders: Multicentre, randomized controlled trial. *Lancet.* 2004;364:597–602. [RCT, n = 2514] [I]
19. Halliday HL, Sweet D. Endotracheal intubation at birth for preventing morbidity and mortality in vigorous, meconium stained infants born at term. *Cochrane Database Syst Rev.* 2009;(1): CD00075320. [Meta-analysis: 4 RCTs, n = 2884]

Malpresentation and malposition

Alexis Gimovsky

KEY POINTS

- **Malpresentation** is **associated** with **uterine anomalies, fibroids, placenta previa, grand multiparity, contracted maternal pelvis, pelvic tumors, prematurity** (the earlier the gestational age (GA), the higher the incidence of malpresentation), **multiple gestation, polyhydramnios, short umbilical cord, fetal anomalies** (e.g., anencephaly, hydrocephalus), **abnormal fetal motor ability, and prior breech delivery.**
- **Complications** of breech presentation include **congenital anomalies, preterm birth (PTB), birth trauma, low Apgar scores and low pH,** regardless of mode of delivery. **Cord prolapse, head hyperextension,** and **head or arm entrapment** are more common with vaginal breech delivery.
- **External cephalic version** (ECV) is a safe and effective intervention for malpresentation. **Urgent cesarean delivery (CD)** for nonreassuring fetal heart rate tracing (NRFHT) and placental **abruption** occur in <0.5% of ECV.
- ECV is to be avoided with **any contraindications to vaginal delivery** such as placenta **previa,** or **prior classical uterine incision.** ECV is relatively contraindicated in rupture of membranes, oligohydramnios, known uterine or fetal anomaly, unexplained uterine bleeding, or active phase of labor.
- **ECV reduces the incidences of noncephalic birth by 54%** and **CD by 37%.** Because ECV is associated with a very low incidence of adverse events and with a significant decrease in CD, **all women at or near term with nonvertex presentations should be offered an ECV. Success rates** range **between 50% and 70%.** Success is increased with **higher parity, transverse or oblique lie, nonengaged presenting part, relaxed uterus, palpable fetal head, and maternal weight less than 65 kg.**
- There is **insufficient evidence** to assess the best GA at which to perform ECV. **Compared with ECV at term, ECV before term** (e.g., 34–35 weeks) reduces noncephalic presentation at birth but does not reduce the rate of CD, and may be associated with an increase in the incidence of **PTB.** About *36 weeks is generally* considered to be the optimal time for attempted ECV.
- Tocolysis with **betamimetics** prior to attempt at ECV is associated with **fewer failures of ECV** and **less CDs.**
- **Anesthetic dose neuraxial blockade** (usually with spinal) **is associated with a 44% increase in the success rate of ECV.**
- ECV should be performed, after appropriate counseling and consent, in a facility with ready availability for ultrasound and for emergency CD.
- **There is inconsistent evidence that moxibustion** at point BL67 alone or in combination with acupuncture, **is associated with higher success rates of ECV,** especially when performed in China.
- Compared with planned vaginal delivery, **planned CD** for the **term breech** fetus is associated with **a decrease in perinatal death and a reduction in serious neonatal morbidity, but no difference in death or neurodevelopmental delay at 2 years after delivery.**
- There is **insufficient evidence** to assess whether outcomes of the **preterm** breech presenting fetus are affected by mode of delivery.
- There is **insufficient evidence** to assess the best mode of delivery for the **nonvertex second twin.** Vaginal delivery of the second nonvertex twin by breech extraction is a reasonable management option by expert operator, possibly by breech extraction.
- There is insufficient evidence to assess any intervention for malposition.

DEFINITIONS
- *Presentation:* Fetal body part that is in the lower uterine segment (lowest in the uterus and closest to the cervix).
- *Malpresentation:* Fetus presenting with the fetal head not in the lower uterine segment.

MALPRESENTATION
Symptoms
Maternal impression of fetal presentation based on fetal movement is suggestive but overall unreliable for predicting fetal presentation.

Epidemiology/Incidence
Breech presentation complicates 3%–4% of all pregnancies at term (≥37 weeks) [1]. Its incidence is inversely proportional to GA, with an incidence of about 25% at 28 weeks, 11% at 32 weeks, and 5% at 34 weeks [2]. In 2003, **87% of all breech presentations resulted in CD;** this is similar to 1990, (90%), but much increased from 1970 (12%) [3,4]. Breech as an indication for CD accounts for 15% of all cesarean deliveries and adds 1.4 billion dollars to U.S. obstetrical costs [4].

Classifications
Breech
Fetus presents in longitudinal lie with head not in the lower uterine segment.
    Fetal breech presentation is further classified as follows:
- *Complete*—Flexion of the fetal hips and knees
- *Incomplete*—Extension of one or both hips (includes footling)
- *Frank*—Flexion at the hips and extension at the knees

Transverse
The fetal longitudinal axis is perpendicular to the long axis of the uterus. The fetus can either present "back up" (fetal small parts present to the cervix) or "back down" (fetal spine or shoulder present to the cervix).

Oblique
The fetal longitudinal axis is diagonal to the long axis of the uterus.

Face
The fetal head is hyperextended so that the fetal occiput is in contact with the fetal back and the mentum (chin) is presenting. The fetal chin may be anterior or posterior relative to the maternal pubic symphysis.

Brow
The presenting part is the portion of the fetal head between the orbital ridge and the anterior fontanelle. The fetal head is positioned midway between full flexion and extension.

Compound
Simultaneous presentation of a prolapsing fetal extremity and the presenting part.

Risk Factors/Associations
Both maternal and fetal factors can lead to malpresentation, including **uterine anomalies, fibroids, placenta previa, grand multiparity, contracted maternal pelvis, pelvic tumors, prematurity** (the earlier the GA, the higher the incidence of malpresentation), **multiple gestation, polyhydramnios, short umbilical cord, fetal anomalies** (e.g., anencephaly, hydrocephalus), **abnormal fetal motor ability, and prior breech delivery.** There is a 9% risk of recurrence of malpresentation in subsequent pregnancies following a prior breech delivery.

Complications
Incidence of **congenital anomalies** (up to 6%), **PTB, birth trauma, low Apgar scores, and low pH** are increased with breech presentation compared with vertex presentation, **regardless of mode of delivery.** Breech presentation may be both a sign and a consequence of fetal compromise, regardless of delivery mode. Incidence of **cord prolapse** is the same with frank breech as with vertex presentations (<1%), 5% with complete breech, 15% with footling breech, and is inversely proportional to GA. **Head hyperextension** (associated with spinal cord injury) and **head or arm entrapment** are associated with breech presentation, particularly with vaginal breech delivery. Presentation at birth does not seem to affect adult intellectual performance. Cesarean or vaginal delivery for breech presentation do not differ in terms of long-term adult intellectual performance [5].

Workup
Fetal presentation should be assessed by Leopold's maneuvers at each prenatal visit starting at ≥ 34 weeks of gestation. If the clinician is unsure, a vaginal examination, or even better, if still unclear, an ultrasound may be indicated to assess fetal presentation.

External Cephalic Version
Definition
Procedure performed by application of pressure and maneuvers to the maternal abdomen with the goal to turn the fetus to a cephalic presentation, thus increasing the likelihood of vaginal delivery (Figure 24.1) [1].

Complications
While the rate of short-term fetal bradycardia can be as high as 20%, the rate of need for **urgent CD** for NRFHT after an ECV is about 1/600 [6]. Placental **abruption** (<1%) and **onset of labor** are uncommon complications. Rare fetal deaths following attempts at version have not been determined to be a result of the procedure [1]. Femur fracture has been reported. In a meta-analysis, there was a **risk of 4.7% for transient abnormal cardiotocography, 0.21% risk of abnormal cardiotocography leading to emergency CD** (with good neonatal outcomes), and **0.35% risk of emergency CD.** Other risks included 0.24% risk of stillbirth, 0.18% risk of placental abruption, 0.18% risk of cord prolapse, and 0.19% risk of fetal death. These complications were not found to be directly related to the ECV procedure. Vaginal bleeding related to ECV occurred in 0.34% of patients and rupture of membranes related to ECV occurred in 0.22% of patients [7].

Contraindications
Any **contraindications to vaginal delivery** such as placenta **previa** or **prior classical uterine incision** are considered contraindications to ECV. There are no trials on ECV in **multiple gestations,** so the safety and efficacy of this procedure cannot be assessed in this population. Relative contraindications are **rupture of membranes, oligohydramnios, known uterine or fetal anomaly, unexplained uterine bleeding, or active phase of labor** [1,8]. ECV in women with prior cesarean deliveries are associated with comparable success rates to those of women without prior cesarean deliveries, but there is insufficient data to assess the safety of this management [9].

Efficacy
Compared with no ECV, **ECV at term** is associated with a statistically significant and clinically meaningful 58% **reduction in noncephalic birth** (relative risk [RR] 0.42, 95% confidence interval [CI] 0.29–0.61) and a 42% **decrease in CD** (RR 0.58, 95% CI 0.40–0.82) [10]. There are no significant differences in Apgar score ratings <7 at 5 minutes (RR 0.63, 95% CI 0.29–1.36), low umbilical artery pH levels (RR 0.65, 95% CI 0.17–2.44), neonatal admission (RR 0.80, 95% CI 0.48–1.34), perinatal death (RR 0.39, 95% CI 0.09–1.64), or time from enrollment to delivery, compared with no ECV [10]. Because ECV is associated with a very low incidence of adverse events and with a significant decrease in CD, **all women at or near term with nonvertex presentations should be offered an ECV.**

Success rates of ECV average **58%,** with a range of 25% to 80% [1]. Success is increased with **higher parity** and with **transverse or oblique lie** (vs. breech). Lower amniotic fluid volume, anterior placenta, and high maternal BMI might decrease the success rate [1]. A meta-analysis showed that **multiparity, non-engagement of the breech, a relaxed uterus, a palpable fetal head, and maternal weight less than 65 kg** were predictors of successful ECV [11]. There is no scoring system to accurately predict the probability of success of ECV. After successful ECV, the chance of spontaneous version to breech is low, but understudied. The chance of spontaneous version after failed ECV is about 6.6% in one study [12].

Timing of Version
Compared with no ECV, **ECV before term reduces noncephalic births** [13–16].

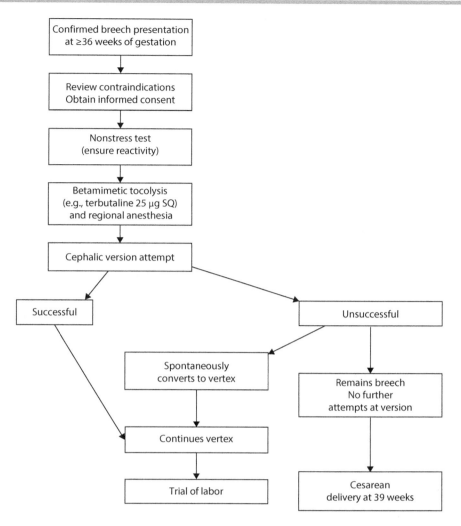

Figure 24.1 Suggested management of breech presentation. *Note:* SQ, subcutaneously. (Adapted from American College of Obstetricians and Gynecologists, *ACOG Clinical Management Guidelines for Obstetrician-Gynecologists Number 13: External Cephalic Version*, Washington, DC: ACOG, 2000.)

Compared with ECV at term, ECV before term reduces noncephalic presentation at birth, but does not reduce the rate of CD, and may be associated with an increase in the incidence of PTB. There is **insufficient evidence to assess the best GA** at which to perform ECV. In general, the later the GA, the lower the success rate, but there are reports of successful ECV in women in term labor. About **36 weeks is generally considered to be the optimal time for attempted version.** At 36 weeks, there is felt to be adequate room to turn the fetus while minimizing the risk of return to breech presentation following a successful ECV. Additionally, if delivery becomes necessary, a 36-week infant has a low rate of respiratory distress syndrome or other complications of prematurity compared with a fetus of <36 weeks GA. Compared with ECV at 37 0/7–38 0/7 weeks, ECV at 34 0/7–36 0/7 weeks is associated with nonsignificant trends for slightly lower (57% vs. 66%) noncephalic presentation at birth and slightly lower (65% vs. 72%) CD [13–16]. In the largest randomized controlled trial (RCT) to date, compared with ECV at >37 weeks, ECV at 34 0/7–35 6/7 weeks was associated with a decrease in the incidence of noncephalic presentation at birth (41% vs. 49%; RR 0.84, 95% CI 0.75–0.94), but no difference in rates of CD (52% vs. 56%; RR 0.93, 95% CI 0.85–1.02) or risk of PTB (6.5% vs. 4.4%; RR 1.48, 95% CI 0.97–2.26) [17].

Tocolysis
Tocolysis with **betamimetics** prior to attempting ECV is associated with 30% **fewer ECV failures,** a 32% reduction in noncephalic presentations at birth, and 23% *less* CDs [18]. A common tocolytic used is terbutaline with a dose of 25 mg subcutaneously once, 10–15 minutes before ECV. Other different betamimetics have been used with no evidence as to the best one or its dosage/timing [18]. One RCT of adjusted doses of intravenous salbutamol tocolysis prior to ECV increased success rates, decreased CD rate, and was well tolerated [19]. Tocolysis can also be used with success in a second ECV attempt after a first ECV attempt has failed [20].

Nifedipine as a uterine relaxant for ECV has also been evaluated. In a randomized, double-blind, placebo-controlled trial of 320 participants, nifedipine **did not significantly improve the success of ECV** [21]. In two RCTs evaluating oral nifedipine versus subcutaneous terbutaline tocolysis for ECV there was higher ECV success with terbutaline (52.2%–58.1% for terbutaline vs. 34.1%–39.5% for nifedipine), less CDs and no difference in neonatal outcomes, although more side effects were noted (maternal palpitations and tachycardia) [22–24].

Nitroglycerin has been studied as an agent to improve ECV success rates. In four small trials, sublingual nitroglycerin was associated with significant side effects and was **not** found to be **effective** [18]. One RCT demonstrated that treatment with intravenous nitroglycerin increased the rate of successful ECV in nulliparous women (24% compared with 8%, $p = .04$) but not in multiparous women [25]. In one trial terbutaline 25 mg subcutaneous 5 minutes prior to ECV was found to have a significantly higher ECV success rate than nitroglycerin [26].

Fetal Acoustic Stimulation
Fetal acoustic stimulation to the fetal head for 1–3 seconds in midline fetal spine positions is associated with fewer failures of ECV at term in a very small study [18,27]. Eleven of 12 ECVs were successful following stimulation [27]. The crossover arm (patients who failed version without stimulation) were then stimulated and 8 of 10 patients were successfully verted, for a total of 19 of 22 successful versions (86%) [26]. The success rate in the control group in this study was lower than expected (8%) [26]. The **evidence is limited and is insufficient** to make a recommendation.

Anesthesia
There is evidence that regional anesthesia affects ECV success. ECV failure, non-cephalic births, and cesarean deliveries were reduced in two trials with epidural but not in three trials with spinal analgesia [18]. ECV success rates increased from 33% to 59% with epidural in one study and from 32% to 69% in another [4,28]. Potential bias in both studies lies in that the care provider was not blinded to placement of epidural [4,28]. It is important to note that **the control groups had lower success rates than expected,** as the average success rate in the literature, which is mostly without anesthesia, is about 58%. All patients in both studies received terbutaline prior to attempt at ECV. It has been postulated that large volume preloading with epidural may increase the amniotic fluid volume [18]. The use of spinal anesthesia has not been associated with any benefit in the success of ECV in some RCTs [8,18]. However, a meta-analysis including seven RCTs, of which five used spinal and two used epidural anesthesia for ECV versus controls, demonstrated **anesthetic dose neuraxial blockade (usually spinal) is associated with a 44% increase in the success rate of external fetal version** [29]. There are no trials to evaluate the potential effects of hydration or transabdominal amnioinfusion on the success rate of spontaneous version or ECV.

Systemic Opioids
There is limited evidence that systemic opioids improve success rates for ECV. One RCT of 60 women showed that the frequency of CD was similar in the opioid (remifentanil) group versus placebo (RR 0.9, 95% CI 0.20–4.27) [18]. In one RCT comparing spinal anesthesia, systemic opioid (remifentanil) and control (no anesthesia/analgesia) for ECV success, ECV was most successful in the spinal anesthesia group (83%) versus opioid (64%) and control (64%). Pain relief was highest with spinal anesthesia, followed by opioid and then control. Incidence of CD for fetal bradycardia was similar amongst groups [30].

Hypnosis
There is one RCT on hypnosis versus neurolinguistic programming for pain relief during ECV and both groups reported a similar degree of relief [18].

ECV Procedure
Given the possible complications, it is prudent to perform ECV in a **facility** with ready availability of emergency CD. **Consent** should be obtained after **counseling** regarding possible complications, alternatives (CD), prognosis and explanation of the actual procedure. A **nonstress test** should be performed before and after ECV. Anesthesia is usually not necessary and has not been absolutely proven to benefit outcomes. **Betamimetic** prophylactic tocolysis should be given (e.g., terbutaline 25 μg subcutaneously 5–10 minutes prior to procedure). There are no trials comparing other technical aspects of ECV. One or two operators can be used. Frequent if not continuous **ultrasound** guidance to assess for fetal well-being and presentation is suggested. Rh-negative women should receive anti-D immunoglobulin. There is no evidence to support immediate induction after successful ECV.

Moxibustion and/or Acupuncture
Moxibustion is a form of traditional Chinese medicine that uses heat generated by burning herbs, most often *Artemisia vulgaris,* to stimulate the acupuncture point BL67 (Zhiyin in Chinese) [31–35]. There is **inconsistent evidence** to assess whether the use of moxibustion converts a breech to a cephalic presentation. Differences in interventions (e.g., moxibustion alone or with acupuncture) make it difficult to perform a satisfactory meta-analysis. Moxibustion may reduce the need for ECV by 53% and reduce the incidence of nonvertex presentation at term by 35%–70%, in Chinese trials [32,33]. In two trials performed in Italy, moxibustion was not well tolerated by 22% of women and therefore not effective [34]; or effective when used with acupuncture [35]. Moxibustion may decrease the use of oxytocin before or during labor for women who had vaginal deliveries and might reduce non-cephalic presentation at birth and CD compared with acupuncture [31]. A meta-analysis performed compiling data from six studies of both Western and Chinese databases shows that **moxibustion at point BL67, alone or in combination with acupuncture, is associated with higher rates of cephalic version of 72.5%,** compared with 53.2% in the control group (RR 1.36, 95% CI 1.17–1.58). This data should be viewed with caution given the high degree of heterogeneity of the studies [36]. Also, there were no significant differences found in safety of moxibustion compared with other techniques. A recent RCT of 328 women showed **no beneficial effect of moxibustion to facilitate ECV** compared with controls when looking at the percent of fetuses in breech presentation at 37 weeks (72.0% vs. 63.4%; RR 1.13, 95% CI 0.98–1.32) [37]. It might be that acupuncture and not moxibustion (especially not at home) is beneficial [35].

Maternal Change in Posture
Maternal changes in position such as knee–chest and others has been suggested as a means to correct breech presentation in pregnancy. There is **insufficient evidence** from the small trials reported so far to support the use of postural management for breech presentation [38]. Meta-analysis could not be undertaken since study designs and outcomes measured were different [39]. Postural management is not associated with a significant effect on the rate of noncephalic births, either for the subgroup in which no ECV was attempted, or for the group overall (RR 0.98, 95% CI 0.84–1.15). No differences were detected for cesarean deliveries (RR 1.10, 95% CI 0.89–1.37). To date **there is no solid evidence for this practice** [38,39].

Delivery Outcomes
It is important to note that the rate of CD after ECV is still about double that of pregnancies presenting with spontaneous cephalic presentation due to higher incidences of dystocia and NRFHT after successful ECV [40].

MODE OF DELIVERY
Singleton
Term Breech
Three RCTs [41], including one large study (the Term Breech Trial) [42], have compared a policy of planned CD to a policy of planned trial of labor to attempt a vaginal delivery. CD occurs in about 45% of women allocated to a vaginal delivery protocol and >90% in those allocated to a CD protocol.

At 4–6 weeks after delivery, compared with planned vaginal delivery, **planned CD is associated with a 67%) decrease in perinatal or neonatal death** (RR 0.33, 95% CI 0.19–0.56) (excluding fetal anomalies) **or serious neonatal morbidity** [41]. This reduction is less for countries with high national perinatal mortality rates [42]. Planned CD is associated with a 71% reduction (from 1.15% to 0.26%) in perinatal or neonatal death (excluding fetal anomalies) [41]. This reduction was similar for countries with low and high national perinatal mortality rates. One death could be prevented for every 112 CDs planned [41]. A secondary analysis [43] of the short-term outcomes of the Term Breech Trial [42] looked at factors associated with adverse outcomes. The lowest morbidity was found in patients with planned CD prior to the onset of labor. In a planned vaginal breech delivery labor augmentation and a second stage greater than 60 minutes are associated with less optimal outcomes [43]. Factors not shown to affect outcome included induction, parity, use of continuous electronic fetal monitoring, or epidural [43]. A "skilled clinician" at the delivery was associated with lower adverse outcomes. "Skilled clinician" was best described by the clinicians themselves rather than by years of experience or being a licensed obstetrician [43].

Three months after delivery, women allocated to the planned CD group reported 38% **less urinary incontinence;** 89% **more abdominal pain;** and 68% **less perineal pain** [44].

Two years after delivery, there was **no difference in the combined outcome "death or neurodevelopmental delay."** Of 463 vaginal delivery patients followed at 2 years, there were only six deaths and seven children with neurodevelopmental delay (2.8%), compared with 2 and 12 of 457 patients (3.1%) in the CD group [45]. The authors postulate that there was no difference seen at the 2-year follow-up (vs. immediate neonatal outcome) because the study was underpowered, the predictive value was low for an association of measures of early morbidity with later death and adverse neurodevelopmental outcomes, and because planned CD is perhaps only reducing the risk of perinatal mortality/morbidity associated with fetal hypoxemia [45]. **Maternal outcomes at 2 years** were also very **similar,** with **constipation** significantly more **common** in the **CD** group (27% vs. 20%), while self-reported incontinence was nonsignificantly different (18% vs. 22%) [46]. Incontinence was different (16% vs. 25%) if comparing women who actually planned and had a CD versus those who planned and had a vaginal delivery [46].

These results are mostly from the Term Breech Trial [42] and its secondary analyses and follow-up [42–45]. These outcomes are based on deliveries done by "clinicians who were regarded as experienced at vaginal breech delivery" [42–46]. As the number of vaginal breech deliveries decreases, physician skill will continue to diminish, with the potential to make vaginal delivery less safe. While it is estimated that >90% of babies presenting nonvertex are currently delivered by CD, there might still be a small role for vaginal delivery for the woman who declines scheduled CD or who presents in advanced labor. The American College of Obstetricians and Gynecologists (ACOG) in 2014 supported the decision that the of mode of delivery depends on the experience of the health care provider [47]. CD is the preferred mode due to the limited experience of most physicians, but planned vaginal delivery of a term singleton fetus may be considered under specific hospital protocols. **All women with breech presentation with a large fetus (>3500 g estimation), unfavorable pelvis, hyperextended head, incomplete or footling breech presentation, NRFHT, severe fetal growth restriction, or lack of experienced obstetrical and anesthesiological operators should have a CD.**

Technical aspects
Cesarean breech delivery: There are no trials to assess technical aspects of breech (or other malpresentation) CD. There is insufficient evidence to assess whether intra-abdominal version during CD before uterine incision affects outcomes.

Vaginal breech delivery: There are several technical suggestions for assisting a vaginal breech delivery; none are based on trials. There is insufficient evidence to assess whether clinical/radiologic pelvimetry affects outcomes in the management of breech presentation. A double setup is suggested: a vaginal delivery should be organized in the operating room and ready for possible CD.

Some other suggestions are as follows: minimal intervention until the abdomen up to the umbilical cord, is delivered; prevention of head extension, with prophylactic Mauriceau maneuver and proper use of Pipers forceps, if necessary. There is not enough evidence to evaluate the effects of expedited vaginal breech delivery (breech delivery from umbilicus to delivery of the head within one contraction) on perinatal outcomes [48].

The same management options exist for transverse/oblique lie as for breech. Fetal ECV, and CD if persistent malpresentation, are the standards of care, with limited trial evidence.

Preterm Breech
There is **insufficient evidence** to assess whether outcomes of the preterm breech presenting fetus are affected by mode of delivery. Very little prospective data, mostly nonrandomized, exists regarding vaginal versus CD of the premature breech infant [1]. Two trials aimed to assess this question failed to randomize the planned sample sizes. After 17 months of patient recruiting at 26 different hospitals, only 13 women had been randomized making it impossible to confer any conclusions in one study [49]. The Iowa premature breech trial was somewhat more successful, recruiting 38 patients over 5 years, but had insufficient data for meaningful conclusions [50]. Outcomes in premature breech infants are mainly related to prematurity and/or fetal anomaly, with unclear effect of mode of delivery [51].

Twins
Breech Second Twin
(See also Chapter 44 in *Maternal-Fetal Evidence Based Guidelines*)

Pregnancies at ≥35 weeks with vertex/breech presentation in twin gestations <7 cm dilation have similar Apgar scores and incidence of neonatal morbidity in the second twin delivered by vaginal or cesarean birth [52]. There was no incidence of birth trauma or intraventricular hemorrhage in any of the 27 breech deliveries of the second twin [52]. Maternal febrile morbidity and length of stay was increased in the CD group [52]. In the largest RCT that randomized women with twin pregnancies to planned CD or planned vaginal delivery, there was a large number of women with non-cephalic second twin. There was no statistically significant difference seen in composite fetal or neonatal morbidity, even when evaluating for interaction with fetal presentation, comparing perinatal morbidity in planned CD versus planned vaginal delivery (odds ratio [OR] 1.16, 95% CI 0.77–1.74). Morbidity included birth trauma, seizures and assisted ventilation. There were also no significant differences noted in serious maternal morbidity (OR 0.86, 95% CI 0.65–1.13) [53]. **Vaginal delivery of the second nonvertex twin is a reasonable management option.** Attempt at vaginal twin delivery of the second twin, especially for a second twin with an estimated fetal weight (EFW) of >1500 g, should be performed with adequate experience of the obstetrician, as well as with continuous availability of expert anesthesia, in or very close to, an operating room. **Total breech extraction of the second twin** is associated with shorter maternal stay, lower neonatal pulmonary disease, infection, and intensive care nursery stay compared with cephalic version [49,54]. There are no trials for twins presenting with **first twin nonvertex** (about 26% of twins). Recommendation for CD under this circumstance is based mostly on data from singleton gestations. Because vaginal delivery of **triplets** is usually associated with an increased risk for stillbirth or neonatal and infant deaths, as compared with CD, **CD is the route of choice,** even if some small series have recently reported similar outcomes for trial of labor or CD for triplets.

Preterm Twins
There are no RCTs of planned CD versus vaginal delivery of preterm twins less than 34 weeks with malpresentation of the second twin. There is insufficient data to make a recommendation.

MALPOSITION
Definitions
Position: Relationship of presenting part (usually occiput for head) to pelvic outlet.
   Malposition: Fetal position that is not occiput-anterior (or sacrum anterior).
   Synclitism of the fetal head is the specific malposition in which neither of the parietal bones precedes the sagittal suture into the maternal birth canal. The situation when one of the parietal bone precedes the sagittal suture is called *asynclitism* [55].

Epidemiology/Incidence
Occiput posterior (OP) is the most common fetal malposition. Only 5% of term fetuses are OP at time of delivery, but about 23% were OP at the beginning of labor [56].

Risk Factors/Associations
OP position is associated with African American race, advanced maternal age, post term pregnancy, birth weight >4000 g, and epidural anesthesia [57]. In a meta-analysis evaluating epidural versus no-epidural/analgesia in labor, malposition was higher in women in the epidural group (RR 1.40, 95% CI 0.98–1.99), although this was not statistically significant [58].

Diagnosis
Fetal malposition can be detected by provider digital examination as well as by transabdominal ultrasound. One prospective RCT found a **difference in digital vaginal examination and transabdominal ultrasonographic examination of fetal head position during the second stage of labor in 20% of the cases evaluated, promoting the use of transabdominal ultrasound to locate the position of the fetal head** [59].

Management
Hands and Knees Posture
There is **insufficient evidence** for assessing the effect of **hands and knees posture** to correct malposition. This has been evaluated **both before (for prevention) and during labor.**

There are two trials on the effect of hands and knees posture *before labor* [60]. Compared with a sitting position, 10 minutes in the hands and knees position is associated with a lower likelihood of malposition of the presenting part of the fetus in a small trial, but assuming the hands and knees posture for 10 minutes twice daily in the last weeks of pregnancy had **no effect on the baby's position at delivery** or any of the other pregnancy outcomes measured in a larger trial [60].

One study evaluated the use of hands and knees position **in labor** involving 147 women in labor at term who assumed the hands and knees position for a period of at least 30 minutes. There was **no significant reduction** in occiput-posterior or occiput-transverse positions at delivery or reduction of operative deliveries. However, there was a significant reduction in back pain [61].

Manual Rotation
Persistent fetal OP position is a risk factor for prolonged labor and higher rate of CD. There is **insufficient evidence** evaluating the use of manual (also called digital) rotation in reducing the prevalence of persistent occiputposterior position and its consequences. In a retrospective cohort study, in women with a fetus in persistent occiput posterior or transverse position in the second stage of labor, manual rotation was associated with lower rates of CD, perineal lacerations, postpartum hemorrhage, and chorioamnionitis, but a higher rate of cervical lacerations [62]. A prospective (but not randomized) study of singletons with occiput-posterior position reported an increase in fetuses delivered in occiput-anterior position (93% vs. 15%) and in spontaneous vaginal delivery (77% vs. 27%) compared with no manual rotation using historic controls [63] (see Chapter 8).

Operative Delivery from Malposition (OP)
There is insufficient evidence to make a recommendation,

Ultrasound
In a recent RCT that evaluated the influence of ultrasound on diagnosis of fetal head malposition and subsequent mode of delivery, using transabdominal ultrasound in active labor did not improve management of labor, increased the incidence of operative delivery (CD + operative vaginal delivery) (RR 1.24, 95% CI 1.08–1.43) and did not decrease maternal and neonatal morbidity [64].

ANESTHESIA
For vaginal breech delivery, an anesthesiologist skilled at the pharmacology of uterine relaxation (e.g., nitric oxide) should be present.

REFERENCES
1. American College of Obstetricians and Gynecologists. *ACOG Clinical Management Guidelines for Obstetrician-Gynecologists Number 13: External Cephalic Version.* Washington, DC: ACOG, 2000. [Review]
2. Hill LM. Prevalence of breech presentation by gestational age. *Am J Perinatol.* 1990;7(1):92–93. [II-3]
3. Martin JA, Hamilton BE, Sutton PD, et al. Births: Final data for 2002. *Natl Vital Stat Rep.* 2003;52(10):1–113.
4. Mancuso KM, Yancey MK, Murphy JA, et al. Epidural analgesia for cephalic version: A randomized trial. *Obstet Gynecol.* 2000;95(5):648–651. [RCT, $n = 108$]
5. Eide MG, Oyen N, Skjaerven R, et al. Breech delivery and intelligence: A population-based study of 8,738 breech infants. *Obstet Gynecol.* 2005;105(1):4–11. [II-2]
6. Dyson DC, Ferguson JE, Hensleigh P. Antepartum external cephalic version under tocolysis. *Obstet Gynecol.* 1986;67(1):63–68. [II-2]

7. Grootscholten K, Kok M, Oei SG, et al. External cephalic version-related risks: A meta-analysis. *Obstet Gynecol.* 2008;112(5):1143–1151. [Meta-analysis: 84 studies, n = 12,955]
8. Dugoff L, Stamm CA, Jones OW, et al. The effect of spinal anesthesia on the success rate of external cephalic version: A randomized trial. *Obstet Gynecol.* 1999;93(3):345–349. [RCT, n = 102]
9. Flamm BL, Fried MW, Lonky NM, et al. External cephalic version after previous cesarean section. *Am J Obstet Gynecol.* 1991;165(2):370–372. [II-2]
10. Hofmeyr GJ, Kulier R. External cephalic version for breech presentation at term. *Cochrane Database Syst Rev.* 2015;(2):CD000083. [8 RCTs, n = 1308]
11. Kok M, Cnossen J, Gravendeel L, et al. Clinical factors to predict the outcome of external cephalic version: A meta-analysis. *Am J Obstet Gynecol.* 2008;199(6):630.e1–630.e7. [Meta-analysis, 53 studies, n = 10,149]
12. Ben-Meir A, Elram T, Tsafrir A, et al. The incidence of spontaneous version after failed external cephalic version. *Am J Obstet Gynecol.* 2007;196(2):157.e1–157.e3. [II-2]
13. Hutton EK, Hofmeyr GJ. External cephalic version for breech presentation before term. *Cochrane Database Syst Rev.* 2015;(1):CD000084. [Meta-analysis: 5 RCTs, n = 2187]
14. Hutton EK, Kaufman K, Hodnett E, et al. External cephalic version beginning at 34 weeks' gestation versus 37 weeks' gestation: A randomized multicenter trial. *Am J Obstet Gynecol.* 2003;189(1):245–254. [RCT, n = 233]
15. Mensink WF, Huisjes HJ. Is external version useful in breech presentation? *Ned Tijdschr Geneeskd.* 1980;124(43):1828–1831. [RCT, n = 102]
16. Van Veelen AJ, Van Cappellen AW, Flu PK, et al. Effect of external cephalic version in late pregnancy on presentation at delivery: A randomized controlled trial. *Br J Obst Gynaecol.* 1989;96(8):916–921. [RCT, n = 180]
17. Hutton EK, Hannah ME, Ross SJ, et al. Early ECV2 Trial Collaborative Group. The Early External Cephalic Version (ECV) 2 trial: An international multicentre randomised controlled trial of timing of ECV for breech pregnancies. *Br J Obstet Gynecol.* 2011;118(5):564–577. [RCT, n = 1543]
18. Hofmeyr GJ. Interventions to for helping to turn breech babies to head first presentation when using external cephalic version. *Cochrane Database Syst Rev.* 2015;(1):CD000184. [17 RCTs c tocolysis, n = 1876; 1 acoustic stimulation, n = 26, 6 RCTs regional anesthesia, n = 554; 1 systemic opiod, n = 60, 1 hypnosis, n = 80]
19. Vani S, Lau SY, Lim BK, et al. Intravenous salbutamol for external cephalic version. *Int J Gynaecol Obstet.* 2009;104(1):28–31. [RCT, n = 114]
20. Impey L, Pandit M. Tocolysis for repeat external cephalic version in breech presentation at term: A randomised, double-blinded, placebo-controlled trial. *Br J Obstet Gynecol.* 2005;112(5):627–631. [RCT, n = 124]
21. Kok M, Bais JM, van Lith JM, et al. Nifedipine as a uterine relaxant for external cephalic version: A randomized controlled trial. *Obstet Gynecol.* 2008;112(2 Pt 1):271–276. [RCT, n = 32]
22. Mohamed Ismail NA, Ibrahim M, Mohd Naim N, et al. Nifedipine versus terbutaline for tocolysis in external cephalic version. *Int J Gynaecol Obstet.* 2008;102(3):263–266. [RCT, n = 86]
23. Collaris R, Tan PC. Oral nifedipine versus subcutaneous terbutaline tocolysis for external cephalic version: A double-blind randomised trial. *Br J Obstet Gynecol.* 2009;116(1):74–80. [RCT, n = 90]
24. Wilcox CB, Nassar N, Roberts CL. Effectiveness of nifedipine tocolysis to facilitate external cephalic version: A systematic review. *Br J Obstet Gynecol.* 2011;118(4):423–428. [3 RCTs, n = 496]
25. Hilton J, Allan B, Swaby C, et al. Intravenous nitroglycerin for external cephalic version: A randomized controlled trial. *Obstet Gynecol.* 2009;114(3):560–567. [RCT, n = 82]
26. El-Sayed YY, Pullen K, Riley ET, et al. Randomized comparison of intravenous nitroglycerin and subcutaneous terbutaline for external cephalic version under tocolysis. *Am J Obstet Gynecol.* 2004;191(6):2051–2055. [RCT, n = 59]
27. Johnson RL, Strong TH, Radin TG, et al. Fetal acoustic stimulation as an adjunct to external cephalic version. *J Reprod Med.* 1995;40(10):696–698. [II-3]
28. Schorr SJ, Speights SE, Ross EL, et al. A randomized trial of epidural anesthesia to improve external cephalic version success. *Am J Obstet Gynecol.* 1997;177(5):1133–1137. [RCT, n = 69]
29. Lavoie A, Guay J. Anesthetic dose neuraxial blockade increases the success rate of external fetal version: A meta-analysis. *Can J Anesth.* 2010;57(5):408–414. [Meta-analysis: 7 RCT, n = 681]
30. Khaw KS, Lee SW, Kee WD, et al. Randomized trial of anaesthetic interventions in external cephalic version for breech presentation. *Br J Anaesth.* 2015;114(6):944–950. [RCT, n = 189, I]
31. Coyle ME, Smith CA, Peat B. Cephalic version by moxibustion for breech presentation. *Cochrane Database Syst Rev.* 2012;(2):CD003928. [Meta-analysis: 8 RCTs, n = 1346]
32. Cardini F, Weixin H. Moxibustion for correction of breech presentation: A randomized controlled trial. *JAMA.* 1998;280(18):1580–1584. [RCT, n = 260, in China]
33. Li Q, Wang L. Clinical observation on correcting malposition of fetus by electro-acupuncture. *J Tradit Chin Med.* 1996;16(4):260–262. [RCT, n = 111]
34. Cardini F, Lombardo P, Regalia AL, et al. A randomised controlled trial of moxibustion for breech presentation. *Br J Obstet Gynecol.* 2005;112(6):743–747. [RCT, n = 123, in Italy]
35. Neri I, Airola G, Contu G, et al. Acupuncture plus moxibustion to resolve breech presentation: A randomized controlled study. *J Matern Fetal Neonatal Med.* 2004;15(4):247–252. [RCT, n = 240, in Italy]
36. Vas J, Aranda JM, Nishishinya B, et al. Correction of nonvertex presentation with moxibustion: A systematic review and meta-analysis. *Am J Obstet Gynecol.* 2009;201(3):241–259. [Meta-analysis: 6 RCTs, n = 1087]
37. Coulon C, Poleszczuk M, Paty-Montaigne MH, et al. Version of breech fetuses by moxibustion with acupuncture: A randomized controlled trial. *Obstet Gynecol.* 2014;124(1):32–39. [RCT, n = 328, I]
38. Hofmeyr GJ, Kulier R. Cephalic version by postural management for breech presentation. *Cochrane Database Syst Rev.* 2000;(3):CD000051. [Meta-analysis: 6 RCTs, n = 417]
39. Founds SA. Maternal posture for cephalic version of breech presentation: A review of the evidence. *Birth.* 2005;32(2):137–144. [Meta-analysis: 4 RCTs, n = 346, but could not be performed because of flaws in RCTs]
40. Vezina Y, Bujold E, Varin J, et al. Cesarean delivery after successful external cephalic version of breech presentation at term: A comparative study. *Am J Obstet Gynecol.* 2004;190(3):763–768. [II-2, n = 602]
41. Hofmeyr GJ, Hannah ME. Planned caesarean section for term breech delivery. *Cochrane Database Syst Rev.* 2015;(3):CD000166. [Meta-analysis: 3 RCTs, n = 2396]
42. Hannah ME, Hannah WJ, Hewson SA, et al. Term Breech Trial Collaborative Group. Planned caesarean section versus planned vaginal birth for the breech presentation at term: A randomised multicentre trial. *Lancet.* 2000;356(9239):1375–1383. [RCT, n = 2088]
43. Su M, McCleod L, Ross S, et al. Term Breech Trial Collaborative Group. Factors associated with adverse perinatal outcome in the Term Breech Trial. *Am J Obstet Gynecol.* 2003;189(3):740–745. [Secondary analysis of RCT, n = 2083]
44. Hannah ME, Hannah WJ, Hodnett ED, et al. Term Breech Trial 3-Month Follow-up Collaborative Group. Outcomes at 3 months after planned cesarean vs planned vaginal delivery for breech presentation at term: The international randomized Term Breech Trial. *JAMA.* 2002;287(14):1822–1831. [RCT analysis of 3-months questionnaire follow-up, n = 1596]
45. Whyte H, Hannah ME, Saigal S, et al.; Term Breech Trial Collaborative Group. Outcomes of children at 2 years after planned cesarean birth versus planned vaginal birth for breech presentation at term: The international randomized Term Breech Trial. *Am J Obstet Gynecol.* 2004;191(3):864–871. [2-year follow-up of children of RCT, n = 923]

46. Hannah ME, Whyte H, Hannah WJ, et al. Term Breech Trial Collaborative Group. Maternal outcomes at 2 years after planned cesarean section versus planned vaginal birth for breech presentation at term: The international randomized Term Breech Trial. *Am J Obstet Gynecol.* 2004;191(3):917–927. [2-year maternal follow-up of RCT, $n = 917$]
47. ACOG Committee on Obstetric Practice. ACOG Committee Opinion 340: Mode of term singleton breech delivery. *Obstet Gynecol.* 2006;108(1):235–237. [III; Expert opinion]
48. Hofmeyr GJ, Kulier R. Expedited versus conservative approaches for vaginal delivery in breech presentation. *Cochrane Database Syst Rev.* 2015;(2):CD000082. [Meta-analysis: no RCTs]
49. Penn ZJ, Steer PJ, Grant A. A multicentre randomised controlled trial comparing elective and selective caesarean section for the delivery of the preterm breech infant. *Br J Obstet Gynecol.* 1996;103(7):684–689. [RCT, $n = 13$; stopped recruitment]
50. Zlatnik FJ. The Iowa premature breech trial. *Am J Perinatol.* 1993;10(1):60–63. [RCT, $n = 38$]
51. Cibils LA, Karrison T, Brown L. Factors influencing neonatal outcomes in the very-low-birth-weight fetus (<1500 grams) with a breech presentation. *Am J Obstet Gynecol.* 1994;171(1):35–42. [II-2]
52. Rabinovici J, Barkai G, Reichman B, et al. Randomized management of the second nonvertex twin: Vaginal delivery or cesarean section. *Am J Obstet Gynecol.* 1987;156(1):52–56. [RCT, $n = 60$]
53. Barrett FR, Hannah ME, Hutton EK, et al. A randomized trial of planned cesarean or vaginal delivery for twin pregnancy. *N Engl J Med.* 2013;369:1295–1305. [RCT, $n = 1398$, I]
54. Mauldin JG, Newman RB, Mauldin PD. Cost-effective delivery management of the vertex and nonvertex twin gestation. *Am J Obstet Gynecol.* 1998;179(4):864–869. [II-2]
55. Malvasi A, Barbera A, Di Vagno G, et al. Asynclitism: A literature review of an often forgotten clinical condition. *J Matern Fetal Neonatal Med.* 2015;28(16):1890–1894. [Review, III]
56. Vitner D, Paltieli Y, Haberman S, et al. Who delivers in occipito-posterior? A multicentric prospective ultrasound-based measurements of fetal station and position throughout labor in a population of 595 women. *Ultrasound Obstet Gynecol.* 2015;46(5):611–615. [Cohort, II-2]
57. Cheng YW, Shaffer BL, Caughey AB. Associated factors and outcomes of persistent occiput posterior position: A retrospective cohort study from 1976 to 2001. *J Matern Fetal Neonatal Med.* 2006;19(9):563. [Cohort, II-2]
58. Amin-Somuah M, Smyth RM, Jones L. Epidural versus non-epidural or no analgesia in labour. *Cochrane Database Syst Rev.* 2011;(12):CD000331. [Meta-analysis, $n = 9658$, I]
59. Dupuis O, Ruimark S, Corinne D, et al. Fetal head position during the second stage of labor: Comparison of digital vaginal examination and transabdominal ultrasonographic examination. *Eur J Obstet Gynecol Reprod Biol.* 2005;123(2):193–197. [II-2]
60. Hofmeyr GJ, Kulier R. Hands and knees posture in late pregnancy or labour for fetal malposition (lateral or posterior). *Cochrane Database Syst Rev.* 2005;(2):CD001063. [Meta-analysis: 2 RCTs, $n = 2647$]
61. Hunter S, Hofmeyr GJ, Kulier R. Hands and knees posture in late pregnancy or labour for fetal malposition (lateral or posterior). *Cochrane Database Syst Rev.* 2007;(4):CD001063. [Meta-analysis: 3 RCT, $n = 2794$]
62. Shaffer BL, Cheng YW, Vargas JE, et al. Manual rotation to reduce caesarean delivery in persistent occiput posterior or transverse position. *J Matern Fetal Neonatal Med.* 2011;24(1):65–72. [II-2]
63. Reichman O, Gdansky E, Latinsky B, et al. Digital rotation from occipito-posterior to occipito-anterior decreases the need for cesarean section. *Eur J Obstet Gynecol Reprod Biol.* 2008;136(1):25–28. [RCT, $n = 61$]
64. Popowski T, Porcher R, Fort J, et al. Influence of ultrasound determination of fetal head position on mode of delivery: A pragmatic randomized trial. *Ultrasound Obstet Gynecol.* 2015;46:520–525. [RCT, $n = 959$, I]

Shoulder dystocia

Sean C. Blackwell

KEY POINTS

- Risk factors for shoulder dystocia include prior shoulder dystocia (recurrence risk ~1%–15%); maternal diabetes mellitus, obesity, postterm, labor induction, epidural anesthesia, labor abnormalities (e.g., prolonged second stage), operative vaginal delivery, and fetal macrosomia (Table 25.1).
- In 50% of shoulder dystocia cases, no risk factors are identified. Therefore, clinicians should be ready for possible shoulder dystocia at every delivery.
- In 40%–60% of shoulder dystocia cases, birth weight is <4000 g.
- Maternal complications of shoulder dystocia include serious vaginal laceration (third or fourth degree) and postpartum hemorrhage.
- A perinatal complication of shoulder dystocia is brachial plexus impairment (BPI), which occurs in 4%–40% of shoulder dystocia cases; over 90% are transient. Approximately one-half of cases of BPI occur without documented shoulder dystocia.
- Other perinatal complications of shoulder dystocia include fractures, hypoxic–ischemic encephalopathy, long-term neurologic disability, and even death.
- Preconception prevention of maternal obesity and diabetes, as well as prenatal prevention of excessive weight gain, decrease the incidence of shoulder dystocia, mainly by prevention of fetal macrosomia.
- In women with **prior shoulder dystocia,** clinicians should review recurrence risk (7%–15%), which risk factors (Table 25.1) are present in the current pregnancy, and also possible complications. If several significant risk factors are still present, the woman may opt for cesarean delivery. If risk factors are not present (except for prior shoulder dystocia), the woman may decide after counseling for either trial of labor or cesarean delivery.
- **Induction of labor at term for suspected fetal macrosomia (estimated fetal weights [EFW] ≥4000 g) in women without diabetes is associated with a similar incidence of cesarean or operative vaginal delivery compared with expectant management, a significant decrease in fetal fractures,** and higher incidences of hyperbilirubinemia and phototherapy. **Induction at ≥38 weeks** would prevent the neonatal complications, and **can be considered.**
- In pregnancies with **EFW > 5000 g in nondiabetic and >4500 g in diabetic women,** The American Congress of Obstetricians and Gynecologists (ACOG) **suggests planned cesarean delivery (without labor attempt) may be considered to avoid shoulder dystocia.**
- In women with EFW >3800 g, **prophylactic McRobert's maneuver and suprapubic pressure** are associated in one randomized controlled trial (RCT) with *significantly fewer instances of shoulder dystocia.*
- Initial responses to shoulder dystocia involve asking for help, and, as first maneuvers, use of McRobert's maneuver and suprapubic pressure (Figure 25.1).
- Second line maneuvers include direct fetal manipulation such as delivery of the posterior arm, or then rotation of fetal shoulders. One-third of shoulder dystocia cases require use of more than two maneuvers. See Figure 25.1 for suggested management of shoulder dystocia.

DIAGNOSIS/DEFINITION

Shoulder dystocia is diagnosed when additional obstetrical maneuvers are required following failure of gentle downward traction on the fetal head to effect delivery of the shoulders [1]. Shoulder dystocia pertains only to vertex presentation.

A quantitative definition of shoulder dystocia has been proposed as a prolonged head-to-body delivery time >60 seconds [2]. This definition categorized 10% of vaginal deliveries as having shoulder dystocia while only 25%–45% of these cases were diagnosed as such by the delivery provider [3]. However, these diagnostic criteria have not been adopted and shoulder dystocia remains a subjective clinical diagnosis by the delivering provider. This may account for some of the variability in the frequency of reported shoulder dystocia across various populations and different studies.

SIGNS

1. Retraction of the delivered fetal head against the maternal perineum (turtle sign).
2. Inability to deliver the fetal shoulders with routine traction in the "axial" direction.

EPIDEMIOLOGY/INCIDENCE

The incidence of shoulder dystocia is about 1% (range 0.6%–1.4%, depending on definition used).

ETIOLOGY/BASIC PATHOPHYSIOLOGY

Shoulder dystocia results from size discrepancy between the fetal shoulders and the pelvic inlet that results in impaction of the anterior shoulders behind the maternal pubis symphysis or the posterior shoulder on the sacral promontory (uncommon), or both (rare) [4]. Persistent anterior–posterior location of the fetal shoulders at the pelvic brim occurs most often due to: increased resistance between the fetal skin and vaginal walls (e.g., fetal macrosomia), a large fetal chest relative to the biparietal diameter (e.g., infants of diabetic mothers), and when truncal rotation does not occur (e.g., precipitous labor).

Table 25.1 Factors Associated with Shoulder Dystocia

Antepartum	Intrapartum
Multiparity	Labor induction and/or augmentation
Postterm gestation	
Maternal obesity	Labor abnormalities
Maternal diabetes	Prolonged first stage
Prior shoulder dystocia	Short second stage
Prior macrosomic child	Prolonged second stage
Excessive gestational weight gain	Epidural
Fetal macrosomia	Operative vaginal delivery (forceps or vacuum)

Source: American College of Obstetricians and Gynecologists, *Obstet Gynecol*, 100(5 Pt 1), 1045–1050, 2002.

Table 25.2 Relationship between Increasing Birth Weight and Maternal Diabetes and the Development of Shoulder Dystocia

Birth Weight (g)	No Diabetes (%)	Maternal Diabetes (%)
4000–4250	5.25	12.2
4250–4500	9.1	16.7
4500–4750	14.3	27.3
4750–5000	21.1	34.8

Source: Nesbitt TS et al., *Am J Obstet Gynecol*, 179(2), 476–480, 1998.

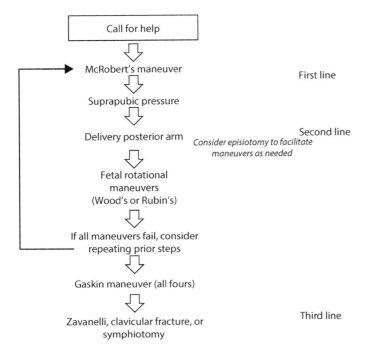

Figure 25.1 Suggested management algorithm for shoulder dystocia.

<4000 g, and of deliveries with birth weight >4000 g only 3.3% develop shoulder dystocia [4,6,7].

Although recognized as a risk factor associated with shoulder dystocia, multiple studies including those using advanced statistical models and techniques have been unable to discriminate labor patterns (e.g., prolonged first and/or second stage) in a manner that improves intrapartum management to predict and avoid shoulder dystocia [8–12]. Dyachenko et al. studied 498 cases of shoulder dystocia (including 90 cases with neonatal injury) versus 622 controls with vaginal delivery assessing for whether a combination of maternal and fetal factors could reasonably predict outcomes. The statistical model that best predicted shoulder dystocia with injury included maternal height and weight, gestational age, parity, and birth weight identified 50.7% of cases with a false positive rate of 2.7%.

COMPLICATIONS
Maternal
Although maternal complications can occur, these are most often mild and not associated with long-term morbidities. The most common complications involve postpartum blood loss and vaginal laceration (Table 25.3).

Perinatal
The most common major complication of shoulder dystocia is **neonatal BPI** which occurs in 4%–40% of cases of shoulder dystocia. In one of the largest series, the rate was 16.8% (Table 25.3) [13]. Most cases of BPI are unilateral (right > left) and involve the C5–C6 roots (Erb–Duchenne's palsy) (Table 25.4). Most bony injuries (clavicle or humerus), although always concerning, are not serious and heal promptly without long-term sequelae. Approximately 1/3 BPIs have a concomitant bony fracture. Fortunately <10% of BPIs are permanent. Most fully recover with physical therapy and, in some situations, respond to neurosurgical treatment. **Permanent BPI is very rare and occurs in 1–2 out of every 10,000 births.** Signs and symptoms are a limp or unmoving paralyzed arm, lack of muscle control in the arm, hand, or wrist, and lack of feeling or sensation in the arm or hand. Neonatal BPIs can occur without shoulder dystocia. In fact, it is estimated that one half of all BPIs occur in the absence of shoulder dystocia and up to 4% of BPIs are associated with cesarean delivery [14,15]. Two studies provide evidence that BPI (both transient and permanent) can occur with cesarean delivery. Gherman et al. [6,16] reported the finding of 17 cases of BPI (six with permanent) associated with cesarean delivery with longer term follow-up (12–29 months). Chang et al. described 30 cases of BPI with cesarean delivery (out of total 387 cases) where 60% were persistent at 1 year [17]. In a recent

RISK FACTORS/ASSOCIATIONS
Table 25.1 lists antepartum and intrapartum risk factors associated with shoulder dystocia. These risk factors have poor predictive value (whether in isolation or in combination with other factors), making them not very useful for clinical decision making. In 50% of cases of shoulder dystocia, no risk factors are identified.

The two risks factors for shoulder dystocia most studied are **maternal diabetes and fetal macrosomia.** The frequency of shoulder dystocia increases with higher birth weight [5] (Table 25.2).

Although there is a consistent relationship regarding birth weight and the risk for shoulder dystocia, it should also be remembered that 40%–60% of cases occur with birth weight

Table 25.3 Maternal and Newborn Complications of Shoulder Dystocia Reported at Single Large Tertiary Care Center

Complication	Frequency (%)
Maternal	
Postpartum hemorrhage	11
Fourth degree laceration (either extension of episiotomy or extension of laceration)	3.8
Vaginal lacerations	19.3
Cervical tear	2
Perinatal	
Any fetal injury	24.9
Brachial plexus injury	16.8
Clavicular fracture	9.5
Humeral fracture	4.2

Sources: Gherman RB et al., *Am J Obstet Gynecol*, 176(3), 656–661, 1997; Gherman RB et al., *Am J Obstet Gynecol*, 178(6), 1126–1130, 1998.

Table 25.4 Types of Brachial Plexus Impairments

Palsy	Description	Level	Frequency (%)
Erb's palsy (also known as Erb–Duchenne's palsy)	Paralysis of flexion, abduction, internal and external rotation of the forearm	C5, C6	>98
Klumpke's palsy	Paralysis of the thumb, fingers, and pronation of the forearm	C8, T1	<1
Complete brachial plexus palsy	Both Erb's and Klumpke's	C5, T1	<1

literature review of neonatal BPP with and without shoulder dystocia, approximately 45% of NPP cases in the United States and 47% outside the United States were not associated with shoulder dystocia at delivery [18]. Table 25.4 describes most common palsies associated with shoulder dystocia.

These data indicate that some cases of neonatal BPIs are unrelated to clinician-applied forces and due to a combination of mechanisms such as endogenous labor forces, the impaction and pressure effects of the shoulder dystocia itself and/or in utero compression or maladaptation [19,20]. External maneuvers such excessive lateral traction are most likely responsible for some cases of BPP from shoulder dystocia, but not all.

Fractures of the clavicle and humerus have also been associated with shoulder dystocia (up to 10.4%), and the maneuvers to resolve it. Nondisplaced fractures of the clavicle can be missed at birth while most humeral fractures involve the upper one third of the bone. Both fractures heal-well with conservative therapy [21].

The effects of shoulder dystocia on **umbilical artery blood gases** have been studied. In a study of 134 cases of shoulder dystocia, mean umbilical pH was not clinically different than cases without shoulder dystocia and there was no association between head-to-body delivery intervals and umbilical pH, base excess, or 5-minute Apgar scores [22]. However, another study done by Leung et al. of 200 cases of shoulder dystocia noted that the umbilical artery pH dropped 0.01 per minute for the head-to-body delivery interval (HBDI). They found an overall 2.5% rate of hypoxic ischemic encephalopathy (the risk was 0.5% if HBDI was <5 minutes compared with 23.5% if HBDI ≥5 minutes) [23].

In a review of 56 cases of fatal shoulder dystocia reported to the Confidential Inquiry into Stillbirths and Deaths in Infancy between 1994 and 1995 from England, Northern Wales, and Ireland the approximate incidence of **fatal shoulder dystocia** is 0.025 per 1000 deliveries. In 47% of these cases, the head-to-body ratio was less than 5 minutes and greater than 10 minutes in 20% [24].

MANAGEMENT
Principles

Shoulder dystocia is an obstetrical emergency and cannot be reliably predicted. Thus prompt recognition and response are essential to optimizing outcomes once it develops. Obstetricians should be trained and ready to manage this complication at every delivery. Therefore, it is imperative that shoulder dystocia training occurs early, and that at least one clinician experienced in the management of shoulder dystocia is present at every delivery.

Prevention
Preconception

Preconception prevention of maternal obesity and diabetes, as well as prenatal prevention of excessive weight gain, decrease the incidence of shoulder dystocia, mainly by prevention of fetal macrosomia.

Antepartum

Since clinical risk factors (Table 25.1) do not accurately predict who will develop shoulder dystocia, few preventive strategies have been proven effective. Nonetheless, avoidance, prevention or proper control of maternal obesity, diabetes, excessive weight gain, and fetal macrosomia would prevent the increased risk of shoulder dystocia associated with these conditions. Women with **prior shoulder dystocia** have about a 1%–15% [25,26] risk of recurrence. In women with a prior shoulder dystocia, counseling should include review of prior delivery events including severity of injury of prior child, which risk factors (Table 25.1) are present in the current pregnancy, and also possible short-term and long-term complications of cesarean delivery. If several significant risk factors are still present, the woman may opt for cesarean delivery. However, given at least 85% of women will not have a recurrent shoulder dystocia and cesarean delivery does have certain surgical risks (especially in setting of maternal comorbidities) a woman with a prior shoulder dystocia after counseling may choose to pursue vaginal delivery [1].

Strategies to perform **cesarean delivery** without a labor attempt, due solely to suspected fetal macrosomia, are neither cost-effective nor practical due to poor prediction abilities [27,28]. This is complicated by the known limitations of prenatal ultrasound to accurately estimate fetal weight, especially with increased fetal size [29,30]. Only at very high estimated fetal weights **(>5000 g in nondiabetic and >4500 g in diabetic women) does ACOG suggests planned cesarean delivery (without labor attempt) may be considered to avoid shoulder dystocia** [29].

Labor induction for women with suspected macrosomia as an intervention to decrease the rate of shoulder dystocia has been tested in four clinical trials, including 1190 women [31–34,35] Women who were randomized to labor induction had a similar incidence of cesarean delivery (26.6% vs. 29.4%;

relative risk [RR], 0.90, 95% confidence interval [CI] 0.75–1.09), operative vaginal delivery (13.0% vs. 15.2%; RR 0.86, 95% CI 0.65–1.13), spontaneous vaginal delivery (60.3% vs. 55.4%; RR 1.09, 95% CI 0.99–1.20), shoulder dystocia (2.4% vs. 4.2%; RR 0.57, 95% CI 0.30–1.08), intracranial hemorrhage (0.6% vs. 0.4%; RR 1.48, 95% CI 0.20–12.57), brachial plexus palsy (0.0% vs. 0.3%; RR 0.21, 95% CI 0.01–4.28), Apgar score <7 at 5 minutes (0.7% vs. 0.5%; RR 1.51, 95% CI 0.25–9.02), cord blood pH<7 (0.2% vs. 0.4%; RR 0.44, 95% CI 0.06–2.97), and mean birth weight (mean difference [MD] –134.41 g, 95% CI –317.27 to 48.46) compared with women expectantly managed. Induction group had a significantly lower time to delivery (MD –7.55 days, 95% CI –8.20 to –6.89), birth weight ≥4000 g (30.7% vs. 61.8%; RR 0.50, 95% CI 0.42–0.59), birth weight ≥4500 g (3.2% vs. 14.8%; RR 0.21, 95% CI 0.11–0.39), incidence of fetal fractures (0.3% vs. 2.0%; RR 0.17, 95% CI 0.03–0.79) and a significantly higher incidence of hyperbilirubinemia (8.8% vs. 2.9%; RR 3.03, CI 1.60–5.74) and phototherapy (11.0% vs. 6.6%; RR 1.68, CI 1.07–2.66) compared with expectant management group [34].

In summary, **induction of labor at term for suspected fetal macrosomia (EFW ≥4000 g) in women without diabetes is associated with a similar incidence of cesarean or operative vaginal delivery compared with expectant management, a significant decrease in fetal fractures**, and higher incidences of hyperbilirubinemia and phototherapy. **Induction at ≥38 weeks** would prevent the neonatal complications, and **can be considered.**

Data regarding the effects on labor induction in women with diabetes to reduce shoulder dystocia are limited to one trial involving 200 women. There was no statistically significant differences in the rate of shoulder dystocia between labor induction and expectant management (0/100 vs. 3/100; RR 0.14 [95 CI 0.01–2.73]) [31].

Intrapartum

Prophylactic McRobert's maneuver, prior to the development of shoulder dystocia, has not been shown to decrease subsequent shoulder dystocia in women at low-risk for this complication [36]. In a small RCT, in 40 women, compared with lithotomy position, the use of the McRobert's maneuver was associated with the same incidence (7.1% vs. 7.7%) of shoulder dystocia in both prophylactic and lithotomy groups. The forced used in traction of the fetal head during vaginal delivery was the same in each group [36].

In another RCT, in 185 women likely to give birth to a large baby (EFW >3800 g), compared with no prophylactic maneuvers, the McRobert's maneuver and suprapubic pressure were associated with a **trend for a lower rate of shoulder dystocia** compared with controls (9% vs. 21%; RR 0.44, 95% CI 0.17–1.14). There were significantly more cesarean sections in the prophylactic group, and when these were included in the results, **significantly fewer instances of shoulder dystocia were seen in the prophylactic group** (RR 0.33, 95% CI 0.12–0.86). In this study, 13 (18%) women in the control group required therapeutic maneuvers after delivery of the fetal head compared with 3 (5%) in the treatment group (RR 0.31, 95% CI 0.09–1.02). One infant in the control group had a brachial plexus injury (RR 0.44, 95% CI 0.02–10.61), and one infant had a 5-minute Apgar score less than seven (RR 0.44, 95% CI 0.02–10.61) [37,38].

Training

Three nonrandomized studies have shown benefits of shoulder dystocia training. In a single center "before and after" study conducted in Jamaica, NY, between 2003 and 2006 (pre) to 2006 and 2009 (post), shoulder dystocia training decreased the rate of BPI associated with shoulder dystocia from 30% (pre) to 10.67% (post) even after adjusting for confounding factors [39]. Another "before and after" study in the United Kingdom showed a reduction in neonatal injury at birth after shoulder dystocia: (9.3% vs. 2.3%; RR 0.25; 95% CI 0.11–0.57) [40]. Finally, in a university hospital setting in Chicago, IL, the effects of a shoulder dystocia protocol was studied in three time periods (6 months prior to training, 6 months during training, and 6 months posttraining). Over the three time periods complete and consistent documentation improved (14%, to 50%, to 92%; $p < .001$), decrease BPI at delivery (10.1%, to 4%, to 2.6%; $p = .03$) and BPI at neonatal discharge (7.6%, to 3%, to 1.3%; $p = .04$). Both the Joint Commission in the United States and the Royal College of Obstetricians and Gynecologists recommend such training.

Recognition

After diagnosis of shoulder dystocia, whether done via recognition of the "turtle sign" or lack of fetal progression with gentle traction, the delivery provider should **"call for help."** This includes utilizing the assistance of other care givers present in the delivery room as well as alerting other obstetrical, pediatric and/or anesthesia providers on the labor and delivery unit.

Therapy

There are no interventional trials in human subjects that compare the safety or effectiveness of various shoulder dystocia therapeutic maneuvers [38]. Thus guidelines are based on observational data and/or expert opinion. The most important feature of the response to shoulder dystocia is that it should be a coordinated and orderly application and progression of obstetrical maneuvers (Figure 25.1) [1, 41]. Table 25.5 describes maneuvers employed to relieve shoulder dystocia [4, 42].

Most authorities recommend **McRobert's as the initial maneuver** since it is easy to perform, is effective, and has a low complication rate. McRobert's alone is effective in 40%–90% of cases. Suprapubic pressure is often done in direct conjunction by nursing personnel. In a series of 134 cases, more than one third of patients required more than two maneuvers to relieve the shoulder dystocia [22]. Another series of 231 shoulder dystocia cases, 57.9% of cases responded to McRobert's and suprapubic pressure alone and had a median duration of 29 seconds [43].

If McRobert's combined with suprapubic pressure are not successful, direct fetal manipulation is attempted next. In a very large series, **delivery of the posterior shoulder was associated with the highest rate of delivery (84%) compared with all other maneuvers (24%–72%)** [44]. These authors have suggested considering using delivery of the posterior arm if delivery is not achieved with McRobert's maneuver and suprapubic pressure. The need of additional maneuvers is associated with higher rates of neonatal injury; 10% with three maneuvers, 16% with four maneuvers, and 23% with five or more [44].

Since shoulder dystocia is a bony dystocia, routine episiotomy is not advised. In a systematic literature review including 14 studies of 9769 cases of shoulder dystocia, there was no reported benefit of episiotomy to prevent or assist with the management of shoulder dystocia [45]. In situations where delivery of the posterior arm is being tried, episiotomy or procto-episiotomy may give the delivery attendant additional room to grab the posterior fetal arm. Other helpful fetal manipulation interventions are either the Wood's corkscrew (Figure 25.2) or Rubin's maneuver (Figure 25.3).

Table 25.5 Description of Various Obstetrical Maneuvers to Resolve Shoulder Dystocia

Maneuver	Maternal or Fetal Manipulation	Type	Description
McRobert's	Maternal	First line	Hyperflexion and abduction of the maternal hips (knee to abdomen position). This causes cephalad rotation of the symphysis pubis, and flattening of the lumbar lordosis, freeing the impacted shoulder.
Suprapubic pressure	Maternal	First line	Pressure directed posteriorly in an attempt to force the anterior shoulder under the symphysis pubis. It also may include lateral pressure from either side of the maternal abdomen or alternating between sides using a rocking pressure. It works by reducing the fetal bisacromial diameter and rotating the anterior shoulder into oblique pelvic diameter.
Delivery of posterior arm	Fetal	Second line	The delivery attendant places his/her hands in the vagina and applies pressure at the antecubital fossa in order to flex the fetal forearm. The arm is subsequently swept out over the infant's chest and delivered over the perineum. Rotation of the fetal trunk to bring the posterior arm anteriorly is sometimes required. Fracture of the humerus can occur with grasping and pulling directly on the fetal arm, as well as application of pressure onto the midhumeral shaft.
Rubin's	Fetal	Second line	Pressure is applied to the posterior surface of the most accessible part of the fetal shoulder to effect shoulder adduction. It works by rotating the fetal shoulder into the oblique pelvic diameter.
Wood's	Fetal	Second line	Pressure is applied onto the anterior surface of the posterior shoulder in order to abduct the posterior shoulder. It works by rotating the fetal shoulder into the oblique pelvic diameter.
Gaskin (knee–chest or all fours)	Maternal	Second line	Patient is rolled from her existing position onto her hands and knees. It works through the downward force of gravity and/or a favorable change in pelvic diameters, which causes disimpaction of the fetal shoulder.
Intentional fracture of clavicle	Fetal	Third line	This works by decreasing the fetal bisacromial diameter.
Zavanelli (cephalad replacement)		Third line	Cephalic replacement of the fetal head from the vagina back into the uterus and then delivery by cesarean section.
Symphysiotomy	Maternal	Third line	Surgical or traumatic separation of the pubis symphysis to facilitate disimpaction of the fetal shoulders.

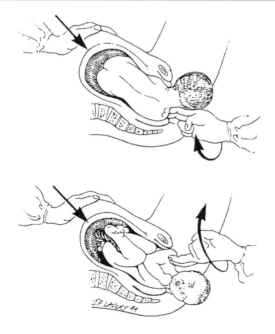
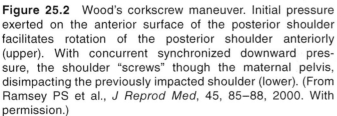

Figure 25.2 Wood's corkscrew maneuver. Initial pressure exerted on the anterior surface of the posterior shoulder facilitates rotation of the posterior shoulder anteriorly (upper). With concurrent synchronized downward pressure, the shoulder "screws" though the maternal pelvis, disimpacting the previously impacted shoulder (lower). (From Ramsey PS et al., *J Reprod Med*, 45, 85–88, 2000. With permission.)

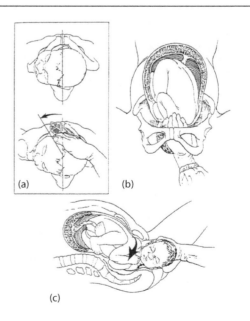

Figure 25.3 Rubin's maneuver. (a) and (b) Pressure is exerted on the posterior surface of the most accessible part of the shoulder to facilitate abduction and disimpaction of the anterior shoulder. (c) Further rotation and adduction toward the fetal chest educes the bisacromial diameter and results in the movement of the shoulders in a transverse position, facilitating passage of the anterior side of the shoulder beneath the pubic arch. (From Ramsey PS et al., *J Reprod Med*, 45, 85–88, 2000. With permission.)

Shoulder Dystocia Delivery Note Addendum

1. Antepartum documentation:
    a. Prior shoulder dystocia? Yes no
    b. Estimated fetal weight _____
2. Mode of vaginal delivery
    a. Spontaneous
    b. Vacuum
    c. Forceps
3. How was the shoulder dystocia diagnosed? Turtle sign
    Failure to deliver shoulders with gentle downward pressure
    Other _____
4. Time fetal head delivered? _____
5. Time body delivered? _____
6. Total duration of shoulder dystocia (in minutes and seconds): _____
7. What shoulder was under the pubis symphysis (anterior) at delivery: Left   Right   Unknown
8. Please describe the obstetrical maneuvers attempted, their order, and who performed:

Maneuver	Order	By whom
McRobert's (Hip flection)	1 2 3 4 5 6 7 8	_____
Suprapubic	1 2 3 4 5 6 7 8	_____
Delivery of posterior arm	1 2 3 4 5 6 7 8	_____
Rubin's (Anterior scapula)	1 2 3 4 5 6 7 8	_____
Wood's (Posterior scapula)	1 2 3 4 5 6 7 8	_____
Episiotomy	1 2 3 4 5 6 7 8	_____
Extension of Episiotomy	1 2 3 4 5 6 7 8	_____
Gaskin's (Knee-chest, all fours)	1 2 3 4 5 6 7 8	_____
Other _____	1 2 3 4 5 6 7 8	_____
Other _____	1 2 3 4 5 6 7 8	_____
Other _____	1 2 3 4 5 6 7 8	_____

Additional delivery comments: _____
_____

9. Was fundal pressure preformed: Yes   No

If yes, by whom and what was reason: _____

10. Who were the health care providers present at delivery?

Primary delivery attendant: _____
CNM: _____
Resident (s) [include PGY year]: _____
Nurse 1: _____
Nurse 2: _____
Nurse 3: _____
Pediatrician: _____
Anesthesiology: _____
Other providers (please add name and role): _____

11. Birth weight (grams) _____
12. Was baby moving his/her extremities: Left   Right   Comment: _____
13. Was X-ray ordered for evaluation any bony fractures?   Yes   No
14. Were umbilical cord gases ordered?   Yes   No
15. Confirm that notes (e.g. medical, nursing, anesthesia, etc.) are consistent   Yes   No
16. Has delivery note been dictated?   Yes   No
17. Family counseled   Yes   No
18. Debriefing with appropriate personnel involved   Yes   No
19. Follow-up about condition of neonate in nursery   Yes   No

Signatures:

_____ _____ _____
Primary delivery provider   Primary delivery nurse   Other care providers in attendance

Figure 25.4 Suggested checklist for the documentation of delivery complicated by shoulder dystocia. CNM, certified nurse midwife.

If these steps all fail, one can repeat the sequence of initial maneuvers and/or attempt placement of the patient in the "all fours" position (Gaskin maneuver) (Figure 25.1). More aggressive, "heroic" maneuvers, which have very high frequency of maternal and fetal complications, may be considered after repeat failure of these first and second line interventions. Third-line maneuvers include intentional fracture of the fetal clavicle, Zavanelli (cephalic replacement), and symphysiotomy. In cases of intractable shoulder dystocia, a technique called posterior axilla sling traction (PAST) has been described. The PAST technique makes use of a sling (e.g., suction catheter or firm urinary catheter) that is placed around the posterior axilla and then used to use traction to either deliver the posterior shoulder or rotate it [46]. Fundal pressure should always be avoided in shoulder dystocia, as it may worsen impaction of fetal shoulder(s).

Counseling and Documentation

After completion of all necessary medical interventions (e.g., repair of maternal lacerations or treatment of hemorrhage), the delivery provider should sit down with patient and her family to review the delivery events, the management steps performed, and need for close newborn follow-up to evaluate for any neonatal injuries especially bony fracture and symptoms of BPI. Open and honest communication with the mother and family after delivery is recommended.

It is important to document in the medical record all maneuvers used in detail, including which shoulder was anterior, and the time from delivery of head to completion delivery of the body (Figure 25.4) [47, 48]. Introduction of a shoulder dystocia protocol has been associated not only with better documentation, but also with less incidence of brachial plexus palsy [47].

Anesthesia

An anesthesiologist should be present during cases of shoulder dystocia to ensure adequate analgesia, and prompt preparation for cesarean delivery if needed.

Neonatal/Infant Follow-Up

Table 25.4 describes most common palsies associated with shoulder dystocia. It is important to underscore that causation has never been proven between shoulder dystocia and palsies, and many palsies develop in babies delivered without shoulder dystocia. Erb's palsy is by far the most common, and the one with the best prognosis. Occasionally BPI occurs on the posterior shoulder. Over 90% of neonates with Erb's palsy with shoulder dystocia recover within 1 year, with most recovery already evident at 3–6 months. Erb's palsy without shoulder dystocia has only a 60% recovery rate, and in about 68% of cases involves the posterior shoulder. Only about 40% of babies with Klumpke's palsy recover by 1 year. If permanent injury (5%–8%) occurs, there is insufficient evidence to assess if surgery is effective.

RESOURCES

American College of Obstetricians and Gynecologists. *Neonatal Brachial Plexus Palsy*, 2014.

REFERENCES

1. American College of Obstetricians and Gynecologists. ACOG practice bulletin no. 40: Clinical management guidelines for obstetrician–gynecologists. *Obstet Gynecol*. 2002;100(5 Pt 1):1045–1050. [Guideline]
2. Spong CY, Beall M, Rodrigues D, et al. An objective definition of shoulder dystocia: Prolonged head-to-body delivery intervals and/or the use of ancillary obstetric maneuvers. *Obstet Gynecol*. 1995;86(3):433–436. [II-2]
3. Beall MH, Spong C, McKay J, et al. Objective definition of shoulder dystocia: A prospective evaluation. *Am J Obstet Gynecol*. 1998;179(4):934–937. [II-2]
4. Gherman RB, Chauhan S, Ouzounian JG, et al. Shoulder dystocia: The unpreventable obstetric emergency with empiric management guidelines. *Am J Obstet Gynecol*. 2006;195(3):657–672. [III; Review]
5. Nesbitt TS, Gilbert WM, Herrchen B. Shoulder dystocia and associated risk factors with macrosomic infants born in California. *Am J Obstet Gynecol*. 1998;179(2):476–480. [II-2]
6. Gherman RB, Ouzounian JG, Goodwin TM. Brachial plexus palsy: An in utero injury? *Am J Obstet Gynecol*. 1999;180(5):1303–1307. [II-2]
7. Gherman RB, Goodwin TM, Souter I, et al. The McRoberts' maneuver for the alleviation of shoulder dystocia: How successful is it? *Am J Obstet Gynecol*. 1997;176(3):656–661. [II-2]
8. McFarland M, Hod M, Piper JM, et al. Are labor abnormalities more common in shoulder dystocia? *Am J Obstet Gynecol*. 1995;173(4):1211–1214. [II-2]
9. Gemer O, Bergman M, Segal S. Labor abnormalities as a risk factor for shoulder dystocia. *Acta Obstet Gynecol Scand*. 1999;78(8):735–736. [II-2]
10. Lurie S, Levy R, Ben-Arie A, et al. Shoulder dystocia: Could it be deduced from the labor partogram? *Am J Perinatol*. 1995;12(1):61–62. [II-2]
11. Mehta SH, Bujold E, Blackwell SC, et al. Is abnormal labor associated with shoulder dystocia in nulliparous women? *Am J Obstet Gynecol*. 2004;190(6):1604–1607; discussion 1607–1609. [II-2]
12. Dyachenko A, Ciampi A, Fahey J, et al. Prediction of risk for shoulder dystocia with neonatal injury. *Am J Obstet Gynecol*. 2006;195(6):1544–1549. [II-2]
13. Gherman RB, Ouzounian JG, Goodwin TM. Obstetric maneuvers for shoulder dystocia and associated fetal morbidity. *Am J Obstet Gynecol*. 1998;178(6):1126–1130. [II-2]
14. Gherman RB, Ouzounian JG, Miller DA, et al. Spontaneous vaginal delivery: A risk factor for Erb's palsy? *Am J Obstet Gynecol*. 1998;178(3):423–427. [II-2]
15. Sandmire HF, DeMott RK. Erb's palsy without shoulder dystocia. *Int J Gynaecol Obstet*. 2002;78(3):253–256. [Review]
16. Gherman RB, Goodwin TM, Ouzounian JG, et al. Brachial plexus palsy associated with cesarean section: An in utero injury? *Am J Obstet Gynecol*. 1997;177(5):1162–1164. [Review]
17. Chang KW, Ankumah NE, Wilson TJ, et al. Persistence of neonatal brachial plexus palsy associated with maternally reported route of delivery: Review of 387 cases. *Am J Perinatol*. 2016;33(8):765–769. [II-2]
18. Chauhan SP, Blackwell SB, Ananth CV. Neonatal brachial plexus palsy: Incidence, prevalence, and temporal trends. *Semin Perinatol*. 2014;38(4):210–218. [Review]
19. Sandmire HF, Demott RK. Controversies surrounding the causes of brachial plexus injury. *Int J Gynaecol Obstet*. 2009;104(1):9–13. [Review]
20. Sandmire HF, DeMott RK. Erb's palsy causation: Iatrogenic or resulting from labor forces? *J Reprod Med*. 2005;50(8):563–566. [Review]
21. Dajani NK, Magann EF. Complications of shoulder dystocia. *Semin Perinatol*. 2014;38(4):201–204. [II-2]
22. Stallings SP, Edwards RK, Johnson JW. Correlation of head-to-body delivery intervals in shoulder dystocia and umbilical artery acidosis. *Am J Obstet Gynecol*. 2001;185(2):268–274. [II-2]
23. Leung TY, Stuart O, Sahota DS, et al. Head-to-body delivery interval and risk of fetal acidosis and hypoxic ischaemic encephalopathy in shoulder dystocia: A retrospective review. *BJOG*. 2011;118(4):474–479. [II-1]
24. Hope P, Breslin S, Lamont L, et al. Fatal shoulder dystocia: A review of 56 cases reported to the confidential enquiry into stillbirths and deaths in infancy. *Br J Obstet Gynaecol*. 1998;105(12):1256–1261. [II-3]

25. Bingham J, Chauhan SP, Hayes E, et al. Recurrent shoulder dystocia: A review. *Obstet Gynecol Surv*. 2010;65(3):183–188. [Review]
26. Mehta SH, Sokol RJ. Risk of shoulder dystocia in second delivery: Does a history of shoulder dystocia matter? *Am J Obstet Gynecol*. 2010;202(3):e11–e12; author reply e12. [II-2]
27. Rouse DJ, Owen J, Goldenberg RL, et al. The effectiveness and costs of elective cesarean delivery for fetal macrosomia diagnosed by ultrasound. *JAMA*. 1996;276(18):1480–1486. [Cost-effectiveness analysis]
28. Rouse DJ, Owen J. Prophylactic cesarean delivery for fetal macrosomia diagnosed by means of ultrasonography—A Faustian bargain? *Am J Obstet Gynecol*. 1999;181(2):332–338. [Review]
29. American College of Obstetricians and Gynecologists. ACOG technical bulletin no. 159: Fetal macrosomia. *Int J Gynaecol Obstet*. 1992;39(4):341–345. [Guideline]
30. Mehta SH, Blackwell SC, Hendler I, et al. Accuracy of estimated fetal weight in shoulder dystocia and neonatal birth injury. *Am J Obstet Gynecol*. 2005;192(6):1877–1880; discussion 1880–1871. [II-2]
31. Boulvain M, Stan C, Irion O. Elective delivery in diabetic pregnant women. *Cochrane Database Syst Rev*. 2001(2):CD001997. [Meta-analysis of RCTs]
32. Irion O, Boulvain M. Induction of labour for suspected fetal macrosomia. *Cochrane Database Syst Rev*. 2000(2):CD000938. [Meta-analysis of RCTs]
33. Gonen O, Rosen DJ, Dolfin Z, et al. Induction of labor versus expectant management in macrosomia: A randomized study. *Obstet Gynecol*. 1997;89(6):913–917. [RCT]
34. Magro-Malosso ER, Saccone G, Chen M, et al. Induction of labor for macrosomia at term: A systematic review and meta-analysis of randomized controlled trials. *BJOG*. 2016; in press. [Meta-analysis, 4 RCTs, n = 1,190]
35. Boulvain M, Senat MV, Perrotin F, et al. Induction of labour versus expectant management for large-for-date fetuses: A randomised controlled trial. *Lancet*. 2015;385(9987):2600–2605. [RCT]
36. Poggi SH, Allen RH, Patel CR, et al. Randomized trial of McRoberts versus lithotomy positioning to decrease the force that is applied to the fetus during delivery. *Am J Obstet Gynecol*. 2004;191(3):874–878. [RCT]
37. Beall MH, Spong CY, Ross MG. A randomized controlled trial of prophylactic maneuvers to reduce head-to-body delivery time in patients at risk for shoulder dystocia. *Obstet Gynecol*. 2003;102(1):31–35. [RCT, n = 185]
38. Athukorala C, Middleton P, Crowther CA. Intrapartum interventions for preventing shoulder dystocia. *Cochrane Database Syst Rev*. 2006(4):CD005543. [Meta-analysis; 2 RCTs, n = 225]
39. Inglis SR, Feier N, Chetiyaar JB, et al. Effects of shoulder dystocia training on the incidence of brachial plexus injury. *Am J Obstet Gynecol*. 2011;204(4):322.e1–322.e6. [II-3]
40. Draycott TJ, Crofts JF, Ash JP, et al. Improving neonatal outcome through practical shoulder dystocia training. *Obstet Gynecol*. 2008;112(1):14–20. [II-3]
41. Royal College of Obstetricians and Gynaecologists. RCOG Green-top Guideline No. 42: Shoulder dystocia. 2005:1–13. [Guideline]
42. Gherman RB. Shoulder dystocia: Prevention and management. *Obstet Gynecol Clin N Am*. 2005;32(2):297–305, x. [Review]
43. Spain JE, Frey HA, Tuuli MG, et al. Neonatal morbidity associated with shoulder dystocia maneuvers. *Am J Obstet Gynecol*. 2015;212(3):353.e351–353.e355. [II-2]
44. Hoffman MK, Bailit JL, Branch DW, et al. A comparison of obstetric maneuvers for the acute management of shoulder dystocia. *Obstet Gynecol*. 2011;117(6):1272–1278. [II-1]
45. Sagi-Dain L, Sagi S. The role of episiotomy in prevention and management of shoulder dystocia: A systematic review. *Obstet Gynecol Surv*. 2015;70(5):354–362. [Review]
46. Cluver CA, Hofmeyr GJ. Posterior axilla sling traction for shoulder dystocia: Case review and a new method of shoulder rotation with the sling. *Am J Obstet Gynecol*. 2015;212(6):784.e781–784.e787. [II-3]
47. Grobman WA, Hornbogen A, Burke C, et al. Development and implementation of a team-centered shoulder dystocia protocol. *Simul Healthc*. 2010;5(4):199–203. [II-2]
48. Deering SH, Tobler K, Cypher R. Improvement in documentation using an electronic checklist for shoulder dystocia deliveries. *Obstet Gynecol*. 2010;116(1):63–66. [II-2]
49. Ramsey PS, Ramin KD, Field CS, et al. Shoulder dystocia. Rotation maneuvers revisited. *J Reprod Med*. 2000;45:85–88. [III]

Postpartum hemorrhage, retained placenta, and uterine inversion

Jennifer Salati and Jorge E. Tolosa

KEY POINTS
- The most common complications of the third stage of labor are postpartum hemorrhage (PPH), retained placenta, and uterine inversion. Timely diagnosis, adequate physical examination, intravenous (IV) access, anesthesia, adequate use of blood products, nursing support and team work are important for the management of third-stage complications.
- In cases of PPH, one should perform uterine massage, explore for and repair any vaginal or cervical lacerations, and manually explore the uterus.
- **Oxytocin** 20–80 international units (IU) in 500–1000 cc normal saline given as a fast IV infusion, or 10 IU intramuscular (IM), should be used as a primary uterotonic for PPH.
- **Methergine** (except in women with hypertension) and **prostaglandin F2α** (except in women with asthma) are beneficial in the treatment of PPH. **Misoprostol** is also helpful as an adjunctive treatment of primary PPH.
- There is insufficient evidence with randomized controlled trials (RCTs) to assess all other interventions for treatment of PPH.
- There is **insufficient evidence with RCTs to recommend pharmacologic agents for the treatment of retained placenta.**

POSTPARTUM HEMORRHAGE
Definitions
The American College of Obstetrics and Gynecology (ACOG) defines PPH as an estimated blood loss (EBL) of ≥500 mL for a vaginal delivery, or ≥1000 mL for a cesarean delivery. Primary PPH is defined as blood loss within 24 hours of delivery exceeding 500 cc for vaginal deliveries and 1000 cc for cesarean delivery. Secondary PPH is defined as excessive blood loss after 24 hours and <12 weeks postpartum. There is no single definition for PPH that has been agreed upon internationally, and multiple guidelines from various national and expert authorities exist (Table 26.1). Recent initiatives have focused on reassessing the existing PPH definitions in an effort to improve clinical management and outcomes [1,2].

Incidence
Approximately 5%–15% of deliveries are complicated by PPH.

Etiology
Common:
- Uterine atony—lack of efficient uterine contraction (most common, accounts for 80%)
- Retained placenta
- Genital tract trauma—vaginal, cervical, and vulvar

Less common:
- Uterine rupture
- Uterine inversion
- Consumptive coagulopathy
- Inherited or acquired bleeding disorders

Risk Factors
At term, the uteroplacental circulation has a blood supply of 600–800 cc/minute. The blood volume expansion of 1.5–2.0 L in pregnant women provides a physiologic reserve for blood loss at delivery. **Cessation of placental site blood flow is due mostly to effective myometrial contractions.** Most major hemorrhage occurs within the first hour postpartum. Risk factors that contribute to decreased myometrial contractions include the following:

- Maternal factors:
  - First pregnancy
  - Maternal obesity
  - Previous PPH—10% recurrence risk
  - High parity
  - Coagulopathy
  - Thrombocytopenia
- Antepartum bleeding—placenta previa, abruption
- Chorioamnionitis
- Uterine fibroids
- Overdistension—macrosomia, multiple gestation, polyhydramnios
- Uterine tocolytics—magnesium, nitroglycerin, anesthetic gas
- Labor factors:
  - Precipitous delivery
  - Prolonged labor—first stage >24 hours
  - Prolonged oxytocin use, and/or maximum of ≥40–50 cc/minute (prolonged labor)

Complications
The most reliable estimates of global **mortality** for mothers in childbirth are reported to be between 250,000 and 300,000 annually [3]. This number has decreased significantly over the past two decades. Many of these deaths result from complications of the third stage of labor [3]. Ninety-nine percent of maternal deaths occur in low and middle-income countries where maternal mortality remains unacceptably high. In sub-Saharan Africa, the risk of maternal death is very high at 1:31, with at least 25% of those deaths due to hemorrhage [4], while in high income countries a woman's lifetime risk of death during or following pregnancy is 1:4300. Secondary PPH is a significant contributor to maternal death mainly, but not only, in

Table 26.1 Definitions for Postpartum Hemorrhage

Guidelines	Postpartum Hemorrhage Definition
ACOG reVITALize Initiative (2014)	Blood loss ≥1000 mL or blood loss with sign/symptoms of hypovolemia in 24 hours after birth (includes intrapartum loss)
World Health Organization (2012)	Blood loss of ≥500 mL in 24 hours after birth Severe PPH-blood loss ≥1000 mL in 24 hours after birth
American College of Obstetricians and Gynecologists (2013)	Blood loss ≥500 mL following vaginal delivery or ≥1000 mL following cesarean delivery
Royal Australian and New Zealand College of Obstetricians and Gynaecologists (2014)	Blood loss ≥500 mL during puerperium Severe postpartum hemorrhage ≥1000 mL
Royal College of Obstetrician and Gynaecologists (2011)	Primary PPH-blood loss of 500–1000 mL in the absence of clinical signs of shock Major PPH-blood loss of ≥1000 mL
Society of Obstetricians and Gynaecologists of Canada (2009)	Any amount of bleeding threatening hemodynamic instability

Abbreviations: ACOG, American College of Obstetricians and Gynecologists; PPH, postpartum hemmorhage.

low income countries. PPH has other serious complications including **hypovolemic shock, disseminated intravascular coagulopathy (DIC), renal failure, hepatic failure, and adult respiratory distress syndrome (ARDS).**

Diagnosis

Regardless of the PPH definition being utilized, the appropriate management of PPH relies upon the clinician's assessment of risk for PPH (Table 26.2) and timely recognition of excessive blood loss. However, the assessment of peripartum blood loss has **classically been determined by a provider's subjective visual estimation of blood loss.** Visual EBL has consistently been shown to result in underestimation of large volume blood loss (>1000 mL) by up to 30%–50%, and overestimation of small volume of blood loss [5,6]. These types of EBL errors have been shown to occur similarly among providers at all levels of training [6]. Formal training in visual blood loss estimation improves accuracy for a period of time, but skills tend to decline after several months [7].

Some obstetric centers have adopted **gravimetric methods for quantifying blood loss,** including **weighing of pads and sponges,** and the use of **calibrated under-buttock drapes.** One study demonstrated that visual assessment of blood loss underestimated that calculated by weighing of pads and sponges by approximately 30% [8]. Another RCT showed that in a simulated environment, **visual blood loss estimation using noncalibrated drapes resulted in underestimation by 15%–40%** (greater error with larger volumes), whereas **use of calibrated drapes resulted in <15% error at all volumes** [9].

Blood loss calculators can be utilized by care teams to facilitate accurate quantification of blood loss after both cesarean and vaginal deliveries. Examples of calculation tools that can be integrated into an electronic medical record system can be found through the California Maternal Quality Care Collaborative (CMQCC) website (www.cmqcc.org/resources-tool-kits/toolkits/ob-hemorrhage-toolkit) and obstetrics (OB) hemorrhage toolkit resources.

Management

Primary PPH. The management of PPH begins with **diagnosis** of PPH and obtaining **help in a multidisciplinary fashion,** including obstetricians, nurses (including charge nurse), anesthesia, and the blood bank (Figure 26.1). The early identification of risk factors is the first step to facilitating increased surveillance, adequate preparation and a more rapid response

Table 26.2 Example of Stratification System by Maternal Risk Factors for PPH

PPH Risk	Risk Factors	Preparation
Low	No previous CD Singleton pregnancy Three prior VD No bleeding disorder No prior PPH	Clot only or type and screen
Medium	Prior CD Multiple gestation ≥4 prior VD Chorioamnionitis Polyhydramnios Macrosomia Abruption Prolonged labor (>24 hours) Prior PPH Large uterine fibroids	Type and screen or type and cross-match
High	Placenta previa Suspected placenta accrete Coagulopathy Platelets <50,000 Multiple risk factors (see above)	Type and cross-match Consider alerting blood bank

Source: Modified from California Maternal Quality Care Collaborative, OB Hemorrhage Toolkit, 2015, available at https://www.cmqcc.org/resources-tool-kits/toolkits/ob-hemorrhage-toolkit. Accessed on November 3, 2015.
Abbreviations: CD, cesarean delivery; VD, vaginal delivery.

to hemorrhage if it does occur (Table 26.2). Risk factors should be evaluated in the prenatal period, and reassessed throughout the intrapartum and postpartum course.

A common accepted approach to the treatment of primary PPH includes:
Logistics:

- Obtain help
- Ensure adequate access with large bore IV (may need two sites)
- Monitor vital signs serially
- Consider placing Foley catheter to empty bladder and monitor urine output
- Obtain laboratory tests—complete blood count with platelets, blood type, antibody screen, fibrinogen, fibrin split products, prothrombin time, and partial prothrombin time

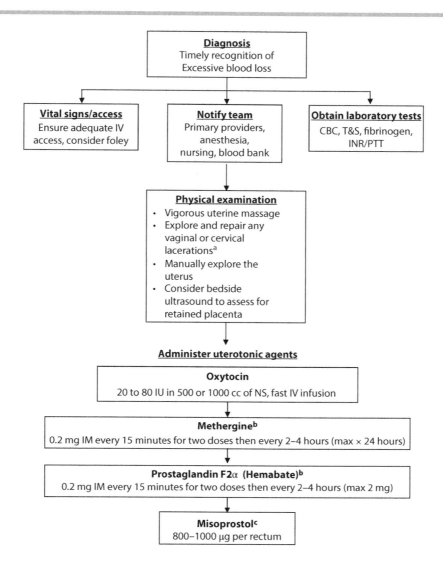

Figure 26.1 Suggested management protocol for primary postpartum hemorrhage. *Notes:* CBC, complete blood count; IM, intramuscular; INR/PTT, international normalized ratio/partial thromboplastin time; IU, international units; IV, intravenous; T&S, type and screen. [a]Consider transfer to operating room for complicated vaginal repairs or any cervical laceration requiring repair. [b]Consider contraindications to methergine (hypertension) and prostagladin F2α (asthma). [c]Can be considered first-line in resource poor settings, no IV access or if contraindications to other medications, and also as an adjunct to first-line oxytocin in high risk cases.

Treatment:

- Vigorous uterine massage until firm
- Explore and repair any vaginal or cervical lacerations
- Manually explore the uterus
- Administer uterotonic drugs
  - Oxytocin 20–80 IU in 500 or 1000 cc of normal saline, fast IV infusion or 10 IU IM
  - Methergine 0.2 mg IM every 15 minutes for two doses, then every 2–4 hours—consider contraindications including hypertension
  - Prostaglandin F2α (carboprost tromethamine, Hemabate) 0.25 mg IM every 15–90 minutes up to eight doses (maximum 2 mg)—consider contraindications including asthma
  - Misoprostol 800–1000 μg per rectum (side effects chills, fever)

Little evidence exists on which to base a protocol **with respect to the order of administration of uterotonics for the treatment of PPH** following vaginal delivery. It is also important to note that the literature on management of intraoperative and postpartum hemorrhage at the time of cesarean section is limited compared with vaginal delivery. Findings have been generalized to cesarean deliveries based on the assumption that they are likely to be beneficial.

Traditionally, oxytocin and ergot alkaloids (e.g., methergine) are used as first-line agents, due to their pharmacokinetic profile and speed of action, with prostaglandin F2α and misoprostol employed as adjunctive therapies. There are few high-quality RCTs directly comparing oxytocin, ergot alkaloids, and prostaglandin F2α, to either placebo or to each other for treatment of PPH. Based on a recent systematic analysis, the addition of misoprostol to conventional injectable uterotonics conferred no added benefit with an increase in side effects [10]. Compared with oxytocin, misoprostol is less effective in primary treatment of PPH. Studies comparing misoprostol to ergot alkaloids have demonstrated conflicting results and the studies are small and heterogeneous.

Thus, there is no compelling evidence to suggest an alteration in uterotonic management at this time. However, it is important to note that **in certain circumstances, rectal misoprostol may be a useful "first-line" therapy for the treatment of PPH.** It may be a more appropriate *first-line agent in the setting of no IV access, patients with contraindications to other uterotonics, or in resource-poor settings.*

Other possible treatments include:

- Uterine curettage if retained placental products cannot be removed manually
- Transfusion of blood and blood products as necessary (Table 26.3)
- Hemostatic drugs
  - Factor VIIa—A single RCT demonstrated that recombinant human FVIIa may reduce the need for surgical intervention for severe PPH that has failed medical management [11]. This RCT was small and not placebo-controlled or blinded. Thus, larger blinded and placebo-controlled trials are needed to assess efficacy and safety
  - Tranexamic acid—Evidence for the use of tranexamic acid for treatment of PPH is limited and mixed. One randomized, open-label trial demonstrated decreased blood loss and morbidity associated with high-dose tranexamic acid [12]. Another historically controlled study did not demonstrate benefit [13]. Neither of these studies was large enough to assess effect on mortality, need for hysterectomy or safety
- If stable, consider pelvic arterial embolization done by interventional radiology (IR)
- If unstable (there are **no high-quality RCTs** investigating the following techniques)
  - Uterine tamponade—gauze packing, Bakri tamponade balloon catheter, or Foley catheter
  - Consider massive transfusion protocol (see Figure 26.2)
  - Laparotomy—uterine artery ligation, B-Lynch or square suture for compression, internal iliac artery ligation
  - Bimanual uterine compression
  - Aortic compression (temporary) and pelvic packing
  - Hysterectomy
  - Nonpneumatic antishock garment (NASG) is a neoprene compression suit fastened around the body to reduce bleeding and reverse shock, to be used as a hemodynamic temporizing measure during transfer to a higher level treatment facility

Secondary PPH There is insufficient evidence to make recommendations for management of secondary PPH [14]. Management similar to that for PPH is suggested, with high suspicion for retained placenta.

RETAINED PLACENTA
Definition
Placenta undelivered ≥30 minutes after infant delivery.

Incidence
Between **0.5% and 3%**.

Complications
Hemorrhage, infection, and genital tract trauma.

Etiology
- Preterm birth—inversely proportional to gestational age.
- Cord avulsion—incidence up to 3% with controlled cord traction, especially by inexperienced operators.
- Placenta accreta (see Chapter 28).

Management
- Obtain adequate anesthesia
- Attempt manual placental extraction
  - One hand is placed over the abdomen to stabilize the uterine fundus, while the other hand is placed through the cervix into the uterus. The placenta is gently separated from the uterus starting at the superior placental edge. If possible, the placenta should be removed intact
- Consider ultrasound to ascertain all placental tissue has been removed
  - The ultrasonographic appearance of the uterus immediately following delivery is variable. **The sensitivity and positive predictive value of ultrasound for the detection of retained products of conception relatively low** (44% and 58%, respectively). The specificity and negative predictive value are better (92% and 87%, respectively) [15]
- Palpate and massage the fundus until firm
- Proceed to operating room for curettage **under ultrasound guidance** if unsuccessful extraction or excessive bleeding
- Consider diagnosis of placenta accreta

Pharmacologic Agents
In the past, pharmacologic interventions have been used in the management of retained placenta. The rationale was that stimulating uterine contractions with oxytocin or prostaglandins, or cervical relaxation with nitroglycerin, would facilitate spontaneous placental delivery and avoid further invasive interventions. However, a recent systematic analysis incorporating 16 RCTs and 1683 patients identified **no differences in the need for manual placental extraction with oxytocin (intraumbilical), prostaglandins** (e.g., F2α, E2, or misoprostol) *or* **nitroglycerin** [16]. The greatest number of

Table 26.3 Blood Products

Product	Volume (mL)	Contents	Effect (Per Unit)
Packed red blood cells	250–400	RBC, WBC, plasma	Increase Hgb by 1g/dL or Hct by 3%
Platelets	50	Platelets, RBC, WBC, plasma	Increase platelet count by 5,000–10,000 mm^3
Fresh frozen plasma	200–250	Fibrinogen, Antithrombin III, clotting factors, plasma	Increase fibrinogen by 5–10 mg/dL
Cryoprecipitate	20–40	Fibrinogen, factor VIII, vWF, factor XIII	Increase fibrinogen by 5–10 mg/dL

Abbreviations: Hct, hematocrit; Hgb, hemoglobin; RBC, red blood cells; WBC, white blood cells; vWF, Von Willebrand factor.

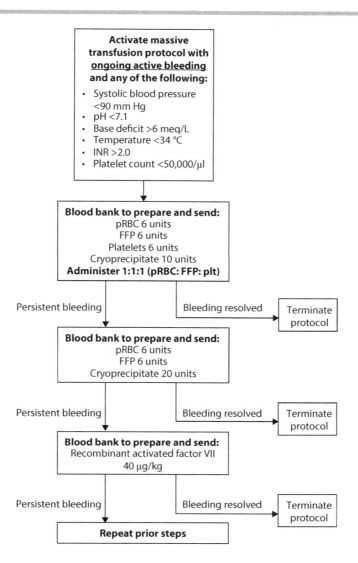

Figure 26.2 Suggested massive transfusion protocol. FFP, fresh frozen plasma; pRBC, packed red blood cells.

studies [10] investigated intraumbilical administration of oxytocin. They concluded that there is **no evidence supporting the use of intraumbilical oxytocin for retained placenta,** and that there has not been adequate evaluation of other pharmacologic interventions by RCT. Therefore, there is **insufficient evidence to recommend pharmacologic agents for the treatment of retained placenta.**

Antibiotics
There is **insufficient evidence** to assess the effects of prophylactic use of antibiotics following manual removal of the placenta [17]. The World Health Organization (WHO) recommends single-dose penicillin or first-generation cephalosporin based on one retrospective study [18,19].

UTERINE INVERSION
Definition
The collapse of the uterine fundus into the uterine cavity.

Incidence
Approximately 1 in 2500 deliveries.

Risk Factors
- Excessive umbilical cord traction
- Fundal pressure
- Fundal cord insertions
- Abnormal placentation

Management
There are no randomized trials to determine the optimal management for uterine inversion. Suggested management may include the following:

- Obtain assistance from other obstetricians or experienced providers and nursing staff
- Obtain adequate anesthesia
- Consider immediate transfer to the operating room
- Obtain large bore IV access
- IV fluid therapy
- If placenta has not yet delivered, avoid separation to reduce bleeding
- **Consider uterine relaxing agents**
  - Nitroglycerin 50–500 mg orally or inhaled per anesthesia—usually preferred as first line

- Magnesium sulfate 4–6 grams IV bolus
- Terbutaline IV 0.25 subcutaneously (SQ)
- **Manual manipulation of the uterus**
  - Manually reduce the uterine fundus by placing the hand through the cervix into the uterine cavity and applying gentle pressure to the inverted fundus. Cup the uterus in palm with fingers posteriorly and thumb anteriorly (no use of fist).
  - Once the fundus has been manually replaced, administer uterotonic therapy (oxytocin) followed by methergine to maintain uterine tone and prevent reinversion.
- **Surgical intervention—laparotomy (rarely needed)**
  - Huntington procedure—clamps are placed on the round ligaments 2 cm deep in the inversion and gentle upward traction applied. Repeat clamping as necessary.
  - Haultain procedure—vertical incision is made in the posterior portion of the inversion ring to increase its size and to reposition the uterus.
  - Uterotonic agents when uterus repositioned.
- If present, treat PPH or retained placenta as described above.

REFERENCES

1. Menard MK, Main EK, Currigan SM. Executive summary of the reVITALize initiative: Standardizing obstetric data definitions. *Obstet Gynecol*. 2014;124(1):150–153. [III]
2. Abdul-Kadir R, McLintock C, Ducloy AS, et al. Evaluation and management of postpartum hemorrhage: Consensus from an international expert panel. *Transfusion*. 2014;54: 1756–1768. [III]
3. Lozano R, Wang H, Foreman K, et al. Progress towards Millennium Development Goals 4 and 5 on maternal and child mortality: An updated systemic analysis. *Lancet*. 2011;378(9797):1139–1165. [II–1]
4. Hogan MC, Foreman KJ, Naghavi M. Maternal mortality of 181 countries, 1980-2008: A systemic analysis of progress towards Millennium Development Goals 5. *Lancet*. 2010;375(9726):1609–1623. [Review]
5. Stafford I, Dildy G, Clark S, Belfort M. Visually estimated and calculated blood loss in vaginal and cesarean delivery. *Am J Obstet Gynecol*. 2008;199(5):519.e1–519.e7. [II-3]
6. Dildy GA, Paine AR, George NC, Velasco C. Estimating blood loss: Can teaching significantly improve visual estimation? *Obstet Gynecol*. 2004;104(3):601–606. [II-3]
7. Toledo P, Eosakul ST, Goetz K, et al. Decay in blood loss estimation skills after web-based didactic training. *Simul Health*. 2012;7(1):18–21. [II-3]
8. Al Kadri HM, Anazi BK, Tamim HM. Visual estimation versus gravimetric measurement of postpartum blood loss: A prospective cohort study. *Arch Gynecol Obstet*. 2011;283(6):1207–1213. [II-2]
9. Toledo P, McCarthy RJ, Hewlett BJ, et al. The accuracy of blood loss estimation after simulated vaginal delivery. *Anesth Analg*. 2007;105(6):1736–1740. [II-1]
10. Mousa HA, Alfirevic Z. Treatment for primary postpartum haemorrhage. *Cochrane Database Syst Rev*. 2014;(1):CD003249. [Meta-analysis: 14 RCTs, $n = 4052$] [I]
11. Lavigne-Lissalde G, Aya AG, Mercier FJ, et al. Recombinant human FVIIa for reducing the need of invasive second-line therapies in severe refractory postpartum hemorrhage: A multicenter, randomized, open controlled trial. *J Thromb Haemost*. 2015;13:520–529. [RCT, $n = 84$] [I]
12. Ducloy-Bouthors AS, Duhamel JB, Broisin F, et al. High-dose tranexamic acid reduces blood loss in postpartum hemorrhage. *Crit Care*. 2011;15(2):R117. [RCT, $n = 144$] [I]
13. Bouet PE, Ruiz V, Legendre G, et al. High-dose tranexamic acid for treatment postpartum hemorrhage after vaginal delivery. *Br. J. Anaesth*. 2015;144(2):339–341. [II-1]
14. Alexander J, Thomas PW, Sanghera J. Treatments for secondary postpartum haemorrhage. *Cochrane Database Syst Rev*. 2002;(1):CD002867. [Meta-analysis: no RCTs]
15. Carlan SJ, Scott WT, Pollack R, Harris K. Appearance of the uterus by ultrasound immediately after placental delivery with pathologic correlation. *J Clin Ultrasound*. 1997;25(6):301–308.
16. Duffy JM, Mylan S, Showell M, et al. Pharmacologic intervention for retained placenta. *Obstet Gynecol*. 2015;(125):711–718. [Meta-analysis: 16 RCTs, $n = 1683$] [I]
17. Chongsomchai C, Lumbiganon P, Laopaiboon M. Prophylactic antibiotics for manual removal of retained placenta in vaginal birth. *Cochrane Database Syst Rev*. 2014;(10):CD004904. [Meta-analysis: 0 RCTs]. [I]
18. World Health Organization (WHO). *WHO Guidelines for the Management of Postpartum Haemorrhage and Retained Placenta*. France: WHO, 2009. [Review]
19. Criscuolo JL, Kibler MP, Micholet S, et al. The value of antibiotic prophylaxis during intrauterine procedures during vaginal delivery. A comparative study of 500 patients. *J Gynecol Obstet Biol Reprod*. 1990;19(7):909–918. [RCT, $n = 500$] [I]

Late-term and postterm pregnancies

Rebecca Jackson

KEY POINTS
- **Postterm pregnancy** is defined as a pregnancy that has lasted until ≥42 weeks, or ≥294 days.
- **Late-term pregnancy** is defined as a pregnancy that has lasted **41 0/7–41 6/7 weeks of gestation**.
- Late-term and postterm pregnancies have twofold increase in risk of macrosomia, and subsequent increase in labor dystocia, operative vaginal delivery, cesarean delivery, perineal injury, and shoulder dystocia.
- Postterm neonates are at increased risk for seizures, meconium aspiration, 5-minute Apgar scores less than 4, and admission to neonatal intensive care unit. Postterm pregnancies are also at increased risk for intrauterine infection, oligohydramnios, nonreassuring fetal heart testing (NRFHT), low umbilical artery pH, and perinatal mortality.
- **Pregnancies with risk factors** such as maternal (e.g., hypertension and diabetes) and fetal (growth restriction) diseases should be delivered at term or as described in the **pertinent guidelines**.
- **Prevention** of postterm pregnancy can be achieved with accurate dating by **routine first-trimester ultrasound** and with serial membrane stripping starting at 38 weeks.
- There is insufficient evidence to assess the efficacy of antepartum testing for pregnancies after their due date. Twice-weekly fetal testing with nonstress test (NST), or NST and maximum vertical pocket (MVP) of amniotic fluid volume (AFV), or biophysical profile (BPP), has been proposed, starting at 41 weeks.
- Routine **induction of labor at ≥41 weeks reduces perinatal mortality, due to a decrease in fetal and neonatal deaths.** Routine induction of labor in this setting is also associated with a **significant 11% decrease in the incidence of cesarean delivery,** and a significant 50% decrease in meconium aspiration syndrome. **Therefore, pregnancies reaching 41 weeks should be recommended induction at 41 0/7–41 6/7 weeks, unless contraindications for induction exist and/or a cesarean is indicated.**
- In women with a prior cesarean delivery, induction of labor is associated with an increase in uterine rupture in comparison to an unscarred uterus and in comparison to spontaneous labor. Nonetheless, induction of labor after appropriate counseling is feasible (e.g., with balloon catheter) in pregnancies ≥41 weeks with a prior cesarean.

DIAGNOSIS/DEFINITION
Postterm pregnancy is defined as pregnancy that has lasted until **≥42 weeks**, or ≥294 days, or ≥14 days after the due date (estimated date of confinement [EDC]) [1]. **Late-term pregnancy** can be defined as a pregnancy that has lasted until **≥41 weeks**, or ≥287 days, or ≥7 days after the due date (EDC) [1]. The term "postdates" can signify a pregnancy that lasted until ≥40 weeks, or ≥280 days, but is often defined differently in the literature and should be avoided [1]. All these definitions may have slightly different meanings in the literature, so it is important to be clear when using these terms. These definitions and this guideline pertain to *singleton gestations*. For multiple gestations, please refer to Chapter 44 in *Maternal-Fetal Evidence Based Guidelines*.

EPIDEMIOLOGY/INCIDENCE
In 2014, in the United States, the **incidence** of late-term pregnancy was 6.31% and of postterm pregnancy was 0.41% [2]. These incidences have significantly decreased in the last few years.

ETIOLOGY/BASIC PATHOPHYSIOLOGY
The most frequent cause of postterm pregnancy is an **error in dating** [1,3]. See Chapter 4 for accurate dating criteria and their benefits, as well as the following sections.

RISK FACTORS/ASSOCIATIONS
Poor (wrong) dating; prior postterm pregnancy; obesity; nulliparity; long (>28 days) cycles without early ultrasound; placental sulfatase deficiency; anencephaly; and male fetus. Obesity appears to be one preconceptionally modifiable risk factor for postterm pregnancy [4].

COMPLICATIONS
Perinatal
Many epidemiological studies have shown that fetal and neonatal complications increase with gestational age after 41 weeks. **Meconium aspiration, intrauterine infection, oligohydramnios, macrosomia, NRFHT, low umbilical artery pH, and low 5-minute Apgar score** have all been associated with postterm pregnancy. **Perinatal mortality** (fetal and neonatal deaths) is twice as high at ≥42 weeks and six times as high at ≥43 weeks compared with the rate for pregnancies delivered between 39 and 40 weeks [1,5].

Two markers of **immediate neonatal morbidity**, umbilical artery pH <7 and base excess ≥12, have been shown to increase in a continuous manner in pregnancies beyond 40 weeks, and increase by odds ratio (OR) 1.65 for pH <7 for pregnancies between 41 and 42 weeks [6].

Neonatal mortality of normal-weight infants appears to be higher for infants born between 41 and 0 days and 41 weeks and 6 days compared with infants born between 38 weeks and 40 weeks and 6 days (OR 1.37, 95% confidence interval [CI] 1.08–1.73) [7].

These data are, however, mixed and may vary based on whether risk factors such as intrauterine growth restriction (IUGR) are included in the analysis. In a review of epidemiological studies published between 1990–2004, 7 out of 11 studies demonstrated an increased stillbirth risk with postterm pregnancies and four suggested that other issues such as IUGR or fetal anomalies had a greater contribution to the stillbirth rate than did prolonged pregnancy [8].

Postmaturity syndrome is present in about 10%–20% of neonates born postterm. These fetuses have decreased subcutaneous fat and lack of vernix and lanugo. Postmature neonates are also more likely to have meconium staining of the amniotic fluid, skin, membranes and umbilical cord. [1].

Maternal

Women giving birth late-term and postterm are at increased risk of **perineal injury, infection, postpartum hemorrhage, and cesarean delivery** [1].

PREGNANCY CONSIDERATIONS

Every woman should be counseled early in pregnancy that up to 50% of gestations, especially in nulliparous women, last until past the due date. This is physiologic and natural for humans. The incidence of fetal death is significantly higher than that of neonatal death at ≥283 days (≥40 weeks and 3 days) [9]. In large series, delivery at 38 weeks is associated with the lowest risk of perinatal death, but this risk is low at <1 to 2/1000 up to 41 weeks and 6 days [10]. **It is important to identify maternal (e.g., hypertension and diabetes) and fetal (e.g., growth restriction) risk factors that would necessitate special management,** as described in the specific chapters in *Maternal-Fetal Evidence Based Guidelines*. The OR for stillbirths and neonatal mortality increases in gestations from 40 weeks onward, and this increase is compounded 7- to 10-fold when the fetus is growth restricted [11].

MANAGEMENT (FIGURE 27.1)
Preconception Counseling

Women with prior postterm pregnancy are at increased risk for recurrent postterm pregnancy. Prevention strategies including weight loss for obese women, appropriate weight gain during the pregnancy, early initiation of prenatal care, and early ultrasound screening should be discussed [3].

Prevention

Routine Early Ultrasound to Reduce Postterm Pregnancies

Accurate assessment of gestational age is extremely important in improving perinatal morbidity and mortality. **First-trimester ultrasound** is the most accurate for pregnancy dating. Early ultrasound also reduces the number of postterm inductions.

Over 40% of women randomized to undergo first-trimester screening had their gestational age adjusted based on the ultrasound measurement of crown–rump length, whereas the corresponding number was only 10.9% for women assigned to second-trimester ultrasound. Furthermore, 4.8% in the first-trimester screening group compared with 13% in the second-trimester ultrasound group had labor induced for a postterm pregnancy (relative risk [RR] 0.37, 95% CI 0.14–0.96), which is a **63% reduction in the induction rate for postterm pregnancy** [11,12]. Compared with no routine early ultrasound, **routine early pregnancy (<20 weeks) ultrasound reduces by 32%–39% the incidence of postterm pregnancy and of induction for postterm pregnancy** [4,12,13] (see also Chapter 4).

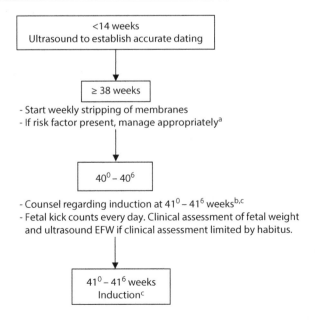

Figure 27.1 Management of late-term pregnancy. *Notes:* 2x/week, twice per week; AFV, amniotic fluid volume; EFW, estimated fetal weight; FGR, fetal growth restriction; NST, nonstress test. [a]Risk factor examples include hypertension, diabetes mellitus, FGR, multiple gestation, etc. Please see guideline pertinent to specific risk factor for management. [b]Suggest induction for all women between 41^0 and 41^6 weeks. [c]See Chapter 21 for effective induction management.

Stripping/Sweeping of Membranes
Compared with no sweeping, **sweeping of the membranes,** performed weekly as a general policy in women at term (e.g., **weekly starting at 38 weeks), is associated with reduced duration of pregnancy** and reduced frequency of pregnancy continuing beyond 41 and 42 weeks [14,15]. To avoid one formal induction of labor, sweeping of membranes must be performed in eight women. **Risk of cesarean section, maternal, or neonatal infection is similar. Serial sweeping of membranes starting at 41 weeks every 48 hours also decreases the risk of postterm pregnancy** from 41% to 23%, with efficacy both in nulliparous and multiparous women [16]. Discomfort during vaginal examination and other adverse effects (bleeding and irregular contractions) are more frequently reported by women allocated to sweeping, but its safety has been confirmed in multiple studies [14–17] (see also Chapter 20).

Breast and Nipple Stimulation to Reduce Postterm Pregnancies
Breast and nipple stimulation daily starting at 39 weeks has not been sufficiently studied to ascertain safety, but it does appear to reduce the incidence of postterm pregnancy by 48% [18,19].

Antepartum Testing
There are insufficient data to assess the best mode of fetal monitoring after the due date, as there are **no trials** to assess the effect of antepartum testing on these pregnancies compared with no testing. Since fetal death rates incrementally increase after the due date, it seems reasonable to test fetuses to assure well-being, especially at ≥41 weeks [1,4,9]. The most used options include NST (also called cardiotocography or CTG), BPP, and modified BPP. Modified BPP includes NST and ultrasound measurement of MVP of AFV. Others have been described, with even less evidence for efficacy. Doppler of any vessel, including the umbilical artery, is not effective in the management of postterm pregnancy. Compared with fetal monitoring using NST and AFV, BPP (computerized cardiotocography, MVP, fetal breathing, fetal tone, and fetal body movements) is associated with increased incidence of inductions and similar outcomes in a small trial in women ≥42 weeks [20]. At ≥41 weeks, **twice-weekly testing** (e.g., with NST and MVP) is recommended [1], but not based on trials (see also Chapter 56 in *Maternal-Fetal Evidence Based Guidelines*). In addition, an effort should be made to **assess fetal weight**, either clinically or, if this assessment is limited, by ultrasound, as the known increase in fetal and neonatal mortality in pregnancies beyond their due date is even higher in IUGR fetuses [11,21].

Interventions
Routine Induction of Labor at ≥41 Weeks
A policy of **labor induction at 41 completed weeks (41–41 6/7) or beyond is associated with significantly fewer perinatal deaths** (1/2814 vs. 9/2785; RR 0.30, 95% CI 0.09–0.99) compared with expectant management, with induction not before 42 weeks [21]. If deaths due to congenital abnormality are excluded, no deaths remain in the labor induction group and eleven deaths remain in the no induction group. There were *fewer cesarean sections* in the induction group (RR 0.89, 95% CI 0.81–0.97). **Labor induction at 41 weeks also significantly reduces the risk of perinatal meconium aspiration syndrome** compared with expectant management (RR 0.50, 95% CI 0.34–0.73). Other maternal and perinatal outcomes are similar between the groups. It is important to recognize, however, that in general the outcomes are very good with both expectant management and induction, with the absolute perinatal death rate/1000 ongoing pregnancies no higher than 1.2/1000 at 42 weeks, increasing up to 6/1000 ongoing pregnancies at 43 weeks [22]. About 410 inductions (95% CI 322–1492) would need to be done at 41 weeks in order to prevent one perinatal death [21].

Routine induction is more cost-effective than expectant management [23]. Several studies have shown that **patient satisfaction is higher with induction of labor** [21–23]. Iatrogenic prematurity should be avoided by careful assessment of gestational age. This risk should be minimal with the advent of widespread early ultrasound use to confirm pregnancy dating. Even planned induction without medical indications at 39 0/7–40 6/7 weeks has been shown not to be associated with an increase with cesarean delivery. [24] See also Chapter 21 for other induction risks and benefits, as well as management of induction.

Women with a favorable cervix. No trials have focused on or included in sufficient numbers pregnancies ≥41 weeks with a favorable cervix (i.e., Bishop score ≥9 or transvaginal ultrasound cervical length [TVU CL] <15 mm). As the complications of induction, particularly a failed induction and unnecessary subsequent cesarean section, are low in women with a favorable cervix, and there appears to be a trend toward decreased perinatal deaths and a statistically significant reduction in meconium aspiration, it seems reasonable to also **recommend induction at 41 0/7–41 6/7 weeks** (41 and 0/7 days) for these women [21,23].

Women with an unfavorable cervix. Cervical ripening is recommended for women with unfavorable cervix prior to labor induction. **If cervical ripening is used, there is no difference in the incidence of cesarean** section in women who were induced or expectantly managed [1,23,25,26]. A discussion about induction of labor after 41 weeks versus expectant management should occur with the patient, and management should include consideration for patient preference and access to antenatal testing (see also Chapter 21). Induction should absolutely be recommended for all patients before 42 0/7 weeks. One hundred and ninety-five inductions would prevent one perinatal death in this group [27].

Women with a prior cesarean delivery. In women with a prior cesarean delivery, induction is associated with a higher incidence of uterine rupture, especially in the nulliparous woman with an unfavorable cervix. The rate of uterine rupture is about 0.4%–0.5% for spontaneous labor, 0.8% for labor induced without prostaglandins, and 2.2% for prostaglandin induced labor [28]. Prostaglandins should, in general, not be used for cervical ripening in a woman with a prior cesarean section. If the woman desires vaginal birth after cesarean (VBAC), it seems reasonable to wait until 40–41 weeks for spontaneous labor. There are insufficient data to assess the risks of trial of labor after cesarean section in a postterm gestation, but if the cervix is favorable, induction can be performed after through discussion of the risks and benefits. **If the cervix is unfavorable, the patient should be apprised of the higher risks of uterine rupture, as well as the risks of a failed induction with an unfavorable cervix. A repeat cesarean section can be offered to decrease these risks** [1,29] (see also Chapter 14).

REFERENCES
1. American College of Obstetricians and Gynecologists. ACOG Practice Bulletin No. 146: Management of late-term and postterm pregnancies. *Obstet Gynecol.* 2014;124(2 Pt1):390–396. [Review].
2. Hamiton BE, Martin JA, Osterman MJ, et al. Births: Preliminary data for 2014. *Natl Vital Stat Rep.* 2015;64(6):1–19. [Epidemiologic data]

3. Neilson JP. Ultrasound for fetal assessment in early pregnancy. *Cochrane Database Syst Rev.* 2005;(3). [Meta-analysis: 9 RCTs, $n = >24,000$]
4. Caughey AB, Stotland NE, Washington AE, et al. Who is at risk for prolonged and postterm pregnancy? *Am J Obstet Gynecol.* 2009;200:683.e1–683.e5. [II–3, $n = 119,162$]
5. Myers ER, Blumrick R, Christian Al. *Management of Prolonged Pregnancy.* Rockville, MD: Agency for Healthcare Research and Quality, 2002. [Review]
6. Caughey AB, Washington AE, Laros RK. Neonatal complications of term pregnancy: Rates by gestational age increase in a continuous, not threshold, fashion. *Am J Obstet Gynecol.* 2005;192:185–190. [II–3, $n = 32,679$]
7. Bruckner TA, Cheng YW, Caughey AB. Increased neonatal mortality among normal-weight births beyond 41 weeks of gestation in California. *Am J Obstet Gynecol.* 2008;199:421.e1–421.e7. [II–3, $n = 1,815,811$]
8. Mandruzzato G, Alfirevic Z, Chervenak F, et al. World Association of Perinatal Medicine. Guidelines for the management of postterm pregnancy. *J Perinatal Med.* 2010;38:111–119. [Meta- analysis]
9. Divon MY, Ferber A, Sanderson M, et al. A functional definition of prolonged pregnancy based on daily fetal and neonatal mortality rates. *Ultrasound Obstet Gynecol.* 2004;23:423–426. [II–2, $n = 656,134$]
10. Smith GCS. Life-table analysis of the risk of perinatal death at term and post term in singleton pregnancies. *Am J Obstet Gynecol.* 2001;184:489–496. [II–2, $n = 700,878$]
11. Divon M, Haglund B, Nisell H. Fetal and neonatal mortality in the postterm pregnancy: The impact of gestational age and fetal growth restriction. *Am J Obstet Gynecol.* 1998;178:726–731. [II–2, $n = 181,524$]
12. Crowley, P. Interventions for preventing or improving the outcome of delivery at or beyond term. *Cochrane Database Syst Rev.* 2005; (4):CD000331. [Meta-analysis: 26 RCTs (variable quality), $n = >25,000$; early ultrasound: 4 RCTs, $n = 21,776$; induction at ≥41 weeks: 19 RCTs, $n = 7925$]
13. Bennett K, Crane J, O'shea P, et al. First trimester ultrasound screening is effective in reducing postterm labor induction rates: A randomized controlled trial. *Am J Obstet Gynecol.* 2003;190:1077–1081. [RCT, $n = 218$]
14. Berghella V, Rogers RA, Lescale K. Stripping of membranes as a safe method to reduce prolonged pregnancies. *Obstet Gynecol.* 1996;87(6):927–929. [RCT, $n = 142$]
15. Boulvain M, Stan C, Irion O. Membrane sweeping for induction of labour. *Cochrane Database Syst Rev.* 2005;(4):CD000451. [Meta-analysis: 22 RCTs, $n = 2797$]
16. de Miranda E, van der Bom JG, Bonsel GJ, et al. Membrane sweeping and prevention of post-term pregnancy in low-risk pregnancies: A randomized controlled trial. *Br J Obstet Gynecol.* 2006;113:402–408. [RCT, $n = 742$]
17. Kashanian M, Akbarian A, Baradaran H, et al. Effect of membrane sweeping at term pregnancy on duration of pregnancy and labor induction: A randomized trial. *Gynecol Obstet Invest.* 2006;62:41–44. [RCT, $n = 122$]
18. Elliott JP, Flaherty JF. The use of breast stimulation to prevent postdate pregnancy. *Am J Obstet Gynecol.* 1984;149:628–632. [RCT]
19. Kadar N, Tapp A, Wong A. The influence of nipple stimulation at term on the duration of pregnancy. *J Perinatol.* 1990;10:164–166. [RCT]
20. Alfirevic Z, Walkinshaw SA. A randomized controlled trial of simple compared with complex antenatal fetal monitoring after 42 weeks of gestation. *Br J Obstet Gynaecol.* 1995;102:638–643. [RCT]
21. Gulmezoglu AM, Crowther CA, Middleton P. Induction of labour for improving birth outcomes for women at or beyond term. *Cochrane Database Syst Rev.* 2012;(6):CD004945. [Meta-analysis: 22 RCTs, $n = 9383$]
22. Heimstad R, Romundstad PR, Hyett J, et al. Women's experiences and attitudes towards expectant management and induction of labor for post-term pregnancy. *Acta Obstet Gynecol Scand.* 2007;86:950–956. [RCT]
23. Hannah ME, Hannah WJ, Hellman J, et al. Canadian Multicenter Post-Term Pregnancy Trial Group. Induction of labour as compared with serial antenatal monitoring in post-term pregnancy. A randomized controlled trial. *N Engl J Med.* 1992;326:1587–1592. [RCT, $n = 3407$]
24. Saccone G, Berghella V. Induction of labor at full term in uncomplicated singleton gestations: A systematic review and meta-analysis of randomized controlled trials. *Am J Obstet Gynecol.* 2015;213(5):629–636. doi:10.1016/j.ajog.2015.04.004. [Meta-analysis of RCTs]
25. Wennerholm U, Hagberg H, Brorsson B, et al. Induction of labor versus expectant management for post-date pregnancy: Is there sufficient evidence for a change in clinical practice? *Acta Obstet Gynecol.* 2009;88:6–17. [Meta-analysis: 14 RCTs, 3 systematic reviews, $n = 6617$]
26. Heimstad R, Skogvall E, Mattsson L, et al. Induction of labor and serial antenatal fetal monitoring in postterm pregnancy. A randomized controlled trial. *Obstet Gynecol.* 2007;109:609–617. [RCT, $n = 508$]
27. Heimstad R, Romundstad P, Salvesen K. Induction of labour for post-term pregnancy and risk estimates for intrauterine and perinatal death. *Acta Obstet Gynecol.* 2008;87:247–249. [II–3, $n = 408,631$]
28. Lydon-Rochelle M, Holt VL, Easterling TR, et al. Risk of uterine rupture during labor among women with a prior cesarean delivery. *N Engl J Med.* 2001;345:3–8. [II–2]
29. American College of Obstetricians and Gynecologists. ACOG Practice Bulletin No. 115: Vaginal birth after previous cesarean delivery. *Obstet Gynecol.* 2010;116:450–463. [Review]

Placental disorders

Moeun Son and William Grobman

Placental disorders include placenta previa, placenta accreta, and vasa previa. For normal or abnormal third stage, including postpartum hemorrhage, retained placenta, and uterine inversion, see Chapters 9 and 26.

KEY POINTS
Placenta Previa
- **Placenta previa** is defined as a placenta that covers the internal os.
- **Low-lying placenta** is defined as a placenta that comes within 0.1–2.0 cm of the internal os but does not cover it.
- **Placental location should be assessed when the fetal anatomic survey ultrasound (usually 18–24 weeks) is performed. If a placenta previa is suspected on transabdominal ultrasound, a transvaginal ultrasound (TVU) should be performed to confirm the diagnosis.**
- The risk that a placenta previa diagnosed in the antepartum period remains a placenta previa at the time of delivery depends on several factors, especially gestational age (GA) at detection, the placental distance from or extent of overlap of the internal os, and the a priori risk of placenta previa related to other risk factors (e.g., prior cesarean delivery). **Most placenta previas diagnosed before the third trimester do not remain placenta previas at the time of delivery.**
- **Women who have the inferior edge of the placenta ≥1 cm from the internal os at around 20 weeks usually do not require further ultrasounds for placental location.**
- **All patients with the inferior placenta edge <1 cm from the internal os or overlying the os at around 20 weeks should be rescanned at least once at approximately 32–35 weeks' gestation to reassess for placental location.**
- All patients with **prior cesarean delivery and placenta previa** that extends anteriorly should have evidence of **placenta accreta** assessed ultrasonographically.
- Women with a **placenta previa** should be delivered by **cesarean**. If the placental lower edge is **within 1–19 mm of the internal os, a trial of labor** can be attempted, but the risk of significant bleeding during labor may be higher, especially in those with a distance of only 1–10 mm.
- The optimal GA for delivery of an asymptomatic woman (i.e., a woman without acute bleeding) with placenta previa is unknown, but **many experts recommend planned cesarean delivery at approximately 36 0/7–37 6/7 weeks.**

Placenta Accreta
- Risk factors for placenta accreta include prior cesarean delivery; placenta previa; prior uterine surgery (e.g., prior myomectomy or prior multiple dilation and evacuations [D&Es]); Asherman's syndrome; submucous leiomyomata; maternal age ≥35 years; multiparity; and smoking.
- **Maternal complications** of placenta accreta include **hysterectomy, injury to other organs, blood transfusion, disseminated intravascular coagulation (DIC), infection,** and **death.** Fetal complications include **preterm birth (PTB) and small for gestational age (SGA).**
- There are **no randomized trials** to assess efficacy of different surgical interventions in or the approaches to the management of placenta accreta. Planned hysterectomy may be beneficial in cases in which the diagnosis is highly suspected, especially for the woman who does not desire further fertility.
- There are no randomized trials to assess the optimal gestation age for delivery of pregnancies with placenta accreta, but The American College of Obstetricians and Gynecologists (ACOG) and Society for Maternal-Fetal Medicine (SMFM) recommend **planned cesarean delivery at around 34 0/7–35 6/7 weeks.**

Vasa Previa
- Vasa previa exists when fetal vessels, unprotected by the umbilical cord or placental tissue, run through the membranes and over the internal os. In this circumstance, rupture of the membranes can lead to rupture of these fetal vessels, with a significant possibility of fetal death. Women with risk factors, such as a velamentous cord insertion, resolved placenta previa, or a succenturiate or bilobed placenta in which intervening vessels may cross the cervix, should have a transvaginal ultrasound (TVU) to detect vasa previa.
- The optimal GA for delivery of an asymptomatic woman (i.e., a woman without acute bleeding) with vasa previa is unknown, but **many experts recommend planned cesarean delivery at approximately 34 0/7–35 6/7 weeks.**

PLACENTA PREVIA
Diagnoses/Definitions
Placenta previa is defined as **a placenta that covers the internal os.** The diagnosis of placenta previa is established by TVU. The terms partial, marginal, complete, or incomplete placenta previa are rooted in preultrasound physical examinations, have been used to signify different conditions, and therefore should be avoided. Moreover, many studies have used these terms to signify different conditions. When the placenta does not cover the internal os, rather than use ambiguous language, it is best to describe the distance of the tip of the placenta from the internal os. **Low-lying placenta** is defined as a placenta that comes within 0.1–2.0 cm of the internal os but does not cover it.

Symptoms
Approximately two-thirds of women with placenta previas have antepartum vaginal bleeding. Therefore, about 33% do not have any symptoms before delivery.

Epidemiology/Incidence
The incidence of placenta previa at term is approximately 0.5% [1]. The frequency of placenta previa is higher earlier in gestation, but many of these cases will resolve. The likelihood of resolution is inversely proportional to GA at the time of examination (Table 28.1) [2].

Risk Factors/Associations
Prior cesarean delivery (Table 28.2), any other uterine surgery (e.g., myomectomy, D&E, dilation and curettage [D&C], and hysteroscopy) involving the uterine cavity, prior placenta previa, and multiparity [3–5].

Complications
Placenta accreta, antepartum and/or postpartum hemorrhage, PTB, and perinatal death [6].

Management
Principles
Placenta location should be assessed at the time of the fetal anatomic survey (usually 18–24 weeks). If placenta previa is suspected by transabdominal examination, a **TVU should be performed for confirmation of the diagnosis** (Figure 28.1). A single antenatal ultrasound that detects a placenta previa, however, may not indicate that a placenta previa will be present at delivery, as the relative position of the placenta with respect to the internal os will change as gestation progresses [2]. The reason for this change in relative position is not placental migration but likely due to the growth and development of the lower uterine segment. Atrophy of placental cells overlying the os also has been postulated as a contributing factor to this apparent positional change. This phenomenon has been cited as the reason that **vasa previa** can be seen in this setting (i.e., when an initially diagnosed placenta previa resolves).

Workup
Examination. Because of the reliability of ultrasound for diagnosis of previa, the technique of double setup examination is unnecessary. If employed, double setup examination should be performed in a setting with the ability to proceed in a prompt fashion with cesarean delivery if indicated.

Ultrasound. **TVU is the gold standard for the diagnosis of placenta previa** (Figure 28.2). It is very safe in these women [3]. The risk that a placenta previa that is diagnosed with ultrasound is present at delivery depends on several factors, including GA at detection, the placental distance from or extent of overlap of the internal os, as well as a woman's a priori risk of placenta previa (e.g., related to a prior cesarean delivery). **Most previas diagnosed before the third trimester resolve** (Table 28.1) [2,7]. If a placenta previa "resolves" but remains proximate to the internal cervical os, a woman still may have an increased risk of third-trimester bleeding, intrapartum hemorrhage, and cesarean delivery [8,9].

Women who have the inferior edge of the placenta **≥1 cm from the internal os at around 20 weeks usually do not require further ultrasounds for placental location** as they are exceedingly unlikely to have a placenta that is low-lying or a previa at delivery. Women who have the inferior placental edge **overlapping the internal os by ≥25 mm at around 20 weeks** have been reported to **usually have persistence of previa even by term** [10,11] (Table 28.1).

All patients with suspected placenta previa in the second trimester should be rescanned at approximately 32–35 weeks' gestation to assess for persistence of placenta previa (Figure 28.1). **Additionally, even if a placenta previa is no longer present, measuring the distance from the placental edge to the internal os in the third trimester can help estimate the risk of bleeding with a trial of labor** [8,9].

All patients with **prior cesarean delivery (or other uterine surgery)** and **placenta previa** that extends anteriorly should have evidence of **placenta accreta assessed ultrasonographically** [5,6] (see the section "Placenta Accreta").

Prenatal Care
All patients with **placenta previa** and **antenatal bleeding** in the third trimester should be advised about **pelvic rest (no vaginal penetration).** Pelvic rest recommendations in women with a placenta that is near but not overlapping the internal os should be individualized and based on bleeding during the pregnancy as well as the distance between the placenta and the internal os. There is insufficient evidence to support the

Table 28.1 Persistence of Placenta Previa until Delivery Stratified by GA at Ultrasound Detection, Type of Previa, and Prior Cesarean Delivery

GA at Detection (weeks)	15–19	20–23	24–27	28–31	32–35
Incomplete previa,[a] no prior cesarean	6	11	12	35	39
Incomplete previa,[a] prior cesarean	7	50	40	38	63
Complete previa, no prior cesarean	20	45	56	89	90
Complete previa, prior cesarean	41	73	84	88	89

Sources: Modified from Dashe JS et al, *Obstet Gynecol*, 99, 692–697, 2002; Becker RH et al., *Ultrasound Obstet Gynecol*, 17, 496–501, 2001; Oppenheimer L et al., *Ultrasound Obstet Gynecol*, 18, 100–102, 2001.
Abbreviation: GA, gestational age.
All data presented as percentages.
[a] Incomplete previa defined as inferior edge of the placenta partially covering or reaching the margin of the internal os.

Table 28.2 Risk of Placenta Previa and/or Accreta Stratified by Number of Prior Cesarean Deliveries

	First CD	Second CD	Third CD	Fourth CD	Fifth CD	≥Sixth CD
Previa	6.4	1.3	1.1	2.3	2.3	3.4
Accreta (no previa)	0.03	0.2	0.1	0.8	0.8	4.7
Accreta (previa)	3.3	11	40	61	67	67

Source: Modified from Silver RM et al., *Obstet Gynecol*, 107, 1226–1232, 2006.
Abbreviation: CD, cesarean delivery.
All data presented as percentage.

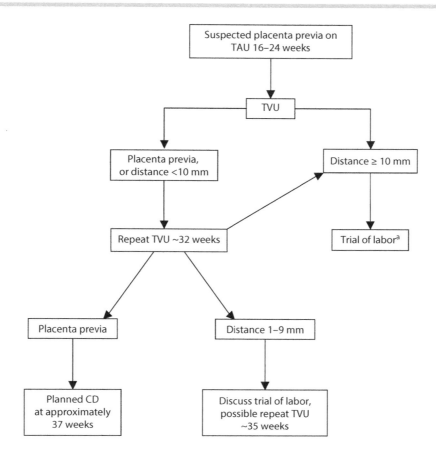

Figure 28.1 Management of suspected placenta previa. CD, cesarean delivery; distance, distance between placental edge to internal cervical os; TAU, transabdominal ultrasound; TVU, transvaginal ultrasound. [a]After discussion with the couple and if no contraindication.

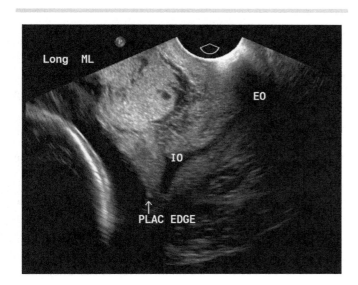

Figure 28.2 Transvaginal ultrasound showing anterior placenta previa, with placental edge covering over the internal os (IO). EO, external os; ML, mediolateral view. (Courtesy of the Division of Maternal-Fetal Medicine, Department of Obstetrics and Gynecology, Northwestern University Feinberg School of Medicine.)

use of routine bed rest in women with placenta previa or to be certain who are optimal candidates, when asymptomatic, for hospitalization [12]. Moreover, while pelvic rest, i.e., nothing per vagina, is often suggested, there is no evidence for its effectiveness. There is no evidence to support the use of autologous blood donation/transfusion for placenta previa [13].

Therapy/Interventions

   Management at home versus hospitalization. There has been no evidence of any clear advantage to a policy of home versus routine hospital care, with **similar maternal and fetal outcomes** demonstrated in the trials that do exist. The only difference is that, compared with hospitalization, management at home, not surprisingly, has been associated with a reduced length of stay in the hospital [12]. There are no data to allow certainty as to who are the optimal candidates for inpatient management. Women who, traditionally, have been **more likely to be managed in the hospital** even though they are not acutely symptomatic are those who **have had recurrent episodes of antepartum hemorrhage (e.g., three or more episodes of bleeding); have other medical complications that increase their risks (e.g., congenital cardiac disease); or are unable to easily access the hospital in an emergency (e.g., lack of telephone at home and far distance from an adequate care facility).**

Often, after an initial antenatal bleeding episode related to placenta previa, if several days of no further bleeding have occurred and there is no other indication for hospitalization, women may be managed as outpatients.

Cervical cerclage. Cervical cerclage has not been proven to be an effective intervention for women with placenta previa [12]. Although the meta-analysis in the Cochrane review that evaluated cervical cerclage in the setting of placenta previa revealed that women randomized to cerclage had a reduced length of inpatient hospitalization, as well as reduced risks of an SGA birth or delivery <34 weeks, the benefits were evident in studies with lower methodological quality, and thus there is not yet sufficient evidence to justify this intervention.

Tocolysis. There is insufficient evidence to assess the benefits of tocolysis for treatment of preterm labor (PTL) specifically in women with a placenta previa. It is reasonable to consider tocolysis, as for women without a placenta previa, if PTL is diagnosed and a course of steroids has not yet been administered [14]. Acute bleeding with instability of the mother or fetus is considered a contraindication to tocolysis.

Antepartum testing. There are insufficient data to assess the usefulness of routine antenatal testing in improving outcomes, and this strategy is presently not indicated.

Delivery

Timing. There is insufficient evidence to be certain of the optimal GA of delivery for women with placenta previa who are not acutely bleeding, although experts have recommended approximately **36 0/7–37 6/7 weeks** [15,16] (Figure 28.1). In the setting of acute bleeding, the timing of delivery depends upon individualization of patient circumstances, taking into account GA, amount of bleeding, and other comorbidities.

Mode. Delivery of women with a placenta previa should be by **cesarean.** Preoperative ultrasonography to assess placental location is useful in determining the optimal place for the uterine incision (Figure 28.1). Those with a placenta not covering the internal os but in the lower segment may have a trial of labor offered, with individual circumstances (e.g., the presence of antepartum bleeding) and the risk of bleeding at delivery taken into consideration. In a recent series, 26/28 (93%) women who had a placental edge to cervical os distance of 1–20 mm and who underwent a trial of labor delivered vaginally [8,17]. Women with a placental edge that is within 1 cm of the internal os can have uncomplicated vaginal deliveries, although their risk of bleeding and requiring a cesarean is higher than in those women whose placenta is 10–20 mm distant from the os (risks of cesarean 75% and 31%, respectively) [8] (Table 28.3). As such, depending upon the distance of the placental edge from the internal os as well as other factors, these patients (i.e., those with a placenta that is not covering the internal os but that is 2 cm or less from the internal os prior to delivery) should have their circumstances discussed and be delivered in facilities with the capacity to perform emergent operative delivery if necessary [18]. In women with the placenta 2 cm or more from the internal os, a trial of labor should be encouraged.

PLACENTA ACCRETA
Diagnosis/Definition

Placenta accreta is defined as a placenta that is abnormally adherent to the uterus. The diagnosis of this condition can be quite difficult, as full ascertainment would require postpartum histologic examination of the entire uteroplacental interface with both placenta and uterus available. Since this is not typically possible, in cases of clinically suspected placenta accreta, failure to demonstrate abnormal villous invasion by pathologic examination cannot always be used to exclude this diagnosis [19]. Therefore, **the diagnosis is often made clinically at delivery**. The antenatal suspicion of placenta accreta can be based on history (e.g., prior cesarean delivery and an anterior placenta previa) or imaging findings (e.g., by ultrasound or magnetic resonance imaging [MRI]), but no method can provide 100% accuracy in antenatal diagnosis.

Epidemiology/Incidence
Traditionally 1/2500 deliveries, although evidence of increasing frequency (3/1000 or more), thought to be related to the increased rate of cesarean delivery, has been reported [20,21].

Etiology/Pathophysiology
Abnormal adherence of chorionic villi to myometrium, associated with total or partial lack of the decidua basalis layer. Cesarean scar pregnancy is diagnosed by ultrasound often in the first trimester, and can be an early sign of later development of placenta accreta [22].

Classification
Abnormally invasive placentas may be categorized according to the depth of their invasion [23].

- **Placenta accreta:** Chorionic villi are attached directly to, but do not invade, the myometrium.
- **Placenta increta:** Placental villi invade into the myometrium.
- **Placenta percreta:** Placental villi invade through the myometrium into the uterine serosa; adjacent organs (e.g., the bladder) may be involved, but this extension is not necessary for the diagnosis.

Risk Factors/Associations
Prior cesarean delivery; placenta previa (Table 28.2); **prior uterine surgery involving the cavity** (e.g., prior myomectomy; D&Es); **Asherman's syndrome; submucous leiomyomata;** cesarean scar pregnancy [5,6,23].

Complications
Maternal. Blood transfusion, infection, DIC, **injury to other organs, hysterectomy, venous thromboembolism, and death** [5,6].

Perinatal. **PTB and SGA** [24].

Table 28.3 Selected Outcomes with Low-Lying Placenta According to Placental Edge to Internal Os Distance

	Distance between Placental Edge and Internal Cervical Os	
	1–10 mm	11–20 mm
Cesarean delivery	75%	31%
Antepartum hemorrhage	29%	3%
Postpartum hemorrhage	21%	10%
Postpartum hemorrhage >1000 mL	8%	10%

Source: Modified from Vergani P et al., *Am J Obstet Gynecol*, 202(6), e10, 2010.

Management

There are **no trials** to assess the comparative effectiveness of different interventions (e.g., planned hysterectomy versus attempted placental extraction for suspected placenta accreta; and preoperative placement versus no preoperative placement of catheters to allow the inflation for internal iliac balloons) in the management of placenta accreta.

Workup

No one imaging modality has been shown to be able to accurately diagnose placenta accreta with 100% sensitivity or specificity. Given the frequency of ultrasonographic imaging during pregnancy, this modality has been most frequently assessed with regard to attempting an antepartum diagnosis (Figure 28.3). Ultrasonographic findings that have been reported in association with placenta accreta are shown in Table 28.4 [23,25–30]. However, even the combination of all these signs is not 100% sensitive for the diagnosis of accreta, and the sensitivity, specificity, positive and negative predictive values for individual signs and combinations of signs have varied substantially in published studies, but have been commonly reported to be about >60%–80% [31,32]. Further imaging modalities to evaluate the possibility of placenta accreta include **MRI** (especially T2 images), which may be informative but also is not considered to be completely diagnostic [28,29]. MRI is not recommended for routine use in suspected accreta. It may useful as an adjunctive tool if the placenta is posterior or to assess invasion of adjacent organs in suspected percreta [33]. Cystoscopy can be considered as an adjunctive tool to assess for the possibility of placenta percreta in cases where bladder invasion is highly suspected due to radiologic studies or to signs such as frank blood in the urine.

Preparations and Plans for Delivery

If placenta accreta is suspected, appropriate counseling and preparations should be made (Table 28.5) [23]. Labor and delivery staff (nursing and anesthesia) as well as blood bank should be notified regarding delivery plans, and the delivery should occur in a location that has the capacity to provide large volumes of blood transfusion and emergent surgery (including hysterectomy). It should be considered whether the particular circumstances would suggest the need for additional surgical services (e.g., gynecologic oncology, urology, general surgery, and vascular surgery). Another potential adjunctive strategy that may be considered is the cell saver. Although multiple other strategies (e.g., ureteral stents, preoperative placement of pelvic artery catheters for potential postpartum embolization and/or balloon inflation) have been utilized, these strategies have not been shown in either prospective trials or retrospective studies to have clear benefits that outweigh risks [23,34–36].

The patient (and family members if available) should be counseled regarding risks, complications, and management. The possible need for **hysterectomy** as a life-saving procedure should be **discussed** with the patient. Plans for future reproduction should be discussed and weighted against the risk of retaining the uterus. Other preventive or therapeutic interventions as described above and below should be discussed.

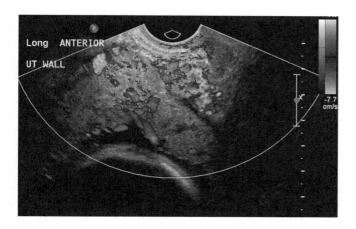

Figure 28.3 Transvaginal ultrasound showing loss of normal hypoechoic retroplacental zone and multiple vascular lacunae with turbulent blood flow within anterior placenta concerning for placenta accreta. UT, uterine. (Courtesy of the Division of Maternal-Fetal Medicine, Department of Obstetrics and Gynecology, Northwestern University Feinberg School of Medicine.)

Table 28.4 Ultrasonographic signs associated with placenta accreta

First trimester
Gestational sac that is located in the lower uterine segment
Multiple irregular vascular spaces noted within the placental bed
Implantation of the gestational sac imbedded into the uterine window at the site of the prior cesarean delivery (cesarean scar ectopic)

Second trimester
Multiple vascular lacunae within the placenta

Third trimester
Loss of the normal hypoechoic retroplacental zone
The presence of multiple vascular lacunae within placenta (Swiss cheese appearance)
Abnormalities of the uterine serosa–bladder interface (interruption of the line, thickening of the line, irregularity of the line, and increased vascularity)
Extension of the villi into the myometrium, serosa, or bladder
Retroplacental myometrial thickness of less than 1 mm
Turbulent blood flow through the lacunae on Doppler ultrasonography
Increased subplacental vascularity
Vessels bridging from the placenta to the uterine margin
Gaps in myometrial blood flow

Sources: Modified from Society for Maternal-Fetal Medicine, and MA Belford, *Am J Obstet Gynecol*, 203, 430–439, 2010; Twickler DM et al., *J Matern Fetal Med*, 9, 330–335, 2000; Palacios Jaraquemada JM and Bruno CH, *Acta Obstet Gynecol Scand*, 84, 716–724, 2005; Warshak CR et al., *Obstet Gynecol*, 108, 573–581, 2006; Silver RM et al., *Am J Obstet Gynecol*, 212, 561–568, 2015.

Table 28.5 Preparations in Cases of Suspected Placenta Accreta

Outpatient procedures
- MFM and Gyn Oncology consultations as outpatient
- Interventional radiology (IR), urology, and anesthesia consultations as outpatient
- Prenatal care and ultrasounds with MFM. Specify:
  - Placenta location
  - Relevant ultrasound findings
  - Relevant MRI findings
  - Obstetric history
  - No. of prior cesarean deliveries
  - Other prior uterine surgery
  - Latest hemoglobin (within 4 weeks of surgery; aim for >10 mg/dL)
- Betamethasone at 33.5 weeks
- Third trimester MRI if posterior placenta or concern for percreta
- Delivery:
  - Timing: 34–35 weeks
  - Designate and make aware primary surgical team (e.g., one MFM and one Gyn Oncology attending, at least)
  - Cesarean hysterectomy in main OR
  - Arrange for cell saver

Inpatient procedures
- Admit the day before
- Type and cross—10 U pRBC, 7 FFP, in room
  - Blood bank to be notified
  - Order the blood products before the case, not same day
- Clear liquid diet/consider bowel preparation if concern for bowel involvement
- Placement of large bore IV
- If IR involved:
  - Fetal heart monitoring before IR
  - Preop for IR by 7 AM first case
  - Heparin 5000 U SQ ×1—needs to be given prior to going to IR
  - Tylenol 95.0 mg, lyrica 150 mg—needs to be given prior to going to IR
  - Preop balloon catheters
  - Fetal heart monitoring after IR
  - Transfer directly from IR suite to main OR
- Unasyn 3 g IV before ureteral stents
- Cell saver in room
- Surgical intensive care unit (SICU) bed on hold

Intraoperative
- Regional anesthesia preferred before delivery of baby; then possibly general anesthesia as per gyn oncology and anesthesia preference
- Positioning: lithotomy in Allen stirrups
- Sequential compression devices (SCDs) placed
- Urology—open-ended ureteral catheters
- Vertical skin incision
- C-section, evaluate need for hysterectomy
- Hysterectomy
- If hysterectomy not done, and placenta left in situ:
  - After OR, to IR for gel foam embolization
  - After discharge will follow with MFM for weekly ultrasounds
  - High potential for infection, need for hysterectomy at a later date

Postoperative
- SICU—if necessary, decide intraoperatively which level of care is appropriate
- Possible post op embolization with IR

Disclaimer: Individual practices and circumstances will vary. This example does not indicate that certain evaluations or consultations are anticipated or expected in all cases.

Abbreviations: FFP, fresh frozen plasma; IV, intravenously; IR, interventional radiology; MFM, maternal-fetal medicine; MRI, magnetic resonance imaging; OR, operating room; pRBC, packed red blood cells; SQ, subcutaneously.

Delivery

Timing. The **optimal GA** for delivery of a woman with placenta accreta is **uncertain**. Many authors recommend a delivery prior to 39 weeks (e.g., 36–37 weeks) in order to avoid an unscheduled delivery and to optimize the capacity for preparation. Fetal maturity testing has been advocated by some and not by others, and one recent decision analysis suggests that it does not help to improve overall health outcomes. This analysis also suggests that in certain high-risk cases (e.g., intermittently bleeding placenta previa with suspected placenta percreta) even earlier delivery (e.g., **34–35 weeks**) may be acceptable [37]. Both the Society for Maternal-Fetal Medicine (SMFM) and the American College of Obstetricians and Gynecologists (ACOG) recommend delivery around 34 0/7–35 6/7 weeks for placenta accreta [23,38]. The final timing for delivery will need to be individualized, and take into account the risks of prematurity to the infant and the risks of major morbidity to the mother.

Technique. General intraoperative considerations include the possibility of a planned vertical skin incision. The uterine incision should be made, if possible, away from the placenta, the position of which can be determined by ultrasound beforehand. **Intraoperative ultrasound** with a sterile cover over the probe placed on the exposed uterus may be helpful if preoperative ultrasound is not informative.

The two most common approaches to management of suspected placenta accreta are hysterectomy without attempt at placental removal versus attempt at placental removal. While there are different potential approaches for managing placenta accreta after delivery of the baby by cesarean, many experts would recommend that **if there is proven placenta accreta** (e.g., placenta directly visualized in the serosa), **highly suspected** accreta by history and radiologic studies (e.g., multiple prior cesarean deliveries, placenta previa, and several ultrasonographic findings of placenta accreta), **or if the mother plans no more childbearing** (e.g., has requested tubal ligation), a reasonable course of action is to **avoid disturbing the implantation of the placenta and proceed with a hysterectomy** while the placenta remains attached [39]. In these controlled situations, maternal morbidity of gravid hysterectomy may be decreased, but fertility is lost.

During hysterectomy, **the uterine serosa overlying the placenta should not be dissected**, including trying to avoid bladder dissection. The blood supply to the placenta is not just from the uterine arteries but also from many collateral vessels. Care should be given to dissection of this extensive blood supply by attempting uterine artery dissection laterally, and then continuing down without incising the placenta. **Total hysterectomy is generally necessary,** as subtotal hysterectomy may leave behind part of the lower segment, where the placenta is abnormally attached and cause bleeding if a previa is present.

If the diagnosis is possible but not certain, and the patient desires to make attempts at avoiding hysterectomy despite having been counseled regarding risks, it is not unreasonable to wait for signs of placental separation, although abnormal adherence or significant hemorrhage should be ascertained and acted upon promptly. If spontaneous placental delivery fails, the operator must decide if either manual placental removal in pieces or hysterectomy is the next intervention, based on several factors, including the degree of invasiveness and amount of bleeding.

If only a small area of the placenta is adherent and a focal area of the placental bed is bleeding, sewing over this area with **sutures can be considered**, but usually these are in the very low uterine segment and cervix and often continue to bleed despite suturing or **uterotonics**. Some have suggested **ligation** of pelvic vessels (such as the internal iliac artery) in the setting of significant hemorrhage, although this may not be beneficial, given the many collateral vessels, and may incur risks as well. Pelvic **packing** has been used in some cases as a measure to temporarily lessen bleeding and allow attainment of hemodynamic stability. Hysterectomy may be necessary if uterine bleeding cannot be controlled, hopefully before massive blood loss and cardiovascular instability. When bleeding is from the lower part of the uterus in the setting of an accreta and placenta implanted low in the uterus (e.g., a previa), total hysterectomy is desirable, as subtotal hysterectomy may not control bleeding. Gravid hysterectomy has been associated with an incidence of maternal mortality of up to 7%, with a 90% incidence of transfusion, 28% incidence of postoperative transfusion, and a 5% incidence of ureteral injuries or fistula formation [19,39].

In some cases, a woman who has not completed childbearing may strongly want to avoid hysterectomy. There are several case reports of expectant (also called "conservative") or medical management in the setting of placenta accreta. In these circumstances, the placenta is left in situ and the cord ligated close to its origin, either with no therapy or with an adjunctive therapy such as **methotrexate and/or arterial embolization**. There is no proven efficacy for methotrexate, or even for embolization. Antibiotic prophylaxis has been suggested given the risk of infection, as have short-term uterotonics for postpartum hemorrhage prevention, but there are no trials of these interventions. Follow-up is also not based on good evidence, but serial ultrasounds (to monitor involution and decrease in placental vascularity) and quantitative human chorionic gonadotrophin (HCG) levels have been proposed. If HCG levels plateau, or uterine size or placental vascularity does not decrease by 72 hours, methotrexate has been given as 1 mg/kg on alternate days for a total of four to six doses, or according to HCG levels and ultrasonographic findings [40]. Women on methotrexate should be monitored with liver function tests (LFTs), platelet counts, and creatinine levels. However, **conservative management, especially for placenta percreta, has been associated with significant morbidity, including infection, delayed hemorrhage, a 42% chance of major morbidity (DIC, major postpartum hemorrhage, pulmonary embolism, sepsis, fistula, AV malformation), and a 58% risk of later hysterectomy (40% of the times emergent) at least up to 9 months postpartum** [41–45] and should be considered only when the woman has been fully apprised of the risks and when no active uterine bleeding is present. In a follow-up study of 96 women with successful conservative management, about 9% had Asherman's syndrome, and 25% had subsequent pregnancies, with 29% recurrent accretas, and 62% third trimester deliveries [46].

Postpartum
Consider reservation of intensive care unit bed for postpartum care.

VASA PREVIA
Diagnosis/Definition
Fetal blood vessels, unprotected by the umbilical cord or placental tissue that run through the membranes and over the internal os. Two types have been described: Type I when there is a velamentous cord insertion, and Type II when the placenta contains a succenturiate lobe or is multilobed and fetal vessels connecting the two placental lobes course over or near the internal os [47].

Symptoms
Asymptomatic unless membranes rupture, at which time vaginal bleeding may be noted.

Epidemiology/Incidence
Approximately 1/2500–1/5000 deliveries [1].

Risk Factors/Associations
Placenta in the lower uterine segment (e.g., low-lying, or previa earlier in pregnancy), velamentous cord insertion, succenturiate or bilobed placenta, and multiple gestations [48].

Complications
Perinatal morbidity (e.g., neonatal anemia) and mortality (up to 56%) due to acute fetal hemorrhage [49].

Management
Principles
Timing of bleeding with antenatally diagnosed vasa previa is variable and impossible to predict. Since the fetal vessels are not protected by placental tissue or Wharton jelly, compression may lead to reduced fetal blood flow and bradycardia, and rupture of membranes with subsequent vessel laceration may result in rapid fetal exsanguination. It's paramount to make the diagnosis of vasa previa antepartum, and not intrapartum.

Workup
TVU with color Doppler is the standard for diagnosis of vasa previa (Figure 28.4). **Women with risk factors that are judged to increase their risk of vasa previa (see above) should be screened with TVU for this condition.** Vasa previa is diagnosed if a vessel is visualized over the cervix with color Doppler demonstrating a rhythm consistent with the fetal heart rate. The American Institute of Ultrasound in Medicine (AIUM) and ACOG recommend that **the placental cord insertion site be documented** whenever technically possible [50]. A recent systematic review showed a high accuracy of TVU color Doppler (median detection rate of 93% and specificity of 99%), but also noted that the quality of the available studies was relatively poor [51]. Thus, not all vasa previa will be detected prenatally, even by adequate examinations and experienced operators using color Doppler. Women whose vasa previa has been **diagnosed prenatally have been reported to have lower perinatal mortality than those with vasa previas that are undiagnosed** (3% vs. 56%) [49].

The Apt test may be used to distinguish between fetal and maternal sources of vaginal bleeding, although this test may be of little use in many clinical situations with bleeding from a vasa previa, as bleeding can lead to rapid deterioration of the fetal status and require urgent delivery before an Apt test can be completed.

Therapy
Level 1 data to guide the management of antenatally diagnosed vasa previa are currently lacking. While some experts suggest that hospitalization at some time after viability may be reasonable, this strategy is unsupported by any adequately powered trials. Many admit women with proven vasa previa around 28–32 weeks. It is reasonable to consider administration of **antenatal corticosteroids** at 28–33 weeks of gestation,

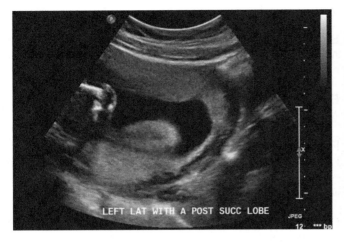
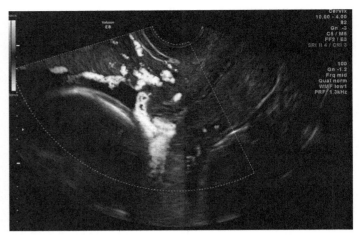
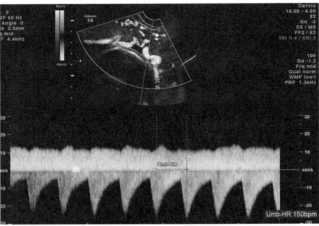

Figure 28.4 Ultrasound images showing vasa previa. (A) Left lateral (LAT) placenta with a posterior succenturiate lobe; (B) transvaginal ultrasound with color Doppler showing vessels visualized over the cervix; and (C) color Doppler of vessel overlying the cervix demonstrates a rhythm consistent with the fetal heart rate. (Courtesy of the Division of Maternal-Fetal Medicine, Department of Obstetrics and Gynecology, Northwestern University Feinberg School of Medicine.)

if indications do not develop prior, in case of the need for urgent preterm delivery [52]. **Women with vasa previa should be delivered by cesarean** at a center capable of providing immediate neonatal blood transfusion if needed [53]. Timing of delivery is controversial, with suggestions for cesarean delivery anywhere **between 34 0/7 and 35 6/7 weeks**, although earlier when preterm premature rupture of membranes (PPROM), PTL, or significant bleeding occurs [1].

REFERENCES

1. Oyelese Y, Smulian JC. Placenta previa, placenta accreta, and vasa previa. *Obstet Gynecol.* 2006;107:927–941. [Review]
2. Dashe JS, McIntire DD, Ramus RM, et al. Persistence of placenta previa according to gestational age at ultrasound detection. *Obstet Gynecol.* 2002;99:692–697. [II–2]
3. Ananth CV, Smulian JC, Vintzileos AM. The association of placenta previa with history of cesarean delivery and abortion: A meta-analysis. *Am J Obstet Gynecol.* 1997;177:1071–1078. [Meta-analysis]
4. Gilliam M, Rosenberg D, Davis F. The likelihood of placenta previa with greater number of cesarean deliveries and higher parity. *Obstet Gynecol.* 2002;99:976–980. [II–2]
5. Silver RM, Landon MB, Rouse DJ, et al. Maternal morbidity associated with multiple repeat cesarean deliveries. *Obstet Gynecol.* 2006;107:1226–1232. [II–2]
6. Grobman WA, Lai Y, Landon MB, et al. Pregnancy outcomes for women with placenta previa in relation to the number of prior cesareans. *Obstet Gynecol.* 2007;110:1249–1255. [II–2]
7. Becker RH, Vonk R, Mende BC, et al. The relevance of placental location at 20–23 weeks gestational weeks for prediction of placenta previa at delivery: Evaluation of 8650 cases. *Ultrasound Obstet Gynecol.* 2001;17:496–501. [II–2]
8. Vergani P, Ornaghi S, Pozzi I, et al. Placenta previa: Distance to internal os and mode of delivery. *Am J Obstet Gynecol.* 2009;201:266.e1–266.e5. [II–2]
9. Bronsteen R, Valice R, Lee W, et al. Effect of a low-lying placenta on delivery outcome. *Ultrasound Obstet Gynecol.* 2009;33:204–208. [II–2]
10. Oppenheimer L, Simpson P, Holmes N, et al. Diagnosis of low-lying placenta: Can migration in the third trimester predict outcome? *Ultrasound Obstet Gynecol.* 2001;18:100–102. [II–2]
11. Oyalese Y. Placenta previa and vasa previa: Time to leave the Dark Ages. *Ultrasound Obstet Gynecol.* 2001;18:96–99. [Review]
12. Neilson JP. Interventions for suspected placenta praevia. *Cochrane Database Syst Rev.* 2010. [Meta-analysis]

13. Dinsmoor MJ, Hogg BB. Autologous blood donation with placenta previa: Is it feasible? *Am J Perinatol.* 1995;12:382–384. [II–2]
14. Sharma A, Suri V, Gupta I. Tocolytic therapy in conservative management of symptomatic placenta previa. *Int J Gynaecol Obstet.* 2004;84:109–113. [II–2]
15. Zlatnick MG, Little SE, Kohli P, et al. When should women with placenta previa be delivered? *J Reprod Med.* 2010;55:373–381. [Decision analysis]
16. Spong CY, Mercer BM, D'alton M, et al. Timing of indicated late-preterm and early-term birth. *Obstet Gynecol.* 2011;118(2 Pt 1):323–333. [Review]
17. Vergani P, Ornaghi S, Ghidini A. Placenta previa (reply). *Am J Obstet Gynecol.* 2010;202(6):e10; author reply e10. [Letter to the Editor]
18. Royal College of Obstetricians and Gynaecologists. *Clinical Green-Top Guideline No. 27: Placenta Praevia: Diagnosis and Management.* London, United Kingdom: RCOG Press, 2001. [Guideline]
19. Jacques SM, Qureshi F, Trent VS et al. Placenta accreta: Mild cases diagnosed by placental examination. *Int J Gynecol Pathol.* 1996;15:28–33. [II–2]
20. Miller DA, Chollet JA, Goodwin TM. Clinical risk factors for placenta previa-placenta accreta. *Am J Obstet Gynecol.* 1997;177:210–214. [II–2]
21. Wu S, Kocherginsky M, Hibbard JU. Abnormal placentation: Twenty-year analysis. *Am J Obstet Gynecol.* 2005;192:1458–1461. [II–2]
22. Timor-Tritsch E, Monteagudo A, Cali G et al. Cesarean scar pregnancy and early placenta accreta share common histology. *Ultrasound Obstet Gynecol.* 2014;43:383–395 [II–2]
23. Society for Maternal-Fetal Medicine, Belford MA. Placenta accreta. *Am J Obstet Gynecol.* 2010;203:430–439. [Review]
24. Gielchinsky Y, Mankuta D, Rojansky N, et al. Perinatal outcome of pregnancies complicated by placenta accreta. *Obstet Gynecol.* 2004;104:527–530. [II–2]
25. Chou MM, Ho ES, Lee YH. Prenatal diagnosis of placenta previa accreta by transabdominal color Doppler ultrasound. *Ultrasound Obstet Gynecol.* 2000;15:28–35. [II–2]
26. Comstock CH, Love JJ Jr., Bronsteen RA, et al. Sonographic detection of placenta accreta in the second and third trimesters of pregnancy. *Am J Obstet Gynecol.* 2004;190:1135–1140. [II–2]
27. Twickler DM, Lucas MJ, Balis AB, et al. Color flow mapping for myometrial invasion in women with a prior cesarean delivery. *J Matern Fetal Med.* 2000;9:330–335. [II–2].
28. Palacios Jaraquemada JM, Bruno CH. Magnetic resonance imaging in 300 cases of placenta accreta: Surgical correlation of new findings. *Acta Obstet Gynecol Scand.* 2005;84:716–724. [II–2]
29. Warshak CR, Eskander R, Hull AD, et al. Accuracy of ultrasonography and magnetic resonance imaging in the diagnosis of placenta accreta. *Obstet Gynecol.* 2006;108:573–581. [II–2]
30. Silver RM, Fox KA, Barton JR, et al. Center of excellence for placenta accreta. *Am J Obstet Gynecol.* 2015;212:561–8. [IV]
31. Bowman ZS, Eller AG, Kennedy AM, et al. Accuracy of ultrasound for the prediction of placenta accreta. *Am J Obstet Gyneol.* 2014;211:177.e1–177.e7 [II-2].
32. D'Antonio F, Iacovella C, and Bhide A. Prenatal identification of invasive placentation using ultrasound: Systematic review and meta-analysis. *Ultrasound Obstet Gynecol.* 2013;42:509–517. [Meta-analysis]
33. Silver R. Abnormal placentation: Placenta previa, vasa previa, and placenta accreta. *Obstet Gynecol.* 2015;126:654–668. [Review]
34. Levine AB, Kuhlman K, Bonn J. Placenta accreta: Comparison of cases managed with and without pelvic artery balloon catheters. *J Matern Fetal Med.* 1999;8:173–176. [II–2]
35. Greenberg JI, Suliman A, Iranpour P, et al. Prophylactic balloon occlusion of the internal iliac arteries to treat abnormal placentation a cautionary case. *Am J Obstet Gynecol.* 2007;197:470.e1–470.e4. [III]
36. Sewell MF, Rosenblum D, Ehrenberg H. Arterial embolus during common iliac balloon catheterization at cesarean hysterectomy. *Obstet Gynecol.* 2006;108:746–748. [III]
37. Robinson BK, Grobman WA. Effectiveness of timing strategies for delivery of patients with placenta previa and accreta. *Obstet Gynecol.* 2010;116(4):835–842. [Decision analysis]
38. American College of Obstetricians and Gynecologists. *ACOG Committee Opinion No. 266: Placenta accreta. Int J Gynaecol Obstet.* 2002;77(1):77–78. [Review]
39. O'Brien JM, Barton JR, Donaldson ES. The management of placenta percreta: Conservative and operative strategies. *Am J Obstet Gynecol.* 1996;175:1632–1638. [II–2]
40. Hundley AF, Lee-Parritz A. Managing placenta accreta. *OBG Manag.* 2002;14(8):18–33. [Review]
41. Alkazaleh F, Geary M, Kingdom J, et al. Elective non-removal of the placenta and prophylactic uterine artery embolization postpartum as a diagnostic imaging approach for the management of placenta percreta: A case report. *J Obstet Gynaecol Can.* 2004;26:743–746. [III]
42. Butt K, Gagnon A, Delisle MF. Failure of methotrexate and internal iliac balloon catheterization to manage placenta percreta. *Obstet Gynecol.* 2002;99:981–982. [III]
43. Teo SB, Kanagalingam D, Tan HK, et al. Massive postpartum hemorrhage after uterus-conserving surgery in placenta percreta: The danger of the partial placenta percreta. *Br J Obstet Gynecol.* 2008;115:789–792. [III]
44. Pather S, Strockyi S, Richards A, et al. Maternal outcome after conservative management of placenta percreta at cesarean section: A report of three cases and a review of the literature. *Aust N Z J Obstet Gynecol.* 2014;54:84–87. [III]
45. Clausen C, Lönn L, Langhoff-Roos J. Management of placenta percreta: A review of published cases. *Acta Obstet Gynecol Scand.* 2014;93:138–143. [III]
46. Sentilhes L, Kayem G, Ambroselli C, et al. Fertility and pregnancy outcomes following conservative treatment for placenta accreta. *Hum Reprod.* 2010;25:2803–2810. [II–2]
47. Catanzarite V, Maida C, Thomas W, et al. Prenatal sonographic diagnosis of vasa previa: Ultrasound findings and obstetric outcome in ten cases. *Ultrasound Obstet Gynecol.* 2001;18:109–115. [III]
48. Baulies S, Maiz N, Munoz A, et al. Prenatal ultrasound diagnosis of vasa praevia and analysis of risk factors. *Prenat Diagn.* 2007;27:595–599. [II–2]
49. Oyelese Y, Catanzarite V, Prefumo F, et al. Vasa previa: The impact of prenatal diagnosis on outcomes. *Obstet Gynecol.* 2004;103:937–942. [II–2]
50. American Institute of Ultrasound in Medicine. AIUM practice guideline for the performance of obstetric ultrasound examinations. *J Ultrasound Med.* 2013;32:1083–1101. [Guideline]
51. Ruiter L, Kok N, Limpens J, et al. A systematic review on the diagnostic accuracy of ultrasound in the diagnosis of vasa previa. *Ultrasound Obstet Gynecol.* 2015;45:516–522. [Meta-analysis]
52. Gagnon R, Morin L, Bly S, et al. Guidelines for the management of vasa previa. *J Obstet Gynaecol Can.* 2009;31:748–760. [Guideline]
53. Society for Maternal-Fetal Medicine (SMFM) Publications Committee, Sinkey RG, Odibo AO, et al. SMFM Consult Series No. 37: Diagnosis and management of vasa previa, *Am J Obstet Gynecol.* 2015;213:615–619. doi: 10.1016/j.ajog.2015.08.031. [Review]

Abruptio placentae

John F. Visintine

KEY POINTS
- Approximately 0.2%–1% of all pregnancies are complicated by placental abruption.
- **Nearly 50% of women with placental abruption have no identifiable risk factors.** Risk factors include abruption in a prior pregnancy, maternal hypertensive disorders, smoking, cocaine, polyhydramnios, multiple gestation, preterm and term premature rupture of membrane, chorioamnionitis, elevated maternal serum alpha-fetoprotein (MS-AFP), pregnancy-associated plasma protein-A (PAPP-A) ≤5th percentile, leiomyoma, subchorionic hematoma, vaginal bleeding <20 weeks, previous cesarean delivery, abdominal trauma, subclinical hypothyroidism, antithyroglobulin and antithyroperoxidase antibodies. The association with thrombophilias has for the most part not been confirmed by prospective studies.
- Complications include antepartum and postpartum hemorrhage, disseminated intravascular coagulopathy (DIC), and acute renal failure, as well as growth restriction, preterm delivery, fetal hypoxia and/or exsanguination, and perinatal mortality.
- **The diagnosis of placental abruption is primarily clinical.** History, physical examination, laboratory and ultrasonographic studies guide management. Ultrasound is primarily useful in ruling out other causes of third-trimester bleeding.
- **Placental pathology** has been shown to confirm the presence of abruption in 25% of those with an **acute clinical abruption,** and **60%** of those with a **chronic clinical abruption.**
- There are no trials to assess any intervention for prevention of abruption or its complications.
- **Prompt delivery is indicated if the pregnancy is late-preterm or term.** However, if less than 34 weeks, expectant management for mild (grade 1) abruptions may allow time for glucocorticoid administration. Maternal or fetal compromise may necessitate delivery. A decision-to-delivery interval of 20 minutes or less is associated with a substantial reduction of neonatal morbidity and mortality in placental abruption with nonreassuring fetal heart testing.
- Mode of delivery is dependent primarily on the condition of the mother and fetus.
  - In most cases, for mild abruption (grade 1, no evidence of maternal or fetal compromise), **vaginal delivery** is indicated.
  - For moderate abruption (grade 2, evidence of fetal nonreassuring testing), rapid delivery typically by **cesarean** is indicated.
  - For severe abruption (grade 3, fetal demise, often with DIC), **vaginal delivery** is indicated.

DEFINITION/DIAGNOSIS
Placental abruption (also called abruptio placentae) is defined as a premature separation of a normally implanted placenta. The diagnosis is a clinical diagnosis of exclusion, based usually on vaginal bleeding in the second or third trimester unexplained by other etiologies (see also section "Etiology/Basic Pathophysiology").

SIGNS AND SYMPTOMS
Signs and symptoms are shown in Table 29.1 [1,2]. About 10%–31% of abruptions present with only concealed (occult) bleeding. Occasionally the presenting sign is fetal death.

EPIDEMIOLOGY/INCIDENCE
- Approximately **0.2%–1%** of all pregnancies are complicated by placental abruption [3–5]. The incidence in the United States has increased, especially in the African-American population, the ethnic group at highest risk, in particular for severe (or grade 3) abruption [3].
- About 60% of abruptions occur preterm, and 50% occur prior to labor.
- The incidence of abruption is possibly highest at 24–26 weeks (up to 9 per 100 births) [6].
- There is over a 5% recurrence risk in a subsequent pregnancy for women with a history of an abruption [4].

GENETICS
A genome wide association study identified several candidate genes associated with placental abruption. The strongest association was with the FLI-1 gene (a megakaryocyte-specific transcription factor). Genes involved in lipid metabolism, cell signaling, mitochondrial biosynthesis, and oxidative phosphorylation are also associated with the risk of placental abruption [7]. The association with thrombophilias has not been confirmed in prospective studies. See section "Risk Factors/Associations" and Chapter 27 in *Maternal-Fetal Evidence Based Guidelines.*

ETIOLOGY/BASIC PATHOPHYSIOLOGY
The etiology is not completely understood but appears to occur as the result of two mechanisms: mechanical separation or as the end result of **defective deep placentation** [8]. Placental separation occurring in association with **mechanical trauma or rapid decompression of a distended uterus** is believed to occur due to shearing forces resulting from a change in surface area of a relatively elastic uterine wall in relation to an inelastic placenta. Blunt trauma to the uterus resulting in abruption or rupture of membranes with rapid decompression of an over distended uterus resulting in abruption are examples of this mechanism.

Table 29.1 Clinical Findings in Women with Placental Abruption

Clinical Findings	%
Vaginal bleeding	67–78
Uterine tenderness or abdominal/back pain	52–66
Nonreassuring fetal testing/Category II or III	60–78
Uterine contractions >5/10 minutes	17

Sources: Hurd WW et al., *Obstet Gynecol*, 61(4), 467–473, 1983; Kasai M et al., *J Obstet Gynaecol Res*, 41(6), 850–856, 2015.

Evidence in support of a defective deep placentation mechanism comes from placental bed biopsies from cases of placental abruption, which show an **absence of physiologic trophoblastic invasion, dilated vessels, and recent thrombosis of spiral arteries** [9]. These changes are seen not only in abruption but also in preeclampsia, intrauterine growth restriction (IUGR), and preterm premature rupture of membranes (PPROM), suggesting that placental abruption represents one **manifestation of a long-standing pregnancy disorder** [8]. Moreover, abnormalities in circulating angiogenic factors have been observed in women who subsequently developed placental abruption. In a nested case–control study, serum levels of the proangiogenic factor placental growth factor (PlGF) were lower, and levels of the potent inhibitor of PlGF, soluble fms-like tyrosine kinase 1 (sFlt-1), were increased [10].

Gross pathology findings associated with placental abruption include **adherent retroplacental clot with depression or disruption of the underlying placental tissue.** Microscopic changes associated with abruption resulting in perinatal mortality include **thrombosed arteries and necrosis of the decidua basalis, and large recent infarcts and stromal fibrosis** in the terminal villi of the placental parenchyma [11]. Severe cases of abruption can result in hemorrhagic infiltration between myometrial fibers that extends to the serosal surface giving the uterus a **dark purple discoloration, also known as Couvelaire uterus** in honor of the French obstetrician who first described this pathologic finding in the early twentieth century [12]. **The pathologic diagnosis of a placental abruption often does not correlate with the clinical diagnosis.** In a large series of placental pathologic evaluations, a placental abruption defined as an adherent clot with disruption of the underlying tissue was demonstrated in 3.8% of specimens, which is higher than the generally accepted incidence based on a clinical diagnosis (0.2%–1%) [13]. Most of those "abruptions" called by pathologists do not have clinical diagnosis of abruption, and many clinical abruptions have no pathologic evidence of abruption. We have structured the chapter around a clinical definition of abruption. A retrospective review of abruption cases diagnosed on clinical grounds or by pathologic criteria were analyzed based on risk factors, acute (cocaine use, trauma <12 hours from delivery) or chronic (hypertension, preeclampsia, acute chorioamnionitis, trauma occurring >12 hours prior to delivery). **Placental pathology confirmed the presence of abruption in only 25% of those with acute risk factors for abruption and 60% of those with a chronic risk factors for abruption** [14].

CLASSIFICATION

A uniformly accepted classification system for placental abruption does not exist. The clinical classification system originally published by Page in 1954 has been used by some authors as a means of grouping placental abruptions in those that can be potentially managed conservatively (grade 1) and those that require more aggressive management (grades 2 and 3) [15] (Table 29.2). A more recent classification defines **severe abruption** as at least one maternal (disseminated intravascular coagulation, hypovolemic shock, blood transfusion, hysterectomy, renal failure, or in-hospital death), fetal (nonreassuring fetal status, intrauterine growth restriction, or fetal death), or neonatal (fetal growth restriction, preterm birth) complication. Using these criteria, **two-thirds of placental abruptions are defined as severe** (overall abruption rate 9.6/1000, severe abruption 6.5/1000) [5]. It should be noted that the definition of placental abruption in this study does not include abruptions only identified through pathologic evaluation of the placenta (grade 0).

RISK FACTORS/ASSOCIATIONS

Nearly 50% of women with placental abruption have no identifiable risk factors (Table 29.3) [16].

- History of an **abruption in a prior pregnancy:** The risk of recurrence is about 5%–17% [17]. After two abruptions, the risk of recurrence is about 25%.
- Maternal **hypertensive disorders:** associated with up to almost 50% of grade 3 abruption cases. In particular, chronic hypertension (incidence 1.5%–2.5%, odds ratio [OR] 2.8), superimposed preeclampsia (about 3%), and severe preeclampsia (OR 4.1) are associated with placental abruption [18,19].
- **Abdominal trauma** is a recognized cause of placental abruption but is responsible for only 1% of cases [20]. See also Chapter 39 in *Maternal-Fetal Evidence Based Guidelines*.
- **Smoking:** 90% increase in abruption in women who smoke compared with controls. Smoking is responsible for 15%–25% of episodes of abruption [18].
- **Cocaine:** 1.9% rate of abruption [21].
- *Previous cesarean* delivery is associated with an increased risk of abruption in subsequent pregnancies (OR 1.3) [22].
- **Polyhydramnios** has been associated with placental abruptions in patients >37 weeks' gestation [23].
- **Multiple gestation:** 1.2% risk of abruption in twins, 1.5% in triplets [24].
- **PPROM:** OR 3.5 [25]. Evidence of old decidual hemorrhage can be found in nearly 40% of placentas from patients with PPROM [26].
- **Chorioamnionitis:** OR 9 [25]. Neutrophil infiltration of the fetal membranes and cervix is seen in premature rupture of membranes (PROM), and chorioamnionitis is associated with placental abruption [27].
- **Leiomyomas** detected at second-trimester ultrasound are associated with a small increase in the risk of abruption (OR 2.1) [28].
- **Ultrasound-detected subchorionic hemorrhage** before 22 weeks of gestation results in an increased risk of placental abruption (OR 2.6) [28].
- **Vaginal bleeding <20 weeks** is associated with an increased risk of abruption (RR 1.6) [29].
- Unexplained **elevated MS-AFP** in the second trimester: OR 6–10 for placental abruption [30,31].
- **PAPP-A** ≤5th percentile in the first trimester is associated with placental abruption (OR, 1.9) [32].
- **Inherited thrombophilias** have been associated with abruption in case–control studies [33,34]. However, **most prospective studies have shown no increased risk of abruption** [35–37]. A retrospective cohort study

Table 29.2 Classification of Placental Abruption

Grade[a]	Clinically Evident Bleeding	Uterine Tenderness	Maternal Hypotension	Maternal Coagulopathy	Fetal Distress
0	No	No	No	No	No
1	Yes	Yes or no	No	No	No
2	Yes or no	Yes	No	Rare	Yes
3	Yes or no	Yes	Yes	Often	Death

Source: Adapted from Sholl JS, Am J Obstet Gynecol, 156(1), 40–51, 1987.
[a]Grade 0: Diagnosis based on examination of the placenta.

Table 29.3 Risk Factors for Placental Abruption

Prior abruption
Chronic hypertension
Severe preeclampsia
Smoking
Cocaine
Chorioamnionitis
Unexplained elevated MS-AFP
PAPP-A levels ≤5th percentile
(P)PROM
Subchorionic hemorrhage
Leiomyoma
Vaginal bleeding <20 weeks
Polyhydramnios
Multiple gestation
Trauma
Subclinical hypothyroidism
Thyroperoxidase or thyroglobulin antibodies

Abbreviations: MS-AFP, maternal serum alpha-fetoprotein, PAPP-A, pregnancy-associated plasma protein-A; (P)PROM, preterm premature rupture of membrane.

comparing thromboprophylaxis with heparin for women with an inherited thrombophilia demonstrated no difference in rates of abruption or other adverse outcomes regardless of treatment [38]. But one large prospective cohort study did demonstrate an increased risk of abruption for women with the prothrombin gene mutation 20210A (OR 12), but not for factor V Leiden mutation, MTHFR C677T or A1298C mutations, or the thrombomodulin gene mutation [39].

- **Advanced maternal age:** It is unclear if there is an association with abruption, as the data are conflicting [40,41].
- **Thyroperoxidase antibodies** have been associated with an increased risk of placental abruption in two large cohort studies (OR 1.5–3.4) [42,43]. An association with abruption was also seen with **thyroglobulin antibodies** (OR 1.4–1.7) [43]. The association with abruption was confirmed in a cohort of low risk women with **subclinical hypothyroidism** [44].

COMPLICATIONS
- **Maternal**
  - **Serious maternal complications** (pulmonary edema, acute respiratory failure, acute heart failure, acute myocardial infarction, cardiomyopathy, puerperal cerebrovascular disorder, coma, and amniotic fluid embolism) occur at a higher ratio for women with **severe abruption** (141.7/10,000) compared with those with a **mild abruption** (33.3/10,000) or nonabruption (15.4/10,000 births) [5].
  - **Antepartum hemorrhage** remains a leading cause of maternal mortality. For pregnancies ending in stillbirth, hemorrhage related to placental abruption is the leading cause of maternal mortality [45].
  - **DIC** was first reported to occur in association with placental abruption by De Lee in 1901 [46]. The development of DIC is thought to be due to a release of thromboplastins, as well as consumption of coagulation factors secondary to an enlarging hematoma. Nearly 30% of patients who present with a severe (grade 3) abruption develop DIC.
  - **Acute renal failure** is a potential maternal complication associated with abruption. Fortunately the incidence of acute renal failure appears to be decreasing, possibly due to improved medical management.
  - **Postpartum hemorrhage secondary to uterine atony** is associated with abruption, as is postpartum anemia and *infection*.
- **Perinatal**
  - **Perinatal mortality** (both fetal and neonatal deaths) varies from 4 to 12/1000 [47]. This high perinatal mortality with abruption is attributable, in part, to its association with **preterm delivery.**
  - Of the excess perinatal deaths, about 55% can be attributed to prematurity. The other is associated with **fetal hypoxia** and/or **exsanguination**, or **growth restriction.**
  - Among abruption cases from a large multicenter case–control study, 60% were found to be small for gestational age; the authors concluded that this association was primarily due to preterm birth [48].
  - Of children with spastic quadriplegic or dyskinetic cerebral palsy, 5.7% are associated with placental abruption [49].

MANAGEMENT
Unfortunately there are **no trials to assess any intervention for management of abruption or its complications** [50]. Recommendations for management are primarily based on expert opinion or at best retrospective case–control studies (Figure 29.1).

Prevention
- A reduction in the risk of placental abruption was demonstrated with **prenatal vitamin C and E supplementation in smokers** (relative risk (RR) 0.09; 95% confidence interval [CI] 0.00–0.87) but not in nonsmokers (RR 0.92; 95% CI 0.52–1.62) [51].
- The use of **magnesium sulfate for women with preeclampsia** was shown to reduce the risk of placental abruption (RR 0.64; 95% CI 0.5–0.83) [52].
- **Smoking cessation counseling, avoidance of cocaine,** and, if possible, **avoidance of other risk factors** may prevent placental abruption.

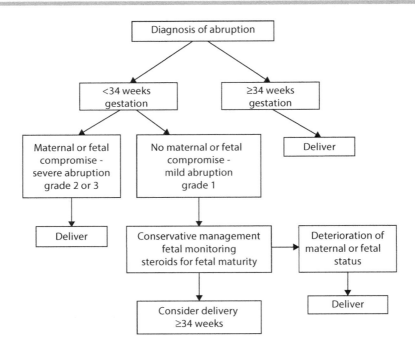

Figure 29.1 Management of abruption placentae.

Preconception Counseling
Women with risk factors should be counseled regarding the risk factors (Table 29.3) and complications of placental abruption, as well as interventions for its prevention.

Workup
- The diagnosis of an abruption is made clinically (vaginal bleeding, abdominal pain/uterine tenderness, nonreassuring fetal testing, or uterine tachysystole). Pathologic evaluation of the placenta may confirm the diagnosis in some cases (25% of acute and 60% of chronic abruptions), but the absence of pathologic findings does not exclude an abruption [14]. Placental abruptions may be occult. At times presenting as preterm labor, they may go undiagnosed until after delivery with examination of the placenta. If a **pathologic** diagnosis (rather than clinical diagnosis) of placental abruption is used the incidence of placental abruption is 3.8% [13] compared with around 1% in epidemiologic studies that employ a clinical diagnosis.
- **History and physical examination**, as well as appropriate **laboratory and ultrasonographic studies**, guide management. Routine assessment should be conducted including **vital signs, oxygenation status, and urine output. Laboratory** assessment may include a **hematocrit, platelet count, coagulation studies** (prothrombin time **[PT], partial** thromboplastin time **[PTT], and fibrinogen), blood type and screen, or cross-match, serum creatinine, and a drug screen.** Other causes of third-trimester bleeding must be excluded. The **differential diagnosis** includes placenta previa, vasa previa, cervical lesions (for example, malignancy) and vaginal lesions.
- An **ultrasound examination** is useful primarily in the exclusion of placenta previa or vasa previa. The sensitivity and specificity of ultrasound in the diagnosis of placental abruption were 24% and 96%, respectively [53]. Of note, a placental abruption was defined in this study by clinical signs or symptoms or by placental examination. So **while ultrasound is very helpful in ruling out other causes of third-trimester bleeding, it lacks the sensitivity needed to reliably detect placental abruption** [53]. The echogenicity of the collection of blood of an abruption depends on the time the ultrasound was performed relative to the onset of symptoms [54]. Acute hemorrhage is hyperechoic to isoechoic compared with the placenta. Resolving hematomas become hypoechoic within 1 week and sonolucent within 2 weeks.
- **Computed tomography (CT)** has been used to identify abruptions in trauma patients. A retrospective study of pregnant trauma patients who were evaluated with CT found a high sensitivity (86%) and specificity (98%) in the detection of placental abruption [55]. In a retrospective review of pregnant trauma patients, **as placental enhancement on CT imaging decreased the presence of clinical findings of placental abruption were found to increase.** The authors found that clinical signs and/or symptoms of abruption were significantly more likely with placental enhancement on CT imaging <50%, and that the likelihood of delivery for abruption increased as the placental enhancement decreased to less than 25% [56].
- **Magnetic resonance (MR)** imaging has also been used to identify placental abruption. In a prospective series of 60 consecutive patients with clinical suspicion of abruption ultrasound imaging and MR imaging were compared. Placental abruption (defined as adherent clot or fibrin by placental examination at delivery) was found in 19 patients. Abruption was identified in 10 of the 19 patients (52%) with ultrasound and in all 19 (100%) with MR imaging ($p = .002$) [57]. This study underscores the relative ability of imaging modalities to identify retroplacental collections, but the presence of absence of adherent placental clot does not always correlate with a clinical abruption.

- A **vaginal speculum examination** should be performed to rule out cervical or vaginal sources of bleeding.
- **Laboratory findings**: A prolonged PT, prolonged PTT, hypofibrinogenemia, and thrombocytopenia can occur in women with abruption for whom DIC develops. D-dimer, a fibrin degradation product, has been evaluated as a diagnostic tool for abruption in two small studies with conflicting results [58,59]; at present the data do not support its routine use. The Kleihauer–Betke (KB) test for fetal red cells in the maternal circulation appears to be a low yield test for women with abruption. In a recent retrospective study of women with a clinical abruption who were screened with a KB, only 3 of 65 were positive (sensitivity 4.4%) [60]. An earlier retrospective study reported **no positive** KB tests out of 27 cases of abruption confirmed by pathology [61].

General Principles

Once the diagnosis of placental abruption has been made, attention should be focused on ensuring maternal and fetal well-being. **Maternal status** should be addressed with attention paid to signs or symptoms of hemorrhage, hypovolemic shock, and DIC. The frequency of repeated evaluations is dependent primarily on the acuity and severity of the abruption. Preparations should be made in anticipation of potential maternal complications. This should include **intravenous access; two large-bore peripheral lines** will allow for rapid fluid or blood component replacement. The **availability of blood** or blood components may be life saving; therefore, close cooperation with blood banking services is essential.

Fetal status is typically assessed with **continuous electronic fetal monitoring,** at least in the acute setting. For women with a chronic abruption, once clinically stable, intermittent monitoring may be a consideration.

Timing of Delivery

Late-Preterm or Term Placental Abruption: ≥34 Weeks
Prompt delivery is indicated if the pregnancy is ≥34 weeks [62–64]. Fortunately rapid labor often ensues as a result of the abruption (Figure 29.1).

Preterm Abruption: <34 Weeks
Maternal or fetal compromise necessitates delivery. In selected patients with mild (grade 1) abruption, with no evidence of maternal or fetal compromise, expectant management may allow time for glucocorticoid administration and appears to be a safe option [1,15,64]. Tocolysis should in general not be used. Antepartum testing should be frequent, and at least initially, continuous fetal monitoring is indicated.

Mode of Delivery

Deciding on the method of delivery is dependent primarily on the condition of the mother and fetus.

Mild Abruption (Grade 1): No Evidence of Maternal or Fetal Compromise
With close monitoring of the mother and fetus, **vaginal delivery** may be accomplished. In studies of women with mild (or grade 1) abruptions, those who delivered vaginally had a similar perinatal mortality rates compared with those with a cesarean delivery [62].

Moderate Abruption (Grade 2): Evidence of Fetal Compromise
Rapid delivery: typically **cesarean delivery** is indicated. In a study of placental abruption complicated by fetal bradycardia, a decision-to-delivery interval of ≤20 minutes was associated with substantially reduced neonatal morbidity and mortality [65].

Severe Abruption (Grade 3): Fetal Death, Often with DIC
Vaginal delivery is preferred in this group as a cesarean delivery may exacerbate maternal hemorrhage. If present, DIC will typically resolve with evacuation of the uterus, with possible improvement in clotting parameters even prior to delivery [66,67].

Anesthesia

No specific suggestions. Anesthesia support is particularly important with DIC, hemorrhagic shock, and massive transfusion cases.

Postpartum

Attention should be paid to hemodynamic state and possible late hemorrhage from uterine atony after abruption.

REFERENCES

1. Hurd WW, Miodovnik M, Hertzberg V, et al. Selective management of abruptio placentae: A prospective study. *Obstet Gynecol.* 1983;61(4):467–473. [II-2]
2. Kasai M, Aoki S, Ogawa M, et al. Prediction of perinatal outcomes based on primary symptoms in women with placental abruption. *J Obstet Gynaecol Res.* 2015;41(6):850–856. [II-2]
3. Ananth CV, Oyelese Y, Yeo L, et al. Placental abruption in the United States, 1979 through 2001: Temporal trends and potential determinants. *Am J Obstet Gynecol.* 2005;192(1):191–198. [Epidemiological review]
4. Ruiter L, Ravelli AC, de Graaf IM, et al. Incidence and recurrence rate of placental abruption: A longitudinal linked national cohort study in the Netherlands. *Am J Obstet Gynecol.* 2015;213(4):573.e1–8. [II-2]
5. Ananth CV, Lavery JA, Vintzileos AM, et al. Severe placental abruption: Clinical definition and associations with maternal complications. *Am J Obstet Gynecol.* 2016;214(2):272.e1–272.e9. [II-2]
6. Oyelese Y, Ananth CV. Placental abruption. *Obstet Gynecol.* 2006;108(4):1005–1016. [Review]
7. Workalemahu T, Enquobahrie DA, Moore A, et al. Genome-wide and candidate gene association studies of placental abruption. *Int J Mol Epidemiol Genet.* 2013;4(3):128–139. [II-2]
8. Brosens I, Pijnenborg R, Vercruysse L, Romero R. The great obstetrical syndromes are associated with disorders of deep placentation. *Am J Obstet Gynecol.* 2011;204(3):193–201. [Review]
9. Dommisse J, Tiltman AJ. Placental bed biopsies in placental abruption. *Br J Obstet Gynaecol.* 1992;99(8):651–654. [II-3]
10. Signore C, Mills JL, Qian C, et al. Circulating angiogenic factors and placental abruption. *Obstet Gynecol.* 2006;108(2):338–344. [II-2]
11. Naeye RL, Harkness WL, Utts J. Abruptio placentae and perinatal death: A prospective study. *Am J Obstet Gynecol.* 1977;128(7):740–746. [II-3]
12. Couvelaire A. Classic pages in obstetrics and gynecology: Alexandre Couvelaire. *Am J Obstet Gynecol.* 1973;116(6):875. [II-3]
13. Gluck L, University of Califorha, San Diego, Department of Pediatrics, Johnson & Johnson Baby Products Company. Institute for Pediatric Service. *Intrauterine Asphyxia and the Developing Fetal Brain.* xvii, 507 p. 2–3. Chicago, IL: Year Book Medical Publishers, 1977.
14. Heller DS, Keane-Tarchichi M, Varshney S. Is pathologic confirmation of placental abruption more reliable in cases due to chronic etiologies compared with acute etiologies? *J Perinat Med.* 2013;41(6):701–703. [II-2]
15. Sholl JS. Abruptio placentae: Clinical management in nonacute cases. *Am J Obstet Gynecol.* 1987;156(1):40–51. [II-3]
16. Toivonen S, Heinonen S, Anttila M, et al. Reproductive risk factors, Doppler findings, and outcome of affected births

17. Rasmussen S, Irgens LM, Dalaker K. The effect on the likelihood of further pregnancy of placental abruption and the rate of its recurrence. *Br J Obstet Gynaecol*. 1997;104(11):1292–1295. [II-2]
18. Ananth CV, Smulian JC, Vintzileos AM. Incidence of placental abruption in relation to cigarette smoking and hypertensive disorders during pregnancy: A meta-analysis of observational studies. *Obstet Gynecol*. 1999;93(4):622–628. [Meta-analysis: 13 studies, n = 1,358,083]
19. Sibai BM, Lindheimer M, Hauth J, et al. Risk factors for preeclampsia, abruptio placentae, and adverse neonatal outcomes among women with chronic hypertension. National Institute of Child Health and Human Development Network of Maternal-Fetal Medicine Units. *N Engl J Med*. 1998;339(10):667–671. [II-2 secondary analysis of RCT data]
20. Higgins SD, Garite TJ. Late abruptio placenta in trauma patients: Implications for monitoring. *Obstet Gynecol*. 1984;63(3 Suppl):10S–12S. [II-2]
21. Dombrowski MP, Wolfe HM, Welch RA, Evans MI. Cocaine abuse is associated with abruptio placentae and decreased birth weight, but not shorter labor. *Obstet Gynecol*. 1991;77(1):139–141. [II-2]
22. Getahun D, Oyelese Y, Salihu HM, Ananth CV. Previous cesarean delivery and risks of placenta previa and placental abruption. *Obstet Gynecol*. 2006;107(4):771–778. [II-2]
23. Sheiner E, Shoham-Vardi I, Hallak M, et al. Placental abruption in term pregnancies: Clinical significance and obstetric risk factors. *J Matern Fetal Neonatal Med*. 2003;13(1):45–49. [II-2]
24. Salihu HM, Bekan B, Aliyu MH, et al. Perinatal mortality associated with abruptio placenta in singletons and multiples. *Am J Obstet Gynecol*. 2005;193(1):198–203. [II-2, n = 1.6 million births]
25. Ananth CV, Oyelese Y, Srinivas N, et al. Preterm premature rupture of membranes, intrauterine infection, and oligohydramnios: Risk factors for placental abruption. *Obstet Gynecol*. 2004;104(1):71–77. [II-2, n = 11,777]
26. Salafia CM, López-Zeno JA, Sherer DM, et al. Histologic evidence of old intrauterine bleeding is more frequent in prematurity. *Am J Obstet Gynecol*. 1995;173(4):1065–1070. [II-2]
27. Lockwood CJ, Toti P, Arcuri F, et al. Mechanisms of abruption-induced premature rupture of the fetal membranes: Thrombin-enhanced interleukin-8 expression in term decidua. *Am J Pathol*. 2005;167(5):1443–1449. [II-2]
28. Stout MJ, Odibo AO, Graseck AS, et al. Leiomyomas at routine second-trimester ultrasound examination and adverse obstetric outcomes. *Obstet Gynecol*. 2010;116(5):1056–1063. [II-2]
29. Ananth CV, Oyelese Y, Prasad V, et al. Evidence of placental abruption as a chronic process: Associations with vaginal bleeding early in pregnancy and placental lesions. *Eur J Obstet Gynecol Reprod Biol*. 2006;128(1–2):15–21. [II-2]
30. Katz VL, Chescheir NC, Cefalo RC. Unexplained elevations of maternal serum alpha-fetoprotein. *Obstet Gynecol Surv*. 1990;45(11):719–726. [II-2]
31. Chandra S, Scott H, Dodds L, et al. Unexplained elevated maternal serum alpha-fetoprotein and/or human chorionic gonadotropin and the risk of adverse outcomes. *Am J Obstet Gynecol*. 2003;189(3):775–781. [II-2]
32. Blumenfeld YJ, Baer RJ, Druzin ML, et al. Association between maternal characteristics, abnormal serum aneuploidy analytes, and placental abruption. *Am J Obstet Gynecol*. 2014;211(2):144.e1–144.e9. [II-2]
33. Kupferminc MJ, Eldor A, Steinman N, et al. Increased frequency of genetic thrombophilia in women with complications of pregnancy. *N Engl J Med*. 1999;340(1):9–13. [II-2]
34. Alfirevic Z, Roberts D, Martlew V. How strong is the association between maternal thrombophilia and adverse pregnancy outcome? A systematic review. *Eur J Obstet Gynecol Reprod Biol*. 2002;101(1):6–14. [II-2]
35. Dizon-Townson D, Miller C, Sibai B, et al. The relationship of the factor V Leiden mutation and pregnancy outcomes for mother and fetus. *Obstet Gynecol*. 2005;106(3):517–524. [II-2]
36. Kjellberg U, van Rooijen M, Bremme K, et al. Factor V Leiden mutation and pregnancy-related complications. *Am J Obstet Gynecol*. 2010;203(5):469.e1–8. [II-1]
37. Silver RM, Zhao Y, Spong CY, et al. Prothrombin gene G20210A mutation and obstetric complications. *Obstet Gynecol*. 2010;115(1):14–20. [II-1]
38. Warren JE, Simonsen SE, Branch DW, et al. Thromboprophylaxis and pregnancy outcomes in asymptomatic women with inherited thrombophilias. *Am J Obstet Gynecol*. 2009;200(3):281.e1–281.e5. [II-2]
39. Said JM, Higgins JR, Moses EK, et al. Inherited thrombophilia polymorphisms and pregnancy outcomes in nulliparous women. *Obstet Gynecol*. 2010;115(1):5–13. [II-2]
40. Kramer MS, Usher RH, Pollack R, et al. Etiologic determinants of abruptio placentae. *Obstet Gynecol*. 1997;89(2):221–226. [II-2]
41. Yogev Y, Melamed N, Bardin R, et al. Pregnancy outcome at extremely advanced maternal age. *Am J Obstet Gynecol*. 2010;203(6):558.e1–558.e7. [II-2]
42. Abbassi-Ghanavati M, Casey BM, Spong CY, et al. Pregnancy outcomes in women with thyroid peroxidase antibodies. *Obstet Gynecol*. 2010;116(2 Pt 1):381–386. [II-2]
43. Haddow JE, McClain MR, Palomaki GE, et al. Thyroperoxidase and thyroglobulin antibodies in early pregnancy and placental abruption. *Obstet Gynecol*. 2011;117(2 Pt 1):287–292. [II-2]
44. Breathnach FM, Donnelly J, Cooley SM, et al. Subclinical hypothyroidism as a risk factor for placental abruption: Evidence from a low-risk primigravid population. *Aust N Z J Obstet Gynaecol*. 2013;53(6):553–560. [II-2]
45. Chang J, Elam-Evans LD, Berg CJ, et al. Pregnancy-related mortality surveillance—United States, 1991–1999. *MMWR Surveill Summ*. 2003;52(2):1–8. [Epidemiological review]
46. Page EW, King EB, Merrill JA. Abruptio placentae: Dangers of delay in delivery. *Obstet Gynecol*. 1954;3(4 SRC - GoogleScholar):385–393. [II-2]
47. Ananth CV, Wilcox AJ. Placental abruption and perinatal mortality in the United States. *Am J Epidemiol*. 2001;153(4):332–337. [II-2, n = 53,371]
48. Nath CA, Ananth CV, DeMarco C, et al. Low birthweight in relation to placental abruption and maternal thrombophilia status. *Am J Obstet Gynecol*. 2008;198(3):293.e1–293.e5. [II-2]
49. Gilbert WM, Jacoby BN, Xing G, et al. Adverse obstetric events are associated with significant risk of cerebral palsy. *Am J Obstet Gynecol*. 2010;203(4):328.e1–328.e5. [II-2]
50. Neilson JP. Interventions for treating placental abruption. *Cochrane Database Syst Rev*. 2003;(1):CD003247. [Systematic review]
51. Abramovici A, Gandley R, Clifton R, et al. Prenatal vitamin C and E supplementation in smokers is associated with reduced placental abruption and preterm birth: A secondary analysis. *BJOG*. 2015;122(13):1740–1747. [I]
52. Duley L, Gulmezoglu AM, Chou D. Magnesium sulphate versus lytic cocktail for eclampsia. *Cochrane Database Syst Rev*. 2010;(9):CD002960. [Systematic review meta-analysis]
53. Glantz C, Purnell L. Clinical utility of sonography in the diagnosis and treatment of placental abruption. *J Ultrasound Med*. 2002;21(8):837–840. [II-2]
54. Nyberg DA, Cyr DR, Mack LA, et al. Sonographic spectrum of placental abruption. *AJR Am J Roentgenol*. 1987;148(1):161–164. [II-2]
55. Manriquez M, Srinivas G, Bollepalli S, et al. Is computed tomography a reliable diagnostic modality in detecting placental injuries in the setting of acute trauma? *Am J Obstet Gynecol*. 2010;202(6):611.e1–611.e5. [II-2]
56. Kopelman TR, Berardoni NE, Manriquez M, et al. The ability of computed tomography to diagnose placental abruption in the trauma patient. *J Trauma Acute Care Surg*. 2013;74(1):236–241. [II-2]

57. Masselli G, Brunelli R, Di Tola M, et al. MR imaging in the evaluation of placental abruption: Correlation with sonographic findings. *Radiology*. 2011;259(1):222–230. [II-2]
58. Nolan TE, Smith RP, Devoe LD. A rapid test for abruptio placentae: Evaluation of a D-dimer latex agglutination slide test. *Am J Obstet Gynecol*. 1993;169(2 Pt 1):265–268; discussion 268–269. [II-2]
59. Neiger R, Krohn HJ, Trofatter MO. Plasma fibrin D-dimer in pregnancies complicated by partial placental abruption. *Tenn Med*. 1997;90(10):403–405. [II-2]
60. Atkinson AL, Santolaya-Forgas J, Matta P, et al. The sensitivity of the Kleihauer–Betke test for placental abruption. *J Obstet Gynaecol*. 2015;35(2):139–141. [II-2]
61. Emery CL, Morway LF, Chung-Park M, et al. The Kleihauer–Betke test. Clinical utility, indication, and correlation in patients with placental abruption and cocaine use. *Arch Pathol Lab Med*. 1995;119(11):1032–1037. [II-2]
62. Knab DR. Abruptio placentae. An assessment of the time and method of delivery. *Obstet Gynecol*. 1978;52(5):625–629. [II-2]
63. Combs CA, Nyberg DA, Mack LA, et al. Expectant management after sonographic diagnosis of placental abruption. *Am J Perinatol*. 1992;9(3):170–174. [II-2]
64. Bond AL, Edersheim TG, Curry L, et al. Expectant management of abruptio placentae before 35 weeks gestation. *Am J Perinatol*. 1989;6(2):121–123. [II-2]
65. Kayani SI, Walkinshaw SA, Preston C. Pregnancy outcome in severe placental abruption. *BJOG*. 2003;110(7):679–683. [II-2]
66. Twaalfhoven FC, van Roosmalen J, Briët E, et al. Conservative management of placental abruption complicated by severe clotting disorders. *Eur J Obstet Gynecol Reprod Biol*. 1992;46(1):25–30. [II-2]
67. Sher G, Statland BE. Abruptio placentae with coagulopathy: A rational basis for management. *Clin Obstet Gynecol*. 1985;28(1):15–23. [II-2]

Postpartum care

Sarah K. Dotters-Katz and Alison M. Stuebe

Postpartum care includes breast-feeding, contraception, postpartum endometritis, postpartum wound complications, and postpartum mood and anxiety disorders.

BREAST-FEEDING
KEY POINTS

- **In normal reproductive physiology, lactation follows pregnancy.** For the infant, use of artificial breast milk substitutes is associated with increased acute and chronic disease risk. For mothers, never or curtailed (e.g., short-term) breast-feeding is associated with increased risks of malignancy and metabolic disease.
- **All major medical organizations recommend 6 months of exclusive breast-feeding**, with continued breast-feeding through 1–2 years, or longer as mutually desired by mother and infant.
- **Infant demand drives maternal milk supply.** To ensure adequate milk production, encourage **frequent, on-demand feeding in response to infant cues, continuing until the infant is satisfied.**
- **Pre- and postnatal lay and/or professional support and evidence-based physician training** improve breast-feeding duration and exclusivity.
- **Maternity care practices affect breast-feeding initiation and duration.** Implementation of the United Nations International Children's Emergency Fund (UNICEF)/World Health Organization (WHO) Baby Friendly Hospital Initiative (BHI) improves breast-feeding duration, intensity, and infant health outcomes.
- Prenatal treatment of inverted nipples does not increase breast-feeding success.
- Distribution of formula company marketing materials and samples adversely affects breast-feeding outcomes. **Formula company materials should not be distributed in healthcare facilities.**
- At birth, early skin-to-skin contact increases breast-feeding duration. **Healthy infants should be placed skin-to-skin on the mother's chest** and remain there, undisturbed, until the first feeding is accomplished.
- Treatment for mastitis begins with frequent removal of milk, hydration, and analgesia. **Healthy term infants can continue to feed on the affected side.** Antibiotics are used if conservative management is ineffective or the patient is acutely ill.
- There is limited evidence that galactogogues increase milk production in placebo-controlled trials. Optimal breast-feeding education can increase milk supply among women with low production.
- Most medications are compatible with breast-feeding, or a safe alternative medication exists. **The physiology of the placenta differs from the breast,** and providers should not extrapolate drug safety information from pregnancy to lactation.
- Breast-feeding is contraindicated in the setting of an infant with classic galactosemia, active maternal use of illicit drugs, maternal medications that are contraindicated in breast-feeding, or maternal infection with human T-cell lymphotropic virus type I or II (e.g., HTLV). Recommendations for breast-feeding in the setting of maternal human immunodeficiency virus (HIV) or tuberculosis vary by region. Women with HIV in the United States are advised not to breast-feed because of the risk of maternal–infant transmission and the availability of safe artificial feeding. Breast-feeding is **temporarily contraindicated** during perinatal maternal varicella infection or from a breast with an active herpetic lesion.

Definition
Breast-feeding is the physiologic form of infant nutrition. Breast-feeding is defined as the infant receiving any amount of human milk. **Exclusive breast-feeding** is defined as receiving human milk alone for nutrition. **Predominant breast-feeding** is defined as receiving human milk and nonformula supplements, and **mixed feeding** is defined as receiving both human milk and infant formula.

Breast-Feeding Physiology
Secretory differentiation occurs during pregnancy, as placental hormones stimulate development of mammary alveoli. After birth, secretory activation occurs, as progesterone levels fall and milk production increases from 50 mL/day to approximately 500 mL/day in the first 2–3 days after birth. **Positive feedback via infant stimulation** of the breast causes secretion of prolactin from the anterior pituitary and oxytocin from the posterior pituitary. **Prolactin** stimulates continuous milk synthesis, whereas **oxytocin** stimulates intermittent milk secretion, when myoepithelial cells contract to transfer milk from the alveoli to the areola. If milk is not removed regularly, negative feedback downregulates prolactin receptors and reduces production [1]. Frequent, on-demand feeding is essential to establish and maintain lactation.

Health Effects of Infant Feeding
Infants who are artificially fed face higher risks of infectious morbidity and chronic disease than infants who are breast-fed. An Agency for Healthcare Research and Quality (AHRQ) meta-analysis of outcomes in developed countries found that **artificially fed infants** faced a 2.0-fold risk of **otitis media**, a 3.6-fold risk of **pneumonia**, and a 2.8-fold risk of **gastrointestinal infection** compared with infants who were exclusively breast-fed [2]. Artificial feeding is also associated with a 1.8- to 3.7-fold [3] risk of **sudden infant death syndrome** (SIDS),

a 1.1- to 1.4-fold [4] risk of **child obesity**, and a 1.5-fold risk of **type 2 diabetes** [4] compared with breast-feeding. Artificial or mixed feeding is also associated with higher risks of **asthma**, odds ratio (OR) 1.2–1.3 [5], compared with exclusive breast-feeding. Among preterm infants, artificial feeding is associated with a 5% absolute increased risk of **necrotizing enterocolitis** compared with being fed mother's milk [2].

For mothers, artificial feeding is similarly associated with increased health risks. Compared with women who have breast-fed, parous women who have never breast-fed or weaned early face **higher rates of breast cancer** [6,7], particularly triple-negative breast cancer [8–10], **ovarian cancer** [11], **retained gestational weight gain** [12,13], **type 2 diabetes** [14–17], **hyperlipidemia** [18], **metabolic syndrome** [19,20], **hypertension** [16,21,22], **and myocardial infarction** [16,23].

Optimal Duration of Exclusive Breast-Feeding

Six months of exclusive breast-feeding, compared with 3–4 months of exclusive breast-feeding with mixed feeding through 6 months, reduces infant risk of gastrointestinal and respiratory tract infections without any adverse effect on infant growth [24]. For mothers, longer exclusive breast-feeding was associated with delayed resumption of menses and, in one small study, with greater maternal weight loss [25].

Infant Feeding Recommendations

All major medical organizations [26–29] *recommend* exclusive breast-feeding for the first 6 months of life. The WHO recommends continued breast-feeding up to 2 years of age or beyond [29]. The American Academy of Pediatrics (AAP) recommends continued breast-feeding for at least the first year of life, continuing for as long as mutually desired by mother and child [30].

Promoting Breast-Feeding

Antenatal interventions can increase breast-feeding initiation and duration (Table 30.1) [31]. Breast-feeding education improves initiation rates among low-income U.S. populations. In subgroup analyses, one-on-one, needs-based, informal education sessions were more effective (relative risk [RR] 2.40, 95% confidence interval [CI] 1.57–3.67) than generic, formal antenatal sessions (RR 1.26, 95% CI 1.00–1.60) [32]. Both lay and professional supports for mothers after birth improve breast-feeding duration and exclusivity, with the strongest effects found with proactive, face-to-face, lay support involving four to eight contacts [33]. An USPSTF review similarly found that interventions to promote and support breast-feeding increase initiation, duration, and exclusivity of breast-feeding (grade B). Interventions that include both prenatal and postnatal components may be most effective [34]. **Proactive, integrated pre- and postnatal support for breast-feeding mothers improves breast-feeding duration and intensity.**

Training of Providers
Breast-feeding education and knowledge among healthcare providers is inconsistent [35–37]. A meta-analysis found that training breast-feeding support personnel using the WHO/UNICEF breast-feeding training course [38] increases duration of exclusive breast-feeding. In a cluster-randomized trial, implementation of a breast-feeding training curriculum for residents improved provider knowledge, practice patterns, and confidence, and increased exclusive breast-feeding rates at 6 months (OR 4.1) compared with control sites [39]. Interventions for hospital staff are similarly associated with improved breast-feeding outcomes [40]. **Healthcare providers who work with mother and infants should receive comprehensive breast-feeding training.**

The Baby Friendly Initiative
Maternity care affects breast-feeding outcomes. The Baby Friendly Initiative (BFI) is WHO-developed set of maternity care recommendations designed to increase initiation and duration of breast-feeding. The BFI requires maternity centers to implement The Ten Steps to Successful Breast-feeding (Table 30.2) [41]. Each country is responsible for establishing processes and procedures for maternity center designation as baby friendly [41]. In a cluster-randomized trial in Belarus, BFI implementation improved breast-feeding exclusivity at 3 months (43.3% vs. 6.4%, $p < .001$) and 6 months (7.9% vs. 0.6%, $p = .01$) and increased any breast-feeding rates at 12 months (19.7% vs. 11.4%). Infants born in intervention hospitals had lower rates of gastrointestinal illness and atopic eczema in the first year of life [42]. Observational studies in the United States have found a dose–response association between implementation of BFI steps and maternal achievement of breast-feeding goals [43,44]. Cohort studies suggest that the Ten Steps are particularly effective among women with lower education, suggesting that BFI maternity care can reduce socioeconomic disparities in breast-feeding [45].

The National Institute for Health and Clinical Excellence (NICE) postnatal care guideline recommends that all healthcare

Table 30.1 Successful Breast-Feeding Recommendations

Offer additional breast-feeding support to women who have had a narcotic/general anesthetic, a caesarean, or delayed contact with their baby.
Ensure breast pumps are available for women who have been separated from their babies, and give instruction on how to use them.
Encourage unrestricted breast-feeding frequency and duration.
Reassure women about breast milk supply and help them gain confidence.
Advise women that babies will stop feeding when satisfied.
Advise women of the signs that a baby is successfully feeding:
- Swallowing is audible and visible.
- There is a sustained rhythmic suck.
- The arms and hands are relaxed.
- The mouth is moist.
- Regular soaked/heavy nappies.

Reassure women that they may feel the following:
- Brief discomfort at the start of feeds in the first few days; this is not uncommon but should not persist.
- Softening of their breast during the feed.
- No compression of the nipple at the end of the feed.
- Relaxed and sleepy.

Attachment and positioning
Advise women of the following signs of good attachment and positioning:
- The baby's mouth is wide open.
- There is less areola visible underneath the chin than above the nipple.
- The baby's chin is touching the breast, the lower lip is rolled down, and the nose is free.
- There is no pain.

If the baby is not attaching effectively, advise teasing the baby's lips with the nipple to open the mouth.

Source: Modified from National Institute for Health and Clinical Excellence, Quick Reference Guide. NICE Clinical Guideline No. 37: Routine Postnatal Care of Women and Their Babies, NICE, London, United Kingdom, 2006.

Table 30.2 Ten Steps to Successful Breast-Feeding

Every facility providing maternity services and care for newborn infants should:
1. Have a written breast-feeding policy that is routinely communicated to all healthcare staff.
2. Train all healthcare staff in skills necessary to implement this policy.
3. Inform all pregnant women abwout the benefits and management of breast-feeding.
4. Help mothers initiate breast-feeding within a half-hour of birth.
5. Show mothers how to breast-feed, and how to maintain lactation even if they should be separated from their infants.
6. Give newborn infants no food or drink other than breast milk unless medically indicated.
7. Practice rooming in—allow mothers and infants to remain together—24 hours a day.
8. Encourage breast-feeding on demand.
9. Give no artificial teats or pacifiers (also called dummies or soothers) to breast-feeding infants.
10. Foster the establishment of breast-feeding support groups and refer mothers to them on discharge from the hospital or clinic.

Source: Modified from World Health Organization, UNICEF, *Baby Friendly Hospital Initiative: Revised, Updated and Expanded for Integrated Care*, World Health Organization, Geneva, Switzerland, 2009.

providers should implement a structured program that encourages breast-feeding, using the BFI as a minimum standard [31] (Table 30.1).

Breast-Feeding in Clinical Care

Antenatal Breast Examination
Clinical guidelines recommend evaluation of breast anatomy as part of prenatal care [27,46]. However, there are no randomized controlled trials (RCTs) regarding the effects of an antenatal breast examination on breast-feeding outcomes or maternal satisfaction [47]. **There is no evidence that antenatal manipulation for inverted nipples improves breast-feeding outcomes [48,49].**

Avoiding Commercial Infant Feeding Materials
In randomized trials, provision of formula company materials and gift packs during prenatal care [50] or during the maternity hospitalization [51–53] reduces exclusive breast-feeding. In a time series design study, changing from formula marketing discharge packs to noncommercial packs was associated with higher breast-feeding rates, but more than one-third of women in the noncommercial cohort received formula samples, demonstrating that policy implementation is challenging [54]. **Formula company marketing materials should not be distributed in the healthcare setting.**

Skin-to-Skin Contact at Birth
Early skin-to-skin contact improves breast-feeding outcomes. Skin-to-skin contact is defined as placing the naked infant prone on the mother's bare chest, with the infant's back covered with a warm blanket, ideally beginning immediately after birth. In a Cochrane meta-analysis, early skin-to-skin contact increased breast-feeding at 1–4 months postbirth (RR 1.27), and increased duration of total breast-feeding by about 6 weeks [55]. Based on these data, the NICE [56], AAP [30], and the American College of Obstetricians and Gynecologists (ACOG) [27] recommend that **all healthy infants should be placed skin-to-skin at birth.** Infants should remain with their mothers for at least 1 hour, and providers should encourage mothers to recognize when the infant is ready to feed and offer help if needed [41]. Routine procedures, such as weighing, bathing, and vitamin K and eye prophylaxis, should be avoided during the first hour, or performed on the mother's chest. Skin-to-skin care during procedures, such as a heel lance, appears to reduce infant pain [57]. Skin-to-skin is also feasible following cesarean section [58].

Anticipatory Guidance to Support Normal Physiology
Human milk production is driven by infant demand. Therefore, **frequent feeding, on demand in response to infant feeding cues, continuing until the infant is satisfied, is a cornerstone of breast-feeding success** [59], although a recent meta-analysis did not identify trials comparing baby-led feeding with scheduled breast-feeding [60]. NICE clinical guidelines have outlined anticipatory guidance for successful breast-feeding (Table 30.1). A small pilot study found that early, limited supplementation with hydrolyzed formula for infants with ≥5% weight loss increased exclusive breast-feeding rates at 1 week and 3 months postpartum [61]; several trials to test whether these findings can be replicated are underway (NCT02313181 and NCT02221167).

Management of Breast-Feeding Complications

Engorgement
Breast engorgement typically occurs between 2 and 5 days postpartum. A meta-analysis found insufficient evidence to support any single treatment strategy for engorgement [62].

Cold packs and cabbage leaves may be helpful, and acupuncture was associated with some improvement in symptoms. NICE guidelines recommend **breast massage, continued breast-feeding, and analgesia** for symptom relief [31].

Mastitis
Mastitis is defined as acute inflammation of connective tissue within the breast, which may or may not be accompanied by infection [63]. Interventions to prevent mastitis have not proven effective [64]. A Cochrane meta-analysis (two RCTs, $n = 125$ patients) concluded that there is insufficient evidence to support treatment with antibiotics [65]. An RCT suggests that lactobacilli strains isolated from breast milk may be effective for treatment of mastitis [66].

Clinical guidelines emphasize **effective milk removal, hydration, and analgesia** as key elements of clinical management of mastitis. Healthy term infants may continue to breast-feed on the affected breast. **If symptoms do not improve with conservative management or the woman is acutely ill, antibiotics are recommended. Penicillinase-resistant penicillins** (e.g., dicloxacillin) **are preferred** [67].

Breast-feeding and Maternal Medications
Most medications are compatible with breast-feeding, or a safe alternative medication exists. The physiology of the placenta differs from that of the maternal breast and infant gut, so the provider should not assume that a drug's pregnancy safety profile applies to breast-feeding. Many drug databases utilized by commercial pharmacies do not contain accurate information on drug safety in lactation [68]. The National Library of Medicine's LactMed database (http://lactmed.nlm.nih.gov/) provides a comprehensive set

of monographs on medication safety in lactation. Decisions about medication use in lactation should consider the risks and benefits of maternal treatment or nontreatment, the risk of drug transfer to the infant, and the risks to mother and infant of discontinuing breast-feeding [69]. Maternal providers should collaborate with the pediatric provider regarding counseling about medication use in breast-feeding.

Milk Expression
If mothers and infants are separated, milk expression is necessary to maintain supply and provide milk to the infant. Evidence suggests that **early initiation of milk expression, simultaneous pumping of both breasts, breast massage, relaxation techniques, and expressing milk after kangaroo (i.e., skin-to-skin) mother care** improve milk production among neonatal intensive care unit (NICU) mothers [70–75].

Galactogogues
There is **limited evidence to support pharmacotherapy for low milk supply** [76,77]. Two small randomized, placebo-controlled, blinded studies have found that domperidone increases milk supply among mothers of preterm infants [78,79]. Domperidone is not approved by the U.S. Food and Drug Administration (FDA) for any indication. Routine use of metoclopramide in the early postpartum period does not improve milk production [80,81]. In two studies among women with low milk supply who received education on optimal breast-feeding [82,83], metoclopramide provided no additional benefit compared with placebo. The AAP notes that galactogogues have a limited role in facilitating lactation; mothers experiencing milk production difficulties should undergo assessment by a lactation specialist and be offered nonpharmacologic measures to increase supply [69].

Maternal Diet during Lactation
In two small trials, maternal dietary restrictions during lactation did not reduce the incidence of atopic eczema or the severity of existing disease [84]. Maternal supplementation with long-chain polyunsaturated fatty acids (LCPUFA) during lactation does not improve infant neurodevelopmental outcomes. In two studies, LCPUFA supplementation increased infant head circumference [85]. A meta-analysis found limited evidence for LCPUFA supplementation during pregnancy and/or lactation to reduce allergic diseases in children [86]. **There is insufficient evidence to recommend LCPUFA supplementation during breast-feeding.**

Contraindications
Breast-feeding is contraindicated in the setting of the following:

- Infant with classic galactosemia (galactose-1-phosphate uridyltransferase deficiency).
- Maternal medications:
  - Mothers with current, active illicit drug use, in absence of a coordinated treatment plan among maternal and infant providers [87].
  - Mothers requiring medications that are contraindicated in breast-feeding.
- Maternal infectious disease:
  - Mothers who are HTLV type I or II positive.
  - Mothers with untreated brucellosis.
  - Mothers with active herpetic lesions on the breast(s). Mothers can continue to breast-feed on the unaffected breast, and provide expressed milk from the affected breast.
  - Mothers with varicella onset within 5 days before until 48 hours after delivery should be separated from their infants, but expressed milk can be provided to the infant.
  - Mothers with HIV infection in settings where safe artificial feeding is available (see below).

Tuberculosis
The AAP lists active, untreated tuberculosis as a contraindication to breast-feeding. According to AAP guidelines, the infant may continue to receive expressed milk while the mother is treated, but mother and infant should be separated until the mother is treated for a minimum of 2 weeks and is documented to be no longer infectious [30]. The WHO recommends continued breast-feeding in the setting of maternal tuberculosis. The infant should be treated with 6 months of isoniazid preventive therapy, followed by immunization with Bacillus Calmette–Guérin (BCG) [88].

Human Immunodeficiency Virus
Artificial infant feeding is efficacious in preventing maternal–child transmission of HIV, but RCTs in regions of the world where access to clean water is limited demonstrate similar mortality and malnutrition among breast-fed and artificially fed infants. If infants are breast-fed, early exclusive breast-feeding and extended antiretroviral prophylaxis reduce the risk of HIV transmission [89].

Women with HIV in the United States are advised not to breast-feed because of the risk of maternal–infant transmission and the availability of safe artificial feeding.

The WHO recommends that national or subnational health authorities determine recommendations regarding infant feeding for HIV-positive mothers, balancing HIV prevention with protection from other causes of child mortality [90]. In countries where breast-feeding is recommended, antiretroviral prophylaxis for mothers and infants reduces HIV transmission. Exclusive breast-feeding is recommended for the first 6 months, continuing through 1 year. When mothers decide to stop breast-feeding, they are advised to wean gradually, over 1 month, and mothers or infants receiving antiretroviral prophylaxis should continue for 1 week after breast-feeding is fully stopped.

CONTRACEPTION
Key Points
- **Postpartum educational interventions can increase contraceptive use and delay repeat pregnancy.**
- **Intrauterine device (IUD)** placement <48 hours postpartum is not associated with infectious morbidity, but expulsion rates are higher than with placement >4 weeks. Since many women do not present for postpartum follow-up, overall IUD **use is highest when inserted in the immediate postpartum period.**
- Postpartum tubal ligation (PPTL) is highly effective. However, risk of regret is higher for PPTL than for interval TL.
- Postpartum placement of the contraceptive implant shows promise as an additional long-acting option for women early in the postpartum period, with potentially less lactogenic effects.
- Lactation amenorrhea is an effective but not perfect method of contraception, until the infant is 6 months old, begins complementary feeding, or the mother's menses resume.

- Barrier methods are preferred during lactation compared with hormonal contraception because of theoretical effects of hormonal methods on milk supply and hormone exposure for the infant.

Background

Sexual activity is resumed by about 53% of women within 6 weeks postpartum, with 41% attempting vaginal sex. By 8 weeks, about 65% attempt vaginal sex. Women with uncomplicated vaginal births resume sex earlier, compared with women who had perineal lacerations, assisted vaginal births, or cesarean deliveries [91]. Two-thirds of women have unmet contraceptive needs after childbirth [92]. Educational interventions during the postpartum hospitalization increase contraceptive use, compared with no intervention. Home visit programs reduce repeat pregnancies among teenagers [93].

Contraceptive Guidelines

A detailed review of contraception is behind the scope of this book. The WHO has published detailed guidelines regarding timing of initiation of postpartum contraception and other relative and absolute contraindications. Postpartum recommendations for healthy women are summarized in Tables 30.3 and 30.4. The full guidelines are available online [94].

Intrauterine Devices

IUDs are highly effective methods of contraception. Unfortunately less than 50% of women who express interest in an IUD postpartum actually receive one [95]. **Immediate postpartum placement** has been shown to be safe, and allows women to access contraception during the maternity hospitalization though is associated with an increased risk of expulsion compared with delayed insertion [96,97]. In an RCT of postplacental versus delayed insertion, women randomized to postplacental insertion were more likely to have a device inserted (98% vs. 90.2%, $p = .20$). There were no differences between groups in IUD use at 6 months postpartum (84.3% vs. 76.5%). However, among women who were ineligible for the study and were advised to follow-up for IUD placement as part of routine postpartum care, only 26.8% were using an IUD at 6 months postpartum [98]. These results were confirmed in a more recent Cochrane review, with IUC use at 6 months twice as likely, though expulsion four times more likely [99]. These results suggest that **women undergoing postplacental placement are more likely to use an IUD than those advised to follow-up for placement during routine postpartum care.**

Postpartum Sterilization

Sterilization is the most commonly used form of contraception worldwide. **Postpartum partial salpingectomy has a 1 year failure rate of 0.6/1000 and a 10-year failure rate of 7.5/1000,** which compares favorably with other sterilization methods [100,101]. In a small RCT, operative times were shorter with postpartum Filshie clip placement compared with the Pomeroy technique, but failure rates were not evaluated [102]. Another larger RCT with 1400 women compared postpartum titanium clips to partial salpingectomy (Pomeroy technique);

Table 30.4 WHO Guidelines for Intrauterine Devices

	Breast-feeding	Not Breast-feeding
LNG-IUD, <48 hours postpartum	2	1
Cu-IUD, <48 hours postpartum	1	1
LNG-IUD or Cu-IUD >48 hours to <4 weeks	3	3
>4 weeks	1	1
Puerperal sepsis	4	4

Source: Modified from World Health Organization, UNICEF, BFHI Section 3: Breastfeeding Promotion and Support in a Baby-Friendly Hospital, a 20-Hour Course for Maternity Staff, World Health Organization, Geneva, Switzerland, 2009. [Guideline]
Abbreviations: CU-IND, copper-bearing intrauterine device; LNG-IUD, levonorgestrel-releasing intrauterine device.
Notes: 1: A condition for which there is no restriction for the use of the contraceptive method; 2: A condition where the advantages of using the method generally outweigh the theoretical or proven risks; 3: A condition where the theoretical or proven risks usually outweigh the advantages of using the method; 4: A condition that represents an unacceptable health risk if the contraceptive method is used.

Table 30.3 WHO Guidelines for Postpartum Contraception: Hormonal Contraception

	Progestin-Only Methods[a]	Combined Hormonal Contraceptives[b]
Breast-feeding		
<6 weeks postpartum	3/2[c]	4
>6 weeks to <6 months postpartum (primarily breast-feeding)	1	3
>6 months postpartum	1	2
Not breast-feeding		
<21 days postpartum	1	(1) Without other risk factors for VTE: 3 (2) With other risk factors for VTE: 3/4
>21 days to 42 days	1	(1) Without other risk factors for VTE: 2 (2) With other risk factors for VTE: 2/3
>42 days	1	1

Source: Modified from World Health Organization, UNICEF, BFHI Section 3: Breastfeeding Promotion and Support in a Baby-Friendly Hospital, a 20-Hour Course for Maternity Staff, World Health Organization, Geneva, Switzerland, 2009.
Abbreviations: VTE, venous thromboembolism; WHO, World Health Organization.
Notes: 1: A condition for which there is no restriction for the use of the contraceptive method; 2: A condition where the advantages of using the method generally outweigh the theoretical or proven risks; 3: A condition where the theoretical or proven risks usually outweigh the advantages of using the method; 4: A condition that represents an unacceptable health risk if the contraceptive method is used.
[a] Progestogen-only pills, levonorgestrel and etonogestrel implants, depot medroxyprogesterone acetate, and norethisterone enanthate.
[b] Combined oral contraceptives, combined contraceptive patch, combined contraceptive vaginal ring, and combined injectable contraceptives.
[c] 3: Depot medroxyprogesterone or norethisterone enanthate, 2: all other Progestogen-only methods.

though this study did not assess operative time, it did find that pregnancy probability at 2 years was .017 and .004 for clips and salpingectomy, respectively ($p = .04$) [103]. Maternal age <30 increases risk of regret and request for tubal reversal [104]. Risk of regret is higher among women undergoing PPTL compared with interval TL. Other risk factors for regret include ligation at the time of C-section, abrupt decision to undergo PPTL, and sterilization performed for obstetrical indications [105].

In a cohort study of women planning postpartum sterilization, one-third did not receive the procedure prior to hospital discharge. Of these women, 47% were pregnant within 1 year, compared with 22% of women who had not planned a postpartum sterilization [106]. Women who desire but do not undergo postpartum sterilization are at high risk for unplanned pregnancy.

Contraception during Breast-Feeding

Breast-feeding reduces fertility and prolongs amenorrhea after childbirth. In the first 6 months after birth, cohort studies suggest that 0%–7.5% of women who are fully breast-feeding and amenorrheic become pregnant [107,108]. To maintain effective protection against pregnancy, another method of contraception must be used as soon as menstruation resumes, the frequency or duration of breast-feeds is reduced, bottle feeds are introduced, or the baby reaches 6 months of age [94].

Nonhormonal methods, such as the copper IUD, and if these are not available, **barrier methods,** including diaphragm, cervical cap, male condom, and female condom, are the **preferred method of contraception during breast-feeding** [109]. The fall in progesterone after birth triggers lactogenesis, raising theoretical concerns that progesterone-containing contraceptives may interfere with lactation, particularly in the early postpartum period. Existing RCTs of hormonal contraception during lactation are of mixed quality, and evidence is insufficient to determine effects on milk production and quality [110]. The WHO medical eligibility criteria for contraceptive use guidelines note that although adverse health effects of exogenous estrogen in infants exposed to combined hormonal contraception have not been reported, existing studies have not been designed to quantify long-term effects. In addition, animal data suggest that progesterone may affect the developing brain, raising questions about the theoretical risks of progestogen-only injectables in the early postpartum period [111]. WHO recommendations regarding hormonal contraception during breast-feeding are listed in Table 30.3. In summary, given the mixed data on hormonal contraception and breast-feeding, the copper IUD or barrier methods are preferred.

WHO guidelines indicate that **breast-feeding women can generally receive the levonorgestrel intrauterine device (LNG-IUD) at <48 hours postpartum** [111]. In a small RCT [112], immediate postpartum placement of an LNG-IUD decreased exclusive breast-feeding rates at 3 and 6 months postpartum compared with insertion at 6–8 weeks. A study comparing insertion at 6–8 weeks of the LNG-IUD with the **Cu T380A IUD** found no differences in breast-feeding outcomes, infant growth, or development [113]. WHO recommendations regarding timing of IUD insertion are listed in Table 30.4.

The **contraceptive implant** is a progesterone-only option that can be placed immediately postpartum. However, theoretical concerns regarding the effect on lactogenesis and lactation exist. In a recent RCT comparing early insertion (1–3 days postpartum) to standard insertion ($n = 69$), there was no difference in hours to lactogenesis (mean difference, −1.4 hours, 95% CI −10.6 to 7.7 hours) or lactation failure (risk difference 0.03, 95% CI −0.02 to 0.08) between the two groups [114]. There was no difference in the percentage of women partially or completely breast-feeding at 3 or 6 months. Women with early insertion were more likely to be contracepting at 3 months. A second small RCT ($n = 24$) used deuterium to index milk ingestion among healthy, term newborns of mothers randomized to immediate postpartum etonogestrel (ENG) implant placement or 6-week placement [115]. Participation was limited to nonobese women who had previously breast-fed for at least 3 months. No differences were found in milk intake.

POSTPARTUM ENDOMETRITIS
Key Points

- The **diagnosis** of postpartum endometritis is based on the presence of ≥2 of the following: fever >100.3°F, at least twice, ≥6 hours apart; fundal tenderness; tachycardia (heart rate >100 beats/minute); and foul-smelling lochia. Endometrial cultures are usually not necessary.
- **Postpartum endometritis is most often associated with cesarean delivery; effective strategies include administration of preoperative antibiotics (either ampicillin or first-generation cephalosporin for just one dose), avoidance of manual placental extraction, nonclosure of both visceral and parietal peritoneum, and suture closure of the subcutaneous tissue when thickness is ≥2 cm.**
- **Gentamicin** and **clindamycin** intravenously, preferably **once daily dosing,** are most effective for the **treatment** of postpartum endometritis.
- Once uncomplicated endometritis has clinically improved with intravenous therapy (usually 24–48 hours afebrile), oral therapy is not indicated.

Diagnosis/Definition
The diagnosis is based on clinical criteria. Table 30.5 describes criteria for diagnosis.

Symptoms/Signs
Those described in Table 30.5, plus abdominal pain, malaise, and elevated white blood cell count.

Epidemiology/Incidence
Endometritis complicates about 1%–3% of vaginal deliveries and 5%–27% of cesarean deliveries [116]. The lower incidence in certain cesarean delivery populations is due to infection precautions at delivery and antibiotic prophylaxis (see Chapter 13). In specific populations such as diabetic, obese, or HIV-positive patients, the risk appears to be higher [117,118].

Etiology/Basic Pathophysiology
Endometritis is an inflammatory process that involves both the endometrium and decidual tissue, secondary to infection. It is surmised that additional factors, (such as host defense, bacterial inoculum, and virulence) other than the presence of bacterial colonization play a role in pathogenesis, since 94% of postpartum patients have positive endometrial samples, but

Table 30.5 Diagnosis of Postpartum Endometritis (≥2 of the Following)

- Fever >100.3°F, at least twice, ≥6 hours apart
- Fundal tenderness
- Tachycardia (heart rate >100 beats/minute)
- Foul-smelling lochia

only a small fraction of these develop the infection. Bacteria usually ascend from the vagina and initially colonize the innermost layer of the endometrial cavity. If this colonization is not treated, infection can spread locally and through the bloodstream, leading to life-threatening complications. The use of prophylactic antibiotics has reduced, but not eliminated, these risks.

Microbiology

Endometrial infection is usually polymicrobial. Isolated bacteria are usually Gram-positive cocci, Gram-negative rods, or anaerobes that might be present in normal female genital tract and presumably reach the endometrium ascending from the vagina (Table 30.6) [119]. A recent systematic review identified isolates from the geneses *Bacteriodes, Staphylococcus, and Streptococcus* as the most common pathogens associated with postpartum endometritis [120]. The presence of these microorganisms and the colonization of the decidua generate multiple microabscesses that trigger invasion of inflammatory cells. These cells release chemical mediators responsible for the different manifestations of endometritis. The presence of two microorganisms in the vagina as assessed by smears or cultures has been associated with postpartum development of endometritis.

Risk Factors/Associations

"Classic" risk factors for postpartum endometritis are shown in Table 30.7 [118,121–127]. Longer labor, longer duration of ruptured membranes, and more frequent vaginal examinations are associated with higher is the risk of infection, as is cesarean or operative vaginal delivery. HIV-positive women with CD-4 count ≤500 cells/mL have similar risks of postpartum endometritis and wound infection as HIV-negative women if they receive prophylactic antibiotics [128,129].

Complications

Treatment failure is uncommon. However, if fevers persist, addition of ampicillin to the primary antibiotic regimen should be considered. When fevers continue to persist, imaging to assess for infected hematoma, pelvic abscess, or septic pelvic thrombophlebitis should be considered. Sepsis is an uncommon complication when endometritis is actively managed. Though rare, endometritis secondary to Group A strep, Clostridium Sordellii, and Staphylococci can lead to necrotizing myometritis, toxic shock syndrome, and multiorgan system failure. Prompt recognition and treatment is imperative when these organisms are present.

Management

Workup

Endometrial cultures are usually not necessary, as the microorganisms identified are usually susceptible to the antibiotic regimens used [130]. Although not a current standard of care [130], some authors recommend the use of endometrial cultures at the time of diagnosis, advocating the need for specific antibiotic coverage [131], but no trials are available to assess their efficacy. Elevation of temperature may be the only sign found in patients with endometritis. Since one single episode of temperature ≥100.4°F (38°C) is commonly present in postpartum patients, and most of them will not develop any infection, **it is recommended that two episodes of temperature elevation outside of the first 24 hours postpartum are identified in order to consider the diagnosis** [132]. Physical examination is the cornerstone for assessment, with midline abdominal pain and uterine tenderness being central findings [133]. Although laboratory studies are not criteria for diagnosis, an increased neutrophil count, as well as elevated proportion of bands, may suggest the presence of an infectious disease [134]. Leukocytosis alone is nonspecific and often physiologic in the postpartum period. However, **urine analysis and culture** should be obtained. The utility of routine **blood cultures** is unclear, though they are useful in immunocompromised patients, those at increased risk for bacterial endocarditis, and for women who present with overt sepsis or fail initial antibiotic therapy [135]. In selected patients, chest X-rays can be taken. Differential diagnosis for a postpartum febrile episode includes atelectasis, pneumonia, viral syndrome, engorgement, mastitis, pyelonephritis, and appendicitis.

Table 30.6 Microorganisms More Frequently Associated with Postpartum Endometritis

Facultative Gram Positive: 51%	Facultative Gram Negative: 28%
Group B streptococci	*Gardnerella vaginalis*
Enterococci	*Escherichia coil*
Staphylococcus epidermidis	*Enterobacter* spp.
Lactobacillus	
Diphtheroids	*Proteus mirabilis*
S. aureus	Others
Others	
Anaerobic: 49%	
Bacteroides bibius	
Peptococcus asaccharolyticus	
Bacteroides spp.	
Peptostreptococcus spp.	
Others	
Veillonella spp.	
Others	

Source: Modified from Rosene K et al., *J Infect Dis*, 153(6), 1028–1037, 1986.

Table 30.7 Risk Factors for Postoperative Endometritis

Cesarean delivery (directly correlated to operative time)
Labor (directly correlated to duration)
Rupture of membranes (directly correlated to duration)
Socioeconomic status
Number of vaginal examinations
Internal fetal monitoring
Manual extraction of placenta
Episiotomy
Operative vaginal delivery
Chorioamnionitis
Preterm delivery
Young age (<17 years old) [121]
Obesity (BMI >30) [122]
Postterm pregnancy
Blood loss [123]
Bacterial vaginosis [124]
GBS colonization [125,126]
Diabetes [118]

Sources: Modified from Diamond MP et al., *Am J Obstet Gynecol*, 155(2), 297–300, 1986; Gibbs RS, *Obstet Gynecol*, 55(5 Suppl); 178S–184S, 1980; Magee KP et al., *Am J Perinatol*, 11(1), 24–26, 1994; Myles TD et al., *Obstet Gynecol*, 100(5 Pt 1), 959–964, 2002; Krohn MA et al., *J Infect Dis*, 179(6), 1410–1415, 1999; Minkoff HL et al., *Am J Obstet Gynecol*, 142(8), 992–995, 1982; Watts DH et al., *Obstet Gynecol*, 75(1), 52–58, 1990.
Abbreviations: BMI, body mass index; GBS, group B streptococcus.

Prevention

Prophylactic antibiotics (either ampicillin or first-generation cephalosporin for just one dose about 30 minutes before skin incision), spontaneous placental removal, nonclosure of both visceral and parietal peritoneum, and suture closure of the subcutaneous tissue when thickness is ≥2 cm should routinely be performed in cesarean delivery (see Chapter 13). Vaginal cleansing with povidone-iodine prior to cesarean delivery, especially in the setting of labor or rupture of membranes should be considered especially if preincision antibiotics cannot be administered [136]. Each of these interventions decreases the incidence of postpartum endometritis and/or fever. In particular, both ampicillin and first-generation cephalosporins have similar efficacy in reducing postoperative endometritis from about 18% to 12%, with no added benefit found in using more broad-spectrum agents [137,138]. In urban, indigenous, mainly Afro-American women with incidence of postpartum endometritis over 24% despite first-generation cephalosporin prophylaxis, the addition of doxycycline 100 mg together with the cephalosporin and azithromycin 1 g orally 6–12 hours postoperatively can decrease the incidence of endometritis to 17%, possibly by targeting *Ureaplasma urealyticum* [139]. The number of vaginal examinations, nulliparity, early gestational age, and cefazolin use were predictors of prophylaxis failure in one study [140]. Cleansing of the vagina with povidone-iodine prior to cesarean delivery has been associated with a reduction in the risk of postpartum endometritis, particularly among women with ruptured membranes [141] (see Chapter 13). In HIV-positive women with a CD4 count less than 500 who had vaginal deliveries, intrapartum cefoxitin reduced the rate of postpartum endometritis by 53% (95% CI 0.24–0.9) [117].

Therapy

Since more than one microorganism is usually involved, a combination of antibiotics is used to assure adequate coverage and prevent resistance. Parenteral, broad-spectrum antibiotics should be initiated and continued until the patient is afebrile. The combination of **gentamicin and clindamycin is appropriate** for the treatment of endometritis [14]. Compared with clindamycin and an aminoglycoside, other regimens have a 1.44 relative risk (RR) of treatment failure [142]. Compared with regimens with **activity against penicillin-resistant anaerobic bacteria**, regimens with poor activity have a 1.94 RR of treatment failure. There was no evidence of difference in incidence of allergic reactions. Cephalosporins were associated with fewer diarrheas. There is no evidence that any one regimen is associated with fewer side effects [142].

In four studies comparing once daily with thrice daily dosing of **gentamicin,** there were fewer failures with **once-daily dosing.** Once-daily gentamicin can be given 5 mg/kg, and once-daily clindamycin phosphate 2700 mg, both intravenously [143]. Thrice-daily dosing consists of clindamycin 900 mg and gentamicin 1.5 mg/kg every 8 hours. It is recommended that levels (peak/trough) of gentamicin should be taken after the third dose, to make sure therapeutic regimens are achieved.

Once uncomplicated endometritis has clinically improved with intravenous therapy (usually 24–48 hours afebrile), oral therapy is not needed; in four trials, there were no differences in outcome with oral therapy versus **no oral therapy** [142].

In low resource setting, where intravenous options are not readily available, alternative regimens should be considered, as untreated infection can lead to sepsis. In a recent systematic review, oral clindamycin with intramuscular genta-mycin was suggested as the first line recommendation, with amoxicillin–clavulanic acid or amoxicillin and metronidazole as alternative regimens [120]. Each of these regimens had at least an 85% cure rate, and they are compatible with breast-feeding.

Response is usually prompt. **If fever persists >48 hours** (<10% of women), the addition of ampicillin can be considered. If fever still persists, pelvic abscess, wound infection, septic pelvic thrombophlebitis (SPT), inadequate antibiotic coverage, and retained placental tissue should be ruled out. SPT, though uncommon, should be suspected when fevers follow a spiking pattern and are unresponsive to antibiotics for more than 5 days [144]. Imaging (CT or MRI) is often used to help aid in the diagnosis of SPT, though no data exist to suggest that one is superior to the other. These modalities can also evaluate for pelvic abscess. Treatment for SPT has been conventionally anticoagulation, though there is no high-quality data to support this. There is one randomized trial with 14 patients that compared antibiotics alone to heparin and antibiotics for women with CT evidence of SPT; the primary outcomes of fever duration and hospital stay did not differ between the two groups [145]. Despite these limited data, expert opinion suggests anticoagulation for women with SPT [144,145]. For women with negative imaging, the likelihood of a resistant organism, a nongenital source of infection (pyelonephritis, pneumonia, and intravenous catheter phlebitis), or noninfectious fever should also be considered [131].

Because of neonatal implications, information on the mother's condition should be provided to the neonate's healthcare provider [130].

Breast-feeding

Most antibiotics, including clindamycin, gentamicin, and penicillin, are considered safe in breast-feeding, although they may cause changes in infant gastrointestinal flora, potentially resulting in diarrhea or thrush [146]. The mother and the pediatric provider should be advised so that they can monitor the infant for side effects.

POSTPARTUM WOUND COMPLICATIONS
Key Points

- Risk factors for post cesarean wound infection are chorioamnionitis, maternal preoperative condition or infection, preeclampsia, higher body mass index (BMI), nulliparity, increased surgical blood loss, and diabetes.
- Prophylactic preincision antibiotics (either ampicillin or first-generation cephalosporin for just one dose), suture closure or drainage of subcutaneous fat in women with ≥2 cm thickness, and suture closure of skin reduce the risk of post cesarean wound infection.
- **Penicillins** are first line antibiotics for wound infection. Wound **drainage and debridement of necrotic tissue** may be necessary.
- Compared with healing by secondary intention, reclosure of the disrupted laparotomy wound after the infection has resolved is associated with success in >80% of women, faster healing times, and fewer office visits.

Diagnosis/Definition

The Centers for Disease Control defines and classifies surgical site infection (SSI) as either superficial, deep or organ/space, as shown in Table 30.8. These criteria should be addressed at the time of diagnosis [147]. The vast majority of significant wound infections in obstetrics are postpartum following cesarean delivery. Breakdown and infection of perineal repair is uncommon.

Table 30.8 Classification of Surgical Site Infection (SSI)

1. **Superficial:** Occurs within 30 days after surgical procedure, involves skin and subcutaneous tissue only, and *at least one* of the following:
   a. Purulent drainage from incision
   b. Organism isolated from culture of fluid or tissue from SSI
   c. At least one of the following: pain, redness, swelling or heat, and superficial incision is deliberately opened by the surgeon
   d. Diagnosis of superficial SSI by surgeon or attending physician
2. **Deep:** Occurs within 30 days from surgical procedure and involves deep soft tissues (fascia, muscle) of the incision, and at least one of the following:
   a. Purulent drainage from incision
   b. Spontaneous dehiscence or deliberately opened by a surgeon when the patient presents at least one of the following: fever, pain, and tenderness
   c. An abscess involving the deep incision is found on direct examination during reoperation, or by histopathologic or radiologic examination
   d. Diagnosis of deep SSI by surgeon or attending physician
3. **Organ/Space:** Occurs within 30 days from surgical procedure and the infection appears to be related to the operation, and infection involves any part of the anatomy (organs, spaces) other than the incision, which was opened or manipulated during an operation, and at least one of the following:
   a. Purulent drainage from a drain placed in the organ/space
   b. Organisms isolated from a culture of fluid or tissue in the organ/space
   c. An abscess involving the organ/space found on direct examination during reoperation or by histopathologic or radiologic examination
   d. Diagnosis of an organ/space SSI by surgeon or attending physician

Symptoms

Wound complications most commonly present with pain, redness, swelling or drainage from the incision site. Fever and purulent drainage may be signs that infection is present. Perineal infection may be associated with malodorous discharge, pain with urination and/or defecation, and dyspareunia.

Epidemiology/Incidence

The incidence of wound infection after cesarean delivery ranges from 2.8%–11.6% to 16.6%–30% in obese patients [148–150]. Perineal wound breakdown occurs between 0.1%–4.6% of deliveries, though actual incidence may be higher due to underreporting [151,152].

Etiology/Basic Pathophysiology

The most common microorganisms identified by cultures from wound infections after cesarean delivery include *Staphylococcus epidermidis, Enterococcus faecalis, S. aureus, Escherichia coli,* and *Proteus mirabilis*. The pathophysiology involves seeding of bacteria either from the uterine cavity or from the skin [148].

Classification

See Table 30.8.

Risk Factors/Associations

Risk factors described are **preoperative remote infection, chorioamnionitis, maternal preoperative condition, preeclampsia, higher BMI, nulliparity, increased surgical blood loss, and staples for skin closure** [122,153–156]. Women with **diabetes** have five times the risk of wound infection compared with women without diabetes [157]. One large case–control study identified subcutaneous hematoma as an additional risk factor for wound infection, (OR 11.6, 95% CI 4.1–33.2) [158]. Risk for wound infection increase with increasing BMI [159]. Staples removed prior to postoperative day 4 are also associated with increased risk of wound complication [160]. Staple closure has been associated with a twofold higher rate of wound infection and complications [155,156].

Risk factors for perineal break down include **third or fourth degree laceration, episiotomy, operative delivery, meconium, and a prolonged second stage.** In one retrospective case–control, an operative delivery with a mediolateral episiotomy was associated with a 6.36-fold increased risk of perineal breakdown or infection, while third/fourth degree laceration and meconium were associated with a 3.7- and 3.22-fold increase risk, respectively [161]. Among women with obstetric anal sphincter injuries, a large prospective study noted at 19.8% infection rate and a nearly 25% breakdown rate, with operative delivery being significantly associated with both outcomes (OR 2.54, 95% CI 1.32–4.87, $p = .008$) [162]. In this study, intrapartum obstetric antibiotics were associated with a decreased risk of wound complications (OR 0.50, 95% CI 0.27–0.94, $p = .03$).

Management

Workup

For women presenting with history concerning for a wound complication, perineal or abdominal, thorough examination of the incision is important. Areas of erythema, induration and fluctuance should be noted, and potentially marked to assess for spread over time. For an abdominal incision, a sterile swab can be used to probe any open areas to assess the dimensions of the separation and to ensure fascial integrity. Observation of any discharge (serosanguinous vs. bloody vs. purulent) may be helpful in diagnosis. Imaging is not indicated unless there is concern for fascial dehiscence or more severe infection.

In early onset wound infection (<48 hours after the procedure), the microorganisms are likely to be either group A streptococcus or *Clostridium*. **A wound culture** can be taken and a Gram stain will depict either Gram-positive cocci or Gram-positive rods, respectively. There are no trials to confirm the efficacy or utility of obtaining a wound culture from abdominal or perineal wounds.

Prevention

Prophylactic antibiotics (either ampicillin or first-generation cephalosporin for just one dose) are associated with a 59% decrease in the incidence of wound infection compared with no antibiotics in women undergoing cesarean delivery [138]. The timing for prophylaxis should be **within 30–60 minutes before the start of procedure,** as while it is not associated with significant change in neonatal outcomes it reduces risk of maternal infectious morbidity (RR 0.59, 95% CI 0.44–0.81) [163–165]. **Suture closure of subcutaneous fat in women with >2 cm thickness** is associated with a significant decrease in wound disruptions, including infections [166] (see also Chapter 13). For incisions closed with staples, removal on or after POD4 also decreases wound complications [155,156]. Based on a the recent meta-analysis and more recent RCT, suture should be strongly encouraged over staples [155,156]. Some centers are using negative pressure wound therapy (NPWT) empirically in morbidly obese patients in an effort to decrease wound complications; early data appear promising [150].

One RCT examining the benefit of prophylactic antibiotics during repair of third and fourth degree lacerations exists. This trial of 147 women did show a difference in perineal wound complication rates between women who received the antibiotics and those who did received placebo (8.4% vs. 24.1%) [167]. This trial used a single dose of intravenous cefoxitin. Further study is needed before recommendations can be made [165,168] (see Chapter 9).

Therapy
For women with perineal wound breakdown, a thorough examination (potentially under anesthesia) is helpful to better characterize the defect and adequately cleanse the wound. There is **insufficient evidence to suggest resuturing or allowing the wound to heal by secondary intent in the absence of infection** [169]. Given the active bacterial ecosystem of the vagina, some providers will assume that a subclinical infection is the reason for the wound breakdown and treat with antibiotics. In the setting of active perineal infection, debridement with antibiotic therapy is indicated. Antibiotic regimens vary, though some experts suggest a 7-day course of 875 mg amoxicillin–clavulanate and 500 mg of metronidazole twice daily [162]. Similar to wound breakdown, insufficient evidence exists regarding repair of the defect versus conservative management in the setting of perineal infection; clinical judgment and patient preferences should be used make this decision [169].

For women with **cesarean delivery,** the onset of the possible abdominal wound infection defines the need for **antibiotics.** For infection arising <48 hours after cesarean, **penicillin** is the drug of choice, based largely on expert opinion. Empiric therapy for cellulitis is reasonable with dicloxacillin, cephalexin, or clindamycin [170]. Wound **drainage and debridement of necrotic tissue** may be necessary. In late-onset wound infection (4–8 days postoperatively), the management consists purely of drainage. Antibiotics are not considered indicated in this setting, unless extensive cellulitis is present, or if the patient does not improve after drainage, in which case necrotizing fasciitis should be considered [131].

Disrupted (Open) Laparotomy Wound, after Infection Has Resolved or If No Infection on Presentation

There are different ways to manage the open wound [171]. Women who present to the clinic or emergency wound with evidence of an abdominal wound separation, hematoma, or seroma without evidence of infection need a thorough evaluation of the incision. The incision should be cleansed with sterile water or saline. When hematoma is present, the wound may need to be partially opened in order to **evacuate the hematoma,** thus decreasing the risk of subsequent infection.

Compared with healing by secondary intention, **reclosure of the disrupted laparotomy wound is associated with success in >80% of women, faster healing times** (16–23 vs. 61–72 days), **and fewer office visits** [172]. No serious morbidity or mortality is associated with either method. There is insufficient evidence to assess optimal timing (probably 4–6 days after disruption if noninfected) and technique (superficial vertical mattress or "en bloc" reclosure of entire wound thickness with absorbable sutures, or adhesive tape) of reclosure, as well as utility of antibiotics. After the wound is free of infection and is granulating properly, local anesthesia can be applied at bedside, and polypropylene mattress stitches can be used to close the skin.

Compared with reclosure using sutures, reclosure using permeable, adhesive tape (Cover-Roll; Biersdorf Inc., Norwalk, CT) was a faster procedure with lower pain scores and similar healing times in a small trial [173]. However, a subsequent study found shorter healing times (16.1 vs. 23.0 days) with suture closure compared with surgical tape [174].

Closure with secondary intention using NPWT, also called vacuum-assisted closure, has not been studied in any trials after cesarean section [175]. A recent meta-analysis in nonpregnant adults found some evidence of improved healing with NPWT but concluded that existing data are insufficient to establish clinical benefit [176].

POSTPARTUM MOOD AND ANXIETY DISORDERS
Key Points

- See Chapter 21 in *Maternal-Fetal Evidence Based Guidelines* for details of management of Mood disorders in pregnancy.
- **One in 7 women experience perinatal depression (PND),** making it the most common complication of pregnancy.
- Risk factors include **history of maternal anxiety or depression, lack of social support traumatic birth experience, infant admission to neonatal intensive care, and breast-feeding problems.**
- Routine screening is recommended **at least once during perinatal care.**
- **Positive screens require additional evaluation**. If depression is diagnosed, referral and follow-up to ensure treatment occurs is essential.

Definition
PND is an episode of moderate or severe major depressive disorder (MDD) beginning either during pregnancy or within 4–6 weeks after delivery [177,178].

Symptoms/Signs
In addition to typical depression symptoms of sadness, despair, disrupted sleep and appetite, women with postpartum depression often experience prominent anxiety symptoms.

Epidemiology/Incidence
Its prevalence is about 15%, affecting one in seven women [179,180].

Risk Factors and Associations
Risk factors for prenatal depression include past history of depression or anxiety, life stressors, lack of social support, unintended pregnancy, lower income or education, domestic violence, and smoking. Additional risk factors for postpartum depression include a traumatic birth experience, infant admission to neonatal intensive care, and difficulties breast-feeding [181].

Complications

During the postpartum period, women with depression are at increased risk of maternal suicide, infanticide, and impaired maternal sensitivity and attachment with the infant [182–185]. Women with depression are also less likely to engage in enriching interactions with the child, such as reading or singing [186]. Anxiety symptoms have been associated with increased maternal healthcare utilization and reduced breast-feeding duration [187,188].

Prevention

Psychosocial and psychological interventions are effective to reduce postpartum depression. In a large meta-analysis, both **lay and professional prevention interventions** reduced postpartum depression symptoms (average RR 0.78, 95% CI 0.66–0.93). Effective strategies included **postpartum home visits, telephone support, and interpersonal psychotherapy.**

Screening

Screening for PND should be performed using a validated instrument, such as the Edinburgh Postnatal Depression Scale (EPDS). Despite the high prevalence and substantial morbidity associated with PND, this condition is under-recognized. Major obstetric and pediatric medical organizations recommend routine screening [3,181]. Although clinicians are generally supportive of screening for PND [189,190], these attitudes do not consistently translate into practice. In the United States, less than half of women are formally screened for PND [191]. Consistent with such efforts, less than 50% of PND cases are detected in routine clinical practice, with antenatal recognition rates reported at 41% [192] and postnatal rates ranging from 29% [193] to 43% [194]. Screening alone does not ensure treatment: in a recent review, one in five women who screened positive had at least one mental health visit [195]. Patient engagement strategies increased the change that women with depression symptoms received mental health care.

Treatment

Both psychotherapy and medications are effective for treating PND. For further details on treatment of postpartum depression, see Chapter 21 in *Maternal-Fetal Evidence Based Guidelines*. As with any patient diagnosed with a health condition, women with postpartum depression should be followed-up to ensure adequate engagement with treatment and response to therapy. Monitoring patient symptoms is essential, just as measurement of blood pressure is necessary to guide treatment of hypertension. A stepped care approach with serial measurement of symptoms with a tool such as the Patient Health Questionnaire 9 (PHQ-9) to inform depression management can increase the likelihood that patients receive adequate therapy [196].

OTHER POSTPARTUM ISSUES

Women report receiving insufficient guidance from their providers about recovery from birth, and feeling unprepared for postpartum concerns is correlated with postpartum mood symptoms [197]. In a randomized trial, **routine provision of guidance about expected symptoms and coping strategies measures reduced depression symptoms** [198] **and increased breast-feeding duration** [199] among black and Latina women.

Table 30.9 Postpartum (Including Postcesarean) Advice Regarding Common Daily Life Activities

Advice	Evidence	Suggested Recommendations
Lifting	Lifting increases intra-abdominal pressure much less than Valsalva, forceful coughing, or rising from supine to erect position [201].	(1) Patients should continue lifting patterns as before prepregnancy. (2) Patients need an adequate postoperative analgesic regimen as necessary.
Climbing stairs	Climbing stairs increases intra-abdominal pressure much less than Valsalva, forceful coughing, or rising from supine to erect position [201].	(1) Patients should continue climbing stairs as before pregnancy. (2) Patients need an adequate postoperative analgesic regimen as necessary.
Driving	No consistent prospective or retrospective evidence.	(1) Patients need an appropriate postoperative analgesic regimen that does not cause a clouded sensorium when driving. (2) Patients may resume driving when comfortable with hand and foot movements required for driving.
Exercise	Limited retrospective and prospective evidence. Forceful coughing increases intra-abdominal pressure as much as jumping jacks [201].	(1) Patients need an appropriate postoperative analgesic regimen as necessary. (2) Patients may resume prepregnancy exercise level. (3) Exercise program may need to be tailored for postpartum women. (4) Preprocedure and postprocedure recommendations should be consistent.
Vaginal intercourse	No retrospective or prospective evidence.	(1) Women and their partners should make the decision to resume intercourse mutually. (2) Women should use appropriate contraception after childbirth. (3) There is insufficient evidence as to when to resume vaginal intercourse.
Returning to work	No consistent retrospective evidence; no prospective evidence.	(1) Women should be encouraged to return to work relatively soon postpregnancy; the usual times in the United States are 6 weeks after vaginal and 8 weeks after cesarean delivery, but these are not based on level 1 evidence. (2) Consider graded return to work, as tolerated.

Source: Adapted from Minig L et al., *Obstet Gynecol*, 114, 892–900, 2009.

There is insufficient evidence for general postpartum advice on common issues such as lifting, climbing stairs, driving, exercise, vaginal intercourse, and return to work. Suggestions based on this limited evidence and mostly expert opinions are shown in Table 30.9 [200,201]. Women are routinely counseled to defer intercourse until 6 weeks postpartum, but there are no data supporting this recommendation. The risk of bleeding or infection is minimal after 2 weeks, and **guidelines recommend that women resume intercourse when it is comfortable and desired**, once the perineum has healed and bleeding has decreased [202]. More than half of women resume sexual intercourse by 6 weeks postpartum, and 90% resume by 12 weeks postpartum [203]. Multiple prospective cohort studies have attempted to identify risk factors for persistent dyspareunia after delivery. Though data are mixed, Connolly, Serati, and Barrett each conducted prospective cohort studies, which failed to implicate mode of delivery, episiotomy, and perineal lacerations as risk factors for postpartum dyspareunia [204–206]. Barrett et al. [204] did note that a history of dyspareunia was a major risk factor for postpartum dyspareunia (OR 4.97).

For other postpartum issues, see also Chapter 1, Chapter 9 (third stage of labor and its complications—includes repair of vaginal lacerations, etc.), Chapter 13 (cesarean delivery—especially for prevention of postpartum endometritis and postpartum wound infection), and chapters pertinent to specific conditions in both this book and its companion *Maternal-Fetal Evidence Based Guidelines*.

REFERENCES

1. Pang WW, Hartmann PE. Initiation of human lactation: Secretory differentiation and secretory activation. *J Mammary Gland Biol Neoplasia*. 2007;12(4):211–221. [Review]
2. Ip S, Chung M, Raman G, et al. Breastfeeding and maternal and infant health outcomes in developed countries. *Evid Rep Technol Asses (Full Rep)*. 2007;153:1–186. [II-2]
3. Hauck FR, Thompson JM, Tanabe KO, et al. Breastfeeding and reduced risk of sudden infant death syndrome: A meta-analysis. *Pediatrics*. 2011;128(1):103–110. [Meta-analysis: 18 case: Control studies, II-2]
4. Horta BL, de Mola CL, Victora CG. Long-term consequences of breastfeeding on cholesterol, obesity, systolic blood pressure, and type-2 diabetes: Systematic review and meta-analysis. *Acta Paediatr*. 2015;104(467):30–37. [Meta-analysis: 105 studies, II-2]
5. Dogaru CM, Nyffenegger D, Pescatore AM, et al. Breastfeeding and childhood asthma: Systematic review and meta-analysis. *Am J Epidemiol*. 2014;179(10):1153–1167. [Meta-analysis: 117 studies]
6. Collaborative Group on Hormonal Factors in Breast Cancer. Breast cancer and breastfeeding: Collaborative reanalysis of individual data from 47 epidemiological studies in 30 countries, including 50302 women with breast cancer and 96973 women without the disease. *Lancet*. 2002;360(9328):187–195. [II-2]
7. Stuebe AM, Willett WC, Xue F, et al. Lactation and incidence of premenopausal breast cancer: A longitudinal study. *Arch Intern Med*. 2009;169(15):1364–1371. [II-2]
8. Work ME, John EM, Andrulis IL, et al. Reproductive risk factors and oestrogen/progesterone receptor-negative breast cancer in the breast cancer family registry. *Br J Cancer*. 2014;110(5):1367–1377. [II-2]
9. Palmer JR, Boggs DA, Wise LA, et al. Parity and lactation in relation to estrogen receptor negative breast cancer in African American women. *Cancer Epidemiol Biomarkers Prev*. 2011;20(9):1883–1891. [II-2]
10. Islami F, Liu Y, Jemal A, et al. Breastfeeding and breast cancer risk by receptor status—A systematic review and meta-analysis. *Ann Oncol*. 2015;26(12):2398–2407. [Review and meta-analysis: 8 cohort studies, 19 case-control studies, 36881 breast cancer cases]
11. Luan NN, Wu QJ, Gong TT, et al. Breastfeeding and ovarian cancer risk: A meta-analysis of epidemiologic studies. *Am J Clin Nutr*. 2013;98(4):1020–1031. [Meta-analysis: 5 prospective studies, 30 case: Control studies]
12. Dewey KG, Heinig MJ, Nommsen LA. Maternal weight-loss patterns during prolonged lactation. *Am J Clin Nutr*. 1993;58(2):162–166. [II-3]
13. Baker JL, Gamborg M, Heitmann BL, et al. Breastfeeding reduces postpartum weight retention. *Am J Clin Nutr*. 2008;88(6):1543–1551. [II-2]
14. Stuebe AM, Rich-Edwards JW, Willett WC, et al. Duration of lactation and incidence of type 2 diabetes. *JAMA*. 2005;294(20):2601–2610. [II-2]
15. Villegas R, Gao YT, Yang G, et al. Duration of breast-feeding and the incidence of type 2 diabetes mellitus in the Shanghai Women's Health Study. *Diabetologia*. 2008;51(2):258–266. [II-2]
16. Schwarz EB, Ray RM, Stuebe AM, et al. Duration of lactation and risk factors for maternal cardiovascular disease. *Obstet Gynecol*. 2009;113(5):974–982. [II-2]
17. Schwarz EB, Brown JS, Creasman JM, et al. Lactation and maternal risk of type 2 diabetes: A population-based study. *Am J Med*. 2010;123(9):863.e861–863.e866. [II-2]
18. Gunderson EP, Lewis CE, Wei GS, et al. Lactation and changes in maternal metabolic risk factors. *Obstet Gynecol*. 2007;109:(3):729–738. [II-2]
19. Ram KT, Bobby P, Hailpern SM, et al. Duration of lactation is associated with lower prevalence of the metabolic syndrome in midlife-SWAN, the study of women's health across the nation. *Am J Obstet Gynecol*. 2008;198:(3):268.e261–268.e266. [II-1]
20. Gunderson EP, Jacobs DR Jr., Chiang V, et al. Duration of lactation and incidence of the metabolic syndrome in women of reproductive age according to gestational diabetes mellitus status: A 20-year prospective study in CARDIA—The coronary artery risk development in young adults study. *Diabetes*. 2010;59(2):495–504. [II-2]
21. Lee SY, Kim MT, Jee SH, et al. Does long-term lactation protect premenopausal women against hypertension risk? A Korean women's cohort study. *Prev Med*. 2005;41(2):433–438. [II-2]
22. Stuebe AM, Schwarz EB, Grewen K, et al. Duration of lactation and incidence of maternal hypertension: A longitudinal cohort study. *Am J Epidemiol*. 2011;174(10):1147–1158. [II-2]
23. Stuebe AM, Michels KB, Willett WC, et al. Duration of lactation and incidence of myocardial infarction in middle to late adulthood. *Am J Obstet Gynecol*. 2009;200(2):138.e131–138.e138. [II-2]
24. Kramer MS, Kakuma R. Optimal duration of exclusive breastfeeding. *Cochrane Database Syst Rev*. 2012;(8):CD003517. [II-2, meta-analysis: 23 studies]
25. Dewey KG, Cohen RJ, Brown KH, et al. Effects of exclusive breastfeeding for four versus six months on maternal nutritional status and infant motor development: Results of two randomized trials in Honduras. *J Nutr*. 2001;131(2):262–267. [2 RCTs, n = 260]
26. American Academy of Family Physicians. Breastfeeding (Position Paper), 2001. Available at: http://www.aafp.org/online/en/home/policy/policies/b/breastfeedingpositionpaper.html. Accessed June 10, 2009. [Guideline]
27. American College of Obstetricians and Gynecologists. Special report from ACOG. Breastfeeding: Maternal and infant aspects. *ACOG Clin Rev*. 2007;12(1 Suppl):1S–16S. [Guideline]
28. Department of Health. Infant Feeding Recommendation, 2003. Available at: http://www.dh.gov.uk/en/Publicationsandstatistics/Publications/PublicationsPolicyAndGuidance/DH_4097197. Accessed December 16, 2010. [Guideline]
29. World Health Organization. *Global Strategy for Infant and Young Child Feeding*. Geneva, Switzerland: World Health Organization, 2003. [Guideline]
30. American Academy of Pediatrics. Breastfeeding and the use of human milk. *Pediatrics*. 2012;129(3):e827–e841. [Guideline]

31. National Institute for Health and Clinical Excellence. Quick Reference Guide. *NICE Clinical Guideline No. 37: Routine Postnatal Care of Women and Their Babies*. NICE, London, United Kingdom, 2006. [Guideline]
32. Dyson L, McCormick F, Renfrew MJ. Interventions for promoting the initiation of breastfeeding. *Cochrane Database Syst Rev*. 2005;(2):CD001688. [Meta-analysis: 11 RCTs, $n = 1553$]
33. Renfrew MJ, McCormick FM, Wade A, et al. Support for healthy breastfeeding mothers with healthy term babies. *Cochrane Database Syst Rev*. 2012;(5):CD001141. [Meta-analysis: 52 studies, 56,451 mother-infant dyads]
34. U.S. Preventative Services Task Force. Primary care interventions to promote breastfeeding: U.S. Preventive Services Task Force Recommendation Statement. *Ann Intern Med*. 2008;149(8):560–564. [Guideline]
35. Freed GL, Clark SJ, Sorenson J, et al. National assessment of physicians' breast-feeding knowledge, attitudes, training, and experience. *JAMA*. 1995;273(6):472–476. [II-2]
36. Walton DM, Edwards MC. Nationwide survey of pediatric residency training in newborn medicine: Preparation for primary care practice. *Pediatrics*. 2002;110(6):1081–1087. [II-2]
37. Pound CM, Williams K, Grenon R, et al. Breastfeeding knowledge, confidence, beliefs, and attitudes of Canadian Physicians. *J Hum Lact*. 2014;30(3):298–309. [Survey; II-2]
38. World Health Organization, UNICEF. *BFHI Section 3: Breastfeeding Promotion and Support in a Baby-Friendly Hospital, a 20-Hour Course for Maternity Staff*. Geneva, Switzerland: World Health Organization, 2009. [Guideline]
39. Feldman-Winter L, Barone L, Milcarek B, et al. Residency curriculum improves breastfeeding care. *Pediatrics*. 2010;126(2):289–297. [Epub July 5, 2010] [Cluster-randomized trial, $n = 417$ residents, 6 interventions, and 7 control sites]
40. Mellin PS, Poplawski DT, Gole A, et al. Impact of a formal breastfeeding education program. *MCN Am J Matern Child Nurs*. 2011;36(2):82–88; quiz 89–90. [Pre/Post intervention study; II-3]
41. World Health Organization, UNICEF. *Baby Friendly Hospital Initiative: Revised, Updated and Expanded for Integrated Care*. Geneva, Switzerland: World Health Organization, 2009. [Guideline]
42. Kramer MS, Chalmers B, Hodnett ED, et al. Promotion of Breastfeeding Intervention Trial (PROBIT): A randomized trial in the Republic of Belarus. *JAMA*. 2001;285(4):413–420. [RCT, $n = 17,046$]
43. Declercq E, Labbok MH, Sakala C, et al. Hospital practices and women's likelihood of fulfilling their intention to exclusively breastfeed. *Am J Pub Health*. 2009;99(5):929–935. [II-2]
44. DiGirolamo AM, Grummer-Strawn LM, Fein SB. Effect of maternity-care practices on breastfeeding. *Pediatrics*. 2008;122(Suppl 2):S43–S49. [II-2]
45. Hawkins SS, Stern AD, Baum CF, et al. Compliance with the baby-friendly hospital initiative and impact on breastfeeding rates. Archives of disease in childhood. *Fetal Neonatal Ed*. 2014;99(2):F138–F143. [II-2]
46. Academy of Breastfeeding Medicine Protocol Committee. Clinical Protocol No. 19: Breastfeeding promotion in the prenatal setting. *Breastfeed Med*. 2009;4(1):43–45. [Guideline]
47. Lee SJ, Thomas J. Antenatal breast examination for promoting breastfeeding. *Cochrane Database Syst Rev*. 2008;(3):CD006064. [Meta-analysis: no RCTs identified]
48. The MAIN Trial Collaborative Group. Preparing for breast feeding: Treatment of inverted and non-protractile nipples in pregnancy. *Midwifery*. 1994;10(4):200–214. [RCT, $n = 463$]
49. Alexander JM, Grant AM, Campbell MJ. Randomised controlled trial of breast shells and Hoffman's exercises for inverted and non-protractile nipples. *BMJ Clin Res*. 1992;304(6833):1030–1032. [RCT, $n = 96$]
50. Howard CR, Howard FM, Lawrence RA, et al. Office prenatal formula advertising and its effect on breast-feeding patterns. *Obstet Gynecol*. 2000;95(2):296–303. [RCT, $n = 547$]
51. Bergevin Y, Dougherty C, Kramer MS. Do infant formula samples shorten the duration of breast-feeding? *Lancet*. 1983;1(8334):1148–1151. [RCT, $n = 448$]
52. Frank DA, Wirtz SJ, Sorenson JR, et al. Commercial discharge packs and breast-feeding counseling: Effects on infant-feeding practices in a randomized trial. *Pediatrics*. 1987;80(6):845–854. [RCT, $n = 343$]
53. Dungy CI, Christensen-Szalanski J, Losch M, et al. Effect of discharge samples on duration of breast-feeding [see comment]. *Pediatrics*. 1992;90(2 Pt 1):233–237. [RCT, $n = 146$]
54. Feldman-Winter L, Grossman X, Palaniappan A, et al. Removal of industry-sponsored formula sample packs from the hospital: Does it make a difference? *J Hum Lact*. 2012;28(3):380–388. [Time series design; II-3]
55. Moore ER, Anderson GC, Bergman N, Dowswell T. Early skin-to-skin contact for mothers and their healthy newborn infants. *Cochrane Database Syst Rev*. 2012;(5):CD003519. [II-2, meta-analysis: 34 RCTs, 2177 mother-baby dyads]
56. National Institute for Health and Clinical Excellence. *NICE Clinical Guideline No. 55: Intrapartum Care: Care of Healthy Women and Babies During Childbirth*. London, United Kingdom: RCOG Press, 2007. [Guideline]
57. Johnston C, Campbell-Yeo M, Fernandes A, et al. Skin-to-skin care for procedural pain in neonates. *Cochrane Database Syst Rev*. 2014;(1):CD008435. [Meta-analysis: 19 studies, $n = 1594$ infants]
58. Hung KJ, Berg O. Early skin-to-skin after cesarean to improve breastfeeding. *MCN Am J Matern Child Nurs*. 2011;36(5):318–324; quiz 325–316. [Time series design study; II-3]
59. De Carvalho M, Robertson S, Friedman A, et al. Effect of frequent breast-feeding on early milk production and infant weight gain. *Pediatrics*. 1983;72(3):307–311. [II-3]
60. Fallon A, Van der Putten D, Dring C, et al. Baby-led compared with scheduled (or mixed) breastfeeding for successful breastfeeding. *Cochrane Database Syst Rev*. 2014;(7):CD009067. [Meta-analyis, no trials found]
61. Flaherman VJ, Aby J, Burgos AE, et al. Effect of early limited formula on duration and exclusivity of breastfeeding in at-risk infants: An RCT. *Pediatrics*. 2013;131(6):1059–1065. [RCT, $n = 40$]
62. Mangesi L, Dowswell T. Treatments for breast engorgement during lactation. *Cochrane Database Syst Rev*. 2010;(9):CD006946. [Meta-analysis: 8 RCTs, $n = 744$]
63. Barbosa-Cesnik C, Schwartz K, Foxman B. Lactation mastitis. *JAMA*. 2003;289(13):1609–1612. [Review]
64. Crepinsek MA, Crowe L, Michener K, et al. Interventions for preventing mastitis after childbirth. *Cochrane Database Syst Rev*. 2010;(8):CD007239. [Meta-analysis: 5 trials, $n = 960$]
65. Jahanfar S, Ng CJ, Teng CL. Antibiotics for mastitis in breastfeeding women. *Cochrane Database Syst Rev*. 2013;(2):CD005458. [Meta-analysis: 2 RCTs, $n = 125$]
66. Arroyo R, Martin V, Maldonado A, et al. Treatment of infectious mastitis during lactation: Antibiotics versus oral administration of lactobacilli isolated from breast milk. *Clin Infect Dis*. 2010;50(12):1551–1558. [RCT, $n = 352$]
67. Amir LH, Academy of Breastfeeding Medicine Protocol Committee. ABM Clinical Protocol No. 4. Mastitis, revised March 2014. *Breastfeed Med*. 2014;9(5):239–243. [Guideline]
68. Akus M, Bartick M. Lactation safety recommendations and reliability compared in 10 medication resources. *Ann Pharmacother*. 2007;41(9):1352–1360. [III]
69. Sachs HC. The transfer of drugs and therapeutics into human breast milk: An update on selected topics. *Pediatrics*. 2013;132(3):e796–e809. [Guideline]
70. Furman LM, Minich N, Hack M. Correlates of lactation in mother of VLBW infants. *Pediatrics*. 2002;109(4):e57. [II-3]
71. Becker GE, McCormick FM, Renfrew MJ. Methods of milk expression for lactating women. *Cochrane Database Syst Rev*. 2008;(4):CD006170. [Meta-analysis: 6 RCTs, $n = 397$]
72. Jones E, Dimmock PW, Spencer SA. A randomised controlled trial to compare methods of milk expression after preterm

73. delivery. *Arch Dis Childhood Fetal Neonatal Ed.* 2001;85(2):F91–F95. [RCT, n = 36]
73. Morton J, Hall JY, Wong RJ, et al. Combining hand techniques with electric pumping increases milk production in mothers of preterm infants. *J Perinatol.* 2009;29(11):757–764. [II-3]
74. Feher SDK, Berger LR, Johnson JD, et al. Increasing breast milk production for premature infants with a relaxation/imagery audiotape. *Pediatrics.* 1989;83(1):57–60. [RCT, n = 71]
75. Acuna-Muga J, Ureta-Velasco N, de la Cruz-Bertolo J, et al. Volume of milk obtained in relation to location and circumstances of expression in mothers of very low birth weight infants. *J Hum Lact J Hum Lact.* 2014;30(1):41–46. [II-2, observational study, n = 26 mother-baby dyads]
76. Anderson PO, Valdes V. A critical review of pharmaceutical galactagogues. *Breastfeed Med.* 2007;2(4):229–242. [Review]
77. Academy of Breastfeeding Medicine. Clinical Protocol No. 9: Use of galactogogues in initiating or augmenting the rate of maternal milk secretion. *Breastfeed Med.* 2011;6(1):41–50. [Guideline]
78. Wan EW, Davey K, Page-Sharp M, et al. Dose-effect study of domperidone as a galactagogue in preterm mothers with insufficient milk supply, and its transfer into milk. *Br J Clin Pharmacol.* 2008;66(2):283–289. [Crossover RCT, n = 6]
79. Campbell-Yeo ML, Allen AC, Joseph KS, et al. Effect of domperidone on the composition of preterm human breast milk. *Pediatrics.* 2010;125(1):e107–e114. [RCT, n = 46]
80. Lewis PJ, Devenish C, Kahn C. Controlled trial of metoclopramide in the initiation of breast feeding. *Br J Clin Pharmacol.* 1980;9(2):217–219. [RCT, n = 20]
81. Hansen WF, McAndrew S, Harris K, et al. Metoclopramide effect on breastfeeding the preterm infant: A randomized trial. *Obstet Gynecol.* 2005;105(2):383–389. [RCT, n = 69]
82. Seema, Patwari AK, Satyanarayana L. Relactation: An effective intervention to promote exclusive breastfeeding. *J Trop Pediatr.* 1997;43(4):213–216. [RCT, n = 50]
83. Sakha K, Behbahan AG. Training for perfect breastfeeding or metoclopramide: Which one can promote lactation in nursing mothers? *Breastfeed Med.* 2008;3(2):120–123. [RCT, n = 20]
84. Kramer MS, Kakuma R. Maternal dietary antigen avoidance during pregnancy or lactation, or both, for preventing or treating atopic disease in the child. *Cochrane Database Syst Rev.* 2006;(3):CD000133. [Meta-analysis: 4 RCTs, n = 334]
85. Delgado-Noguera MF, Calvache JA, Bonfill CX. Supplementation with long chain polyunsaturated fatty acids (LCPUFA) to breastfeeding mothers for improving child growth and development. *Cochrane Database Syst Rev.* 2010;(12):CD007901. [Meta-analysis: 6 RCTs, 1280 women]
86. Gunaratne AW, Makrides M, Collins CT. Maternal prenatal and/or postnatal n-3 long chain polyunsaturated fatty acids (LCPUFA) supplementation for preventing allergies in early childhood. *Cochrane Database Syst Rev.* 2015;(7):CD010085. [Meta-analysis: 8 RCTs, n = 3366 women, 3175 children]
87. Reece-Stremtan S, Marinelli KA. ABM Clinical Protocol No. 21. Guidelines for breastfeeding and substance use or substance use disorder, revised 2015. *Breastfeed Med.* 2015;10(3):135–141. [Guideline]
88. World Health Organization. *Treatment of Tuberculosis: Guidelines.* 4th ed. Geneva, Switzerland: World Health Organization, 2010. [Guidelines]
89. Horvath T, Madi BC, Iuppa IM, et al. Interventions for preventing late postnatal mother-to-child transmission of HIV. *Cochrane Database Syst Rev.* 2009;(1):CD006734. [Meta-analysis: 6 RCTs, 1 cohort intervention study]
90. World Health Organization. *Guidelines on HIV and Infant Feeding: Principles and Recommendations for Infant Feeding in the Context of HIV and a Summary of the Evidence.* Geneva, Switzerland: World Health Organization, 2010. [Guideline]
91. McDonald EA, Brown SJ. Does method of birth make a difference to when women resume sex after childbirth? *BJOG.* 2013;120:823–30. [II-2]
92. Ross JA, Winfrey WL. Contraceptive use, intention to use and unmet need during the extended postpartum period. *Int Family Planning Persp.* 2001;27(1):20–27. [II-3]
93. Lopez LM, Hiller JE, Grimes DA. Education for contraceptive use by women after childbirth. *Cochrane Database Syst Rev.* 2010;(1):CD001863. [Meta-analysis]
94. World Health Organization. *Medical Eligibility Criteria for Contraceptive Use.* 4th ed. Geneva, Switzerland: World Health Organization, 2010. Accessed December 23, 2010. [Review]
95. Ogburn JA, Espey E, Stonehocker J. Barriers to intrauterine device insertion in postpartum women. *Contraception.* 2005;72(6):426–429. [II-2]
96. Sonalkar S, Kapp N. Intrauterine device insertion in the postpartum period: A systematic review. *Eur J Contracept Reprod Health Care.* 2015;20(1):4–18. [Systematic review, II-2]
97. Grimes DA, Lopez LM, Schulz KF, et al. Immediate post-partum insertion of intrauterine devices. *Cochrane Database Syst Rev.* 2010;(5):CD003036. [Meta-analysis: 9 RCTs]
98. Chen BA, Reeves MF, Hayes JL, et al. Postplacental or delayed insertion of the levonorgestrel intrauterine device after vaginal delivery: A randomized controlled trial. *Obstet Gynecol.* 2010;116(5):1079–1087. [RCT, n = 102]
99. Lopez LM, Bernholc A, Hubacher D, et al. Immediate postpartum insertion of intrauterine device for contraception. *Cochrane Database Syst Rev.* 2015;(6):CD003036. [Meta-Analysis: 4 RCTs, n = 210]
100. Peterson HB. Sterilization. *Obstet Gynecol.* 2008;111(1):189–203. [III]
101. Peterson HB, Xia Z, Hughes JM, et al. The risk of pregnancy after tubal sterilization: Findings from the U.S. collaborative review of sterilization. *Am J Obstet Gynecol.* 1996;174(4):1161–1168; discussion 1168–1170. [II-2]
102. Kohaut BA, Musselman BL, Sanchez-Ramos L, et al. Randomized trial to compare perioperative outcomes of Filshie clip vs. Pomeroy technique for post-partum and intraoperative cesarean tubal sterilization: A pilot study. *Contraception.* 2004;69(4):267–270. [RCT]
103. Rodriguez MI, Seuc A, Sokal DC. Comparative efficacy of postpartum sterilisation with the titanium clip versus partial salpingectomy: A randomised controlled trial. *BJOG.* 2013;120(1):108–112. [RCT, n = 1400]
104. Curtis KM, Mohllajee AP, Peterson HB. Regret following female sterilization at a young age: A systematic review. *Contraception.* 2006;73(2):205–210. [Review]
105. Chi IC, Jones DB. Incidence, risk factors, and prevention of poststerilization regret in women: An updated international review from an epidemiological perspective. *Obstet Gynecol Surv.* 1994;49(10):722–732. [Review]
106. Thurman AR, Janecek T. One-year follow-up of women with unfulfilled postpartum sterilization requests. *Obstet Gynecol.* 2010;116(5):1071–1077. [II-3]
107. Van der Wijden C, Manion C. Lactational amenorrhoea method for family planning. *Cochrane Database Syst Rev.* 2015;(10):CD001329. [Meta-analysis: 15 observational studies, II-2]
108. Kennedy KI, Visness CM. Contraceptive efficacy of lactational amenorrhoea. *Lancet.* 1992;339(8787):227–230. [II-2]
109. Berens P, Labbok M, Academy of Breastfeeding Medicine. ABM Clinical Protocol No. 13. Contraception during breastfeeding, revised 2015. *Breastfeed Med.* 2015;10:3–12. [Guideline]
110. Lopez LM, Grey TW, Stuebe AM, et al. Combined hormonal versus nonhormonal versus progestin-only contraception in lactation. *Cochrane Database Syst Rev.* 2015;(3):CD003988. [Mata-analysis: 11 RCTs, n = 1482 women]
111. World Health Organization. *Medical Eligibility Criteria for Contraceptive Use.* Geneva, Switzerland: World Health Organization, 2015. [Guideline]
112. Chen BA, Reeves MF, Creinin MD, et al. Postplacental or delayed levonorgestrel intrauterine device insertion and breast-feeding duration. *Contraception.* 2011;84:499–504. [RCT, n = 96]
113. Shaamash AH, Sayed GH, Hussien MM, et al. A comparative study of the levonorgestrel-releasing intrauterine system

Mirena versus the Copper T380A intrauterine device during lactation: Breast-feeding performance, infant growth and infant development. *Contraception.* 2005;72(5):346–351. [II-1]
114. Gurtcheff SE, Turok DK, Stoddard G, et al. Lactogenesis after early postpartum use of the contraceptive implant: A randomized controlled trial. *Obstet Gynecol.* 2011;117(5):1114–1121. [RCT, n = 69]
115. Braga GC, Ferriolli E, Quintana SM, et al. Immediate postpartum initiation of etonogestrel-releasing implant: A randomized controlled trial on breastfeeding impact. *Contraception.* 2015;92(6):536–542. [RCT, n = 24]
116. Brown CE, Stettler RW, Twickler D, et al. Puerperal septic pelvic thrombophlebitis: Incidence and response to heparin therapy. *Am J Obstet Gynecol.* 1999;181(1):143–148. [II-2]
117. Sebitloane HM, Moodley J, Esterhuizen TM. Prophylactic antibiotics for the prevention of postpartum infectious morbidity in women infected with human immunodeficiency virus: A randomized controlled trial. *Am J Obstet Gynecol.* 2008;198(2):189. e1–189.e6. [RCT, n = 424]
118. Diamond MP, Entman SS, Salyer SL, et al. Increased risk of endometritis and wound infection after cesarean section in insulin-dependent diabetic women. *Am J Obstet Gynecol.* 1986;155(2):297–300. [II-2]
119. Rosene K, Eschenbach DA, Tompkins LS, et al. Polymicrobial early postpartum endometritis with facultative and anaerobic bacteria, genital mycoplasmas, and chlamydia trachomatis: Treatment with piperacillin or cefoxitin. *J Infect Dis.* 1986;153(6):1028–1037. [RCT]
120. Meaney-Delman D, Bartlett LA, Gravett MG, Jamieson DJ. Oral and intramuscular treatment options for early postpartum endometritis in low-resource settings: A systematic review. *Obstet Gynecol.* 2015;125(4):789–800. [Systematic Review II]
121. Magee KP, Blanco JD, Graham JM, et al. Endometritis after cesarean: The effect of age. *Am J Perinatol.* 1994;11(1):24–26. [II-2]
122. Myles TD, Gooch J, Santolaya J. Obesity as an independent risk factor for infectious morbidity in patients who undergo cesarean delivery. *Obstet Gynecol.* 2002;100(5 Pt 1):959–964. [II-2]
123. Wolfe HM, Gross TL, Sokol RJ, et al. Determinants of morbidity in obese women delivered by cesarean. *Obstet Gynecol.* 1988;71(5):691–696. [II-3]
124. Watts DH, Krohn MA, Hillier SL, et al. Bacterial vaginosis as a risk factor for post-cesarean endometritis. *Obstet Gynecol.* 1990;75(1):52–58. [II-2]
125. Krohn MA, Hillier SL, Baker CJ. Maternal peripartum complications associated with vaginal group B streptococci colonization. *J Infect Dis.* 1999;179(6):1410–1415. [II-2]
126. Minkoff HL, Sierra MF, Pringle GF, et al. Vaginal colonization with group B beta-hemolytic streptococcus as a risk factor for post-cesarean section febrile morbidity. *Am J Obstet Gynecol.* 1982;142(8):992–995. [II-2]
127. Gibbs RS. Clinical risk factors for puerperal infection. *Obstet Gynecol.* 1980;55(5 Suppl):178S–184S. [II-2]
128. Ferrero S, Bentivoglio G. Post-operative complications after caesarean section in HIV-infected women. *Arch Gynecol Obstet.* 2003;268(4):268–273. [II-2]
129. Watts DH, Lambert JS, Stiehm ER, et al. Complications according to mode of delivery among human immunodeficiency virus-infected women with CD4 lymphocyte counts of < or = 500/ microL. *Am J Obstet Gynecol.* 2000;183(1):100–107. [II-3]
130. American College of Obstetrians and Gynecologists, American Academy of Pediatrics. *Guidelines for Perinatal Care.* 6th ed. Washington, DC: ACOG, 2007. [Review]
131. Sweet RL, Gibbs RS. *Infectious Diseases of the Female Genital Tract.* Philadelphia, PA: Wolters Kluwer Health/Lippincott Williams & Wilkins, 2009. [Review]
132. Monif GR, Baker DA. *Infectious Diseases in Obstetrics and Gynecology.* 5th ed. New York, NY: Parthenon Publishing, 2004. [Review]
133. Gabbe SG, Niebyl JR, Simpson JL, eds. *Obstetrics: Normal and Problem Pregnancies.* Philadelphia, PA: Churchill Livingstone/Elsevier, 2007. [Review]
134. Chen K. Postpartum endometritis. UpToDate. 2010. http://www.uptodate.com/contents/postpartum-endometritis. Accessed on December 23, 2010. [Review]
135. Kankuri E, Kurki T, Carlson P, Hiilesmaa V. Incidence, treatment and outcome of peripartum sepsis. *Acta Obstet Gynecol Scand.* 2003;82(8):730–735. [III]
136. Haas DM, Morgan S, Contreras K. Vaginal preparation with antiseptic solution before cesarean section for preventing postoperative infections. *Cochrane Database Syst Rev.* 2014;(9):CD007892. [Meta-analysis: 5 RCT, n = 1766]
137. Hopkins L, Smaill FM. Antibiotic prophylaxis regimens and drugs for cesarean section. *Cochrane Database Syst Rev.* 1999;(2):CD001136. Available at: http://www.mrw.interscience.wiley.com/cochrane/clsysrev/articles/CD001136/frame.html. [Meta-analysis]
138. Hofmeyr GJ, Smaill FM. Antibiotic prophylaxis for cesarean section. *Cochrane Database Syst Rev.* 2010;(1):CD000933. Available at: http://www.mrw.interscience.wiley.com/cochrane/clsysrev/articles/CD000933/frame.html. Accessed on December 23, 2010. [Meta-analysis]
139. Andrews WW, Hauth JC, Cliver SP, et al. Randomized clinical trial of extended spectrum antibiotic prophylaxis with coverage for *Ureaplasma urealyticum* to reduce post-cesarean delivery endometritis. *Obstet Gynecol.* 2003;101(6):1183–1189. [RCT, n = 597]
140. Chang PL, Newton ER. Predictors of antibiotic prophylactic failure in post-cesarean endometritis. *Obstet Gynecol.* 1992;80(1):117–122. [II-2]
141. Haas DM, Morgan Al Darei S, Contreras K. Vaginal preparation with antiseptic solution before cesarean section for preventing postoperative infections. *Cochrane Database Syst Rev.* 2010;(3):CD007892. [Meta-analysis: 4 RCTs, n = 1198]
142. French L, Smaill FM. Antibiotic regimens for endometritis after delivery. *Cochrane Database Syst Rev.* 2004;(4):CD001067. Available at: http://www.mrw.interscience.wiley.com/cochrane/clsysrev/articles/CD001067/frame.html. Accessed on December 23, 2010. [Meta-analysis]
143. Livingston JC, Llata E, Rinehart E, et al. Gentamicin and clindamycin therapy in postpartum endometritis: The efficacy of daily dosing versus dosing every 8 hours. *Am J Obstet Gynecol.* 2003;188(1):149–152. [RCT, n = 110]
144. Garcia J, Aboujaoude R, Apuzzio J, Alvarez JR. Septic pelvic thrombophlebitis: Diagnosis and management. *Infect Dis Obstet Gynecol.* 2006;2006:15614. [III]
145. Brown CE, Stettler RW, Twickler D, Cunningham FG. Puerperal septic pelvic thrombophlebitis: Incidence and response to heparin therapy. *Am J Obstet Gynecol.* 1999;181(1):143–148. [II-2]
146. National Library of Medicine. LactMed. Available at: http://toxnet.nlm.nih.gov/cgi-bin/sis/htmlgen?LACT. Accessed November 10, 2015. [Review]
147. Mangram AJ, Horan TC, Pearson ML, et al. Guideline for prevention of surgical site infection, 1999. Hospital Infection Control Practices Advisory Committee. *Infect Control Hosp Epidemiol.* 1999;20(4):250–278; quiz 279–280. [Guideline]
148. Martens MG, Kolrud BL, Faro S, et al. Development of wound infection or separation after cesarean delivery. Prospective evaluation of 2,431 cases. *J Reprod Med.* 1995;40(3):171–175. [II-1]
149. Alanis MC, Villers MS, Law TL, et al. Complications of cesarean delivery in the massively obese parturient. *Am J Obstet Gynecol.* 2010;203(3):271.e1–271.e7. [II-2]
150. Anglim B, O'Connor H, Daly S. Prevena, negative pressure wound therapy applied to closed Pfannenstiel incisions at time of caesarean section in patients deemed at high risk for wound infection. *J Obstet Gynaecol.* 2015;35(3):255–258. [II-2]
151. Goldaber KG, Wendel PJ, McIntire DD, Wendel GD Jr. Postpartum perineal morbidity after fourth-degree perineal repair. *Am J Obstet Gynecol.* 1993;168(2):489–493. [II-2]
152. Ramin SM, Gilstrap LC III. Episiotomy and early repair of dehiscence. *Clin Obstet Gynecol.* 1994;37(4):816–823. [III]

153. Tran TS, Jamulitrat S, Chongsuvivatwong V, et al. Risk factors for postcesarean surgical site infection. *Obstet Gynecol.* 2000;95:(3):367–371. [II-2]
154. Vermillion ST, Lamoutte C, Soper DE, et al. Wound infection after cesarean: Effect of subcutaneous tissue thickness. *Obstet Gynecol.* 2000;95(6 Pt 1):923–926. [II-2]
155. Figueroa D, Jauk VC, Szychowski JM, et al. Surgical staples compared with subcuticular suture for skin closure after cesarean delivery: A randomized controlled trial. *Obstet Gynecol.* 2013;121(1):33–38. [RCT, $n = 398$]
156. Tuuli MG, Rampersad RM, Carbone JF, et al. Staples compared with subcuticular suture for skin closure after cesarean delivery: A systematic review and meta-analysis. *Obstet Gynecol.* 2011;117(3):682–690. [Meta-analysis: 5 RCTs, 1 prospective cohort study, $n = 1487$]
157. Cruse PJ, Foord R. A five-year prospective study of 23,649 surgical wounds. *Arch Surg.* 1973;107(2):206–210. [II-1]
158. Olsen MA, Butler AM, Willers DM, et al. Risk factors for surgical site infection after low transverse cesarean section. *Infect Control Hosp Epidemiol.* 2008;29(6):477–484; discussion 485–476. [II-2]
159. Stamilio DM, Scifres CM. Extreme obesity and postcesarean maternal complications. *Obstet Gynecol.* 2014;124(2 Pt 1):227–232. [II-2]
160. Mackeen AD, Berghella V, Larsen ML. Techniques and materials for skin closure in caesarean section. *Cochrane Database Syst Rev.* 2012;(11):CD003577. [Meta-analysis: 8 RCTs]
161. Williams MK, Chames MC. Risk factors for the breakdown of perineal laceration repair after vaginal delivery. *Am J Obstet Gynecol.* 2006;195(3):755–759. [II-2]
162. Lewicky-Gaupp C, Leader-Cramer A, Johnson LL, et al. Wound complications after obstetric anal sphincter injuries. *Obstet Gynecol.* 2015;125(5):1088–1093. [II-2]
163. Wax JR, Hersey K, Philput C, et al. Single dose cefazolin prophylaxis for postcesarean infections: Before vs. after cord clamping. *J Matern Fetal Med.* 1997;6(1):61–65. [RCT, $n = 90$]
164. Sullivan SA, Smith T, Chang E, et al. Administration of cefazolin prior to skin incision is superior to cefazolin at cord clamping in preventing postcesarean infectious morbidity: A randomized, controlled trial. *Am J Obstet Gynecol.* 2007;196(5):455.e1–455.e5. [RCT, $n = 357$]
165. American College of Obstetricians and Gynecologists. ACOG Practice Bulletin No. 120: Use of prophylactic antibiotics in labor and delivery. *Obstet Gynecol.* 2011;117(6):1472–1483. [Guideline]
166. Anderson ER, Gates S. Techniques and materials for closure of the abdominal wall in caesarean section. *Cochrane Database Syst Rev.* 2004;(4):CD004663. Available at: http://www.mrw.interscience.wiley.com/cochrane/clsysrev/articles/CD004663/frame.html. Accessed on December 23, 2010. [Meta-analysis]
167. Duggal N, Mercado C, Daniels K, et al. Antibiotic prophylaxis for prevention of postpartum perineal wound complications: A randomized controlled trial. *Obstet Gynecol.* 2008;111(6):1268–1273. [RCT, $n = 147$]
168. Buppasiri P, Lumbiganon P, Thinkhamrop J, et al. Antibiotic prophylaxis for third- and fourth-degree perineal tear during vaginal birth. *Cochrane Database Syst Rev.* 2014;(10):CD005125. [Meta-Analysis: 1 RCT, $n = 147$]
169. Dudley LM, Kettle C, Ismail KM. Secondary suturing compared to non-suturing for broken down perineal wounds following childbirth. *Cochrane Database Syst Rev.* 2013;(9):CD008977. [Meta-analysis: 2 observational studies]
170. Baddour L. Cellulitis and erysipelas. UpToDate. 2010. http://www.uptodate.com/contents/cellulitis-and-erysipelas. Accessed on December 23, 2010. [Review]
171. Sarsam SE, Elliott JP, Lam GK. Management of wound complications from cesarean delivery. *Obstet Gynecol Surv.* 2005;60(7):462–473. [Review]
172. Wechter ME, Pearlman MD, Hartmann KE. Reclosure of the disrupted laparotomy wound: A systematic review. *Obstet Gynecol.* 2005;106(2):376–383. [Review]
173. Harris RL, Magann EF, Sullivan DL, et al. Wound dehiscence: Secondary closure with suture versus noninvasive adhesive bandage. *Female Pelvic Med Reconst Surg.* 1995;1(1):88–91. [RCT, $n = 27$]
174. Zaid TM, Herring WP, Meeks GR. A randomized trial of secondary closure of superficial wound dehiscence by surgical tape or suture. *Female Pelvic Med Reconst Surg.* 2010;16(4):246–248. [RCT, $n = 30$]
175. Eginton MT, Brown KR, Seabrook GR, et al. A prospective randomized evaluation of negative-pressure wound dressings for diabetic foot wounds. *Ann Vasc Surg.* 2003;17(6):645–649. [RCT, $n = 10$]
176. Gregor S, Maegele M, Sauerland S, et al. Negative pressure wound therapy: A vacuum of evidence? *Arch Surg.* 2008;143(2):189–196. [Meta-analysis: $n = 602$]
177. American Psychiatric Association. *Diagnostic and Statistical Manual of Mental Disorders (DSM-5).* Arlington, VA: American Psychiatric Publishing, 2013.
178. World Health Organization, ed. *The International Statistical Classification of Diseases and Related Health Problems, 10th revision (ICD-10).* Geneva, Switzerland: World Health Organization, 1992.
179. Gavin NI, Gaynes BN, Lohr KN, et al. Perinatal depression: A systematic review of prevalence and incidence. *Obstet Gynecol.* 2005;106(5 Pt 1):1071–1083.
180. Gaynes BN, Gavin N, Meltzer-Brody S, et al. Perinatal depression: Prevalence, screening accuracy, and screening outcomes. *Evid Rep Technol Assess (Summ).* 2005;119:1–8.
181. American College of Obstetricians and Gynecologists Committee on Obstetric Practice. ACOG Committee Opinion No. 630: Screening for perinatal depression. *Obstet Gynecol.* 2015;125(5):1268–1271. [Guideline]
182. Lindahl V, Pearson JL, Colpe L. Prevalence of suicidality during pregnancy and the postpartum. *Arch Womens Ment Health.* 2005;8(2):77–87.
183. Campbell SB, Brownell CA, Hungerford A, et al. The course of maternal depressive symptoms and maternal sensitivity as predictors of attachment security at 36 months. *Dev Psychopathol.* 2004;16(2):231–252.
184. McLearn KT, Minkovitz CS, Strobino DM, et al. The timing of maternal depressive symptoms and mothers' parenting practices with young children: Implications for pediatric practice. *Pediatrics.* 2006;118(1):e174–e182.
185. Paulson JF, Dauber S, Leiferman JA. Individual and combined effects of postpartum depression in mothers and fathers on parenting behavior. *Pediatrics.* 2006;118(2):659–668.
186. NICHD Early Child Care Research Network. Chronicity of maternal depressive symptoms, maternal sensitivity, and child functioning at 36 months. *Dev Psychol.* 1999;35(5):1297–1310.
187. Paul IM, Downs DS, Schaefer EW, et al. Postpartum anxiety and maternal-infant health outcomes. *Pediatrics.* 2013;131(4):e1218–e1224.
188. Stuebe AM, Grewen K, Meltzer-Brody S. Association between maternal mood and oxytocin response to breastfeeding. *J Womens Health (Larchmt).* 2013;22(4):352–361.
189. Dietrich AJ, Williams JW Jr., Ciotti MC, et al. Depression care attitudes and practices of newer obstetrician-gynecologists: A national survey. *Am J Obstet Gynecol.* 2003;189(1):267–273.
190. LaRocco-Cockburn A, Melville J, Bell M, Katon W. Depression screening attitudes and practices among obstetrician-gynecologists. *Obstet Gynecol.* 2003;101(5 Pt 1):892–898.
191. Seehusen DA, Baldwin LM, Runkle GP, Clark G. Are family physicians appropriately screening for postpartum depression? *J Am Board Fam Pract.* 2005;18(2):104–112.
192. Goodman JH, Tyer-Viola L. Detection, treatment, and referral of perinatal depression and anxiety by obstetrical providers. *J Womens Health (Larchmt).* 2010;19(3):477–490.
193. Fairbrother N, Abramowitz JS. New parenthood as a risk factor for the development of obsessional problems. *Behav Res Ther.* 2007;45(9):2155–2163.

194. Hearn G, Iliff A, Jones I, et al. Postnatal depression in the community. *Br J Gen Pract*. 1998;48(428):1064–1066.
195. Byatt N, Levin LL, Ziedonis D, et al. Enhancing participation in depression care in outpatient perinatal care settings: A systematic review. *Obstet Gynecol*. 2015;126(5):1048–1058. [Meta-analysis: 17 studies]
196. Trivedi MH, Rush AJ, Gaynes BN, et al. Maximizing the adequacy of medication treatment in controlled trials and clinical practice: STAR(*)D measurement-based care. *Neuropsychopharmacology*. 2007;32(12):2479–2489. [Symptoms monitoring protocol for STAR*D effectiveness study of measurement-based treatment for depression in primary care]
197. Howell EA, Mora PA, Chassin MR, Leventhal H. Lack of preparation, physical health after childbirth, and early postpartum depressive symptoms. *J Womens Health (Larchmt)*. 2010;19(4):703–708. [Survey, $n = 720$, II-2]
198. Howell EA, Balbierz A, Wang J, et al. Reducing postpartum depressive symptoms among black and Latina mothers: A randomized controlled trial. *Obstet Gynecol*. 2012;119(5):942–949. [RCT, $n = 540$]
199. Howell EA, Bodnar-Deren S, Balbierz A, et al. An intervention to extend breastfeeding among black and Latina mothers after delivery. *Am J Obstet Gynecol*. 2014;210(3):239.e1–239.e5. [RCT, $n = 540$]
200. Minig L, Trimble EL, Sarsotti C, et al. Building the evidence base for postoperative and postpartum advice. *Obstet Gynecol*. 2009;114:892–900. [Review]
201. Wier LF, Nygaard IE, Wilken J, et al. Postoperative activity restrictions: Any evidence? *Obstet Gynecol*. 2006;107:305–309. [Review]
202. American College of Obstetrians and Gynecologists, American Academy of Pediatrics. *Guidelines for Perinatal Care*. 7th ed. Washington, DC: ACOG, 2012. [Guideline]
203. Leeman LM, Rogers RG. Sex after childbirth: Postpartum sexual function. *Obstet Gynecol*. 2012;119(3):647–655. [Review]
204. Barrett G, Pendry E, Peacock J, et al. Women's sexual health after childbirth. *BJOG*. 2000;107(2):186–195. [II-2]
205. Connolly A, Thorp J, Pahel L. Effects of pregnancy and childbirth on postpartum sexual function: A longitudinal prospective study. *Int Urogynecol J Pelvic Floor Dysfunct*. 2005;16(4):263–267. [II-2]
206. Serati M, Salvatore S, Khullar V, et al. Prospective study to assess risk factors for pelvic floor dysfunction after delivery. *Acta Obstet Gynecol Scand*. 2008;87(3):313–318. [II-2]

31

The neonate

Gary A. Emmett and Swati Murthy

KEY POINTS

- **Necessary equipment** for neonatal stabilization must be available at every delivery.
- **Personnel trained in neonatal resuscitation** should be present at every delivery.
- **An infant who is 37+ weeks of gestation, is crying or breathing, and has good muscle tone does not require resuscitation. Dry the baby, place the baby skin-to-skin with the mother, and cover the baby with dry linen to maintain temperature.**
- Provide routine care, provide warmth, assure open airway, dry, and continuously evaluate color, activity and breathing.
- Neonatal resuscitation begins if child does not proceed through successful transition, not based on a specific Apgar number at any time. Stimulate the baby and open the airway. Routine suctioning is no longer suggested. If further resuscitation is needed, it is frequently due to poor respiratory transition and can usually be resolved with bag-and-mask **support of airway and breathing.**
- **Initial bag-and-mask resuscitation should be with room air.** Oxygen should be titrated with continuous pulse oximetry to maintain the baby within the target saturations (Table 31.6).
- **Low-risk infants** are 37 weeks of gestation or older and have birth weight between 2500 and 4200 g, Apgar scores of 7 or above at 5 minutes, normal vital signs, and no signs of congenital anomalies or respiratory distress.
- A difficult transition may be anticipated by infants who are not low risk and may be due to hypothermia, hypoglycemia, or congenital anomalies.
- **The preterm infant** (especially 35 weeks of gestation or less) is at *greater risk* for complications in the delivery room and in the well nursery. With high-risk infants, there must be immediate access to means of establishing **intravenous (IV) access** and **airway pressure**.
- **Late-preterm infants** are those born at 34 0/7–36 6/7 weeks. While these infants are often the size and weight of some term infants, they are physiologically more immature and at higher risk for complications.
- Every nursery should have preexisting protocols to institute best stabilization practices and should have clear statements of what conditions and degree of illness are appropriate to go to the well-baby nursery.
- **The majority of cases of cerebral palsy do not result from isolated intrapartum asphyxia with resultant hypoxemia and organ damage.**
- The health benefits to circumcision include prevention of urinary tract infection, penile cancer, and transmission of sexually transmitted infections. In the United States, the **benefits are not considered great enough for universal circumcision of males.**

DELIVERY ROOM MANAGEMENT

For management of the normal neonate, see also Chapter 9 (third stage). For management specific to meconium, see Chapter 23. The perinatal period is the riskiest time in a child's life [1–3]. Every newborn has the right to a resuscitation performed at a high level of competence. A competent resuscitation means that the proper equipment and well-trained personnel must be at every delivery. **Necessary equipment** is shown in Table 31.1.

Initiation of Resuscitation

Due to the complex physiologic changes that occur at birth, many newborns will experience apnea or bradycardia that will require opening the airway, stimulation, and ventilation. The need for medication is rare.

The first steps include the following:

- **Thermal management:** Placing the infant under a preheated radiant warmer, drying and stimulating the newborn, and frequently replacing wet blankets with dry ones.
- **Opening the airway:** Because of evidence that suctioning of the nasopharynx can lead to bradycardia during resuscitation, the first step is simply opening the airway. Clearing the airway should be reserved for babies with obvious obstruction of the airway or who require positive pressure ventilation. Most historic methods of removing meconium from the airway (suctioning of the oral pharynx before delivery of the shoulders and elective endotracheal intubation and direct suctioning of the trachea) have not been shown to improve outcomes. There is insufficient evidence to recommend a change in the current practice of endotracheal suctioning of nonvigorous babies with meconium stained amniotic fluid, but if this cannot be done easily and quickly, start bag-mask ventilation, especially if child is bradycardic.
- **Tactile stimulation:** Rubbing the baby's back, trunk, or extremities may occasionally be necessary to stimulate the baby to normal breathing and heart rate. For persistent apnea after tactile stimulation, positive pressure ventilation should be initiated immediately.

Chest compressions may be necessary if there is continued bradycardia (heart rate less than 60 beats/minute) after breathing is adequately supported. On rare occasions, medications are necessary and should be available (refer to Table 31.2 for the full list.). The most commonly used are as follows:

1. *Epinephrine 1:10,000:* 0.1–0.3 mL/kg IV or via endotracheal tube (ETT) given rapidly
2. *Volume expanders:* normal saline, Ringer's lactate, or whole blood. Dose is 10 mL/kg IV over 5–10 minutes

Table 31.1 Necessary Equipment for Neonatal Resuscitation in the Delivery Room

1. Suction equipment:
   a. Bulb syringe
   b. Mechanical suction and tubing
   c. Suction catheters of various sizes (recommended: 5 or 6, 8, 10, and 12 or 14 Fr)
   d. Feeding tubes (8 Fr with 20-mL syringe)
   e. Meconium aspirator
2. Bag mask equipment
   a. Device for delivering PPV such as neonatal resuscitation bag with manometer or T-piece resuscitator
   b. Face masks in newborn and premature sizes
   c. Oxygen and compressed air sources
   d. Oxygen blender with flow meter and tubing
3. Intubation equipment
   a. Laryngoscope with 00, 0, and 1 blades (for preterm and term infants)
   b. Endotracheal tubes (ETT) (2.5–4.0 mm)
   c. Stylet
   d. CO_2 detector
   e. Laryngeal mask airway (for use in the case of a difficult intubation)
4. Other equipment
   a. Clock (Apgar timer)
   b. Alcohol
   c. Stethoscope
   d. Gloves
   e. Scissors
   f. Tape (for securing ETT and lines)
   g. Stopcocks
   h. Syringes (1–20 mL)
   i. Umbilical artery and vein tray with catheters (3.5 and 5 Fr)
   j. Warmer
   k. Needles (25, 21, and 18 gauge)
   l. Pulse oximeter
   m. Food-grade plastic wrap
   n. Transporter

Abbreviations: CO_2, carbon dioxide; PPV, positive pressure ventilation.

Table 31.2 Medications Required for Resuscitation

1. Epinephrine 1:10,000 (0.1 mg/mL)
2. Crystalloid fluids (normal saline or Ringer's lactate)
3. Sodium bicarbonate 4.2% (5 mEq/10 mL)
4. Dextrose 10%
5. Normal saline flushes
6. Naloxone hydrochloride

---

3. *Sodium bicarbonate 0.5 mEq/mL:* 2 mEq/kg IV given over at least 2 minutes
4. *Naloxone hydrochloride 1.0 mg/mL:* 0.1 mg/kg IV or intramuscularly (IM) given rapidly

Delivery Room Resuscitation

The need to treat the newborn is based on frequent evaluation of respirations, heart rate, and oxygenation. The algorithm in Figure 31.1 can be used as a guideline for the resuscitation of a term or late preterm infant. **The Apgar score (outlined in Table 31.3) is a useful tool for communicating an infant's status, but should not be used to guide resuscitation.**

The Difficult Transition

Successful transition to extrauterine life generally occurs over the first hours after birth. Delay in transition can occur for many reasons. Common causes of delayed transition are listed in Table 31.4.

In infants with signs of poor transition (tachypnea, cyanosis, mottled skin or pallor, tremors, and/or jitteriness), additional measurements of the child's vital signs should be considered. These include temperature, blood glucose, and arterial blood saturation (by pulse oximetry or blood gas). Some of the more common reasons for delayed transition are discussed below.

Hypoglycemia

Low blood glucose in the newborn is a common problem often associated with a diabetic mother or with abnormal in utero growth—either too small or too large. A less common cause is congenital abnormalities of the pancreas. The exact definition of hypoglycemia is not agreed upon but all *symptomatic* infants should be treated. Treatment should be initiated immediately. Specific guidelines vary with the institution.

According to the 2011 report by the Committee of Fetus and Newborn of the American Academy of Pediatrics (AAP), treatment should proceed as in Table 31.5. Screening should be limited to term babies who are symptomatic (see Table 31.5), or ones that are at high-risk, which include babies that are less than 37 weeks gestation, small for gestational age (SGA), large for gestational age (LGA), and/or infant or diabetic mother (IDM). Routine screening of blood glucose is not needed in healthy, term newborns after uneventful pregnancy and delivery, except if they are symptomatic. No studies have demonstrated harm from asymptomatic hypoglycemia in the first 12 hours of life. Screening in late preterm infants and SGA infants should continue up to at least 24 hours. After 24 hours, any infant with glucose that is persistently <45 mg/dL should continue to be screened until stable. If glucose is not stable at 24 hours of age, or symptoms continue in spite of treatment, transfer to a higher level of care is necessary [4].

THE NEONATE

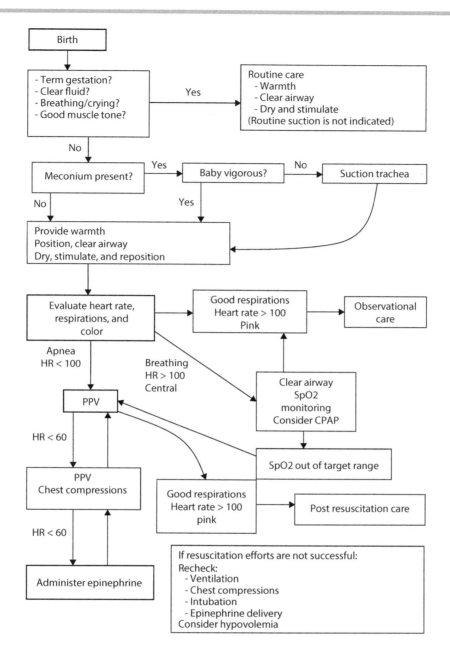

Figure 31.1 Neonatal Resuscitation Program (NRP) guidelines for resuscitation. CPAP, continuous positive airway pressure; HR, heart rate; PPV, positive pressure ventilation.

Table 31.3 Apgar Score

	0	1	2
Color	Blue/pale	Acrocyanosis	Pink
Heart rate	Absent	<100/minute	>100/minute
Reflex/irritability	No response	Grimace	Cry/active withdrawal
Tone	Limp	Some flexion	Active motion
Respirations	Absent	Weak cry/hypoventilation	Good/crying

Meconium

Meconium is the thick, green bowel movement of a newborn infant. All newborns should have a bowel movement within 24 hours of birth. Intrauterine stress or stress during delivery may cause the meconium to pass early. Meconium-stained fluid may be present in 8%–20% of deliveries and is almost exclusively found in term or postterm infants [1]. The fluid may be lightly stained and thin or very dark and thick, but all meconium-stained fluid presents a risk to the baby. The treatment is based on the condition of

Table 31.4 Factors Associated with Delayed Transition

Infant
    Hypothermia
    Hypoglycemia
    Retained pulmonary fluid
    Preterm birth (<37 weeks)
    Multiple births
    Small or large for gestational age (<2500 g or >4200 g)
    Postterm birth (≥42-week gestation)
    Meconium
    Low Apgar scores (i.e., <7 at 5 minutes)
    Congenital problems (i.e., chromosomal abnormalities and structural problems)
    Infection
Mother
    Diabetes
    Hypertension or preeclampsia
    Tocolysis
    Licit or illicit drug
    No prenatal care
    Age greater than 35 years

Table 31.5 Hypoglycemia Management in the Child after 34 Weeks of Gestation at Risk (34–36 Weeks' Gestation, Small for Gestation Age, Infants of Diabetic Mothers, and/or Large for Gestational Age)

Symptomatic* with Serum Glucose <40 mg/dL	Asymptomatic (4–24 Hours of Age)	Asymptomatic (Birth to 4 Hours of Age)
Use IV glucose	Initial feed within 1 hour. screen glucose 30 minutes after first feed. If initial screen is <25 mg/dL, feed and recheck in 1 hour. If repeat glucose is still <25 mg/dL, start IV glucose. If 25–40 mg/dL, refeed and use IV glucose as needed. If repeat glucose, use IV glucose as needed.	Continue feeds every 2–3 hours. Screen glucose prior to each feed. If screen <35 mg/dL, feed and recheck in 1 hour. If repeat glucose is still <35 mg/dL, start IV glucose. If repeat glucose 35–45 mg/dL, refeed and glucose as needed.

Abbreviations: IV, intravenous.
*Symptomatic hypoglycemia: irritability, tremors, jitteriness, exaggerated reflexes, high-pitched cry, seizures, lethargy, floppiness, cyanosis, apnea, and poor feeding.
Note: Target glucose >45 mg/dL before routine feedings. IV infusion, if needed, at 5–8 mg/kg/minute (80–100 mL/kg/24 hours).

the infant at birth. If the baby is vigorous and cries immediately, resuscitation should proceed normally. If the infant is limp or lethargic, he or she should be delivered immediately and placed on the warmer. Meconium suctioning, by intubating the baby and directly suctioning the trachea with a meconium aspirator attached to the ETT, may be helpful if it can be done quickly and easily. If not, simply bag the baby with room air. Current recommendation is to not suction the baby before delivery of the shoulders and to apply mask-and-bag resuscitation with room air as soon as possible to a baby who is not vigorous.

Respiratory Distress
Respiratory distress and/or tachypnea may occur and can be the manifestation of underlying illnesses. Etiologies include abnormalities of the lung (respiratory distress or aspiration syndromes, infections, pneumothorax, and congenital lung abnormalities), structural airway problems (choanal atresia, tracheal-esophageal fistula, and micrognathia), abnormalities of the cardiovascular system (primarily congenital heart disease—cyanotic or not, congestive heart failure, and pulmonary hypertension), abnormalities of the neurologic system (central nervous system [CNS] infections, hypoxic injury, and hydrocephalus), blood dyscrasia (anemia or polycythemia), infections, metabolic problems, or exposure to maternal drugs. Specific treatment should be aimed at the underlying etiology. Screening laboratory tests and imaging studies such as complete blood count (CBC), C-reactive protein (CRP), blood gas, and chest X-ray should be initiated if indicated.

Clear evidence exists that either insufficient or excessive oxygen can be harmful to the newborn infant. Hypoxia/ischemia can result in injury to the brain and other organs, but even brief exposure to excessive oxygen can result in vision or other neurological problems. Newborn babies do not have high levels of blood oxygen until at least 10 minutes after birth, so pulse oximetry below 90 is completely normal just after birth. Also, because of circulation changes at birth, cyanosis does not always mean lack of oxygen and a pink color of the skin does not always mean presence of oxygen in the newborn. When using pulse oximetry on the newborn in the first hour of life, it should be applied preductally (the right, upper extremity).

Resuscitation in newborns 34 weeks and older should always begin with room air. Goals for children not going successfully through transition are presented in Table 31.6 and range from 65% blood oxygenation/pulse oximetry in the first minute of life to 85% or higher after 10 minutes. This major change in the use of oxygen during the initial resuscitation of the newborn will seem dramatic to delivery room personnel and a well-organized educational program where

Table 31.6 Goal Preductal (Right-Hand) Oxygen Saturations after Birth

1 minute	60%–65%
2 minutes	65%–70%
3 minutes	70%–75%
4 minutes	75%–80%
5 minutes	80%–85%
10 minutes	85%–95%

clear posting of the new protocol in every venue where neonates are resuscitated is of the utmost importance.

Transient Tachypnea of the Newborn
In the newborn, tachypnea without respiratory distress may be a benign condition called transient tachypnea of the newborn (TTN). These infants are usually term or near term and will develop tachypnea following birth. They may have respiratory rates up to 120 breaths/minute, nasal flaring, grunting, and retractions, but upon physical examination, they do not appear to be in serious distress. Risk factors include cesarean delivery, precipitous delivery, fetal polycythemia, and delivery to a diabetic mother. There is no clear etiology to this disorder, but it is thought to be due to a combination of delayed resorption of fetal lung fluid from the lymph system, pulmonary immaturity, and a mild surfactant deficiency. Unfortunately, TTN is not easily distinguishable from other causes of tachypnea, such as pneumonia or sepsis. If the condition does not quickly resolve, these infants should have screening laboratory tests, including a CBC, CRP, and blood culture, along with a chest X-ray and a pediatric or neonatal consult. In TTN, the lab work will be normal and the chest X-ray will have increased pulmonary vascular markings and fluid in the fissures. More seriously affected infants may be treated with broad-spectrum antibiotics until infection can be excluded. In addition, those infants with respiratory rates above 60 breaths/minute should not be fed by mouth, and some will require either nasogastric (NG) tube feeds or IV fluids if the tachypnea lasts more than 12 hours.

Common Malformations Affecting Transition
Some congenital abnormalities of the newborn can present as problems in the delivery room. Below is a list of common malformations and best stabilization practices before transfer to a tertiary care nursery.

1. Choanal atresia (blockage of the nasal passageway): Secure an oral airway.
2. Pierre Robin sequence (small mandible with relatively large tongue): Secure an oral airway, but consider intubation if inadequate.
3. Congenital diaphragmatic hernia: At birth, immediate insertion of an NG tube to decompress the stomach and intubation of the airway are required.
4. Abdominal wall defects (omphalocele and gastroschisis): Cover the defect with a silo as soon as possible after birth. Gastroschisis may require prompt surgical correction; therefore, surgery should be called as soon as the baby is born.
5. Neural tube defects: Best emergent management is controversial, but the goal is to keep the area moist and free of contamination. The area may be covered with sterile plastic wrap, or the baby may be placed in a sterile plastic bag to just above the lesion.

Withholding or Discontinuing Resuscitation

There are conditions associated with high mortality and poor outcomes in which withholding resuscitation may be appropriate, particularly when there has been an opportunity for parental agreement. Cases should be addressed on an individual basis with a consistent and coordinated approach by both the obstetric and neonatal teams and in consultation with the parents. Cases where noninitiation of therapy could be considered may vary by region and include:

- Gestational age less than 23 weeks
- Birth weight less than 400 g
- Anencephaly
- Some chromosomal abnormalities, such as Trisomy 13

Resuscitation should always be considered in cases with high rates of survival and acceptable rates of morbidity. This generally includes infants who are 25 weeks gestation and above and most infants with congenital abnormalities. In cases of uncertain prognosis, parental desire should be weighed heavily.

It is reasonable to consider stopping resuscitation in infants who are born without a detectable heart rate, if the heart rate remains undetectable at 10 minutes of life.

TYPE OF NURSERY: LOW- VERSUS ELEVATED-RISK NEONATES

Minimal intervention is needed for the infant with no risks and a normal delivery. Therefore, it is important to distinguish which infants are at low risk and can go to the well baby nursery, and which infants are at high risk and require further evaluation.

Low Risk

These infants can be admitted without pediatric specialist consultation. Low-risk infants are 37 weeks of gestation or older and have birth weight between 2200 and 4200 g, Apgar scores of 7 or above at 5 minutes, normal vital signs, and no signs of congenital anomalies or respiratory distress.

Elevated Risk

Elevated-risk infants require pediatric specialist consultation prior to admission to the well baby nursery. Criteria include infants at risk for neonatal abstinence syndrome, sepsis, rupture of membranes greater than 16 hours, exposure to group B streptococcus (GBS) that was inadequately treated, maternal temperature of greater than 100.4°F (38°C) within 24 hours of delivery, infants of diabetic mothers, infants born outside of the hospital, infants of uncertain gestation, infants 36 weeks' gestation or less, infants less than 2200 g, and infants greater than 4200 g.

Late-preterm infants at 34–36 weeks gestation are of often the size and weight of term infants, but are physiologically immature. They are at increased risk for hypothermia, hypoglycemia, dehydration, and poor feeding. The AAP recommends that late-preterm infants receive special attention prior to discharge and close outpatient follow-up in order to prevent rehospitalization [5].

CARE OF THE WELL NEWBORN AFTER LABOR AND DELIVERY (L&D) CARE

All infants must be observed until they complete transition. A skilled staff member must assess the vital signs every 30 minutes for at least 2 hours and observe that the newborn is completely stable on its own. Completion of transition includes thermostability, respiratory rate less than 60 breaths/minute, heart rate greater than 100 beats/minute, and good muscle tone and sucking reflex.

NEWBORN SCREENING

Neonatal screening has arisen from the politics of medicine and of government, and has not been subject to consistent cost-benefit analysis or evidence-based medicine [6–8]. The required tests vary from state to state, but each state requires screening after 24 hours of life. Both the American College of Medical Genetics and Centers for Disease Control (CDC) have made model screening lists, but there is no single list of tests universally required in 2015. The tests suggested are referenced in Table 31.7.

CIRCUMCISION

The health benefits to circumcision include prevention of urinary tract infection (from about 7–14/1000 to 1–2/1000), **penile cancer** (about 1000 circumcisions needed to prevent one penile cancer), **and transmission of sexually transmitted infections** (about 15% decrease in lifetime human immunodeficiency virus [HIV] risk). **In the United States, the benefits are not considered great enough for universal circumcision of males.** The AAP recommends that circumcision should be **parental choice** and only agreed to after a discussion with a health care provider about the risks and benefits [9]. The World Health Organization encourages circumcision as a method to reduce the risk of acquiring HIV infection in populations at high risk for HIV [10]. Complications of circumcision, which have been reported to range from 0.3% to 20%, include excessive bleeding (1/100–1/1,000), infection (1–6/10,000), penile injury (4/10,000). Circumcision is often a social decision rather than a medical decision. The pediatric practitioner should delay or prevent circumcision in the following cases:

- Suspected sepsis or bacteremia
- Family history of bleeding problems (until the child is fully assessed by hematologist)
- Genital abnormalities, including ambiguous genitalia, micropenis (<2.5 cm from pubic bone to penile tip), hypospadias, epispadias, or chordae.

Performing a Circumcision

Prior to circumcision, infants should have completed transition, voided at least once, and been fasting for 1 hour prior to the procedure. Pain control should be utilized and can include a dorsal penile nerve block, topical analgesic, or subcutaneous ring block. Sucrose water or sweet wine also provides some pain control. Techniques for circumcision include the Mogen™, Plastibell™, and Gomco™. After the procedure, breast- or bottle-feeding is an excellent pain control method. If needed, the dose of acetaminophen is 12–15 mg/kg/dose. A gauze wrap is no longer recommended after the procedure. The area should be kept clean with plain water and covered with lubricant for up to 1 week until completely healed. The parents should be told to expect a white yellow discharge for 5–7 days.

Table 31.7 Disorders Recommended by the American College of Medical Genetics Task Force for Inclusion in Newborn Screening[a]

Disorders of organic acid metabolism
  Isovaleric acidemia
  Glutaric aciduria type 1
  3-Hydroxy-3-methylglutaric aciduria
  Multiple carboxylase deficiency
  Methylmalonic acidemia, mutase deficiency form
  3-Methylcrotonyl-CoA carboxylase deficiency
  Methylmalonic acidemia, Cb1 A and Cb1 B forms
  Propionic acidemia
  Beta-ketothiolase deficiency
Disorders of fatty acid metabolism
  Medium-chain acyl-CoA dehydrogenase deficiency
  Very long chain acyl-CoA dehydrogenase deficiency
  Long-chain L-3-hydroxy acyl-CoA dehydrogenase deficiency
  Trifunctional protein deficiency
  Carnitine uptake defect
Disorders of amino acid metabolism
  Phenylketonuria
  Maple syrup urine disease
  Homocystinuria
  Citrullinemia
  Argininosuccinic acidemia
  Tyrosinemia type 1
Hemoglobinopathies
  Sickle cell anemia
  Hemoglobin S-b-thalassemia
  Hemoglobin SC disease
Other disorders
  Congenital hypothyroidism
  Biotinidase deficiency
  Congenital adrenal hyperplasia
  Galactosemia
  Hearing deficiency
  Cystic fibrosis

Sources: Adapted from Natowicz M, *N Engl J Med*, 353, 867–870, 2005; Watson MS et al., *Newborn Screening: Toward a Uniform Screening Panel and System*, Maternal and Child Health Bureau, Rockville, MD, 2005.
Abbreviations: CoA, coenzyme A; Cb1 A, cobalamin A; Cb1 B, cobalamin B; S-b-thalassemia, sickle beta-thalassemia; SC, sickle cell.
[a]The American College of Medical Genetics Task Force also recommended reporting an additional 25 disorders (secondary targets) that can be detected through screening but that do not meet the criteria for primary disorders (6). At this time, there is a state-to-state variation in newborn screening; a list of the disorders that are screened for by each state is available at http://genes-r-us.uthscsa.edu.

CARE OF THE PRETERM INFANT

The delivery of a preterm infant follows many of the guidelines generated for the term infant [1–3]. These infants born at 36 weeks' gestation or less are at high risk for problems immediately following birth and in the subsequent newborn period. If a preterm delivery is anticipated, the delivery should be attended by a team of neonatal intensive care unit (NICU) personnel (physician, nurse, and respiratory therapist). Management of the infant includes accentuated attention to drying and maintaining thermal stability and close observation of blood glucose, fluid requirements, and respiratory function. **Babies less than 29 weeks gestation should be wrapped in polyethylene in order to prevent evaporative heat loss.**

In high-risk infants, the prophylactic placement of an umbilical venous line should be considered. Also, early institution of positive airway pressure may be necessary to prevent respiratory failure. Preparation for and anticipation of the delivery with the availability of the proper equipment and personnel for stabilization and transport will optimize survival.

A detailed review of the topic of neonatal care of the preterm infant is beyond the scope of this book. Table 31.8 has recent data on survival at very early (22–28 weeks) gestational ages, helpful for obstetric and neonatal counseling [11].

NEONATAL ENCEPHALOPATHY AND CEREBRAL PALSY
Neonatal Encephalopathy

Neonatal encephalopathy (NE) is a clinically defined syndrome of disturbed neurologic function in the earliest days of life in the term infant, manifested by difficulty initiating and maintaining respiration, depression of tone and reflexes, subnormal level of consciousness, and, often, seizures. It can result from a myriad of conditions and may or may not result in permanent neurologic impairment [12,13].

Hypoxic–Ischemic Encephalopathy

Hypoxic–ischemic encephalopathy (HIE) is a subset of neonatal encephalopathy for which the etiology is considered to be a limitation of oxygen and blood flow near the time of birth. A comprehensive assessment of neonatal status, maternal history, obstetric antecedents, intrapartum factors, and placental pathology is required in order to determine if hypoxic–ischemia occurred in close temporal proximity to L&D. The following conditions increase the likelihood that hypoxia-ischemia played a role in causing NE [14]:

- Apgar score of 6 or lower at 5 minutes
- Fetal umbilical artery pH <7.0 or base deficit ≥12 mmol/L
- Magnetic resonance (MR) imaging or MR spectroscopy showing hypoxic–ischemic pattern of cerebral imaging (deep nuclear gray matter or watershed cortical injury)
- Multisystem organ failure
- Sentinel hypoxic/ischemic event immediately before or during labor/delivery (uterine rupture, umbilical cord prolapse, maternal cardiovascular collapse, fetal exsanguination)
- Fetal heart rate pattern suggesting an acute peripartum or intrapartum event
- Lack of other contributing factors such as infection, fetomaternal hemorrhage, or chronic placental lesions
- Development of spastic quadriplegia or dyskinetic cerebral palsy (other types of cerebral palsy are less likely to be associated with acute intrapartum hypoxic-ischemic events)

There are many causes for low Apgar scores outside of HIE, but a 5-minute Apgar score that is 7 or greater makes HIE as a cause of NE unlikely. It is important when considering fetal heart rate to make a distinction between patients who present with an abnormal tracing and those who develop an abnormal tracing during delivery. A heart rate pattern that converts from a Category I tracing to a Category III tracing is suggestive of a hypoxic–ischemic event.

Neonatal encephalopathy can be a result of antenatal factors alone, intrapartum factors alone, or both in combination. Around 25% of infants surviving with NE will have long-term neurologic sequelae [13]. The usual progression of events is shown in Figure 31.2.

Therapeutic Hypothermia

Induced therapeutic hypothermia is recommended for infants 36 weeks and greater with evidence of moderate-to-severe HIE. Several randomized controlled trials have demonstrated lower mortality and less neurodevelopmental disability at 18 months in babies when compared to babies who were not cooled. Therapeutic hypothermia should be administered at institutions with multidisciplinary care and capability for long-term follow-up [3].

Cerebral Palsy

Cerebral palsy is a chronic static neuromuscular disability characterized by aberrant control of movement or posture, appearing early in life and not the result of recognized progressive disease. Cerebral palsy affects 2/1000 live births.

Table 31.8 Survival to Discharge at Very Early (22–28 Weeks) Gestational Ages

Gestational Age (Weeks)	Survival to Discharge (All) (%)	Survival to Discharge without Major Morbidities[a] (%)
22	9	0
23	33	0.75
24	65	6
25	81	20
26	87	26
27	94	47
28	94	56

Source: Data from Stoll BJ et al., JAMA, 314(10), 1039–1051, 2015.
[a]No necrotizing enterocolitis, sepsis, meningitis, bronchopulmonary dysplasia, severe intraventricular hemorrhage, periventricular leukomalacia, and retinopathy of prematurity grade 3 or higher.

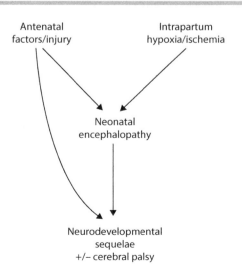

Figure 31.2 Progression of events in neonatal encephalopathy.

Prevention is elusive. **The majority of cases of cerebral palsy do *not* result from isolated intrapartum asphyxia with resultant hypoxemia and organ damage** [13]. Other factors associated with cerebral palsy and/or neonatal encephalopathy are as follows:

- Increasing maternal age
- Family history of seizures or neurologic disease
- Maternal history of infertility treatment or previous neonatal death
- Severe preeclampsia
- Intrauterine growth restriction
- Congenital malformations or genetic abnormalities
- Autoimmune and coagulation disorders
- Infections

Timing of Neonatal Encephalopathy

Estimating the time when neonatal encephalopathy occurred is extremely difficult. Some [12] have reported risk factors related to this condition:

- 69% Only antepartum risk factors
- 25% Both antepartum risk factors and evidence for intrapartum hypoxia
- 4% Intrapartum hypoxia without antepartum risk factors
- 2% No recognized risk factors

Therefore, the incidence of neonatal encephalopathy attributed to intrapartum hypoxia in absence of other preconception or antepartum abnormalities is about 1.6/10,000 infants [12,13].

Seventy-five percent of children with **cerebral palsy** had **normal Apgar scores** at birth [12] (see Table 31.9).

Criticism of the management of labor should not be confused with cerebral palsy causation because the two often may not be linked.

Table 31.9 Apgar Scores and Cerebral Palsy

0–3 at 5 minutes	0.3%–1.0% of babies with cerebral palsy
0–3 at 10 minutes	10% of babies with cerebral palsy (but rates drop to 5% if scores improve at 15 and 20 minutes)
<3 at 15 minutes	53% mortality, 36% of survivors with cerebral palsy
<3 at 20 minutes	60% mortality, 57% of survivors with cerebral palsy

REFERENCES

1. Gomella TL, Cunningham MD, Eyal FG, et al. eds. *Neonatology: Management, Procedures, On-Call Problems, Diseases, and Drugs.* 7th ed. New York, NY: McGraw-Hill, 2013. [Review]
2. Kattwinkel J, ed. *Textbook of Neonatal Resuscitation.* 6th ed. Elk Grove Village, IL: American Academy of Pediatrics, 2011. [Review]
3. Kattwinkel J, Perlman JM, Aziz K, et al. Neonatal resuscitation: 2010 American Heart Association, American Academy of Pediatrics. 2005 American Heart Association Guidelines for Cardiopulmonary Resuscitation and Emergency Cardiovascular Care. *Pediatrics.* 2011;126(5):e1400–e1413. [Review]
4. Adamkin DH, Committee on Fetus and Newborn. Clinical report—Postnatal glucose homeostasis in late-preterm and term infants. *Pediatrics.* 2011;127(3):575–579.
5. Engle WA, Tomashek KM, Wallman C. Committee on fetus and newborn, American Academy of Pediatrics. Late-preterm infants: A population at risk. *Pediatrics.* 2007;120(6):1390–1401. [Review]
6. Natowicz M. Newborn screening—Setting evidence-based policy for protection. *N Engl J Med.* 2005;353:867–870. [Review]
7. Watson MS, Mann MY, Lloyd-Puryear MA, et al.; American College of Medical Genetics Newborn Screening Expert Group. *Newborn Screening: Toward a Uniform Screening Panel and System.* Rockville, MD: Maternal and Child Health Bureau, 2005. [Review]
8. American College of Medical Genetics and Genomics. Medical Genetics: Translating Genes Into Health®. Available at: https://www.acmg.net/ACMG/Publications/Practice_Guidelines_docs/NBS_report.aspx. Accessed August 4, 2015. [Review]
9. American Academy of Pediatrics, Task Force on Circumcision. Circumcision policy statement. *Pediatrics.* 1999;103(3):686–693. [Review; revised September 1, 2012]
10. World Health Organization 2010. *Manual for Early Infant Male Circumcision Under Local Anesthesia.* Geneva, Switzerland: World Health Organization, 2010. Available at: http://apps.who.int/iris/bitstream/10665/44478/1/9789241500753_eng.pdf. Accessed on August 23, 2016.
11. Stoll BJ, Hansen NI, Bell EF, et al for the Eunice Kennedy Shriver National Institute of Child Health and Human Development Neonatal Research Network. Trends in care practices, morbidity, and mortality of extremely preterm neonates, 1993–2012. *JAMA.* 2015; 314(10):1039–1051. doi: 10.1001/jama.2015.10244. [Epidemiologic data]
12. Hankins GD, Speer M. Defining the pathogenesis and pathophysiology of neonatal encephalopathy and cerebral palsy. *Obstet Gynecol.* 2003;102:628–636. [Review]
13. Clark SM, Basraon AK, Hankins GD. Intrapartum asphyxia, neonatal encephalopathy, cerebral palsy, and obstetric interventions in the term and near-term infant. *NeoReviews.* 2013;14(1):e13–e21. [Review]
14. American College of Obstetricians and Gynecologists, Task Force on Neonatal Encephalopathy. Executive summary: Neonatal encephalopathy and neurologic outcome, second edition. *Obstet Gynecol.* 2014;123(4):896–901. [Guideline]

32

The adnexal mass

Lauren Cooper Hand, George Patounakis, and Norman G. Rosenblum

KEY POINTS
- There are **no randomized trials** on interventions for adnexal masses in pregnancy.
- **Ultrasound,** with transvaginal and Doppler capabilities, **is the mainstay of diagnosis and prognosis.**
- **Most adnexal masses are simple cysts and will resolve. The most common persistent adnexal mass in pregnancy is a mature teratoma.**
- **The risk of an adnexal mass representing malignancy is 5%. Half of all ovarian cancers in pregnancy are epithelial and half of those are of low malignant potential.**
- For **a persistent adnexal mass in pregnancy,** early preoperative **consultation with a gynecologic oncologist, anesthesiologist, and neonatologist** is recommended.
- Complications related to the **persistent adnexal mass** in gravid patients may include **severe pain** (5%–26%), **ovarian torsion** (7%–12%), **cyst rupture** (9%), **pelvic impaction and obstruction of labor** (17%), and **ovarian cancer** (5%).
- **CA-125 is nonspecific and can be elevated simply due to pregnancy; between 15 weeks and delivery, levels between** 1,000 and 10,000 units/mL cannot be attributed to pregnancy alone.
- Management in the **first trimester** is almost uniformly **expectant** unless the clinical presentation is acute or malignancy is suspected.
- Although there are no guidelines, **surgery** in pregnancy can be reserved for adnexal masses that persist in the second trimester, and are either ≥**10 cm, symptomatic, or have solid or mixed solid and cystic findings concerning for malignancy.**
- When necessary and feasible, **surgery should be scheduled in the early second trimester** when organogenesis is complete, most spontaneous abortions have occurred, and the risk for premature delivery is low.
- **Intervention** should be considered **at any point** in gestation **if a mass is complex or suspicious for malignancy and increases in size.**
- If a suspicious **adnexal mass is identified incidentally at the time of cesarean section,** it should be *removed* and not simply aspirated.
- **If a malignant neoplasm of the ovary** is found at the time of exploration, the surgeon should consult a gynecologic oncologist to properly **stage the disease.**
- For more advanced ovarian cancer, the degree of cytoreductive surgery and the timing of initiation of chemotherapy will depend on fetal viability and maternal choice.

DEFINITION/DIAGNOSIS
An adnexal mass is any mass in the ovary or tube or attached to them (adnexa). There is an increase in the detection of asymptomatic adnexal masses in pregnancy due to the increase in prenatal ultrasounds. The vast majority (>90%) of adnexal masses in pregnancy are ovarian. Most are benign simple cysts under 5 cm. Table 32.1 outlines the differential diagnosis of an adnexal mass during pregnancy [1]. The diagnosis is most accurately made **by ultrasound,** even if it is possible to diagnose an adnexal mass by bimanual physical examination. A persistent adnexal mass is one that does not resolve by the second trimester.

EPIDEMIOLOGY/INCIDENCE
In earlier studies, approximately 1%–4% of women were diagnosed with an adnexal mass in pregnancy with persistence of only 1 in 200 to 1 in 600 into the second trimester [2,3]. A more recent study of adnexal masses that performed ultrasound of asymptomatic women during nuchal translucency evaluation (11–14 weeks) found an **incidence of almost 25%, with 85% of those resolving during the pregnancy without intervention** [4]. This dramatic increase in incidence is likely secondary to the early prevalence of functional cysts that spontaneously resolve during the pregnancy. Meanwhile, a recent study looking at over 7.7 million deliveries from 2003 to 2011, showed *the* **incidence of ovarian masses to be 0.25% at the time of delivery** [5]. The majority of the adnexal masses are simple cysts such as corpus luteal or other functional cysts. **Most of them** (up to 90%) **when identified during pregnancy will spontaneously regress prior to the second trimester.** The likelihood of regression is inversely related to size. Only 6% of cysts <6 cm compared with 39% of cysts >6 cm persist into the second trimester of pregnancy [6–8]. Two adnexal conditions are specifically associated with pregnancy and spontaneously regress in the postpartum period requiring no further treatment—luteomas of pregnancy and theca lutein cysts. Only **5% of adnexal masses found in the beginning of pregnancy are malignant ovarian tumors** [3]. **The incidence of ovarian cancer in pregnancy is rare, 1 in 18,000 to 1 in 47,000 deliveries** [9,10]. It is the fifth most common cancer diagnosed in pregnancy [11].

CLASSIFICATION
Among persistent adnexal masses diagnosed during pregnancy (age group 18–35 years), **mature teratomas are the most common** followed by benign serous and mucinous cystadenomas (Table 32.2) [12]. Most of the literature on ovarian cancer in pregnancy is based on case reports and series. In one of the largest case series, the most common ovarian cancers found in pregnancy are serous and mucinous tumors of low malignant potential [1].

RISK FACTORS/ASSOCIATIONS
Maternal age is a risk factor for malignancy, but ovarian malignancies can occur at any reproductive age. A study assessing the accuracy of combining patient demographics, serum CA-125,

Table 32.1 Differential Diagnosis of Most Common Adnexal Masses in Pregnancy

Benign	Malignant
Corpus luteum	Germ cell tumor
Simple cyst	Cystadenocarcinoma
Hemorrhagic cyst	Borderline tumors
Dermoid	Sex cord stromal tumor
Endometrioma	Metastatic cancer to ovary
Myoma	
Luteoma	
Hyperstimulated ovary	
Hydrosalpinx	
Theca lutein cyst	
Ectopic/heterotopic pregnancy	
Cystadenoma	
Peritoneal cyst	
Paraovarian/paratubal cyst	

Source: Adapted from Schwartz N et al., *Clin Obstet Gynecol*, 52, 570–585, 2009.

Table 32.2 Relative Frequency of Adnexal Masses Diagnosed in Pregnancy

Diagnosis	Percent
Benign (95%)	
Dermoid	37
Serous or mucinous cystadenoma	24
Corpus luteum	17
Endometrioma	5
Leiomyoma	5
Other (paraovarian, luteoma, theca-lutein)	12
Malignant (5%)	
Epithelial	50
Low malignant potential	66
Invasive	33
Germ cell tumor	30
Sex cord stromal tumor	20

Source: Adapted from Liu JR et al., *Cancer Obstetrics and Gynecology*, Lippincott Williams & Wilkins, Philadelphia, PA, 1999.

and ultrasonographic features in predicting the risk of malignancy of an ultrasonographically confirmed adnexal mass in nonpregnant women found age, menopausal status, weight, tumor morphology, presence of ascites, tumor laterality, tumor diameter, and CA-125 level to be associated with risk of malignancy [13]. Specifically, **age ≤55, premenopausal weight >200 lb, cystic morphology, negative ascites, unilaterality, diameter <10 cm, and CA-125 <35 were associated with benign masses.** None of the cystic tumors in that study were malignant. Furthermore, a large study in postmenopausal women with unilocular cystic masses <10 cm found none to have malignancy [14]. **Assisted reproductive technologies** increase the incidence of enlarged ovaries, cysts, and therefore adnexal masses.

COMPLICATIONS

Many studies show that planned abdominal surgery in pregnancy is safe [11,15–17] Complications related to the persistent adnexal mass in gravid patients include **severe pain** (26%), **ovarian torsion** (1%–22%), **cyst rupture** (0%–9%), and **pelvic impaction and obstruction of labor** (2%–17%) [11,15]. Ovarian torsion, the most common significant complication in pregnancy, occurs usually in less than 15% of the cases and is most common in adnexal masses with sizes between 6 and 8 cm 16]. Approximately 60% of torsion happens between 10 and 17 weeks' gestation and less than 6% happens after 20 weeks' gestation [16]. **Ovarian cancer** is estimated to occur in about 5% of adnexal masses found in the beginning of pregnancy [3]. Most malignancies are either germ cell, stromal, or epithelial tumors of low malignant potential [17].

MANAGEMENT
Principles
There are **no trials** available to assess any intervention in the management of adnexal masses in pregnancy. **As about 90% of these masses resolve and the risk of malignancy is 5%, in general, expectant management with serial ultrasounds is usually appropriate in the vast majority of, but not all, clinical situations.** If malignancy is suspected, the best gestational age for surgery is about 16–18 weeks, as the risk of loss is lowest.

Workup
Ultrasound
Highly skilled ultrasonographers may be able to accurately diagnose complications of adnexal masses in pregnancy (e.g., cancer and torsion) without surgical intervention. Suspicious characteristics of an adnexal mass include **complex** masses consisting of both **solid and cystic components** with nodularity, thick septations, irregular borders, solid masses containing irregular echoes, and papillary projections [18]. While cancer can be present in a cyst of any size, adnexal masses of ≤5 cm have an incidence of malignancy less than 1% [11]. Even unilocular cysts <10 cm in postmenopausal women can be safely followed by serial ultrasounds until they resolve or develop solid and/or wall abnormalities prompting surgical intervention secondary to a high suspicion of malignancy [14]. In addition to routine ultrasonography, color **Doppler** studies may be used to distinguish between malignant and benign adnexal masses [19]. Low pulsatility index of <1.0 and low impedance are associated with ovarian neoplasms. **Transvaginal** ultrasound may also help to better visualize the adnexal mass. The overall sensitivity of high-resolution ultrasound in distinguishing malignant from benign adnexal masses is 96.6%, specificity of 77%, and negative predictive value of 99% [19]. After 20 weeks, adnexal masses are more difficult to see by ultrasound given the larger uterine size. However, definitive diagnosis requires pathologic confirmation.

Magnetic Resonance Imaging
Although ultrasound is usually the extent of preoperative imaging, magnetic resonance imaging (MRI) has been used to characterize adnexal masses. There are insufficient data to assess the effect of MRI on management of adnexal masses in pregnancy, but a review of the topic with respect to each type of adnexal mass and the usefulness of MRI has been published [20]. The conclusions are that **MRI can assist ultrasound** in distinguishing an exophytic leiomyoma, degenerating leiomyoma, an endometrioma, a dermoid cyst, and a decidualized endometrioma, from other masses. Furthermore, it supports the value in MRI of detecting massive ovarian edema and distant findings such as widespread ascites, peritoneal implants, and lymphadenopathy that can help distinguish benign from malignant masses.

Laboratory

Most tumor markers may be elevated in normal pregnancy and are generally **not helpful** in distinguishing between a benign or malignant ovarian mass in pregnancy. For example, up to 16% of pregnant patients may have an elevated **CA-125** [21]. Levels of CA-125 peak in the first trimester (range, 7–251 units/mL), and decrease consistently thereafter. Low-level elevations in pregnancy are typically not associated with malignancy [17]. Levels from 1,000–10,000 units/mL after 15 weeks of gestation are likely to be cancer [3].

Therapy

Treatment planning is dependent upon the timeliness of detection of an adnexal mass in pregnancy. When an adnexal mass is diagnosed in the first trimester, the likelihood of a functional etiology is high, as is the probability of spontaneous resolution. In pregnant women, most simple cysts <6 cm have been shown to spontaneously resolve [22–25]. Given the high obstetrical risk during this period, **the management in the first trimester is almost uniformly expectant when the clinical presentation is not acute** [11]. Similarly, **intervention in the third trimester is typically deferred until delivery or the postpartum period as the risk of delaying therapy rarely outweighs the risk of surgery to the mother and the fetus.** When necessary and feasible, **surgery should be scheduled in the early second trimester** after most functional cysts have resolved, organogenesis is complete, most spontaneous losses have occurred, and the risk for premature delivery is low. Progesterone supplementation is necessary if the corpus luteum is removed prior to 8 weeks [3]. **Intervention should be considered at any point in gestation if a mass is complex or highly suspicious for malignancy and increases in size** (Figure 32.1). In addition to suspected malignancy, **surgical intervention may be indicated if torsion, rupture, or hemorrhage is identified.**

For persistent adnexal masses in pregnancy, **early preoperative consultation with a gynecologic oncologist, anesthesiologist, and neonatologist is recommended** [26]. Consultation at <15 weeks is recommended for better operative planning. Masses present after the first trimester that should be resected include those masses with the following characteristics: greater than 10 cm, symptomatic, or are solid or solid and cystic on ultrasound [27].

Surgery

Removal of adnexal masses can be accomplished via laparoscopy, laparotomy, or at time of cesarean section. When exploration is necessary, all efforts should be made to **avoid unnecessary manipulation of the uterus** to minimize premature uterine contractions. Other intraoperative and postoperative considerations should be kept in mind when operating on a pregnant patient (Table 32.3). Pre- and postoperative fetal doptones are recommended in the first trimester or early second trimester. Continuous fetal heart monitoring can be considered when viability is reached with the ability for an emergent cesarean section if needed [28–30].

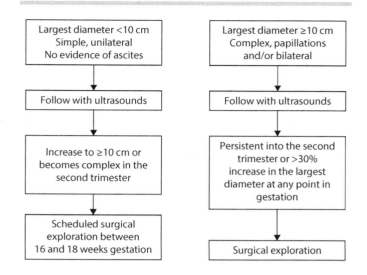

Figure 32.1 Management of the ovarian mass in pregnancy.

While traditionally a laparotomy was the standard recommendation used to explore the abdomen of a pregnant patient with an adnexal mass, **laparoscopy** is currently not only an acceptable alternative (in experienced hands) but also is **preferred in cases with low suspicion of malignancy,** as it offers the benefit of a more expeditious recovery [31–33]. In a Cochrane review on laparoscopy for adnexal tumors in pregnancy, the available case series were too limited for conclusions to be made on risks and benefits of laparoscopy. The need for a randomized controlled study was concluded [34]. However, laparoscopic surgery can be safely performed for ovarian torsion during pregnancy [35,36]. Abdominal surgery during pregnancy, in particular laparotomy, has been associated with higher rates of miscarriage and preterm birth compared with no surgery [11].

If a suspicious adnexal mass is identified incidentally at **the time of cesarean section**, it should be **removed** and not simply aspirated [2]. With aspiration and cytologic evaluation, malignancy could be missed [37].

If a malignant neoplasm of the ovary is suspected prior to surgery, a vertical incision is preferred and a frozen section should be sent. The surgeon's obligation is to consult a gynecologic oncologist in order to properly stage the disease (Table 32.4).

Table 32.3 Preoperative, Intraoperative, and Postoperative Considerations

Preoperative management	Preoperative hydration—to reduce risk of hypotension, uteroplacental insufficiency, and resultant fetal hypoxemia
Placement	15% left lateral tilt if the uterus is >20 weeks to shift the uterus off the inferior vena cava/wedge placement under the right hip
Monitoring	All viable fetuses (≥24 weeks) may be continuously monitored
Anesthesia	Preoxygenation with 100% oxygen administered by face mask for 3–5 minutes
	Halothane, isoflurane, and enflurane decrease uterine tone and may inhibit labor during the operative procedure
	Cocaine hydrochloride is a vasoconstrictor and contraindicated during pregnancy.

Sources: Adapted from Caspi B et al., *Ultrasound Obstet Gynecol,* 7, 275–279, 1996; Granberg S et al., *Gynecol Oncol,* 35, 139–144, 1989; Hata K and Hata T, *J Ultrasound Med,* 15, 571–575, 1996.

Table 32.4 FIGO Staging for Cancer of the Ovary, Fallopian Tube, and Peritoneum (2014)

Stage I—Growth limited to the ovaries or fallopian tubes
    Stage IA—Growth limited to one ovary or fallopian tube, no ascites, no tumor on external surface, and capsule intact
    Stage IB—Growth limited to both ovaries or fallopian tubes, no ascites, no tumor on external surface, and capsule intact
    Stage IC—Tumor limited to one or both ovaries or fallopian tubes with any of the following:
    Stage IC1—Surgical spill intraoperatively
    Stage IC2—Capsule ruptured before surgery or tumor on ovarian or fallopian tube surface
    Stage IC3—malignant cells in the ascites or peritoneal washings
Stage II—Growth involving one or both ovaries, with pelvic extension (below pelvic brim) or peritoneal cancer
    Stage IIA—Extension and/or implants to the uterus and/or fallopian tubes and/or ovaries
    Stage IIB—Extension to other pelvic intraperitoneal tissues
Stage III—Tumor involving one or both ovaries, fallopian tubes, or peritoneal cancer, with cytologically or histologically confirmed peritoneal implants outside the pelvis and/or metastasis to the retroperitoneal lymph nodes
    Stage IIIA—Metastasis to the retroperitoneal lymph nodes with or without microscopic peritoneal involvement beyond the pelvis
    Stage IIIA1—Positive retroperitoneal lymph nodes only (cytologically or histologically proven)
    Stage IIIA1(i)—Metastasis ≤10 mm in greatest dimension
    Stage IIIA1(ii)—Metastasis >10 mm in greatest dimension
    Stage IIIA2—Microscopic extrapelvic (above the pelvic brim) peritoneal involvement with or without positive retroperitoneal lymph nodes
    Stage IIIB—Macroscopic peritoneal metastases beyond the pelvic brim ≤2 cm in greater dimension, with or without metastasis to the retroperitoneal lymph nodes
    Stage IIIC—Macroscopic peritoneal metastases beyond the pelvic brim >2 cm in greater dimension, with or without metastasis to the retroperitoneal lymph nodes[a]
Stage IV—Distant metastases excluding peritoneal metastases
Stage IVA—Pleural effusion with positive cytology
Stage IVB—Metastases to extra-abdominal organs (including inguinal lymph nodes and lymph nodes outside the abdominal cavity)[b]

Abbreviation: FIGO, Federation Internationale de Gynecologie et d'Obstetrique (International Federation of Gynecology and Obstetrics).
[a]Includes extension of tumor to capsule of liver and spleen without parenchymal involvement of either organ.
[b]Parenchymal metastases are stage IVB.

Since most present as stage I disease, a unilateral salpingo-oophorectomy, omentectomy, and limited pelvic and para-aortic lymph node dissection is the procedure of choice. All suspicious lesions should be biopsied, with surface excrescences and ascites being suggestive of malignancy. If benign disease is suspected, cystectomy is preferred over a salpingoophorectomy.

If the disease appears to be confined to the pelvis, comprehensive surgical staging is indicated. The staging procedure includes peritoneal cytology, multiple peritoneal biopsies, omentectomy, and pelvic and paraaortic lymph node sampling. Rarely is a hysterectomy indicated. **For more advanced disease, cytoreductive surgery should be attempted.** The timing of initiation of chemotherapy will depend on fetal viability and maternal choice, and should be managed by a gynecologic oncologist. Returning for staging after completion of pregnancy is not thought to adversely impact survival, though late stage of disease has poor overall survival.

REFERENCES

1. Schwartz N, Timor-Tritsch I, Wang E. Adnexal masses in pregnancy. *Clin Obstet Gynecol.* 2009;52:570–585. [Review]
2. Koonings PP, Platt LD, Wallace R. Incidental adnexal neoplasms at cesarean section. *Obstet Gynecol.* 1988;72:767–769. [II-3]
3. Horowitz NS. Management of adnexal masses in pregnancy. *Clin Obstet Gynecol.* 2011;54(4):519–527. [Review]
4. Yazbek J, Salim R, Woelfer B, et al. The value of ultrasound visualization of the ovaries during the routine 11–14 weeks nuchal translucency scan. *Eur J Obstet Gynecol Reprod Biol.* 2007;132:154–158. [II-3, $n = 2925$]
5. Nazer A, Czuzoj-Shulman N, Oddy L, Abenhaim HA. Incidence of maternal and neonatal outcomes in pregnancies complicated by ovarian masses. *Arch Gynecol Obstet.* 2015 Apr; 292(5):1069–1074. [II-3]
6. Hess LW, Peaceman A, O'Brien WF, et al. Adnexal mass occurring with intrauterine pregnancy: Report of fifty-four patients requiring laparotomy for definitive management. *Am J Obstet Gynecol.* 1988;158:1029–1034. [II-3]
7. Whitecar MP, Turner S, Higby MK. Adnexal masses in pregnancy: A review of 130 cases undergoing surgical management. *Am J Obstet Gynecol.* 1999;181:19–24. [II-3]
8. Beischer NA, Buttery BW, Fortune DW, et al. Growth and malignancy of ovarian tumours in pregnancy. *Aust NZ J Obstet Gynaecol.* 1971;11:208–220. [II-3]
9. Munnell EW. Primary ovarian cancer associated with pregnancy. *Clin Obstet Gynecol.* 1963;6:983–993. [III]
10. Dgani R, Shoham Z, Atar E, et al. Ovarian carcinoma during pregnancy: A study of 23 cases in Israel between the years of 1963 and 1984. *Gynecol Oncol.* 1989;33:326–331. [II-3]
11. Schmeler KM, Mayo-Smith WW, Peipert JF, et al. Adnexal masses in pregnancy: Surgery compared with observation. *Obstet Gynecol.* 2005;105:1098–1103. [II-3]
12. Liu JR, Lilja JF, Johnston C. Adnexal masses in pregnancy. In Trimble EL, Trimble CL, eds. *Cancer Obstetrics and Gynecology.* Philadelphia, PA: Lippincott Williams & Wilkins, 1999: 239–248. [III]
13. McDonald JM, Doran S, DeSimone CP, et al. Predicting risk of malignancy in adnexal masses. *Obstet Gynecol.* 2010;115:687–694. [II-2, $n = 395$]

14. Modesitt SC, Pavlik EJ, Ueland FR, et al. Risk of malignancy in unilocular ovarian cystic tumors less than 10 centimeters in diameter. *Obstet Gynecol.* 2003;102:594–599. [II-2, n = 3259]
15. Struyk AP, Treffers PE. Ovarian tumors in pregnancy. *Acta Obstet Gynecol Scand.* 1984;63:421–424. [II-3]
16. Yen C, Lin S, Murk W, et al. Risk analysis of torsion and malignancy for adnexal masses during pregnancy. *Fertil Steril.* 2009;91:1895–1902. [II-3, n = 174]
17. American College of Obstetricians and Gynecologists. ACOG Practice Bulletin No. 83: Management of adnexal masses. *Obstet Gynecol.* 2007;110:201–214. [Review]
18. Bromley B, Benacerraf B. Adnexal masses during pregnancy: Accuracy of sonographic diagnosis and outcome. *J Ultrasound Med.* 1997;16:447–454. [II-3]
19. Wheeler TC, Fleischer AC. Complex adnexal mass in pregnancy: Predictive value of color Doppler ultrasonography. *J Ultrasound Med.* 1997;16:425–428. [II-2, n = 34]
20. Telischak NA, Yeh BM, Joe BN, et al. MRI of adnexal masses in pregnancy. *Am J Roentgenol.* 2008;191:364–370. [Review]
21. Niloff JM, Knapp RC, Schaetzi E, et al. CA125 antigen levels in obstetric and gynecology patients. *Obstet Gynecol.* 1984;64:703707. [II-3]
22. Hogston P, Lilford RJ. Ultrasound study of ovarian cysts in pregnancy: Prevalence and significance. *Br J Obstet Gynaecol.* 1986;93:625–628. [II-3]
23. Thornton JG, Wells M. Ovarian cysts in pregnancy: Does ultrasound make traditional management inappropriate? *Obstet Gynecol.* 1987;69:717–721. [II-3]
24. Bernhard LM, Klebba PK, Gray DL, et al. Predictors of persistence of adnexal masses in pregnancy. *Obstet Gynecol.* 1999;93:585–589. [II-3]
25. Zanetta G, Mariani E, Lissoni A, et al. A prospective study of the role of ultrasound in the management of adnexal masses in pregnancy. *Br J Obstet Gynecol.* 2003;110:578–583. [II-2, n = 79]
26. American College of Obstetricians and Gynecologists. ACOG Committee Opinion No. 284: Nonobstetric surgery in pregnancy. *Obstet Gynecol.* 2003;102:431. [Review]
27. Hoover K, Jenkins TR. Evaluation and management of adnexal mass in pregnancy. *Am J Obstet Gynecol.* 2011;205(2):97–102. [Review]
28. Caspi B, Appelman Z, Rabinerson D, et al. Pathognomonic echo patterns of benign cystic teratomas of the ovary: Classification, incidence and accuracy rate of sonographic diagnosis. *Ultrasound Obstet Gynecol.* 1996;7:275–279. [II-2, n = 115]
29. Granberg S, Wikland M, Jansson I. Macroscopic characterization of ovarian tumors and the relation to the histological diagnosis: Criteria to be used for ultrasound evaluation. *Gynecol Oncol.* 1989;35:139–144. [II-3]
30. Hata K, Hata T. Intratumoral blood flow analysis in ovarian cancer: What does it mean? *J Ultrasound Med.* 1996;15:571–575. [II-3]
31. Soriano D, Yefet Y, Seidman DS, et al. Laparoscopy versus laparotomy in the management of adnexal masses during pregnancy. *Fertil Steril.* 1999;71:955–960. [II-2, n = 88]
32. Yuen PM, Ng PS, Leung PL, Rogers MS. Outcome in laparoscopic management of persistent adnexal mass during the second trimester of pregnancy. *Surg Endosc.* 2004;18(9):354–357. [II-3]
33. Mathevet P, Nessah K, Dargent D, et al. Laparoscopic management of adnexal masses in pregnancy: A case series. *Eur J Obstet Gynecol Reprod Biol.* 2003;108(2):217–222. [II-3]
34. Bunyavejchevin S, Phupong V. Laparoscopic surgery for presumed benign ovarian tumor during pregnancy. *Cochrane Database Syst Rev.* 2013;(1):CD005459. doi: 10.1002/14651858. CD005459.pub3. [Review]
35. Shalev E, Peleg D. Laparoscopic treatment of adnexal torsion. *Surg Gynecol Obstet.* 1993;176:448–450. [II-3]
36. Cohen SB, Oelsner G, Seidman DS, et al. Laparoscopic detorsion allows sparing of the twisted ischemic adnexa. *J Am Assoc Gynecol Laparosc.* 1999;6:139–143. [II-3]
37. Rodin A, Coltart TM, Chapman MG. Needle aspiration of simple ovarian cysts in pregnancy. Case reports. *Br J Obstet Gynaecol.* 1989;96:994–946. [II-3]

Cervical cancer screening and management in pregnancy

Talia M. Maas and Christine H. Kim

KEY POINTS
- Cervical cancer screening guidelines for nonpregnant women can be followed in pregnant women. These suggest **initiating Pap smear screening at age 21, regardless of onset of sexual activity.** Routine screening intervals have also been extended to every 3 years for women in their twenties without human papillomavirus (HPV) cotesting and every 5 years in women over 30 with the addition of HPV cotesting.
- **The only cervical diagnosis** that is considered **to alter management in pregnancy is invasive cancer.**
- A more **conservative approach should be used to manage cervical intraepithelial neoplasia (CIN).**
- Due to risks of bleeding and premature rupture of membranes, **endocervical curettage (ECC)** is **never recommended in pregnancy.**
- **Diagnostic conization** during pregnancy should **only be considered when** either the biopsy, or cytology is **suggestive of invasive cancer** and the diagnosis of invasion would result in a modification of treatment recommendations, timing, or mode of delivery.
- **In the diagnosis of invasive cancer with a grossly visible lesion, cesarean delivery** is indicated and results in better survival outcomes as well as a decreased risk of obstetrical bleeding in the intrapartum and postpartum periods.
- **If a nonvisible microinvasive lesion** (stage IAI or IA2) is identified, **either the abdominal or vaginal route of delivery is acceptable,** depending on obstetrical and gynecologic circumstances.
- Once the diagnosis of cervical cancer is established, individualized recommendations for the **management of the malignancy** as well as the *pregnancy* are formulated **with consideration for the stage of disease, gestational age at the time of diagnosis, and maternal desires regarding the continuation of her pregnancy.**
- Fertility-sparing surgery and neoadjuvant chemotherapy for earlier stage cervical cancer found in pregnancy may be considered without worsening survival.

HISTORIC NOTES
The cytologic evaluation of the cervix, known as the Pap smear, was developed in the 1940s by George Papanicolaou. The Bethesda System standardized terminology for reporting Pap smear cytology results in 1988 [1] and was subsequently revised in 2001 [2]. In response to the standardization of cytology results, the American Society for Colposcopy and Cervical Pathology (ASCCP) initiated a process that developed comprehensive, evidence-based consensus guidelines to assist clinicians in managing abnormal cervical cytology results. The ASCCP screening guidelines were most recently updated in 2012 [3].

DIAGNOSIS/DEFINITION
Microinvasive cervical cancer is defined as cancer spread to no more than 5 mm into the tissue of the cervix. Invasive cervical cancer is defined as cancer spread from the surface of the cervix to tissue deeper in the cervix, possible spread to part of the vagina, to the lymph nodes, to the other tissues surrounding the cervix, within the pelvis, or beyond the pelvic areas into nearby organs.

EPIDEMIOLOGY/INCIDENCE
The overall rate of an abnormal Pap smear with atypical squamous cells–undetermined significance (ASC-US) or higher in the United States is estimated around 4% from data collected between 2003 and 2010 [4]. The peak age incidence of cervical cancer is in the mid-forties [5]. In low- and middle-income countries, cervical cancer is the second most common cancer among women, the third most common cause of cancer-related death, and the most common cause of mortality from gynecologic malignancy. In contrast, in high-income countries, the success of Pap smear screening has greatly reduced the incidence of disease by accurately detecting preinvasive and early-invasive cervical disease. In the United States, **the incidence of cervical cancer ranges from 1.5 to 12 cases in 100,000 pregnancies** [6]. About 1% of the women who have cervical cancer are pregnant at the time of diagnosis. The likelihood that a pregnant woman with ASC pathology has a detectable high-risk human papillomavirus (HR HPV) is 84% [7].

CLASSIFICATION
The Pap smear report consists of the following [2]:

Specimen Type
- **Conventional Pap smear**: Cells from the transformation zone are sampled and transferred directly onto a slide [8].
- **Liquid-based cytology**: Cells from the transformation zone are placed in a prepared liquid preservative and processed by a laboratory. This is the **method most commonly used in clinical practice** in the United States because of the added benefit of using a single sample for HPV cotesting. The use of liquid-based media can also control for obscuring factors including blood, inflammation, and other processes [8].
- There is no difference in unsatisfactory rates, cytology classifications, and accuracy between conventional and liquid-based cervical cytology [9].

Specimen Adequacy
Satisfactory for Evaluation
- Defined as a minimum of 5,000 well-visualized squamous cells on a liquid-based preparation or 8,000 to 12,000 well-visualized squamous cells on a conventional smear.

- The presence of endocervical cells indicates that the area at risk for neoplasia, the transformation zone, has been adequately sampled [10].
- Samples reported as negative but with absent or insufficient endocervical/transition zone components have raised concern about missed pathology. Prior guidelines have recommended repeat cytology. Recent meta-analysis studies reported that negative cytology (with or without sufficient sampling of the endocervical/transition zone) has both good negative predicative value as well as good specificity. **Current guidelines do not recommend repeat follow-up Pap smears.** Women ages 21–29 are to continue with routine screenings. **Women older than 30 years of age are recommended to undergo HPV cotesting for an added margin of safety. Alternatively if cotesting is unavailable, patients are to undergo repeat testing in 1 year. Pregnant women are recommended to follow the same age depended guidelines** [3].

Unsatisfactory for Evaluation
- Defined as more than 75% of the cells being uninterpretable or an unlabeled specimen.
- Since women with this result are more likely to have intraepithelial lesions or cancer on follow-up than women with satisfactory Pap smears [10], a repeated pap smear in 2–4 months is recommended. If the subsequent Pap smear is unsatisfactory, evaluation with colposcopy and/or biopsies is appropriate [11].

Interpretation/Result

Squamous Epithelial Cell Abnormalities
- ASC of either of the following:
  - Undetermined significance (ASC-US)
  - Suspicious for high-grade squamous intraepithelial lesions (HSILs or ASC-H)
- Low-grade squamous intraepithelial lesions (LSIL)
  - Changes consistent with HPV, mild dysplasia, or grade 1 CIN I
- HSIL
  - HSIL includes moderate or severe dysplasia, CIN II, CIN III, carcinoma in situ (CIS), and should indicate if there are features suspicious for invasive disease. When glandular cell abnormalities are present, it should be noted whether there are changes favoring neoplasia
- Carcinoma

Glandular Cell Abnormalities
- Atypical glandular cells (AGCs) may be of endocervical, endometrial, or other glandular origin
- Endocervical adenocarcinoma in situ (AIS)
- Adenocarcinoma

Human Papillomavirus Testing

HPV testing is now an integral part of cervical cancer screening. Updated ASCCP Consensus guidelines that were most recently validated in 2015 state **HPV cotesting is recommended for all female patients over the age of 30 and for all patients with ASC-US cytology.**

- HPV infection is the leading etiologic agent in the development of premalignant and malignant lower genital tract disease [12].
- **Cotesting should only detect for the presence of high-risk HPV species. There is no role in testing for low-risk genotypes. Detecting low-risk genotypes has been proven to cause unnecessary procedures and testing, therefore decreasing clinical specificity. It is recommended to use only Food and Drug Administration (FDA)-approved HPV DNA detection kits** [8].
- The most well-studied HPV test is the Hybrid Capture 2 HPV DNA Assay (Digene Corporation, Beltsville, MD), which uses a probe mix for high-risk (HR) HPV types 16, 18, 31, 33, 35, 39, 45, 51, 52, 56, 58, 59, and 68 [13].
- A newer assay for detecting HR HPV was approved for FDA use in 2009. Cervista™ HR HPV (Hologic Corporation, Waltham, MA) includes the 13 HPV types above and adds type 66 [8].
- Cervista HPV 16/18 is another diagnostic test that specifies type 16 and 18. These two represent the most common types found in cervical squamous cell carcinomas and adenocarcinomas, respectively.
- Ongoing research looks promising in improving specificity and positive predictive value of screening for CIN2+ by looking at messenger RNA (mRNA) instead of DNA for HR HPV [14].

MANAGEMENT
Pregnancy Considerations

Pregnancy-induced changes in the cervix include hyperemia, eversion of columnar epithelium, more prominent glands, and increased production and volume of mucus. The decidual changes may exaggerate the colposcopic appearance of CIN. A biopsy during pregnancy may cause substantial bleeding [3]. In pregnancy, the general philosophy for the treatment of intraepithelial neoplasia of the cervix has become expectant management after careful diagnosis.

Screening in Pregnancy

The Pap smear is used to screen for cellular abnormalities that are associated with an increased risk for the development of cervical cancer. It selects those women who should have further evaluation, such as HPV DNA testing, colposcopy, and/or biopsy, which then are used for treatment decisions. The National Comprehensive Cancer Network (NCCN) panel has adopted recommendation set forth by the American Cancer Society on initiation and frequency of Pap smear [15]. New recommendations for 2012 include **initiating Pap smear screening at age 21, regardless of onset of sexual activity. Routine screening intervals have also been extended to every 3 years for women in their twenties and should not include routine HPV cotesting unless abnormal cytology is detected. Women greater than 30 years of age should undergo screening every 5 years with both cytology and HPV cotesting. If HPV cotesting is unavailable, cytology alone every 3 years is recommended.** The rationale is that invasive cancer is rare in women under 21 years. The evidence for increasing the interval is based on studies that suggested no statistical difference between annual surveillance and 2- to 3-year intervals.

Annual surveillance is recommended for patients with known immunosuppression from HIV or organ transplantation, women exposed to diethylstilbestrol in utero, or those who have been previously treated for CIN 2, CIN 3, or cervical cancer.

Pap smears are often obtained at the first prenatal visit by many providers, but the **guidelines for nonpregnant women can be followed in pregnant women** [8].

Consultations Required

Consultation with gynecologic oncologists is recommended in cases of cervical cancer [16]. Consultation should occur as early as possible after the diagnosis of cervical cancer for better therapeutic planning. Collaboration with a Maternal-Fetal Medicine specialist is also recommended for management of obstetrical complications and delivery planning.

Indications for Colposcopy and Cervical Biopsy during Pregnancy

As in nonpregnant women, **women with abnormal Pap smears during pregnancy should undergo colposcopy with directed biopsies** of suspicious areas to rule out invasive disease (Figure 33.1) [3].

ASC-US, HPV negative

- No indication for colposcopy at any age. Pregnant patients have to follow age-appropriate routine screening.

LSIL and ASC-US, HR HPV positive

- Ages 21–24 years: women are to undergo repeat Pap smear and cotesting in 12 months. Colposcopy is not recommended.
- Ages >24 years: In pregnant patients, colposcopy is recommended but it is acceptable to defer colposcopy to 6 weeks postpartum.

HSIL or more invasive cytology

- In patients with higher grade lesions noted on cervical screening examinations necessary colposcopically directed cervical biopsies can be safely performed at any time during pregnancy. Many defer biopsy until the second trimester when the risk of incidental pregnancy loss is minimal. Due to risks of bleeding and premature rupture of membranes, **ECC is never recommended in pregnancy.** Cervical biopsies should only be performed if CIN II or above is suspected on colposcopic examination.

CIN1:

- If adequate samples are obtained during colposcopy and invasive disease is not suspected at any point during the pregnancy, it is recommended to defer repeat colposcopy to 6 weeks postpartum.

CIN2/3 and carcinoma in situ (CIS):

- In women with histological diagnosis of CIN2/3 or (CIS) on initial colposcopy, it is recommended to perform repeat colposcopy and cytology every 12 weeks for the duration of the pregnancy. Repeat biopsy is recommended only if the appearance of the lesions worsens or if cytology is concerning for invasive cancer. It is acceptable to defer tissue biopsy to 6 weeks postpartum if no progression of the lesion is noted on colposcopy and cytology [3].

Diagnosis of Invasive Cancer

Once the diagnosis of cervical cancer is established, individualized recommendations for the management of the malignancy as well as the pregnancy are formulated with consideration for the stage of disease, gestational age at the time of diagnosis, and maternal desires regarding the continuation of her pregnancy (see Chapter 42 in *Maternal-Fetal Evidence Based Guidelines*). **The patient should seek consultation by specialists in both maternal-fetal medicine as well as gynecology/oncology.**

Management of the Abnormal Pap Smear

There are **no randomized control trials** assessing any aspect of management of abnormal Pap smear in pregnancy. Most of the recommendations are based on expert opinion and anecdotal experience [16–18]. **The only diagnosis that is considered to alter management in pregnancy is invasive cancer.**

Management of abnormal Pap smears in pregnancy should follow the recommendations delineated in Figure 33.1. Recommendations for **colposcopy** in pregnant patients are similar to those in the nongravid state, with certain exceptions

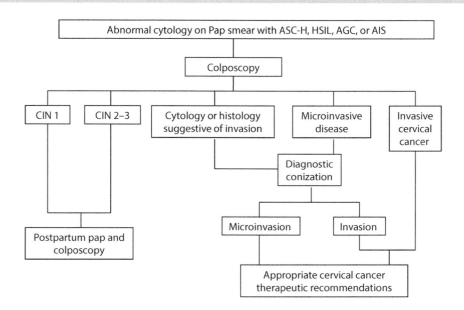

Figure 33.1 Algorithm for the workup of abnormal cytology in pregnancy. AGC, atypical glandular cell; AIS, adenocarcinoma in situ; ASC-H, atypical squamous cells higher; CIN, cervical intraepithelial neoplasia; HSIL, high-grade squamous intraepithelial lesion.

as listed in Table 33.1. Newer guidelines for colposcopy in pregnancy state that colposcopy is preferred for ASC-US associated with positive HR HPV type or LSIL Pap smears, but also that colposcopy can be deferred by the clinician until after pregnancy for these two categories. Colposcopy during pregnancy has as its **primary goal to assess for invasive cancer.** Biopsies should only be performed for women with colposcopic impression of **CIN 3/CIS, AIS, or cancer,** with the purpose to exclude invasive cancer [19].

Repeat Pap and colposcopy is recommended if invasive cancer is suspected but not yet proven, specifically with evidence of CIN2/3 or CIS on cytology or biopsy. Repeat biopsy during pregnancy should only be performed if progression of lesion is suspected. **ECC is not performed** in pregnancy [14,19].

Conization performed during pregnancy is associated with increased morbidity. The most common complications include hemorrhage, abortion, premature delivery, and infection [20]. **Therefore, cervical conization has limited indications in pregnancy** (Table 33.2). In general, diagnostic conization during pregnancy should only be considered **when either the biopsy or cytology is suggestive of invasive cancer or AIS** and the diagnosis of invasion would result in a modification of treatment recommendations, timing, or mode of delivery [19].

Unlike standard recommendations for cervical conization in nonobstetrical patients with inadequate colposcopic biopsies or discordance between Pap smears and colposcopic biopsies [12], pregnant women with these findings can defer further examination until after pregnancy if invasive cancer has been ruled out. If a cervical conization must be performed during pregnancy, this procedure should ideally be performed in the early second trimester.

Management of Cervical Cancer

For staging and management please refer to Table 33.3 and Chapter 42 in *Maternal-Fetal Evidence Based Guidelines* [10] (Figure 33.1). Microinvasive cervical cancer is defined as cancer spread to no more than 5 mm deep into the cervical stroma. Microinvasive disease includes stages IA1 and IA2. Invasive cervical cancer is defined as cancer that has invaded deeper than 5 mm into the cervical stroma, is grossly visible, or involves additional structures. Invasive disease includes Stage IB1 or greater.

Stage IA1:

- **Conization** is recommended for both treatment and diagnosis in patients with evidence of Stage IA1 cancer [21]. To minimize the risk of spontaneous abortion is it optimal to perform conization in the early second trimester [20].
- If conization margins are negative, patients can be managed expectantly for the duration of the pregnancy [20].
- Either abdominal or vaginal delivery routes are expectable for these patients. Mode of delivery should be discussed with a maternal-fetal medicine specialist with consideration of other gynecological and obstetrical circumstances. This should be decided on an individual basis [21].
- If continued fertility is desired, patients can be followed up every 3 months for 2 years and every 6 months for the next 3 years [20].

Stage IA2

- **Conization** with the addition of **pelvic lymphadenectomy** is recommended to rule out high-risk disease. Radical trachelectomy is not recommended given the risk significant blood loss and obstetrical complications resulting from prolonged surgery [21].
- Given the technical complications performing lymphadenectomy after 25 weeks of gestation in patients diagnosed after 25 weeks, it is recommended to delay treatment and full surgical staging until after delivery. If disease progression is suspected, it is recommended to obtain an abdominal and pelvic magnetic resonance imaging (MRI) [20].
- As stated above, patients can undergo either abdominal or vaginal delivery with consideration of other obstetrical circumstances. Delivery can be delayed until fetal maturity at 37 weeks [20].
- Given that IA2 carries a higher risk of nodal metastasis, patients can undergo either classic cesarean delivery with modified radical hysterectomy or surgery can be delayed 6–8 weeks postpartum in the case of vaginal delivery [20].

Stage IB1

- Neoadjuvant **chemotherapy** is recommended until fetal maturity. The goal of therapy is to stabilize the tumor during pregnancy [21]. Postponement of treatment is acceptable if there is no evidence of progression of disease. As stated above, MRI should be obtained if there is any suspicion. Patients should be examined every 2–4 weeks [20].
- Delivery can be delayed until documented fetal lung maturity with amniocentesis. Testing for fetal lung maturity should begin at 32 weeks [20].
- Patient should undergo classic cesarean delivery with modified radical hysterectomy and pelvic lymphadenectomy [20].

Stage IB2 and higher stage tumors

- **Termination** of pregnancy is recommended given high risk of disease progression during pregnancy [21].
- **If pregnancy is desired**, initiation of neoadjuvant **chemotherapy** is recommended. Chemotherapy allows the pregnancy to be continued to an average of 33 weeks. **Early delivery** is recommended to expedite the initiation of standard of care treatment. The practitioner should discuss the initiation of betamethasone therapy and preterm delivery [21].
- The patient should undergo a cesarean delivery followed by initiation of therapy 6 weeks postpartum [20].

Table 33.1 Cervical Screening Considerations During Pregnancy

- Endocervical brush cytology is safe.
- Cervical biopsy is safe.
- Endocervical curettage (ECC) should be avoided.
- For ASC and LSIL, HR HPV positive, colposcopy is preferred but can be done postpartum.
- For CIN 2 or CIN 3, Pap and colposcopy can be repeated postpartum if cancer is not suspected.
- Delay treatment of any level of CIN until postpartum period.
- Cervical conization is recommended if invasion is suspected.

Abbreviations: ASC, atypical squamous cell; CIN, cervical intraepithelial neoplasia; HR HPV, high-risk human papillomavirus; LSIL, low-grade squamous intraepithelial lesion.

Table 33.2 Indications for Conization in Pregnancy

- Histologic presence of microinvasive or invasive disease
- Persistent cytologic impression of invasive cancer (in absence of histologic confirmation)
- Histologic presence of adenocarcinoma in situ

Table 33.3 Staging and Management of Cervical Cancer in Pregnancy

Stage 0	Carcinoma in situ	*Preinvasive* disease—not treated in pregnancy
Stage I	The tumor is confined to the cervix	
	IA Microinvasive disease, with the lesion not grossly visible: no deeper than 5 mm and no wider than 7 mm	*Microinvasive cervical cancer*—not treated during pregnancy
	IA1 invasion ≤3 mm deep and ≤ 7 mm wide	
	IA2 invasion >3 mm but <5 mm deep and ≤7 mm wide	
	IB Larger tumor than in IA2 or grossly visible, confined to cervix	Histologically confirmed, *invasive cervical cancer* is the only indication to treat during pregnancy
	IB1 Clinical lesion ≤4 cm in greatest dimension	
	IB2 Clinical lesion >4 cm in greatest dimension	
Stage II	Tumor extends beyond the cervix but does not involve the pelvic side wall or lower third of the vagina	
	IIA Without lateral extension into the parametrium	
	IIA1 Clinically visible lesion ≤4 cm in greatest dimension	
	IIA2 Clinically visible lesion >4 cm in greatest dimension	
	IIB With lateral extension into parametrial tissue	
Stage III	Tumor extends to the pelvic side wall and/or involves lower third of the vagina and/or causes hydronephrosis or nonfunctioning kidney	
	IIIA Involves the lower third of the vagina without extension to the pelvic side wall	
	IIIB Involves the pelvic side wall and/or hydronephrosis or nonfunctioning kidney	
Stage IV	Extensive local infiltration or has spread to a distant site	
	IVA Involvement of bladder or rectal mucosa	
	IVB Distant metastases	

Recurrence and Follow-Up Treatment

Seventy-five percent of patients with CIN diagnosed during pregnancy have persistent or progressive disease at postpartum evaluation [21]. A regression rate of only 12% is found in pregnant women with CIN III, emphasizing the importance of **reevaluation 6 weeks postpartum** [12,22].

Routine surveillance can be resumed if there is no recurrence after the first 2 years of follow-up, which includes performing two Pap smears at 6-month intervals or HPV testing at 1-year intervals. Postpregnancy surveillance intervals are modified if the Pap smear or colposcopic biopsies reveal CIN 2, CIN 3, or CIS, and are the same as the nonpregnant guidelines [12].

Prevention

HPV-16 vaccine reduces the incidence of both HPV-16 infection and HPV-16-related CIN [23]. Currently, the three licensed HPV vaccines available in the United States include Cervarix (two-valent, types 16,18), Gardisil (four-valent, types 6,11,16,18), and most recently, Gardisil-9 (nine-valent, types 6,11,18,19,31,33,45,52,58). The nine-valent vaccine was recently found to be equivalent to the prior recommended vaccine [24,25].

No HPV vaccine should not be administered during pregnancy (see Chapter 38 in *Maternal-Fetal Evidence Based Guidelines*).

REFERENCES

1. National Cancer Institute Workshop. The 1988 Bethesda System for reporting cervical/vaginal cytological diagnoses. *JAMA*. 1989;262:931. [Review; III]
2. Solomon D, Davey D, Kurman R, et al. The 2001 Bethesda System: Terminology for reporting results of cervical cytology. *JAMA*. 2002;287:2114. [Review; III]
3. Massad SL, Einstein MH, et al. Updated consensus guidelines for the management of abnormal cervical cancer screening tests and cancer precursors. *J Lower Genital Tract Dis*. 2013;17:S1–S27. [Review; III]
4. Katki HA, Schiffman M, Castle PE, et al. Benchmarking CIN 3+ risk as the basis for incorporating HPV and Pap cotesting into cervical screening and management guidelines. *J Low Genit Tract Dis*. 2013;17:S28. [II-3]
5. Insinga RP, Glass AG, Rush BB. Diagnosis and outcomes in cervical cancer screening: A population-based study. *Am J Obstet Gynecol*. 2004;191:105–113. [II-3]
6. Hunter MI, Krishnansu T, Bradley JM. Cervical neoplasia in pregnancy. Part 2: Current treatment of invasive disease. *Am J Obstet Gynecol*. 2008;199:10–18. [Review; III]
7. Lu DW, Pirog EC, Zhu X, et al. Prevalence and typing of HPV DNA in atypical squamous cells in pregnant women. *Acta Cytol*. 2003;47(6):1008–1016. [II-3]
8. ACOG Committee on Practice Bulletins—Gynecology. ACOG Practice Bulletin No. 131: Screening for cervical cancer. *Obstet Gynecol*. 2012;120(5):1222–1238. [Review; III]
9. Davey E, Barratt A, Irwig L, et al. Effect of study design and quality on unsatisfactory rates, cytology classifications, and accuracy in liquid-based versus conventional cervical cytology: A systematic review. *Lancet*. 2006;367:122–132. [Meta-analysis; I]
10. Ransdell JS, Davey DD, Zaleski S. Clinicopathologic correlation of the unsatisfactory Papanicolaou smear. *Cancer*. 1997;81:139. [II-3]
11. American College of Obstetricians and Gynecologists. ACOG Practice Bulletin No. 140: Management of abnormal cervical cancer screening test results and cervical cancer precursors. *Obstet Gynecol*. 2013;122(6):1338–1367. [Review; III]
12. Bosch FX, Manos MM, Munoz N, et al. Prevalence of human papillomavirus in cervical cancer: A worldwide perspective. International Biological Study on Cervical Cancer (IBSCC) study group. *J Natl Cancer Inst*. 1995;87:796. [II-3]
13. Lorincz A. Hybrid capture method of detection of human papillomavirus DNA in clinical specimens. *Papillomavirus Rep*. 1996;7:1–5. [II-3]

14. Burger EA, Kornør H, Klemp M, et al. HPV nRMA tests for the detection of cervical intraepithelial neoplasia: A systematic review. *Gynecol Oncol.* 2011;120(3):430–438; [Epub December 4, 2010]. [Review; III]
15. Saslow D, Solomon D, Lawson HW, et al. American Cancer Society, American Society for Colposcopy and Cervical Pathology, and American Society for Clinical Pathology screening guidelines for the prevention and early detection of cervical cancer. *Am J Clin Pathol.* 2012;137:516–542. [Review; III]
16. ACOG Committee on Obstetric Practice. ACOG Committee Opinion No. 284, August, 2003: Nonobstetric surgery in pregnancy. *Obstet Gynecol.* 2003;102(2):431. [Review; III]
17. Hunter MI, Krishnansu T, Bradley JM. Cervical neoplasia in pregnancy. Part 1: Screening and management of preinvasive disease. *Am J Obstet Gynecol.* 2008;199:3–9. [Review; III]
18. Massad SL, Wright TC, Cox TJ, et al. Managing abnormal cytology results in pregnancy. *J Lower Genital Tract Dis.* 2005;9(3):146–148. [Review; III]
19. Fader AN, Alward EK, Niederhauser A, et al. Cervical dysplasia in pregnancy: A multi-institutional evaluation. *Am J Obstet Gynecol.* 2010;203:113.e1–113.e6. [II-3]
20. Nguygen CC, Montz FJ, Bristow RE, et al. Management of stage I cervical cancer in pregnancy. *Obstet Gynecol Surv.* 2000;10:633. [Review; III]
21. Amant F, Halaska MJ, Fumagalli M, et al. Gynecologic cancers in pregnancy: Guidelines of a second international consensus meeting. *Int J Gynecol Cancer.* 2014;24:394. [Review; III]
22. Palle C, Bangsball S, Andreasson B. Cervical intraepithelial neoplasia in pregnancy. *Acta Obstet Gynecol Scand.* 2000;79:306–310. [II-3]
23. Koutsky LA, Ault KA, Wheeler CM, et al. A controlled trial of a human papillomavirus type 16 vaccine. *N Engl J Med.* 2002;347:1645–1651. [RCT, $n = 2392$; I]
24. Markowitz LE, Dunne EF, Saraiya M, et al.; Centers for Disease Control and Prevention; Advisory Committee on Immunization Practices (ACIP). Quadrivalent human papillomavirus vaccine. Recommendations of the Advisory Committee on Immunization Practices (ACIP). *MMWR Recomm Rep.* 2007;56(RR-2):1–32. [Review; III]
25. Joura E, Giuliano A, Iverson O, et al. A 9-valent HPV vaccine against infection and intraepithelial neoplasia in women. *N Engl J Med.* 2015;372:711–723. [RCT, $n = 14215$; I]

Index

Abdominal decompression, 27
Abdominal distension, 42
Abdominal surgery, in pregnancy, 344
Abdominal trauma, 310
Abdominal wall defects, 339
Abnormal FHR in labor, algorithm for, 120
ABO/Rh (D) type screen test, 19
Abruptio placentae, 235, 309–313
aCGH, see Array comparative genomic hybridization
Acidemia, 111
   FHR monitoring, 117
Acidosis, 111
Acid prophylaxis drugs, 90
ACMG, see American College of Medical Genetics and Genomics
ACOG, see American College of Obstetricians and Gynecologists
Active management of the third stage of labor (AMSTL), 106–107
   algorithm for, 104
   oxytocin, 104–105
Acupressure, 126
Acupuncture, 126, 259
Acute renal failure, 311
Adenosine monophosphate (AMP), 218
Adhering to the as low as reasonably achievable (ALARA) principle, 49
Adhesion formation prevention, for cesarean delivery, 152
Adhesive drapes, for cesarean delivery, 148
Adnexal mass, in pregnancy, 343–346
Advanced maternal age (AMA), 7
AED, see Antiepileptic drug
Aerobic exercise, 22
AFI, see Amniotic fluid index
Agonist/antagonists, 127
AIUM, see American Institute of Ultrasound in Medicine
ALARA principle, see Adhering to the as low as reasonably achievable principle
Alcohol use, 22
AMA, see Advanced maternal age
Ambroxol, 217
Ambulation, 90
American College of Medical Genetics and Genomics (ACMG)
   carrier screening, 79
   direct-to-consumer genetic testing, 82
American College of Obstetricians and Gynecologists (ACOG), 51, 52, 113, 139, 161, 289
   carrier screening, 77, 79
   Committee Opinion, 98
   premature rupture of membranes, 245–246
American Institute of Ultrasound in Medicine (AIUM), 51, 52

Amniocentesis, 65–66, 204, 231
Amnioinfusion, 119, 234, 270
   for prolonging latency, 231
Amniotic fluid index (AFI), 88
Amniotomy, 256, see also Artificial rupture of membranes (AROM)
AmniSure, 243
AMP, see Adenosine monophosphate
Ampicillin, 232–233, 245
Ampicillin-sulbactam, 221
AMSTL, see Active management of the third stage of labor
Analgesia/anesthesia, 109, 125, 189, 222, 234, 287
   emergency, 134–135
   epidural, 127–130
   neuraxial, 126
   for pain control, 107
   spinal, 130
   for vaginal breech delivery, 278
Anembryonic pregnancy, ultrasound diagnosis of, 51–52
Anemia, 43–44
Aneuploidy
   diagnostic tests, 65–66
   microdeletions and duplications, 72–73
   positive screening for, 64–65
   pretest general counseling for, 60–61
Antenatal bleeding, 300
Antenatal breast examination, 319
Antenatal class, 27
Antenatal corticosteroids, 305
Antenatal education program, 86
Antenatal noninvasive aneuploidy screening, 61
Antepartum, 283–284
   hemorrhage, 301, 311
Antepartum testing, 188, 222, 302
   during cervical ripening, 260
Antibiotic prophylaxis, 27, 140
Antibiotics, 218
   for women, 179–180
Antibody screen test, 19
Antiepileptic drug (AED), 11
Antigen avoidance diet, 23
Antiphospholipid syndrome, 187
Anxiety, during labor pain, 89
Appendectomy, for cesarean delivery, 152
Apt test, 305
Aromatherapy, 89, 126
Array comparative genomic hybridization (aCGH), 66
Artificial feeding, 318
Artificial rupture of membranes (AROM), 91
ASD, see Atrial septal defect
Ashkenazi Jewish ancestry, 79–82
Asphyxia, 111

Aspirin therapy, 131
Asthma exacerbation, 42
Asymptomatic bacteriuria, 205
   urine culture for, 19
Atosiban, 221
Atrial septal defect (ASD), 69
Autosomal recessive inheritance, 79
Azithromycin, 232–233

Baby friendly initiative (BFI), 318–319
Back pain, 28
Bacterial vaginosis (BV), 20, 205
Balloon catheter, 253–254
Barusiban, 221
Baths, induction of labor, 260
Before labor interventions, 86
Beta human chorionic gonadotropin, 176
Betamethasone, 147, 216, 232
Betamimetics, 218–219, 221, 275
BFI, see Baby friendly initiative
Biofeedback, 126
Biophysical profile score (BPS), 54
Biparietal diameter (BPD), 50, 64
Birth assistants, training of, 87
Birth centers, 87
Bishop score, 252–253
Bladder catheterization, 92
Bladder flap, for cesarean delivery, 149
Blighted ovum, definition of, 175
Blood pressure, 18
Blood product consent, for Jehovah's Witness patients, 108
Bloom syndrome, 80
Blunt trauma, 309
Body mass index (BMI), 3
BPD, see Biparietal diameter
BPS, see Biophysical profile score
Breast engorgement, 319
Breastfeeding, 28, 107
   contraception during, 322
   education, 318–319
   medications and complications, 319–320
Breast stimulation, 259–260
   to reduce postterm pregnancies, 297
Breech delivery, forceps for, 138
Butorphanol, 120
BV, see Bacterial vaginosis

Caffeine, 24
Calcium channel blockers, 220, 222
Calcium supplements, 26
Calf stretching, 28
Canavan disease, 80
Candida, 205
Carbetocin, 105, 150
Carboprost, 105

INDEX

Carcinoma in situ (CIS), 351
Cardiopulmonary resuscitation, 135
Cardiotocography (CTG), 111, 297
Cardiovascular changes, 35–41
Carrier screening
    Ashkenazi Jewish population, 79–82
    direct-to-consumer genetic testing, 82
    fragile X syndrome, 78
    genetic counseling, 75–77
    hemoglobinopathies, 77–78
    spinal muscular atrophy, 78–79
Castor oil, 260
Category III tracings, 111, 116
Category II tracings, 111, 114–116
Category I tracings, 111, 114
CBC, see Complete blood count
CD, see Cesarean delivery
CDMR, see Cesarean delivery on maternal request
Cell-free fetal DNA screening, 63
Cerclage removal, preterm premature rupture of membranes, 233–234
Cerebral palsy, 341–342
Cerebroventricular hemorrhage, 232
Cervical assessment, 86, 91
Cervical biopsy during pregnancy, 351
Cervical cancer screening, 19, 349–353
Cervical cerclage, 302
Cervical dilation, for cesarean delivery, 151
Cervical examination, 20, 121
Cervical insufficiency (CI), 193
Cervical length (CL), 54–55
    screening, 206
Cervical ripening, 297
    antepartum testing during, 260
    definition of, 249
Cervidil, 257
Cervix, cytologic evaluation of, 349
Cesarean delivery (CD), 98–100, 267, 326
    anesthesia for, 132–134
    delivery timing, 145
    history and epidemiology/incidence, 143
    indication for, 164
    indications for, 144
    labor induction, 250–252, 255
    operative table, preparations on, 147–148
    optimal rate, 144–145
    outcome in, 276
    planning of, 222
    postoperative care, 153–154
    preoperative considerations, 145–147
    rate, 236
    short- and long-term outcomes, 154
    surgical technique, 148–153
Cesarean delivery on maternal request (CDMR), 144
CF, see Cystic fibrosis
CFM, see Continuous fetal monitoring
Chest compressions, 335
Childbirth, fear of, 86
Child obesity, 318
Chlamydia, 230, 233
    screening, 19
Chlorhexidine, 88

Choanal atresia, 339
Cholesterol-lowering diet, 23
Chorioamnionitis, 235, 310
Chorion villus sampling (CVS), 65–66
Choroid plexus cysts (CPCs), 64
Chromosomal abnormalities, 64
    of early pregnancy loss, 176
Chromosomal microarray analysis (CMA), 66
Chronic diseases, 7
CI, see Cervical insufficiency
Circumcision, 340
CIS, see Carcinoma in situ
CL, see Cervical length
Classical forceps, 138
Clindamycin, 324
Clinical pelvimetry, 20
CMA, see Chromosomal microarray analysis
CMV, see Congenital cytomegalovirus; Cytomegalovirus
Coached maternal pushing, 99
Coagulation system, 44–45
Cocaine, 120
Colposcopy, indications for, 351
Combined spinal epidural (CSE), 130–131
Combine first- and second-trimester tests, 62–63
Commercial infant feeding materials, 319
Complete abortion, 175
Complete blood count (CBC), 19, 77, 338–339
Computed tomography (CT), diagnosis of placental abruption, 312
Computerized FHR monitoring, 118
Congenital cytomegalovirus (CMV), 64
Congenital diaphragmatic hernia, 339
Congenital heart disease, 132
Conization, 352
Constipation, 29
Continuous fetal monitoring (CFM), 231
Contraception, 320–322
    during breast-feeding, 322
    intrauterine devices (IUDs), 321
    postpartum sterilization, 321–322
Cord blood collection, 106
Cord drainage, 106
Cord gases, 106
Cord prolapse, 235
Cord traction, 106
Corticosteroids, 120, 216–217
    for fetal/neonatal maturation, 231–232
Couvelaire uterus, 310
COX inhibitors, 220, 222
CPCs, see Choroid plexus cysts
C-reactive protein (CRP), 338–339
Crown-rump length (CRL), 50
CRP, see C-reactive protein
Cryoprecipitate, 135
CSE, see Combined spinal epidural
CTG, see Cardiotocography
CVS, see Chorion villus sampling
Cystic fibrosis (CF), 2, 76–77
Cytomegalovirus (CMV), 20
Cytotec™, see Misoprostol

DCC, see Delayed cord clamping
Defective deep placentation, 309
Dehydroepiandrosterone sulfate (DHEAS), 259
Delayed cord clamping (DCC), 106, 222
Delayed vs. early hospital admission, 88
Delivery mode, 277–278
Delivery room management, neonate
    difficult transition, 336–339
    initiation of resuscitation, 335–336
    resuscitation, 336
    withholding or discontinuing resuscitation, 339
Delivery room resuscitation, newborn, 336–337
Dental support device, during second stage of labor, 99
DES, see Diethylstilbestrol
Dexamethasone sulfate, 259
DHEAS, see Dehydroepiandrosterone sulfate
Diabetes, 7
Diagnostic panty liner, 228–229
Diagnostic tests
    chorion villus sampling and amniocentesis, 65–66
    microarrays and other genetic, 66
Diastolic blood pressure, 18
Diethylstilbestrol (DES), 188
Difficult transition, newborn, 336–339
Di George Syndrome, 72–73
Digital scalp, see Vibroacoustic stimulation
Dihyrolipoamide dehydrogenase (DLD) deficiency, 81
Dilapan, 253
Dinoprostone gel, 257
Direct-to-consumer (DTC) genetic testing, 82
Disrupted laparotomy wound, 154, 326
DLD deficiency, see Dihyrolipoamide dehydrogenase deficiency
Doppler, 53–54
Double-balloon Foley catheters, 254–255
Down's syndrome, genetic ultrasound screening for, 63–65
DTC genetic testing, see Direct-to-consumer genetic testing
Ductus venosus (DV), 54
Duodenal atresia, 63
Duplication, 72–73
DV, see Ductus venosus
Dyspnea, 42
Dystocia, 93

Early cord clamping (ECC), 106
Early deceleration, of fetal heart rate, 112
Early pregnancy loss (EPL)
    definition of, 175–176
    diagnosis of, 176
    management of, 177–180
    patient counseling of, 180
    risk factors of, 177
EASI, see Extra-amniotic saline infusion
EBL, see Estimated blood loss

ECC, see Early cord clamping; Endocervical curettage
Echogenic intracardiac foci, 64
ECV, see External cephalic version
Edema, routine evaluation for, 20
Edinburgh postnatal depression scale (EPDS), 327
EFM, see Electronic fetal monitoring
Elective forceps delivery, 137
Elective repeat cesarean delivery (ERCD), 167
Electronic fetal monitoring (EFM), 111, 117, 118
Electronic FHR monitoring vs. intermittent auscultation, 113–117
Elevated-risk infants, 339
Embryonic demise
 definition of, 176
 ultrasound diagnosis of, See Anembryonic pregnancy, ultrasound diagnosis of
Empiric therapy, 326
Endocervical curettage (ECC), 351
Endocrine, 186
 changes, 42–43
 evaluation, 185–186
Endometrial biopsy, 186
Endometritis, 322–323
Endotracheal intubation, 133, 271
Enemas, 88
 induction of labor, 260
Energy (calorie)/protein supplementation, 23
ENG, see Etonogestrel
EPDS, see Edinburgh postnatal depression scale
Epidural anesthesia
 for cesarean delivery, 132–133
 neuraxial labor analgesia, 127–130
Epidural blood patch, 130
Epidural space, 128
Epinephrine, 335
Episiotomy
 operative vaginal delivery, 140
 during second stage of labor, 100
EPL, see Early pregnancy loss
ERCD, see Elective repeat cesarean delivery
Ergometrine, 105
Ergot alkaloids, 105
Erythromycin/erythromycin alone, 232–233
Estimated blood loss (EBL), 290
Estriol, unconjugated, 62
Estrogen, 259
Etonogestrel (ENG), 322
Euglycemia, 10
Exclusive breast-feeding, 317
Expanded carrier screening, 82
Expectant management
 of early pregnancy loss, 176, 178
 vs. surgical management, 179
Expert Systems (ES), see Computerized FHR monitoring
External cephalic version (ECV), 170, 273–276
External vs. internal FHR monitoring, 118

Extra-amniotic prostaglandins, 257–258
Extra-amniotic saline infusion (EASI), 254
Extraperitoneal vs. transperitoneal cesarean delivery, 149

Failed intubation, 134
False-positive rate, 117
Familial dysautonomia, 80
Familial hyperinsulinism, 81
Fanconi anemia, 80
Fascial closure techniques, 152
Fascial incision, cesarean delivery, 149
Ferning test, 227, 229, 243
Fetal anatomy, 52
Fetal assessment test, 88
Fetal bowel, echogenicity of, 64
Fetal cardiac activity, 51
Fetal compression syndrome, 236
Fetal death, 313
Fetal demise, 236
Fetal echocardiography, 55
Fetal electrocardiogram, 119
Fetal fibronectin (FFN), 215, 228–229, 253
Fetal growth restriction (FGR), 64, 112, 117
Fetal heart rate (FHR)
 disturbances, 170
 patterns, definitions of, 112
 tracing, 88
Fetal heart rate (FHR) monitoring, 111–113, 147
 amnioinfusion, 119
 during cervical ripening, 260
 external vs. internal, 118
 intrauterine resuscitation, 121
 other tests, 118–119
 tocolysis, 120–121
 vs. intermittent auscultation, 113–117
Fetal heart tones, 20
Fetal macrosomia, 165
Fetal maturity
 assessment, 231
 steroids for, 147
Fetal movement, 20
Fetal/neonatal benefit
 antibiotics for, 232–233
 corticosteroids for, 231–232
 tocolysis for, 233
Fetal neuroprotection, magnesium sulfate for, 233
Fetal pulse oximetry, 119
Fetal scalp blood sampling (FSBS), 118
Fetal status, 313
Fetal surveillance, preterm premature rupture of membranes, 231
FFN, see Fetal fibronectin
FGR, see Fetal growth restriction
FHR, see Fetal heart rate
FHR monitoring, see Fetal heart rate monitoring
First stage of labor
 abnormal progression of, 92–93
 active management of, 92
 continuous support in, 89
 maternal position, 90

nutrition in, 89–90
stripping in, 91
First-trimester screening (FTS), 51, 61–63
 "fetal dating" ultrasonography, 21, 295
Fish intake, preterm birth, 197, 200
5p-(Cri-Du-Chat Syndrome), 73
Foley bulbs, 245
Foley catheter, 253–254
Folic acid supplementation, 5, 24–25
Food-borne illnesses, prevention of, 20
Food safety, in pregnancy, 23
Forceps vs. vacuum-assisted delivery, 118, 138–139
47,XXX, 72
Fragile X syndrome, 78
Freestanding birth centers, 87
FSBS, see Fetal scalp blood sampling
FTS, see First-trimester screening
Fundal pressure, during second stage of labor, 99
Future fertility, on early pregnancy loss, 180

GA, see Gestational age
Galactogogues, 320
Gastrointestinal changes, 45
Gastrointestinal infection, infants, 317
Gaucher disease, 80
GBS, see Group B streptococcus
General anesthesia, for cesarean delivery, 133–134
Genetic amniocentesis, 270
Genetic counseling, 75–77
Genetic evaluation, 184–185
Genetic testing, 66
 direct-to-consumer, 82
Genital herpes, 20
Gentamicin, 324
Gestational age (GA), 50–51, 61, 193, 229–230
 and labor induction, 252
Gestational sac, 51–52
Glandular cell, 350
Glucose, urine dipstick for, 19
Glyceryl trinitrate (GTN), 220
Glycogen storage disease, 81
Glycosuria, urine dipstick for, 19
Glycosylated hemoglobin (HgB A1c), 7
Gonorrhea, 230
 screening, 19
Group B streptococcus (GBS)
 colonization, 205
 premature rupture of membranes, 245
 prophylaxis, 88–89
Group prenatal care, 17–18
GTN, see Glyceryl trinitrate

Hair removal, for cesarean delivery, 148
Hands-on vs. hands-poised method delivery, 99
HBsAg screening, 19
hCG, see Human chorionic gonadotropin
Health-care provider, 17
Heartburn, 29
Heart disease, 132
HELLP syndrome, 131

Hemabate, 105
Hematologic changes, 43–45
Hematoma, 130
Hemodynamic changes, in pregnancy, 35–41
Hemoglobinopathies, 77–78
Hemorrhoids, 29
Hepatitis B vaccination, 7
Hepatitis C serology screening, 19
Heritable genetic disorders, 2
Herpes simplex virus (HSV), 230
  screening for, 20
HgB A1c, see Glycosylated hemoglobin
HIE, see Hypoxic–ischemic encephalopathy
HIV, see Human immunodeficiency virus
Homeopathy, 260
Homeostasis changes, 45–46
Home uterine activity monitoring (HUAM), 204, 222
Home vs. in-hospital care, preterm labor, 222
Hormonal contraception, 321
Hospital admission, delayed vs. early, 88
Hospitalization, preterm premature rupture of membranes, 231
HPV testing, see Human papillomavirus testing
HSV, see Herpes simplex virus
HUAM, see Home uterine activity monitoring
Human chorionic gonadotropin (hCG), 188
Human immunodeficiency virus (HIV), 230, 320
  serology screening, 19
Human milk production, 319
Human papillomavirus (HPV) testing, 350
Hyaluronidase, 259
Hydration, 121, 218
Hygroscopic dilators, 253
Hyperemesis gravidarum, 43
Hypertension, 10–11
Hypertensive disorders, 131
Hypnosis, 126
Hypnotherapy, 126
Hypoglycemia, 336
Hypotension, 129, 132, 133
Hypoxemia, 111
Hypoxia, 111
Hypoxic–ischemic encephalopathy (HIE), 118, 169, 341
Hysterectomy, 303

IAI, see Intra-amniotic infection
Iatrogenic PPROM (iPPROM), 237–238
IDM, see Infant/diabetic mother
IGFBP-1, see Insulin-like growth factor–binding protein 1
IM administration, see Intramuscularly administration
Immunologic evaluation, 186
Incomplete abortion, 175
Indomethacin, 200, 204, 221
Induction of labor, see Labor induction
Indwelling bladder catheterization, 148
Infant/diabetic mother (IDM), 336

Infant feeding
  health effects of, 317–318
  recommendations for, 318
Infection precautions, preterm premature rupture of membranes, 230–231
Influenza vaccination, 5
Informed consent, 126
Inherited thrombophilias, 310–311
Inhibin, 62
Instrumental vaginal birth, 117
Insulin-like growth factor–binding protein 1 (IGFBP-1), 227–228, 243
Internal os, 299
International Federation of Gynecology and Obstetrics (FIGO) (2012), 98
Interobserver variability, fetal heart rate monitoring, 117
Intra-abdominal drain, for cesarean delivery, 152
Intra-abdominal irrigation, for cesarean delivery, 152
Intra-amniotic infection (IAI), 265–267
  in women, 215
Intramuscularly (IM) administration, 127
Intraobserver variability, fetal heart rate monitoring, 117
Intraoperative ultrasound, 304
Intrapartum, 284
Intrauterine devices (IUDs), 321
Intrauterine fetal demise (IUFD), 117
Intrauterine growth restriction (IUGR), 204, 295–296
Intrauterine pressure catheter (IUPC), 92, 170
Intrauterine resuscitation, 121
Intravenous (IV)
  administration, 127
  fluids, 90
  prostaglandins, 258
Invasive cancer, diagnosis of, 351
Iodine supplements, 26
iPPROM, see Iatrogenic PPROM
Irondeficiency anemia, 44
Iron supplements, 26
Itching, 28
IUDs, see Intrauterine devices
IUFD, see Intrauterine fetal demise
IUGR, see Intrauterine growth restriction
IUPC, see Intrauterine pressure catheter

Jehovah's witness pregnant woman care, 108–109
Joubert syndrome, 81

Karyotype, 184–185
Karyotype abnormalities
  future pregnancy preconception counseling, 68
  klinefelter syndrome, 71–72
  neonatology management, 67
  trisomy 13, 69–70
  trisomy 21 (down's syndrome), 66–67
  turner syndrome, 70–71
Klinefelter syndrome, 71–72

Labor and delivery (L&D) care, 340
Laboratory screening, follow-up, 21
Laboratory tests, 2
Labor induction, 283–284
  amniotomy, 256
  antepartum testing, 260
  balloon catheter, 253–254
  breast stimulation, 259–260
  cervical assessment, 249
  double-balloon Foley catheters, 254–255
  extra-amniotic saline infusion, 254
  hygroscopic dilators, 253
  indications for, 250–252
  maternal characteristics, 252
  membrane stripping, 255–256
  outpatient vs. inpatient, 260–261
  pharmacologic methods, 256–259
  premature rupture of membrane, 255
Labor pain, 126
Labor stimulant, 121
Lamicel, 253
Laminaria, 253
Large for gestational age (LGA), 336
LAST, see Local anesthetic systemic toxicity
Last menstrual period (LMP), 50
Late deceleration, of fetal heart rate, 112
Late-preterm abruption, 313
Late-preterm infants, 339
Late-term gestation, 86
Late-term pregnancy, 295–297
L&D care, see Labor and delivery care
Left uterine displacement, 126, 135
Leg cramps, 28
Leg edema, 29
Leiomyomas, 310
Leopold's maneuvers, 20
LGA, see Large for gestational age
Liquid-based cytology, 349
LMP, see Last menstrual period
LMWH, see Low-molecular-weight heparin
Local anesthetic, 129
Local anesthetic systemic toxicity (LAST), 134
Long-term morbidities, 236
Low-dose aspirin, 188
Lower uterine segment, ultrasound of, 170
Low-glycemic index diet, 23
Low-lying placenta, 299
Low-molecular-weight heparin (LMWH), 147, 187, 188
Low vs. elevated-risk neonates, 339
Lumbo-sacral sterile water injection, 128
Lung development, phases of, 235

Magnesium sulfate (MgSO$_4$), 120, 220–222
  for neuroprotection, 217
Magnesium supplements, 25
Magnesium vs. magnesium alone, 221
Magnetic resonance (MR) imaging, diagnosis of placental abruption, 312
Major depressive disorder (MDD), 326
Malposition, 278

Malpresentation
    external cephalic version, 274–276
    mode of delivery, 277–278
    moxibustion, 276
Manual rotation, in second stage of labor, 99
Maple syrup urine disease, 81
Markers, 63
MAS, see Meconium aspiration syndrome
Massage therapy, 126
Massive transfusion, 135
Mastitis, 319
Maternal age, 343–344
Maternal analyte screening, 62
Maternal blood pressure, 121
Maternal cardiac disease, 132
Maternal demographics, 163
Maternal diet, during lactation, 320
Maternal-Fetal Medicine Units Network (MFMU Network), 166, 167
Maternal hemorrhage, 135
Maternal hypertensive disorders, 310
Maternal medications, 319–320
Maternal obesity, 132
Maternal oxygen, 97
Maternal position
    during cesarean delivery, 147–148
    first stage of labor, 90
    during second stage of labor, 98
Maternal position change, 121
Maternal serum alpha-fetoprotein (MSAFP), 61
Maternal status, 313
Maternal surveillance, preterm premature rupture of membranes, 231
Mature teratomas, 343
MCA, see Middle cerebral artery
MDD, see Major depressive disorder
Mean sac diameter (MSD), 175
Mechanical trauma, 309
Meconium, 231, 269–271, 337–338
Meconium aspiration syndrome (MAS), 269
Meconium-stained amniotic fluid (MSAF), 269
Medical management of early pregnancy loss, 178
    patient acceptability, preference, counseling, 180
Medical vs. expectant management, 179
Medical vs. surgical management, 178–179
Medications/teratogens, 11
Megaloblastic macrocytic anemia, 44
Meiotic nondisjunction, 68
Membrane stripping, 255–256
Meperidine, 120, 127
Methergine®, 105
Methotrexate, 178
MFMU Network, see Maternal-Fetal Medicine Units Network
Microarrays test, 66
Microdeletion, 72–73
Microinvasive cervical cancer, 349
Middle cerebral artery (MCA), 54
Midwife-led care, 87
Mifepristone, 178, 259

Mild abruption, 313
Milk expression, 320
Milking of cord, 222
Minute ventilation, 41
Misoprostol, 105, 150–151, 179, 245, 256–257
Mixed feeding, 317
Mode of delivery, 277–278
Moderate abruption, 313
Monotherapy, 11
Morphine, 120
Morphine sleep, 88
Morphology ultrasound, 52
Mosaicism, 68, 69
Moxibustion, 276
MSAF, see Meconium-stained amniotic fluid
MSAFP, see Maternal serum alpha-fetoprotein
MSD, see Mean sac diameter
Mucinous tumors, 343
Mucolipidosis, 80–81
Multidisciplinary care, 2
Multifetal reduction, 206
Multiple gestations, 206–207
Multivitamin supplements, 24

Nalbuphine, 120
Naloxone, 127
    hydrochloride, 336
Nasal bone, 62
NASG, see Nonpneumatic antishock garment
Nasopharyngeal suctioning, 270
Nausea, 45
NE, see Neonatal encephalopathy
Negative pressure wound therapy (NPWT), 326
Nemaline myopathy, 81
Neoadjuvant chemotherapy, 352
Neonatal
    consultation, 69
    echocardiogram, 67
Neonatal death rates, 169
Neonatal encephalopathy (NE), 341, 342
Neonatal intensive care unit (NICU), 340
Neonatal management, 267
Neonatal morbidity/mortality, prophylaxis to prevent, 216–217
Neonatal resuscitation, initiation of, 334–335
Neonatal seizures, 113
Neonate
    care of preterm infant, 340–341
    cerebral palsy, 341–342
    delivery room management, 335–339
    labor and delivery care, 340
    low vs. elevated-risk, 339
    neonatal encephalopathy, 341
Neonatology management, karyotype abnormalities, 67
Neural tube defects (NTDs), 5, 61, 339
    maternal serum alpha-fetoprotein screening for, 65

Neuraxial labor analgesia, 126, 127
    combined spinal epidural, 130–131
    contraindications to regional anesthesia, 131
    epidural analgesia, 128–130
Newborn neonatal screening, 340
Nicardipine, 220
Nicotine replacement therapy (NRT), 198
NICU, see Neonatal intensive care unit
Niemann–Pick disease, 81
Nifedipine, 220, 275
Nipple stimulation, to reduce postterm pregnancies, 297
Nitrazine test, 227, 229, 243
Nitric oxide (NO) donors, 221, 259
Nitroglycerine, 221
NO donors, see Nitric oxide donors
Nonmegaloblastic macrocytic anemia, 44
Nonpneumatic antishock garment (NASG), 292
Nonreassuring fetal heart rate (NRFHR), 67, 111–113, 117–121
Nonreassuring fetal heart rate tracing (NRFHT), 97, 144, 273
Nonsteroidal anti-inflammatory drugs (NSAIDs), 153–154, 220
    for perineal pain control, 107
Nontocolytic interventions, for preterm labor, 217–218
    bed rest, 217–218
    hydration, 218
Nonvertex presentation, 86
NPWT, see Negative pressure wound therapy
NRFHR, see Nonreassuring fetal heart rate
NRFHT, see Nonreassuring fetal heart rate tracing
NRT, see Nicotine replacement therapy
NSAIDs, see Nonsteroidal anti-inflammatory drugs
NT, see Nuchal translucency
NTDs, See Neural tube defects
Nuchal fold, 64
Nuchal translucency (NT), 51, 59, 61
Nursery management, karyotype abnormalities, 67–68

Obstetric interventions for periviable birth, 215
Oligohydramnios, 236–237
Omega-3 fatty acids, 197, 201
Omega-3 supplements, 26
Opening the airway, 335
Operative vaginal delivery (OVD), 137–141
Optimal duration of breast-feeding, 318
Oral dexamethasone, 216
Oral health care, 26
Oral misoprostol, 257
Oral prostaglandins, 258
Oro-pharyngeal suctioning, 270
Otitis media, 317
Ovarian cancer, Federation Internationale de Gynecologie et d'Obstetrique staging for, 346

Ovarian cyst rupture, 344
OVD, see Operative vaginal delivery
Oxygen administration, for cesarean delivery, 148
Oxygenation, 121
Oxytocin, 103–105, 150, 244–245, 317
   during first stage of labor, 91–92
   labor stimulation with, 258–259
Oxytocin prophylaxis, 105
Oxytocin receptor antagonists, 221–222

Pain, 125
   labor, 126
PAPP-A, see Pregnancy associated plasma protein-A
Pap smear, 349–353
Paracervical block, 128
Parenteral opioids, 127
Parietal peritoneum, for cesarean delivery, 149
Partial thromboplastin time (PTT), 131
Partogram, 91
Parvovirus, 2
Patient acceptability of early pregnancy loss, 180
Patient-controlled epidural analgesia (PCEA), 129
Patient counseling, of early pregnancy loss, 180
PCEA, see Patient-controlled epidural analgesia; Post-cesarean delivery analgesia
PDPH, see postdural puncture headache
PEIC, see Physical exam-indicated cerclage
Pelvic examination, 18–19
Pelvic lymphadenectomy, 352
Pelvic pain, 28
Pelvic rest, 300
Pelvimetry, 86
Penicillin, 324, 326
Perinatal death rates, 113, 117, 169
Perinatal depression (PND), 326–327
Perinatal mortality, 311
   incidence of, 17
Perineal lacerations, 107
Perineal massage, 27
   during second stage of labor, 99
Perineal pain control, 107
Perineal shaving, 88
Perineal warm packs, during second stage of labor, 99
Periodontal disease, 204
Peripheral nerve blocks, 128
Peritoneal nonclosure, 152
Pessary, 200, 207
PGE2, see Prostaglandin E2
PGF2fα, see Prostaglandin F2fα
PH, see Pulmonary hypoplasia
Pharmacokinetics, 46
Pharmacologic agents, 292–293
pH definitions, 111
Phenobarbital, 217
Physical exam-indicated cerclage (PEIC), 204
Pierre Robin sequence, 339
Piracetam, 121

Pitfalls, 52
PL, see Pregnancy loss
Placenta
   accreta, 302–305
   previa, 299–302
   third stage of labor, 106
Placental abruption, 309, see also Abruptio placentae
   classification of, 311
   clinical findings in women with, 310
   diagnosis of, 312
Placental alpha-microglobulin test, 227, 229
Placental disorders
   placenta accreta, 302–305
   placenta previa, 299–302
   vasa previa, 305–306
Placental pathology, 310
Planned home birth, 86–87
Planned hospital birth, 87
Planned repeat cesarean delivery (PRCD), 167–170
PND, see Perinatal depression
POC, see Products of conception
Polyhydramnios, 310
Post-cesarean delivery analgesia (PCEA), 134
Postdural puncture headache (PDPH), 129, 130, 133
Postmaturity syndrome, 296
Postoperative counseling, after cesarean delivery, 154
Postpartum/breast-feeding, 189, 267
   preterm birth, 223
Postpartum care
   breast-feeding, 317–320
   contraception, 320–322
   endometritis, 322–324
   mood and anxiety disorders, 326–327
   wound complications, 324–326
Postpartum endometritis, 236, 322–324
Postpartum hemorrhage (PPH), 103–105, 289–292
   prevention of, 150–151
   secondary to uterine atony, 311
Postpartum mood disorders, 326–327
Postpartum period depression, 27–28
Postpartum sterilization, 321–322
Postpartum wound complications, 324–326
Postterm pregnancy, 234–235, 295–297
Posture, maternal change in, 276
PPH, see Postpartum hemorrhage
PPROM, see Preterm premature rupture of membranes
PRCD, see Planned repeat cesarean delivery
Precautions, 52
Preconception care, 187, 283
   folic acid supplementation, 5
   for maternal medical disorders, 8–10
   nutrition, weight, and exercise, 3–5
   opportunities for, 1–2
   recommendations, 7
   reproductive health plan, 2–3
   substance abuse/environmental hazards/toxins, 11
   vaccinations, 5–7

Preconception counseling, 108, 312
   preterm birth, 222
   preterm premature rupture of membranes, 229–230
Predominant breast-feeding, 317
Pre-eclampsia, 204
Pregnancy
   cervical biopsy during, 351
   depression, 27–28
   dyspnea of, 42
   induction of labor, 251
   iodine requirements, 43
   and periviable PTB, 216
   physiologic adaptations during, 36–38
   physiologic changes in, 35
   preconception counseling for, 68
   screening in, 350
Pregnancy associated plasma protein-A (PAPP-A), 59
Pregnancy loss (PL), 193
   threatened, 177
Pregnancy-related endocrine alterations, 42
Pregnancy-related hemodynamic changes, 35
Pregnancy-specific hormones, 42
Pregnant women, normal reference ranges in, 39–41
Premature/prelabor rupture of membranes (PROM), 243–246, 265
   diagnostic tests, 229
   labor induction for, 254–255
Prenatal care, 108, 187
   interventions for common pregnancy complaints, 28–29
   organizational issues, 17–21
   preterm labor, 222
Prenatal counseling, 230
Prenatal diagnosis, definition of, 59–60
Prenatal education, 21, 27, 170
Prenatal record, 18
Prepidil, 257
Preterm abruption, 313
Preterm birth (PTB), 1, 214–218
   infections, 205–206
   multiple gestations, 206–207
   prevention, 193–195
   primary prevention strategies for, 195–198
   secondary prevention of, 198–204
Preterm infant care, 340–341
Preterm labor (PTL), 193–194, 229
   calcium channel blockers, 220
   fetal fibronectin, 215
   magnesium sulfate, 220–221
   neonatal morbidity/mortality, 216–217
   nitric oxide donors, 221
   nontocolytic interventions for, 217–218
   postpartum/breast-feeding/counseling, 223
   preconception counseling, 222
   primary tocolysis, 218–220
   tocolysis, 218
   transvaginal ultrasound cervical length, 214–215

Preterm premature rupture of membranes
(PPROM), 194, 227–229, 267
 amniocentesis, 231
 anesthesia, 234
 antibiotics for prolongation of latency,
  232–233
 cerclage removal, 233–234
 corticosteroids for fetal/neonatal
  maturation, 231–232
 iatrogenic, 237–238
 infection precautions, 230–231
 postpartum, 234–235
 preconception counseling, 229–230
 prenatal counseling, 230
 previable, 235–238
 in twin gestations, 238
 vitamin C and E, 233
Preterm uterine contractions, women with,
 215
Previous lumbar surgery, 132
Primary tocolysis, 218–219, 221–222
Probiotics, 23
Products of conception (POC), 186
 karyotype, 184–185
Progesterone, 187–188, 221–222, 233
Prolactin, 317
Prolongation of latency
 antibiotics for, 232–233
 tocolysis for, 233
Prolonged second stage of labour, 100
PROM, see Premature/prelabor rupture of
 membranes
Prompt delivery, 313
Prophylactic antibiotics, 324, 325
 cesarean delivery, 145
Prophylactic tocolysis, 97–98
Prostaglandin E2 (PGE2), 257
Prostaglandin F2α, 105
Prostaglandin F2fα (PGF2fα), 259
Prostaglandins, 105, 258
Proteinuria, screening for, 19
PTB, see Preterm birth
PTL, see Preterm labor
PTT, see Partial thromboplastin time
Pudendal block, 128
Pulmonary hypoplasia (PH), 236
Pushing method, second stage of labor,
 98–99
Pyelectasis, 64

Randomized controlled trials (RCTs), 1, 7, 17,
 61, 103–104, 117–121
Rapid decompression, of distended uterus,
 309
RCTs, see Randomized controlled trials
Rectus muscle cutting, for cesarean delivery,
 149
Rectus muscles, 152
Recurrent pregnancy loss (RPL), 183–184
 anesthesia, 189
 antepartum testing, 188
 negative workup, 187–188
 preconception care, 187
 screening tests, 184–186

Regional anesthesia, 128, 131
Relaxation techniques, 126
Relaxin, 259
Renal system changes, 45–46
Reproductive health plan, 2–3
Resealing techniques, preterm premature
 rupture of membranes, 237
Respiratory changes, 41–42
Respiratory complications rates, 169
Respiratory depression/arrest, 130
Respiratory distress, 338–339
Retained placenta, 103, 236, 292–293
Retinal hemorrhages, 139
Ritgen's maneuver, 99
ROM, see Rupture of membranes
Rotational forceps, 138
Routine induction, of labor, 297
Routine platelet count, 131
Routine vs. selective ultrasound
 examination, 50
RPL, see Recurrent pregnancy loss
Rubella antibody, 19
Rupture of membranes (ROM), 119

Screening tests
 anatomic evaluation, 185
 endocrine evaluation, 185–186
 genetic evaluation, 184–185
 immunologic evaluation, 186
 for infections, 218
 vs. diagnostic tests, 60
Second stage of labor
 management, 98–100
 prolonged second stage, 100
 prophylactic interventions, 97–98
Second-trimester "fetal anatomy"
 ultrasound, 21
Second-trimester screening (STS), 52,
 62–63
Seizure disorders, 11
Sepsis calculator, 267
17 α-hydroxyprogesterone caproate (17P),
 206
 vs. cerclage, 203
Severe abruption, 313
Sexual intercourse, 260
SGA, see Small for gestational age
Short humerus, 64
Shoulder dystocia, 281–283
 anesthesia, 287
 antepartum, 283–284
 intrapartum, 284
 preconception, 283
 therapy, 284–287
SIDS, see Sudden infant death syndrome
Single antenatal ultrasound, 300
Skin cleansing, for cesarean delivery, 148
Skin incision techniques, for cesarean
 delivery, 148–149
Skin-to-skin contact, 319
Sleep, morphine, 88
Slow-release pessary (vaginal insert), 257
SMA, see Spinal muscular atrophy (SMA)
Small for gestational age (SGA), 336

SMFM, see Society for Maternal-Fetal
 Medicine
Smoking cessation programs, 11, 198
Society for Maternal-Fetal Medicine
 (SMFM), 54–55
Sodium bicarbonate, 336
Specimen adequacy, 349–350
Spinal anesthesia
 for cesarean delivery, 133
 neuraxial labor analgesia, 130
Spinal muscular atrophy (SMA), 78–79
Spontaneous abortion, 175
Spontaneous labor, prediction of onset, 86
Spontaneous PPROM, 230
Squamous epithelial cell, 350
SSI, see Surgical site infection
Standard ultrasound, 52
Sterile water, injections of, 128
Steroids
 for fetal maturity, 147
 neonatal benefits, 246
Stillbirth rates, 169
Stretch marks, 28
Stripping/sweeping of membranes, 297
STS, see Second-trimester screening
Subcutaneous tissue, for cesarean delivery,
 149, 152–153
Sublingual misoprostol, 257
Sudden infant death syndrome (SIDS), 65, 317
Surgical intervention, 294
Surgical management of early pregnancy
 loss, 178
Surgical site infection (SSI), 324–325
SVR, see Systemic vascular resistance
Symphyseal-fundal height measurement, 20
Syncope, 41
Syntocinon®, 103–105
Syntometrine, 105
Syphilis screening, 19
Systemic vascular resistance (SVR), 35

TA, see Tranexamic acid
TA cerclage, see Transabdominal cerclage
Tachysystole, 111
Tactile stimulation, 335
TAP block, see Transversus abdominis plane
 block
Tay–Sachs disease, 80
TCD, see Trans-cerebellar diameter
Teamwork training, 87
TENS, see Transcutneous electrical nerve
 stimulation
Teratogens, 11
Terbutaline, 120
 pump, 221
Termination of pregnancy (TOP), 197, 235
Term placental abruption, 313
Term Prelabor Rupture of Membranes Study
 (Term PROM), 266, 267
Term PROM, see Term Prelabor Rupture of
 Membranes Study
Tetanus vaccination, 7
Therapeutic hypothermia, 341
Therapeutic ultrasound, for perineal pain, 107

Therapy of an adnexal mass, in pregnancy, 345–346
Thermal management, 335
Third stage of labor
  active management of, 106–107
  definition of, 103
    perineal pain control and breast-feeding, 107
    umbilical cord and placenta, 106
    uterotonics, 103–106
Third trimester, 52–53
Third-trimester "fetal growth" ultrasound, 21
Three-dimensional ultrasound, 55
Three-tier FHR interpretation system, 111, 113
Thrombocytopenia, 44
Thrombophilia, 186, 187
Thyroid-binding globulin, 43
Thyroid gland, functions of, 43
Thyroid homeostasis, 43
Thyroid-stimulating hormone (TSH) level, 10
Thyroperoxidase antibodies, 311
Thyrotropin-releasing hormone (TRH), 217
Tocolysis, 120–121, 302, *see also* Tocolytic therapy
Tocolytic therapy, 218–219
Tocomonitoring, 121
TOLAC, *see* Trial of labor after cesarean
TOP, *see* Termination of pregnancy
Topical anesthetics, 107
Total spinal, 134
Toxins, 11
Toxoplasmosis, 20
Tractocile, *see* Atosiban
Training of providers, breast-feeding, 318
Tranexamic acid, 292
Tranexamic acid (TA), 105, 106, 151
Transabdominal amnioinfusion, 119
Transabdominal amnioinfusions, 228–229, 237
Transabdominal (TA) cerclage, 202
Trans-cerebellar diameter (TCD), 50
Transcervical amnioinfusion, 119
Transcervical chorion villus sampling technical instrument, 66
Transcutaneous electrical nerve stimulation (TENS), 127
Transient tachypnea of the newborn (TTN), 339
Translocations, 68, 69
Transperitoneal cesarean delivery, extraperitoneal *vs.*, 149
Transvaginal cervical length, 253
Transvaginal scanning, 51
Transvaginal ultrasound (TVU), 51, 176, 299, 344
Transvaginal ultrasound cervical length (TVU CL), 214–215
Transversus abdominis plane (TAP) block, 134
TRH, *see* Thyrotropin-releasing hormone
Trial of labor after cesarean (TOLAC)
  benefits and least morbidity of, 167–169
  candidates for, 163
  definitions, 162

historical perspectives, 161–162
labor factors, 165
management of, 169–170
maternal demographics, 163
obstetric history, 163–165
uterine rupture, 165–167
Trichomonas vaginalis, 205
Trimester, ultrasound examinations by, 51–53
Triple screen, 62
Trisomy 13, 69–70
Trisomy 18 (Edward syndrome), 68–69
Trisomy 21 (Down's syndrome), 66–67
TSH level, *see* Thyroid-stimulating hormone level
TTN, *see* Transient tachypnea of the newborn
Tuberculosis, 20
  breast-feeding, 320
Turner syndrome, 70–71
TVU, *see* Transvaginal ultrasound
TVU CL, *see* Transvaginal ultrasound cervical length
TVU CL screening, 54–55
Twin pregnancies, with PPROM, 238
Twins, screening for aneuploidies in, 65
Type 2 diabetes, 318

UFH, *see* Unfractionated heparin
UIC, *see* Ultrasound-indicated cerclage
Ultrasound
  biophysical profile score, 54
  cervical length, 54–55
  Doppler, 53–54
  gestational age dating, in pregnancy, 50–51
  informed consent, 49–50
  during labor, 92
  of lower uterine segment, 170
  to reduce postterm pregnancies, 296
  routine *vs.* selective use of, 50
  safety of, 49
  three-dimensional, 55
  by trimester, 51–53
Ultrasound examination
  diagnosis of placental abruption, 312
  induction of labor, 251
Ultrasound-indicated cerclage (UIC), 200
Umbilical artery, 53–54, 283
Umbilical cord, third stage of labor, 106
Unfractionated heparin (UFH), 147, 187, 188
Ureaplasma urealyticum, 324
Ureoplasma urealyticum colonization, 205–206
Urgent cesarean delivery (CD), 273
Urinary tract infections (UTI), 145
Urine culture, for asymptomatic bacteriuria, 19
Urine dipstick for protein, 19
Usher syndrome, 81
Uterine artery, 54
Uterine atony, prevention of, 150–151
Uterine cavity, 187
Uterine cleaning, 151
Uterine cooling, 151
Uterine enlargement, 42

Uterine exteriorization, 151
Uterine incision, 149–151
Uterine inversion, 103, 293–294
Uterine massage, 106, 151
Uterine rupture, 162, 165–167
Uterine stapling, 149–150
Uterotonics, 103–106, 305
UTI, *see* Urinary tract infections

Vaccinations, 5–7, 26
Vacuum application, 140
Vacuum-assisted delivery, forceps *vs.*, 138–139
Vacuum extractors, 138
Vaginal birth after cesarean (VBAC), 117, 161, 162
Vaginal bleeding, 310
Vaginal delivery, 313
Vaginal insert
  misoprostol, 256
  PGE2 (Cervidil), 257
Vaginal irrigation, 148
Vaginal misoprostol, 256
Vaginal prostaglandins, 244
Vaginal speculum examination, 313
Valsalva *vs.* spontaneous pushing method, 98–99
Valvular heart disease, 132
Vancomycin, 245
Variable deceleration, of fetal heart rate, 112
Varicella, 20
Varicosities, 29
VAS, *see* Visual analog scale
Vasa previa, 305–306
VBAC, *see* Vaginal birth after cesarean
Venous thromboembolism, prophylactic agents to prevent, 147
Ventricular septal defect (VSD), 68
Vibroacoustic stimulation, 118
Visual analog scale (VAS), 127
Vitamin A supplements, 25
Vitamin B6 (pyridoxine) supplements, 25
Vitamin C, 233
Vitamin C supplements, 25
Vitamin D supplements, 25
Vitamin E, 233
Vitamin E supplements, 25
Vitamin K, 217
Vomiting, 45
VSD, *see* Ventricular septal defect

Walker–Warburg syndrome, 81–82
Water immersion, 126
Water immersion, during labor, 90
Withholding or discontinuing resuscitation, 339
Wound culture, 325
Wound debridement, 326
Wound drainage, 326

X-inactive specific transcript (XIST), 71
XIST, *see* X-inactive specific transcript

Zidovudine, 120
Zinc supplements, 26